R. Luchetti · P. Amadio (Eds.) Carpal Tunnel Syndrome

R. Luchetti · P. Amadio (Eds.)

Carpal Tunnel Syndrome

With 374 Figures in 543 Parts and 49 Tables

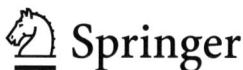
Springer

Riccardo Luchetti, M.D.
Via Pietro da Rimini 4, 47900 Rimini, Italy

Peter Amadio, M.D.
Mayo Clinic, 200 First Street SW, Rochester, Minnesota 55905, USA

This Work is an updated and revised version edited by Riccardo Luchetti and Peter Amadio of the original Italian edition of *Sindrome del tunnel carpale*
Copyright © 2002 Verduci Editore, Roma

ISBN 3-540-22387-8   Springer-Verlag Berlin Heidelberg New York

Library of Congress Control Number: 2005932251

This work is subject to copyright. All rights are reserved, whether the whole or part of the material is concerned, specifically the rights of translation, reprinting, reuse of illustrations, recitation, broadcasting, reproduction on microfilm or in any other way, and storage in data banks. Duplication of this publication or parts thereof is permitted only under the provisions of the German Copyright Law of September 9, 1965, in its current version, and permission for use must always be obtained from Springer-Verlag. Violations are liable to prosecution under the German Copyright Law.

Springer is a part of Springer Science+Business Media
http://www.springer.com

© Springer-Verlag Berlin Heidelberg 2007

Printed in Germany

The use of general descriptive names, registered names, trademarks, etc. in this publication does not imply, even in the absence of a specific statement, that such names are exempt from the relevant protective laws and regulations and therefore free for general use.

Product liability: The publishers cannot guarantee the accuracy of any information about the application of operative techniques and medications contained in this book. In every individual case the user must check such information by consulting the relevant literature.

Editor: Gabriele Schröder
Desk Editor: Irmela Bohn
Production Editor: Joachim W. Schmidt

Cover design: eStudio Calamar, Spain

Typesetting: FotoSatz Pfeifer GmbH, D-82166 Gräfelfing
Printed on acid-free paper – 24/3150 – 5 4 3 2 1 0

Dedication

We dedicate this work to our fathers, Mario Luchetti and Peter Amadio, Jr., who died as we were editing this work. Their love, support, and example have made all that we have done possible. We hope that the final product would have met with their approval.

           Ciao, papà   *Riccardo Luchetti*
                         Peter C. Amadio

Foreword

Although carpal tunnel syndrome has been recognized as a clinical reality for only about 50 years, it represents today a very substantial problem with high impact on life quality for a large number of patients and with important socio-economic consequences for society. The signs and symptoms are often puzzling, with pain and sensory disturbances not only in the hand but sometimes also involving the whole extremity. Although the basic etiology is a compression lesion of the median nerve at wrist level, this lesion has an impact on the whole length of the neurons – from finger tips to the dorsal root ganglia and spinal cord level.

The literature on carpal tunnel syndrome is enormously diversified and very difficult to grasp. Dr. Luchetti has undertaken a very impressive task to summarize, in one volume, current concepts regarding the pathophysiology and diagnosis of this syndrome as well as basic anatomy, treatment options, complications from surgery, and what we should do when things go wrong. He also addresses the difficulties in evaluating and assessing the results from treatment.

Editing a multiauthor volume is not an easy task and the result in the past literature has often been a recapitulation of old data and already-published illustrations. However, this volume is a striking exception. New original drawings and photographs are being mixed with some classic illustrations, which results in a very attractive book at a high educational level. It is an important contribution to the already existing literature on carpal tunnel syndrome, and it adds considerably to our understanding of this puzzling condition as well as nerve compression syndromes in general.

Göran Lundborg

Preface

Carpal tunnel syndrome is the most common hand problem, affecting as much as 5% of the adult population; yet in the large majority of cases, the condition is idiopathic. While surgical treatment often results in improvement, residual loss of function and some persistence of symptoms are common. Clinicians still disagree as to diagnostic criteria, the relation of carpal tunnel syndrome to work, the best way to evaluate the results, and the proper treatment. Yet despite the ubiquity of the condition, and the thousands of scientific papers and hundreds of lay publications discussing it, the extant medical texts which summarize all this for the clinician are few, often out of date, and tend to focus on a single perspective, whether that be etiology, evaluation, or an illustration of a particular surgical method.

It is clear that a comprehensive text, summarizing existing knowledge of carpal tunnel syndrome from a multidisciplinary perspective, is long overdue. For that reason, we are very happy to bring this volume on carpal tunnel syndrome to publication. In it, we present the assembled thoughts of more than 80 international experts on carpal tunnel syndrome and its treatment, covering medical, surgical, and rehabilitation specialties. It represents what we consider to be the best current thinking on the pathology, diagnosis, and treatment of carpal tunnel syndrome, including the latest options for primary carpal tunnel release and revision surgery. While many of these chapters appeared in an earlier, Italian language version, all have been updated, and there are new chapters on pathology, objective evaluation, and new strategies for reoperation. We believe that this text will fill an important void in the current literature, in summarizing the vast and complex literature on a common and often troublesome condition.

Of course, while we are happy to have assembled this book, and hope that its contents prove as educational for the reader as they have been for us, the work has been the cooperative effort of a large international group of coworkers. We wish to thank especially our many professional colleagues, who were so willing to contribute their expertise; our families, for their understanding, in allowing us the time to edit the volume; and our editors at Springer-Verlag, Gabriele Schröder and Irmela Bohn. We hope that you agree with us that the product was worth the effort.

Peter Amadio
Riccardo Luchetti

Foreword to the Italian Edition

When my friend Dr. Riccardo Luchetti asked me to write an introduction for his book I asked myself:

Once again, why write a book on carpal tunnel syndrome, especially since pages and pages have already been written concerning this subject. But, actually, it is exactly this topic about which there are still many questions that need to be answered and areas of grey which need to be made much more clear.

Carpal tunnel syndrome – should it always be operated on, in all cases? I personally have colleagues who have operated on over a thousand cases, and other colleagues, who, over the years, have operated on only a handful of cases. It is difficult to determine why! Maybe this syndrome pool varies greatly depending on the specific type of patients that visit a particular outpatient clinic or the type of industry that surrounds a certain region. It may also be due to the very variable surgical indications, which need to be scrutinized and revised.

Traditional Standard Surgery or Endoscopic?
The positive and negative factors associated with these two techniques do not go hand in hand with each other. But will they ever? Of course we must also take into consideration the learning curve, not to mention the ligament; should we leave it open or re-suture it?

What about residual symptoms and last resort surgical interventions to remedy previously unsuccessful surgery?

If for some hand surgeons these questions have absolute answers, (with some modifications depending upon individual cases) for other surgeons, the responses to these questions still hold some doubt.

Therefore, Dr. Luchetti's initiative to write, once again, a book regarding carpal tunnel syndrome has been courageous, since not everyone will be convinced of its necessity.

"De captu lectoris habent sua fata libelli." I can only hope this publication will capture the interest of many a reader.

G. Brunelli

Preface to the Italian Edition

Carpal tunnel syndrome (CTS) surgery is currently the most commonly performed hand surgery. One can easily find a significant amount of scientific literature specifically on this topic. Being that it is a very well-known pathology, there has been a constant evolution concerning its treatment and associated surgical techniques. In the last 10 years the introduction of surgical endoscopy has revolutionized the method of CTS treatment by demonstrating its effective or even superior clinical results than those rendered by a classical surgical technique. This surgical approach has also led us to research and publish the associated complications that can arise from using these new surgical techniques, as well as to scrutinize the various methods that can be used with these newly proposed instruments. Nevertheless, the advent of this technique has left hand surgeons perplexed as to technique/outcome results and urged the experts of this pathology to re-evaluate and statistically analyze surgical outcome results of each surgeon's CTS technique, for both its advantages and disadvantages. Competitive research, at an international level, has been initiated in order to improve each surgical treatment technique and to accurately publish scientific information concerning each technique's surgical outcome. The idea of dedicating, not just a chapter but an entire book to CTS surgery and its treatment, comes from the necessity to excel in a specific surgical field. This book is a scientific contribution, providing the reader accurate CTS pathology data research. The goal of this book is to specify the existence of various surgical techniques and to determine their validity in the accurate treatment of CTS. Each author has carefully described the surgical technique that they use, along with its particularities. A CD accompanies the book so that the reader can visually observe these particularities that are associated with each chapter's technique, allowing for a clearer and more explicit description.

In addition, both conservative preoperative CTS treatments have been included in the book, as well as postoperative rehabilitation protocols.

Since CTS postoperative complications tend to be on the rise, a precise recognition of why these complications are occurring needs to be documented. The majority of this book is dedicated to each surgical technique proposed and its possible complications.

At the end of the book there is a chapter dedicated to a study on the evaluation of surgical data results. This topic has been included since it is no longer sufficient to evaluate one's treatment results only from a clinical point of view; it is also necessary to evaluate patient satisfaction and determine if their expectations have been satisfied. Recently, this evaluation method has been greatly enhanced by the use of generic, specific, and pathology-based questionnaires.

This book is indicated:

For those surgeons who are interested in specializing in this sector (hand surgeons, orthopedic surgeons, plastic surgeons, physiatrists, and physical and occupational therapists) young and old.

For the younger surgeons, the book has been set up in such a way that one can easily refer to a specific surgical technique regarding this pathology and at the same time be informed of alternative treatment methods, even those that are noninvasive. The reader is well informed of each technique's complications and their respective treatments.

For those surgeons who already have CTS surgical treatment experience, the book is an opportunity to deepen one's knowledge in this pathology and its accompanying surgical technique. Once read completely, it becomes quite clear that CTS and its surgical treatment has been quite underestimated. An incorrect surgical treatment of CTS can render the patient not only dissatisfied, but also unable to correctly use their hand in activities of daily living, not to mention manual labor activities.

This specific book is geared towards addressing the questions that all physicians and medical students may have concerning this pathology and its associated complications.

Riccardo Luchetti

Contents

Part I – General

1. History of Carpal Tunnel Syndrome
   P.C. AMADIO 3
   References 8

2. Anatomy of the Carpal Tunnel
   P. YUGUEROS, R.A. BERGER 10
   References 12

3. Normal Anatomy and Variations of the Median Nerve in the Carpal Tunnel
   H.-M. SCHMIDT 13
   Carpal Tunnel 13 / Flexor Retinaculum 13 / Median Nerve 15 / Median
   Nerve Branches 17 / References 19

4. Etiopathogenesis
   R. LUCHETTI 21
   Introduction 21 / Idiopathic Forms 21 / Secondary Form 22 / Summary
   of CTS Causes 25 / References 25

5. The Pathophysiology of Median Nerve Compression
   R. LUCHETTI 28
   Introduction 28 / Anatomy Notes 28 / Pathophysiology 32 / Stages
   of Compressive Nerve Injuries 38 / Conclusion 39 / References 40

6. Ischemia-Reperfusion Injury as a Common Etiology of "Idiopathic" Carpal
   Tunnel Syndrome: Biochemical and Immunohistochemical Evidence
   A.E. FREELAND, M.A. TUCCI, V. SUD 42
   Introduction 42 / Anatomic Factors 42 / Pathophysiologic Factors 42 / Bio-
   chemical Factors 43 / Histologic Factors 45 / Discussion 46 / References 46

7. Carpal Canal Pressure Measurements: Literature Review
   and Clinical Implications
   R. LUCHETTI, R. SCHOENHUBER 49
   Initial Studies 49 / Clinical Studies 49 / Dynamic Evaluation 52 / Centimetric
   Evaluation of Endocanal Pressure 52 / Endocanalar Pressure, Wrist Posturing
   Splints Used During Activities of Daily Living 55 / Conclusion 57 / Clinical
   Implications 58 / References 58

Part II – Diagnosis

8. Clinical Diagnosis
   M. CERUSO, R. ANGELONI, G. LAURI, G. CHECCUCCI 63
   References 67

9. Neurophysiological Assessment of Carpal Tunnel Syndrome
   R. SCHOENHUBER, L. CAPONE, R. GENTILE, R. PENTORE 69
   Introduction 69 / The Neurophysiological Examination 70 / Median Nerve
   Sensory Conduction Studies 70 / Comparison Methods: Sensory Median

to Ulnar and Median to Radial Nerve Fibers 71 / Median Nerve Motor Conduction Studies 71 / Needle Electromyography 72 / Conclusions 73 / References 73

10. Diagnostic Imaging
    E. Cerofolini 75
    Magnetic Resonance 75 / Postsurgery Findings 77 / Ultrasound Studies 78 / References 80

11. Quantitative Assessment of Historical and Objective Findings:
    A New Clinical Severity Scale of CTS
    F. Giannini 82
    Introduction 82 / Objective Findings 82 / Historical Findings 84 / A New Clinical Scale: Validation of the Measurement 85 / Conclusions 87 / References 87

12. Differential Diagnosis of Carpal Tunnel Syndrome
    P.C. Amadio 89
    References 93

13. Carpal Tunnel Syndrome: Rare Causes
    A. Landi, A. Leti Acciaro, N. Della Rosa, A. Pellacani 95
    Anatomic Anomalies 95 / Traumatic Lesions 96 / Congenital Deformities and Anomalies 96 / Recurrent Focal Neuropathies 97 / Connective Tissue Disorders 97 / Endocrine Disorders 98 / Infectious Diseases 98 / Metabolic Diseases 98 / Blood Coagulation Disorders 99 / Tumors 99 / References 100

Part III – Treatment

14. Conservative Care for Carpal Tunnel Syndrome
    J.S. Brault 105
    Introduction 105 / Activity/Ergonomic Modification 105 / Splinting 105 / Exercise/Modalities 107 / Oral Medication 107 / Corticosteroid Injections 108 / Conclusion 109 / References 109

15. The Cutaneous Innervation of the Palm and Its Implications During Carpal Tunnel Release Surgery
    M.M. Tomaino 111
    Introduction 111 / Incision Selection: Historical Review 111 / Current Anatomical Studies and Implications on Incision Selection 111 / Summary 113 / References 113

16. Traditional Technique: Wrist-Palm Incision
    G. Cristiani, M. Marcialis 115
    Introduction 115 / Surgical Technique 115 / Indications 116 / Contraindications 119 / Complications 119 / Author's Suggestions 119 / Postoperative Care 120 / Rehabilitation Protocol 120 / References 120

17. Palmar Incision
    R. Luchetti 121
    Introduction 121 / Author's Preferred Technique 122 / Additional Technical Procedure 127 / Summary and Suggestions 128 / References 129

18. Open Carpal Tunnel Release with a Short Palmar Incision and No Specialized Instruments Combined with a Rehabilitation Program for Early Return to Activity
    P.A. Nathan 130
    Implementation of OCTR with Short Palmar Incision 130 / Indications/Contraindications and Complications 130 / Surgical Anesthesia 131 / Instrumentation and Surgical Technique 131 / Immediate Postoperative Rehabilitation 132 / Return-to-Work Intervals 133 / Summary 133 / References 134

19. The Mini-Invasive Technique for Carpal Tunnel Release: Open Approach with Converse Fiberoptic Light Retractor
    P. Di Giuseppe 135
    Introduction 135 / Mini-Invasive Technique 136 / Operative Technique 136 / Comments and Conclusions 138 / References 138

20. The Indiana Tome for Carpal Release
    B.J. Wilhelmi, W.P. Andrew Lee 140
    History 140 / Indications 141 / Technique 141 / Advice 145 / Complications 145 / Rehabilitation 145 / Conclusion 145 / References 146

21. Alternative Techniques and Variants: Double Approach – Proximal and Distal Mini-Incisions
    M. Corradi 147
    Introduction 147 / Technique 147 / Discussion 149 / References 150

22. Anatomic Landmarks for Endoscopic Carpal Tunnel Release
    T.K. Cobb, W.P. Cooney 151
    Introduction 151 / Anatomy 151 / Technique 152 / References 155

23. Endoscopic Carpal Tunnel Release
    J.C.Y. Chow, A.A. Papachristos 156
    History of the Endoscopic Release of Carpal Ligament 156 / Chow Technique 156 / Alternative Chow Technique 164 / 17 Years' Experience and Clinical Results 164 / References 164

24. Endoscopic Technique: The Gilbert Technique (or Technique by Two Different Portals)
    F. Brunelli, C. Spalvieri, A. Gilbert, M. Merle 166
    History 166 / Technique 166 / Indications and Contraindications 168 / Results and Complications 168 / Advice and Tricks 168 / Conclusion 169 / References 170

25. Endoscopic Carpal Tunnel Release
    C.A. Peimer, R.K. Brown 171
    Indications and Contraindications 171 / Anatomy 171 / Single-Portal Technique (Modified from Agee) 172 / Efficacy 174 / Complications 174 / Authors' Recommendations 175 / References 175

26. Endoscopic Carpal Tunnel Release: Menon's Technique
    P.G. Castelli, A. Dell'Uomo, C. Ferrari 177
    Instrumentation 177 / Surgical Anatomy 178 / Surgical Technique 179 / Postoperative Treatment 183 / Results 183 / Complications 183 / Discussion 184 / References 184

27. The Distal Single Incision Scope-Assisted Carpal Tunnel Release – Thirteen-Year Follow-Up Results
    M. A. Mirza, M.K. Reinhart 186
    Introduction 186 / Study Protocol 186 / Operative Technique 186 / Results 189 / Complications 192 / Discussion 192 / Conclusion 193 / References 193

28. Carpal Tunnel Release with Limited Visualization
    C. Panciera, P. Panciera 194
    Introduction and History 194 / Technique Description 194 / Indications – Contraindications 198 / Complications 198 / Results 199 / Conclusions 199 / References 199

29. Closed Technique With Paine Retinaculotome and Modified Retinaculotome MDC
   A. Mantovani, L. De Cristofaro, A. Ciaraldi 200
   Introduction 200 / Technique 200 / Indications and Contraindications 205 / Complications and Results 206 / The Modified Retinaculotome MDC 207 / References 209

30. Closed Carpal Tunnel Release Technique with GRS
   A. Atzei, M.D. Putnam, S. Tognon, L. Cugola 211
   Introduction 211 / Surgical Anatomy and Skin Incision Landmarks 211 / Control of Correct Position of the Guide 213 / Surgical Technique 214 / Postoperative Treatment 218 / Discussion 218 / References 219

31. Carpal Tunnel Syndrome Release Using the Chiena Technique
   V.P. De Tullio 220
   Introduction 220 / Surgical Technique 220 / Material and Method 224 / Conclusions 225 / References 225

32. Reconstruction of the Flexor Retinaculum
   A. Lluch 226
   Morphological Changes of the Carpal Tunnel After Division of the Flexor Retinaculum 226 / Function of the Flexor Retinaculum as a Flexor Tendon Pulley 227 / Loss of Grip Strength After Carpal Tunnel Release 228 / Palmar Scar Pain 228 / Methods of Reconstructing the Flexor Retinaculum 229 / Personal Technique for Reconstruction of the Flexor Retinaculum 231 / Results After the Reconstruction of the Flexor Retinaculum 235 / Secondary Reconstruction of the Flexor Retinaculum 235 / Conclusions 236 / References 237

33. Critical Appraisal of Transverse Carpal Ligament Reconstruction. Theoretical, Experimental, and Clinical Considerations
   M. Altissimi 239
   Introduction 239 / Evaluation of Results of Ligament Reconstruction 240 / References 240

34. Comparison of Grip Strength Evolution After Carpal Tunnel Release by Three Different Techniques
   G. Foucher, G. Pajardi, L. Van Overstraeten, J. Braga Da Silva 241
   Introduction 241 / Material and Methods 241 / Results 242 / Discussion 244 / Conclusion 245 / References 245

35. Median Nerve Compression Secondary to Fractures of the Distal Radius
   A. Badia 247
   References 251

Part IV – Rehabilitation

36. Postoperative Treatment of Carpal Tunnel Syndrome After Median Nerve Decompression (Open Field or Endoscopic Technique)
   T. Fairplay, G. Urso 255
   Introduction 255 / Postoperative Treatment 255 / Recovery of Finger Range of Motion and Differential Gliding Exercises for the Finger Flexor Tendons 256 / Retrograde Massage and Increasing Venous Return 257 / Shoulder Exercises 258 / Splint Removal 259 / Suture Removal 259 / Scar Treatment; Remodeling, and Desensibilization (When Necessary) 259 / Wrist Range of Motion Exercises 260 / Transcutaneous Electric Stimulation (T.E.N.S.) or Microcurrent Stimulation 260 / Median Nerve Gliding Exercises 261 / Strengthening Exercises 262 / Sensory Evaluation and Re-education 262 / Ergonomic Therapy (Work Hardening) 263 / Conclusion 264 / References 265

Part V – Complications

37. Carpal Tunnel Syndrome Surgical Complications
    P. BEDESCHI 269
    Introduction 269 / Classification of CTS Surgery Complications 269 / Analysis of the Complications 270 / Conclusions 285 / References 287

38. Complications Following Endoscopic Treatment
    G. PAJARDI, G. PIVATO, L. PEGOLI, D. PISANI 290
    Introduction 290 / Complications of the Endoscopic Treatment 290 / Analysis of Complications Using Bedeschi's Classification 290 / Conclusions 295 / References 297

39. Role of Neurosensory Testing in Differential Diagnosis of Failed Carpal Tunnel Syndrome
    J. H. COERT, A. L. DELLON 299
    Introduction 299 / Patient Examples of Neurosensory Testing 299 / Discussion 299 / Summary 306 / References 306

40. Secondary Carpal Tunnel Surgery
    T.H.H. TUNG, S.E. MACKINNON 307
    Complications Following Carpal Tunnel Surgery 308 / Clinical Evaluation of the Patient with Failed Carpal Tunnel Release 313 / Surgical Techniques in Secondary Carpal Tunnel Surgery 314 / Conclusion 317 / References 317

41. Hypothenar Fat-Pad Flap
    R. GIUNTA, U. FRANK, U. LANZ 319
    Introduction 319 / Historical Background 319 / Technique 319 / Rehabilitation 320 / Indications/Contraindications 320 / Results 321 / Complications 322 / Tips and Tricks 322 / References 322

42. Management of Recurrence of Carpal Tunnel Syndrome by Using the Abductor Digiti Minimi Muscle Flap to Cover the Median Nerve
    J. H. COERT, A. L. DELLON 324
    Introduction 324 / Surgical Approach and Example Cases 324 / Discussion 326 / References 326

43. Protection of the Median Nerve with the Pronator Quadratus and Palmaris Brevis Muscle Flaps
    B. BATTISTON, P. TOS, R. ADANI 327
    Introduction 327 / Pronator Quadratus Muscle Flap 327 / Palmaris Brevis Muscular Flap 329 / Discussion 331 / References 332

44. Vein Wrapping of the Median Nerve
    D.G. SOTEREANOS, N.A. DARLIS 333
    Introduction 333 / Basic Science 333 / Preoperative Assessment 334 / Operative Technique 334 / Results 336 / References 336

45. Synovial Flap Plasty as a Treatment of Recurrent Carpal Tunnel Syndrome
    D. ESPEN 338
    Introduction 338 / Definition of "Recurrence" 338 / Method 338 / Surgical Technique 338 / Postoperative Management 341 / Evaluation 341 / Different Treatment Options for Recurrence 341 / Discussion 341 / References 341

46. Reverse Island Forearm Flaps for the Coverage of the Median Nerve in Recurrent Carpal Tunnel Syndrome
    M. RICCIO, A. BERTANI, W.A. MORRISON 343
    Introduction 343 / The Forearm Radial Artery Flap 345 / The Retrograde Radial Forearm Flap 349 / The Forearm Ulnar Artery Flap 350 / The Posterior Interosseous Flap 353 / Clinical Case Reports 355 / Results 356 / Discussion 357 / Patient Selection for Surgery 357 / Conclusions 358 / References 359

47. The Ulnar Fascial-Fat Flap for the Treatment of Scarred Median Nerve in Recalcitrant Carpal Tunnel Syndrome
A. Vigasio, I. Marcoccio 361
Introduction 361 / Surgical Technique 363 / Results 365 / Conclusions 367 / References 368

48. Protective Covering of the Nerve by the "Vela Quadra" Flap
A. Pagliei, F. Catalano, F. Fanfani 369
Introduction 369 / Anatomy 369 / Surgical Technique 369 / Clinical Applications 373 / Conclusions 374 / References 374

49. Free Vascularized Omental Transfer for the Treatment of Recalcitrant Carpal Tunnel Syndrome
R. J. Goitz, J.B. Steichen 376
Introduction 376 / Technique 377 / Results 377 / Discussion 378 / References 379

Part VI – Evaluation of Results

50. Outcomes Assessment Protocols
R. Padua, E. Romanini, R. Bondì 383
Introduction 383 / Outcome Analysis 383 / Subjective Assessment Questionnaires (Patient-Oriented) 384 / Assessment Protocol in Carpal Tunnel Syndrome 384 / Conclusion 385 / Appendix: The SF-36 Questionnaire 386 / References 391

51. Carpal Tunnel Syndrome: Multicenter Studies with Multiperspective Assessment – Results of the Italian CTS Study Group
L. Padua 392
Introduction 392 / Study Design 392 / Definition of Cases and Data Collection 392 / Patient-Oriented Data – Boston Carpal Tunnel Questionnaire 392 / Dissociation Between Clinical-Neurophysiological Findings and Patient Symptoms 393 / Evolution of Untreated Carpal Tunnel Syndrome 395 / Symptoms and Neurophysiological Picture of Carpal Tunnel Syndrome in Pregnancy 396 / Evolution of Carpal Tunnel Syndrome in Pregnancy 396 / Diagnostic Pathway and Differences Between the Populations Enrolled in the Northern, Central, and Southern Regions of Italy 397 / Occurrence of Carpal Tunnel Syndrome in Males and Females 397 / The Usefulness of Segmental and Comparative Tests 398 / Italian CTS Study Group – Participating Members 398 / References 399

Subject Index 401

Contributors

Maurizio Altissimi, M.D., Ph.D.
Università degli Studi di Perugia
S. C. Chirurgia della Mano e Microchirurgia, Azienda Ospedaliera "S. Maria" Terni
chirurgia.mano@aospterni.it

Peter Amadio, M.D.
Mayo Clinic, 200 1st Street SW, Rochester, MN 55905, USA
amadio.peter@mayo.edu
pamadio@mayo.edu

Andrea Atzei, M.D.
Policlinico "G B Rossi", UO Chirurgia della Mano Via delle Menegone 10,
37134 Verona, Italy
andreatzei@libero.it
atzei@borgoroma.univr.it

Alejandro Badia, M.D., FACS.
Miami Hand Center, Chief of Hand Surgery
Baptist Hospital, Miami, Florida, Co-founder, Da Vinci learing center
8905 SW 87th Avenue, Suite 100, Miami, FL 33176, USA
alex@surgical.net

Bruno Battiston, M.D.
Ospedale C.T.O., Via Zuretti 29, 10126 Torino, Italy
brunob@alma.it

Professor Paolo Bedeschi
Surgery, University of Modena, Italy
Honorary President, Italian Society for Surgery of the Hand
Casa di Cura Fogliari, Chirurgia della Mano, Via Lana 1, 41100 Modena, Italy
paolobedeschi@tin.it

Richard A. Berger, M.D., Ph. D.
Mayo Clinic, 200 1st Street SW, Rochester, MN 55905, USA
berger.richard@mayo.edu

Jeffrey Brault, M.D.
Mayo Clinic, 200 1st Street SW, Rochester, MN 55905, USA

Francesco Brunelli, M.D.
Institut de la Main, Clinique Jouvenet
6, Square Jouvenet, 75016 Paris, France
BRUNELLFRA@aol.com
francescobrunelli@hotmail.com

Pier Giorgio Castelli, M.D.
Ospedale degli Infermi, Divisione di Ortopedia
ASL 12, 13900 Biella (BI), Italy

Emilio Cerofolini, M.D.
Policlinico, Servizio di Radiologia 2, 41100 Modena, Italy
emilio.cerofolini@libero.it

Massimo Ceruso, M.D.
UO Chirurgia della Mano, Azienda Ospedaliera Careggi
Largo Palagi 1, 50139 Firenze, Italy
cerusom@tin.it

James C. Y. Chow, M.D.
Orthopaedic Center of Southern Illinois, 4121 Veterans Memorial Drive
Mt. Vernon, IL 62864, USA
ocmtv@midwest.net

William P. Cooney, M.D.
Mayo Clinic, 200 1st Street SW, Rochester, MN 55905 USA
cooney.william@mayo.edu

Maurizio Corradi, M.D.
Università degli Studi di Parma, Istituto di Clinica Ortopedica e Traumatologica
43100 Parma, Italy
mcorradi@ipruniv.cce.unipr.it
maurizio.corradi@libero.it

Guido Cristiani, M.D.
Hesperia Hospital, 41100 Modena, Italy
guidocristiani@libero.it

Vincenzo Paolo De Tullio, M.D.
Ospedale Morgagni, UO Ortopedia e Traumatologia 47100 Forli, Italy

Piero Di Giuseppe, M.D.
Ospedale G. Fornaroli, Divisione di Chirurgia Plastica e Centro di Chirurgia
della Mano, Via Al Donatore di Sangue, 20013 Magenta (Milano), Italy
piero.digiuseppe@fastwebnet.it

David Espen, M.D.
Ospedale Generale, Divisione Ortopedia – Traumatologia
Via L. Böhler 5, 39100 Bolzano, Italy
davidespen@hotmail.com

Tracy Fairplay LPT
Via Molinelli 45, 40141 Bologna, Italy
zangbzan@tin.it

Guy Foucher, M.D.
4, Boulevard de President-Edwards (Bd. de l'Orangerie),
67000 Strasbourg, France
IFSSH@aol.com

Fabio Giannini, M.D.
Istituto di Clinica delle Malattie Nervose e Mentali Policlinico „Le Scotte"
Viale Bracci, 53100 Siena, Italy
gianninif@unisi.it

Robert J. Goitz, M.D.
University of Pittsburgh Medical School, Department of Orthopaedic Surgery
3471 5th Avenue, Suite 911, Pittsburgh, PA, 15213, USA
goitzrj@upmc.edu

Antonio Landi, M.D.
Policlinico, UO Chirurgia della Mano e Microchirurgia Azienda Ospedaliera
41100 Modena, Italy
landi.a@policlinico.mo.it, landi_antonio@virgilio.it

W. P. Andrew Lee, M.D.
University of Pittsburgh, School of Medicine, Scaife Hall 690, 3550 Terrace Street,
Pittsburgh, PA 15261, USA
leewpa@upmc.edu

Alberto Lluch, M.D., Ph.D.
Institut Kaplan, Paseo Bonanova 9, 08022 Barcelona, Spain
alluch@telefonica.net, lluch@filnet.es

Riccardo Luchetti, M.D.
Via Pietro da Rimini 4, 47900 Rimini, Italy
rluc@adhoc.net

Alberto Mantovani, M.D.
Ospedale di Legnago, Divisione di Ortopedia e Traumatologia
AULSS 21 Regione Veneto, Verona, Italy
alberto_mantovani@tin.it

M. A. Mirza, M.D.
290 E. Main Street, Suite 200, Smithtown, NY 11787, USA
AMSURGICAL@aol.com, npreinhart@yahoo.com

Peter Nathan, M.D. †
Portland Hand Surgery & Rehabilitation Center, 2455 NW Marshall, Suite 1
Portland, OR 97210-2997 USA

Roberto Padua, M.D.
GLOBE, Divisione di Ortopedia, Ospedale S. Giacomo
Via Canova 29, 00100 Roma, Italy
rpadua@mclink.it

Luca Padua, M.D.
Università Cattolica, Divisione di Neurologia Largo
A. Gemelli 8, 00168 Roma, Italy
padual@tin.it, lpadua@mclink.it

Antonio Pagliei, M.D.
Via Filippo Corridoni 19, 00195 Roma, Italy
chir.mano@tin.it

Professor Giorgio Pajardi
Policlinico Multimedica, Chirurgia della Mano, Università di Milano
Via Milanese 300, S. S. Giovanni, Milano, Italy
gpajardi@centrostudimano.it

Cesare Panciera, M.D.
Via Amalfi 19, 31100 Treviso, Italy
panciera@tin.it

Professor Clayton A. Peimer, M.D.
Northwestern University, Orthopaedic Surgery Evanston Northwestern Healthcare
1000 Central Street, Suite 880, Evanston, IL 60201, USA
peimer@northwestern.edu, Cpeimer@enh.org

Professor Michele Riccio, M.D.
Ospedale Riuniti, Via Conca 71 – Torrette, 60121 Ancona, Italy
michriccio@libero.it
m.riccio@ao-umbertoprimo.marche.it

Professor Dr. Hans-Martin Schmidt
Universität Bonn, Anatomisches Institut, Nussallee 10, 53115 Bonn, Germany
h.-m.schmidt@uni-bonn.de

Professor Dr. Rudolf Schoenhuber
Ospedale Generale Regionale, Divisione di Neurologia
Via Böhler 5, 39100 Bolzano, Italy
rschoenh@tin.it

Dean G. Sotereanos, M.D.
University of Pittsburgh, Department of Orthopaedic Surgery
3471 Fifth Ave., Suite 1010, Pittsburgh, PA 15213, USA

Professor Matthew M. Tomaino, M.D.
University of Pittsburgh, Department of Orthopaedic Surgery
3471 Fifth Avenue, Suite 1010, Pittsburgh, PA 15213, USA
tomainomm@msx.upmc.edu,
mtomaino@uoi.upmc.edu

Thomas H. H. Tung, M.D.
Division of Plastic and Reconstructive Surgery, Suite 17424, East Pavilion
One Barnes-Jewish Hospital Plaza, St. Louis, Missouri 63110, USA
tungt@msnotes.wustl.edu

Adolfo Vigasio, M.D.
Istituto Clinico Città di Brescia, Via Gualla 15, 25123 Brescia, Italy
avigasio@libero.it

Part I
General

History of Carpal Tunnel Syndrome

P.C. Amadio

Carpal tunnel syndrome is the most common condition surgically treated by hand surgeons. It is interesting to note this condition was only definitively described in the years after World War II. Retrospectively, however, this condition did not appear suddenly at that time but was known under a variety of different names in the past. Patients who appear to have suffered from carpal tunnel syndrome are clearly depicted in the surgical literature going back at least to the mid-1800s. The evolution of the clinical understanding that led to the current knowledge of carpal tunnel syndrome is an interesting one and represents a pattern that may be typical for many medical conditions. Specifically, early on there was confusion as to the pathophysiology, resulting in a variety of etiological theories, which in turn resulted in a variety of apparently different diagnoses being applied to the same clinical entity. Only later did the clinical threads merge and result in a single coherent clinical picture.

For carpal tunnel syndrome there were three major threads which needed to unite in order to establish our current understandings. Specifically, these were the threads of acroparesthesia, thenar neuritis, and median neuropathy after wrist fracture. The earliest of these threads was actually median neuropathy after wrist fracture, known at least since 1836 when Gensoul [1] described a case of the median nerve entrapped in an open fracture of the radius. In 1854 Paget [2] described two cases of median neuropathy after fracture of the distal radius. One case was treated by amputation and the other by splinting. Coming closer to our current understanding and therapeutic regimen, Bouilly, in 1884, described a 17-year-old with a Colles fracture and median neuropathy treated by excision of prominent palmar callus [3]. Additional cases were reviewed by Blecher in 1908 [4] and Kirchheim in 1909 [5]. By 1926 Dickson was describing a case of causalgia after Colles fracture, relieved by median neurolysis [6]. Finally, in 1933 Abbott and Saunders, in their classic cadaver study, injected dye into the carpal tunnel and noticed increased resistance to dye flow with wrist flexion [7]. As a result of this they condemned the Cotton-Loder position (Fig. 1.1), which had been commonly used up until that time for the treatment of Colles fracture. Bunnell later stated that it was this paper by his San Francisco colleagues, Abbott and Saunders, which prompted his own interest in what later came to be known as carpal tunnel syndrome [8]. The problem of carpal tunnel syndrome after Colles fracture continues, of course, to remain an important clinical problem (Fig. 1.2).

A related thread was that of median neuropathy associated with lunate dislocation. Speed reported three

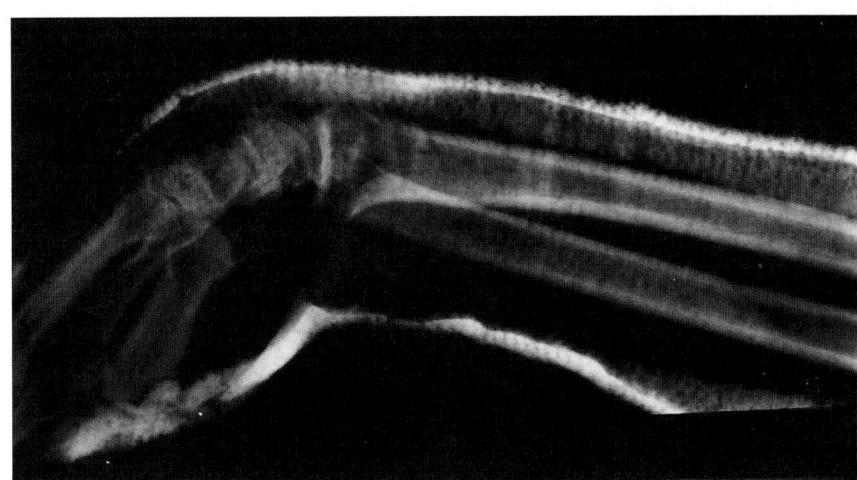

Fig. 1.1. The Cotton-Loder position of wrist flexion to maintain reduction after Colles fracture has been justifiably condemned

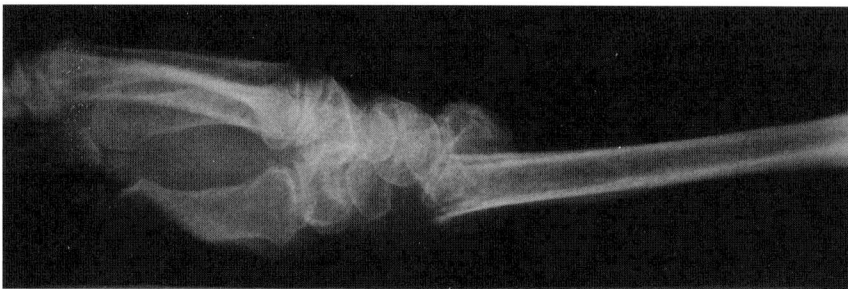

Fig. 1.2. Displaced Colles fractures are still a common cause of posttraumatic carpal tunnel syndrome

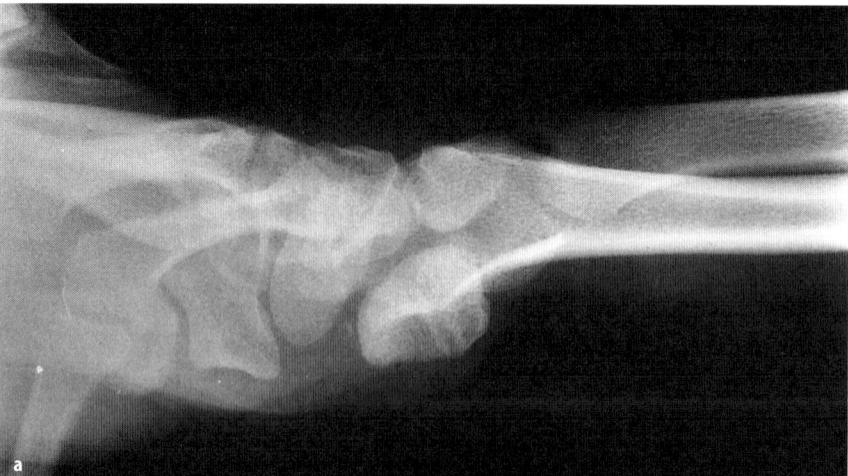

Fig. 1.3. a,b Chronic lunate dislocation remains a classic cause of carpal tunnel syndrome, and is still treated by lunate excision. **a** Chronic lunate dislocation associated with symptoms of carpal tunnel syndrome. **b** Complete relief of symptoms after excision of the dislocated lunate

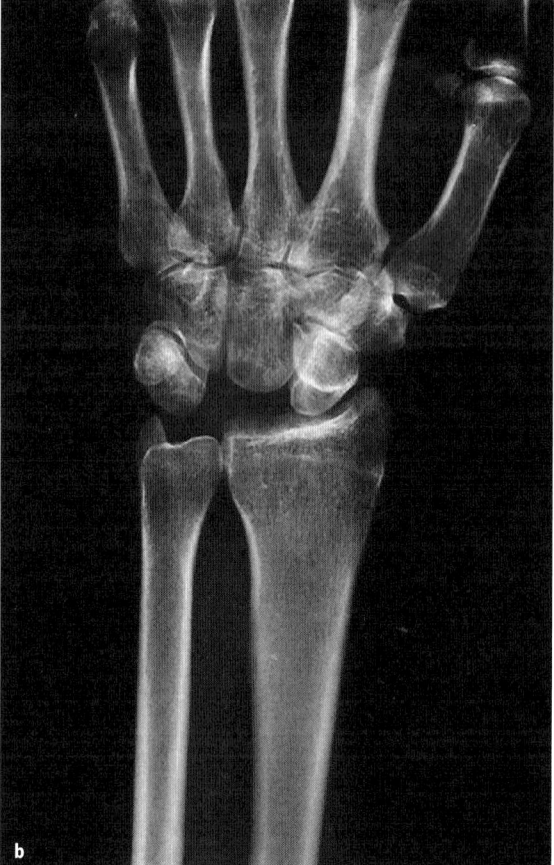

cases in 1922 [3], which improved with excision of the lunate. Watson-Jones in 1927 [9] and Meyerding in 1927 [10] also reported excellent restoration of median nerve function after removal of the dislocated lunate bone. The problem of chronic lunate dislocation and its treatment by lunate excision, of course, remains relevant to the present day (Fig. 1.3).

The second major thread, historically speaking, was that of acroparesthesias. Initially, there was no thought that acroparesthesias and median neuropathy associated with wrist fractures might actually share a final common anatomic bottleneck, namely the flexor retinaculum at the wrist. In 1862 Raynaud postulated that there was a vasomotor origin for these acroparesthesias [35]. Nonetheless he described what appears to be fairly classical symptoms of carpal tunnel syndrome: "a depressing sense of numbness and tingling...the tactile sense may be so much impaired that it is difficult for the fingers to retain small objects." Certainly this is a common complaint among carpal tunnel syndrome patients even to this day. In 1880 Putnam, in Boston, reported on 37 patients, mostly women, who had nocturnal paresthesias. He noted that "simply letting the arm hang out of the bed or shaking it about...[or the use of] prolonged rubbing would relieve the symptoms." He also noted "certain fingers were more severely affected...often it's those supplied by the median nerve" [12]. Again, classic symptoms for present-day carpal tunnel syndrome patients, yet despite what appears to be clear evidence pointing at the median nerve as the culprit, and the wrist as a likely level, Putnam thought that "alterations of the blood supply of the median nerve" were the cause and suggested galvanism, amyl nitrate, or cannabis as recommended treatments. Ormerod, in 1883, coined the term acroparesthesias to describe the numbness and tingling of the fingertips that Raynaud and Putnam had previously characterized [13]. In 1906 Farquhar Buzzard, physician extraordinary to King Edward VII of England, postulated that acroparesthesias were due to problems at the brachial plexus level, most often related to a cervical rib [14, 15]. He recommended first rib resection as a treatment. This therapy was subsequently popularized in the USA by W. W. Keene [14], a surgeon who again had high political connections: he had treated the head and neck cancer of U.S. President Grover Cleveland some years previously. Unfortunately for patients with carpal tunnel syndrome, this hypothesis of brachial plexopathy as etiology for acroparesthesias became quite popular, and resulted in a variety of misdirected surgical therapies up until the late 1940s [16, 17]. Walsh in 1944 [18] was still promoting the theory of acroparesthesias as a brachial plexopathy and Behrman in 1945 [19] noted the common acroparesthesias associated with pregnancy and again blamed them on compression at the brachial plexus. Ultimately, as we know now, these hypotheses as to the etiology of acroparesthesias represented errors in diagnosis, and ultimately a blind alley.

A second blind alley was the theory of thenar neuritis, i.e., that the problem of thenar atrophy (Fig. 1.4) was separate from the problem of acroparesthesias. This is even a bit more difficult to understand; why would one would postulate that the numbness in the median nerve distribution was due to a problem in the brachial plexus while the motor atrophy of the thenar muscles was due to a focal problem of the motor branch in the hand? Certainly, Occam's razor would suggest a single common diagnosis, namely compression at the carpal tunnel. Nonetheless, Hunt in the early 1900s coined the term median thenar neuritis and suggested an occupational cause [20]. He de-emphasized the sensory symptoms and Moersch in 1938 again reiterated the possibility of isolated thenar involvement [21]. Ultimately, again, this was a blind alley.

Who had the first thought that the numbness of the fingertips might represent a low median neuropathy is of course impossible to know. A review of the Mayo Clinic medial records showed that as early as 1910, Henry Plummer, an outstanding diagnostician of his day, had diagnosed idiopathic low median neuropathy in a 66-year-old man [10]. He offered no treatment, however. In 1913 Pierre Marie and Charles Foix in a report to the French Neurological Society described an autopsy case of an 80-year-old woman [22]. A large pseudoneuroma was found with distal demyelination of the median nerve. They suggested that "perhaps in a case in which the diagnosis is made early enough…-transection of the ligament could stop the development of these phenomena." Prescient words, but unfortunately, apparently few people read or thought about Marie's and Foix's observation, as the next appearance in the literature of treatment focusing on the carpal tunnel is a report by Learmonth, published in 1933 [23]. In this report he describes two cases, one patient operated on in 1929 in which he divided the flexor retinaculum in order to treat a median neuropathy secondary to scaphoid nonunion, and another case in 1930 where he treated a patient with median neuropathy by

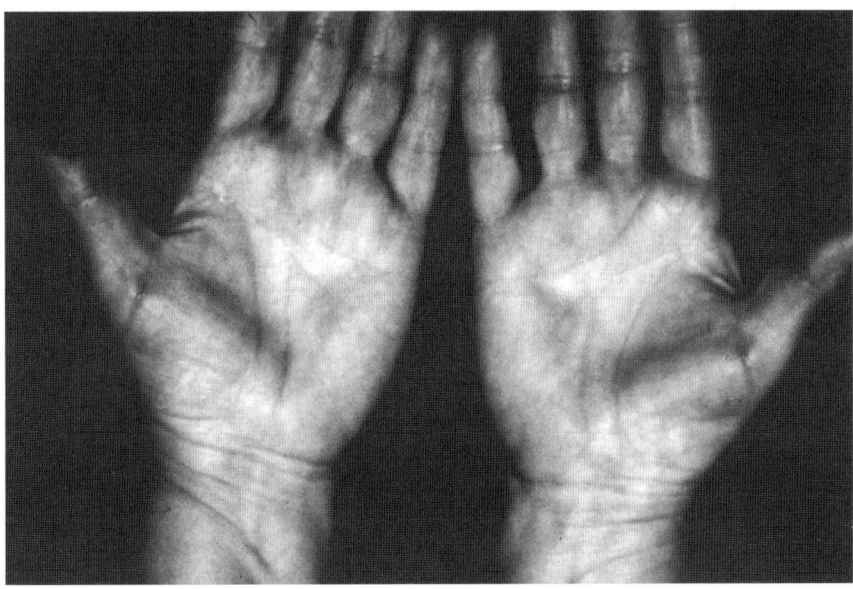

Fig. 1.4. Thenar wasting such as this was once believed to be due to an isolated constriction of the motor branch of the median nerve. The associated paresthesias were thought to be due to a brachial plexopathy. Today we understand that both are consequences of the same cause, carpal tunnel syndrome

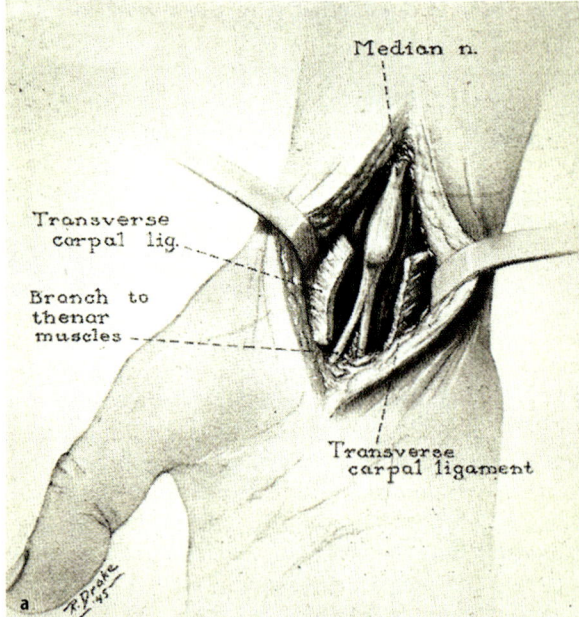
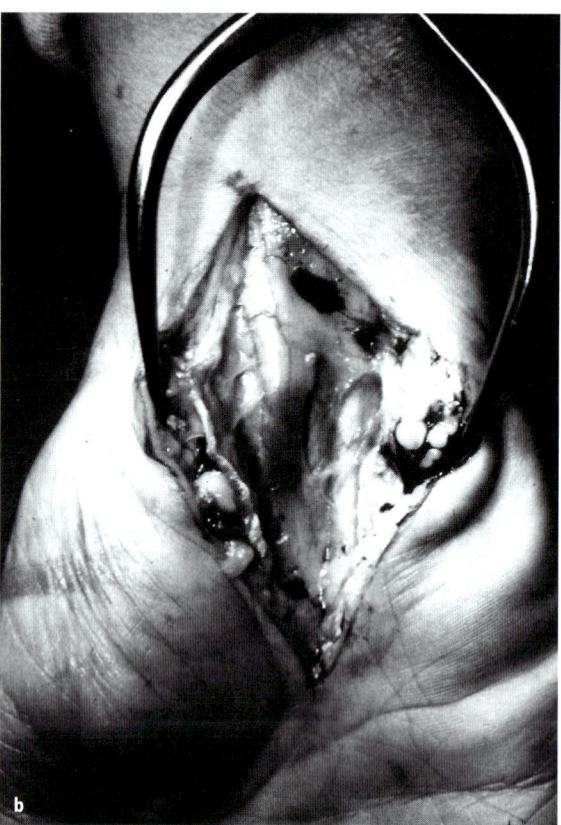

Fig. 1.5. a This illustration from Cannon and Love's article accurately represents **b** the anatomy of carpal tunnel syndrome and carpal tunnel release surgery. (Artwork copyright Mayo Foundation, previously reproduced in the *Journal of Bone and Joint Surgery*, with permission)

division of the flexor retinaculum in a case associated with wrist arthritis but without any specific carpal injury. This is getting much closer to our current understanding of carpal tunnel syndrome, although Learmonth again apparently thought that the condition was rare. In 1935 Zabriskie thought that "the sensation of tingling suggests more than the thenar branch is affected" [24]. In 1939 Wartenberg wrote that "one point completely ignored by Hunt...the paresthesias of which most patients complained" [25], again, attempting to join the threads of thenar neuritis and acroparesthesias into the final common pathway of carpal tunnel syndrome: Zachary, in 1995, had similar thoughts [26]. Finally, in 1946 Cannon and Love published 38 cases of surgical division of the flexor retinaculum for treatment of distal median neuropathy [27]. This landmark article also included the first accurate description of a surgical technique (Fig. 1.5).

Brain is usually described as having written the landmark paper in carpal tunnel syndrome, but as seen above there was considerable literature already existing pointing in the direction before Brain wrote his classic Lancet paper in 1947 [28]. In that paper he described acroparesthesias and thenar neuritis as variable manifestations of median neuropathy due to compression at the flexor retinaculum. He emphasized that this is "caused ONLY by a median nerve lesion, and not a lesion involving the brachial plexus." Unfortunately, the illustration accompanying Brain's article was misleading and suggested that the flexor retinaculum was located proximal to the wrist flexion crease (Fig. 1.6). This may have led to some misunderstanding with regard to the proper treatment of the condition [29], and may have led to the popularity in some circles of incisions for carpal tunnel release in the distal forearm rather than the palm.

The name most associated with the popularization of carpal tunnel syndrome is certainly that of George Phalen. In classic papers published in 1950 [30], 1951 [8], and 1957 [31], he wrote of his clinical experience in literally hundreds of surgical cases. He specifically cited Brain as a prime influence on him [32], although Phalen was also a close associate of Bunnell during World War II and was a student at Mayo Clinic in the 1930s, and thus a contemporary there of Moersch and Learmonth.

The source of the name "carpal tunnel syndrome" is unclear. It was first used in print in 1953 by Kremer et al. [33]. They credited, however, a 1949 personal communication by M.J. McArdle.

We now understand the pathogenesis of carpal tunnel syndrome to be related to synovial thickening and increased pressure in the carpal canal. This etiology was emphasized by Phalen in the early 1950s [8, 30, 31], but was also noted by Woltman in 1941 [34]. Brain [28] and Denny-Brown [35] emphasized ischemia due to ex-

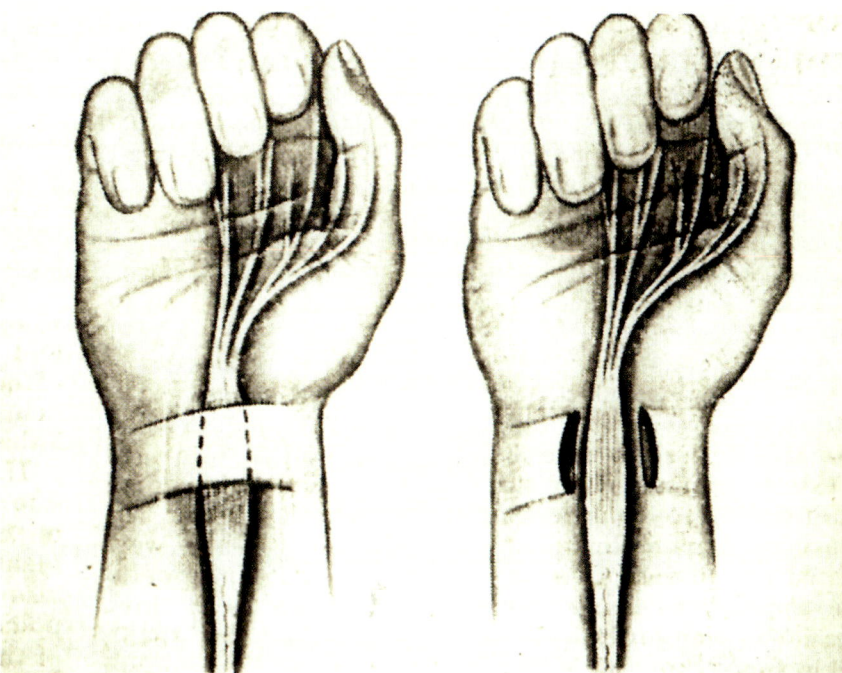

Fig. 1.6. The illustration from Brain's article represents the anatomy inaccurately, indicating that the flexor retinaculum is located proximal to the wrist crease rather than distal to it. (with permission, *Lancet*)

Fig. 1—Case I : median nerve flattened and enlarged under carpal ligament.

ternal compression. As previously mentioned, Raynaud [11] and Putnam [12] thought that ischemia of small nerve fibers, due to pathology in the intrinsic vascularization of the median nerve, was the most likely etiology. This is certainly a factor in the etiology of carpal tunnel syndrome in some cases of diabetic polyneuropathy, but is not considered to be the most common cause of the condition.

The work association of carpal tunnel syndrome was postulated even before the condition was well described. In 1873 Poore [36] described what appears to be carpal tunnel syndrome and called it writer's cramp. In the early 1900s Hunt was readily ascribing the etiology of thenar neuritis to occupational activities. Further elucidation of the epidemiology of carpal tunnel syndrome had to await the study of Stevens et al. in 1980 [37], which reviewed all cases of carpal tunnel syndrome in a single community in the USA. There was roughly one new medically diagnosed case per thousand population during the years 1960 to 1980. Subsequent studies have suggested that there is a considerable reservoir of untreated and undiagnosed carpal tunnel syndrome in the community [38]. The best current estimate of the prevalence of carpal tunnel syndrome in a community, whether medically diagnosed or not, is in the range of 2% to 5% [39].

For many years it was considered that Learmonth (Fig. 1.7) did the first flexor retinaculum release for a diagnosis of median neuropathy. It is difficult to know for certain, but a case identified in a review of Mayo Clinic

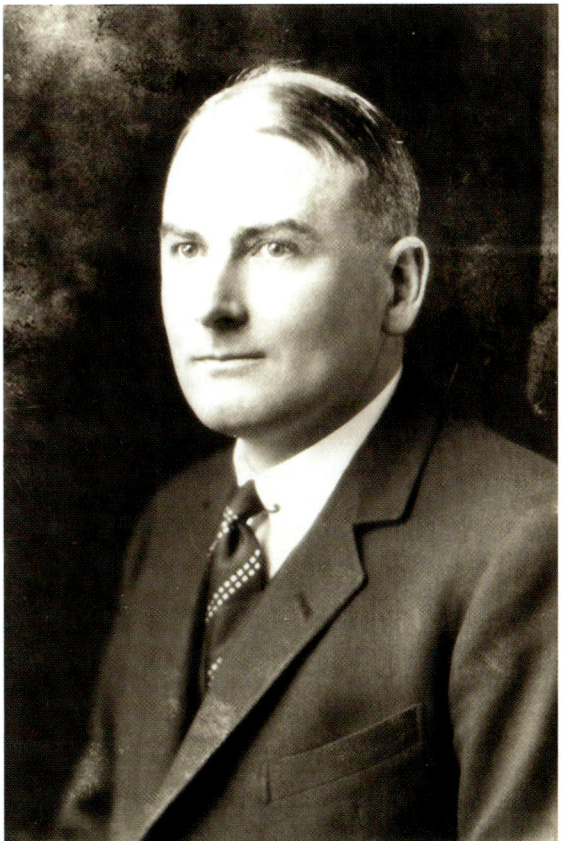

Fig. 1.7. James R. Learmonth. (photo copyright Mayo Foundation, reproduced with permission)

medical records suggest that Herbert Galloway, a Canadian orthopedic surgeon, and one of the early presidents of the American Orthopedic Association, did explore a median nerve at the wrist for a postcrush median neuropathy, and released the flexor retinaculum in 1924 [40]. To date, no earlier cases have been identified.

Steroid injection is a common treatment for carpal tunnel syndrome. It is hard to know again when steroids were first used but as early as 1954, the Mayo Clinic medical records document the use of steroid injections for the treatment of carpal tunnel syndrome [10]. Phalen and Kendrick were the first to publish their experience, in 1957 [31].

As noted above, the association of carpal tunnel syndrome with pregnancy was recognized early on. Putnam associated acroparesthesias with pregnancy in 1888 [12]. Kremer postulated that fluid retention was the most likely etiology in 1953 [33]; his opinion is still the standard explanation.

Simpson in 1956 reported on the use of neurophysiological testing in carpal tunnel syndrome [41]. There have been considerable publications since, and the American Academy of Electrodiagnostic Medicine has published standards for the electrophysiological diagnosis of carpal tunnel syndrome [42].

As this historical review demonstrates, carpal tunnel syndrome has been the focus of considerable discussion in the medical literature, but our understanding continues to evolve. Recently, the literature has focused on the work relationship of carpal tunnel syndrome [43]; the effectiveness of endoscopic therapy [39]; the mechanisms by which steroid therapy has its benefit [44]; the utility of diuretics, nonsteroidal anti-inflammatory medication, and vitamins in the therapy of carpal tunnel syndrome [43]; and the diagnostic criteria for carpal tunnel syndrome [45]. Is carpal tunnel syndrome a clinical condition, diagnosed on the basis of symptoms and physical examination? Is it a physiological condition that can only be diagnosed on the basis of electrophysiological abnormalities? Most people believe that carpal tunnel syndrome is a clinical diagnosis, based on a presumed physiological abnormality, specifically of median nerve function at the level of the flexor retinaculum. As such, electrophysiological diagnostic testing is a powerful confirmatory study, but is neither sufficient to make the diagnosis nor, if normal, to rule out the diagnosis. It seems clear that there are many people who have electrophysiological slowing of median nerve conduction at the wrist with absolutely no symptoms [38]. These would appear not to be carpal tunnel syndrome, and as best as can be determined from the limited epidemiological studies that are available, most of these cases do not evolve into carpal tunnel syndrome over time [38]. On the other hand, patients who have symptoms consistent with carpal tunnel syndrome, even in the presence of normal electrophysiological testing, appear to respond like those with electrophysiological abnormalities to the various treatments that are offered, including surgical decompression [46]. This would tend to confirm that the diagnosis of carpal tunnel syndrome should be a clinical one.

In summary, carpal tunnel syndrome is a useful example of the evolution of a medical idea: the joining of seemingly disparate trains of thought, the frustration of blind alleys, and finally the rapid dissemination of a coherent clinical pathological picture.

References

1. Gensoul (1836) Arch gén de méd XL: 187
2. Paget J (1854) Lectures on Surgical Pathology. Philadelphia, Lindsay and Blakistone
3. Lewis D, Miller EM (1922) Peripheral nerve injuries associated with fractures. Trans Am Surg Assoc 40:489–580
4. Blecher (Dr) (1908) Die Schädigung des Nervus medianus als Komplikation des typischen Radiusbruches. Dtsch Z Chir 93:34–45
5. Kirchheim T (1910) Ueber Verletzungen des N. medianus bei Fractura radii an klassicher Stelle. Thesis. Berlin, Friedrich-Wilhelm Universität zu Berlin
6. Dickson FD (1926) South M J xix:37
7. Abbott LC, Saunders JB del M (1933) Injuries of the median nerve in fractures of the lower end of the radius. Surg Gynecol Obstet 57:507–516
8. Phalen GS (1951) Spontaneous compression of the median nerve at the wrist. JAMA 145:1128–1132
9. Watson-Jones R (1929) Carpal semilunar dislocations and other wrist dislocations with associated nerve lesions. Proceedings of the Royal Society of Medicine 22:1071–1086
10. Amadio PC (1992) The Mayo Clinic and carpal tunnel syndrome. Mayo Clin Proc 67:42–48
11. Raynaud M (1888) De l'asphyxie locale et de la gangrène symétrique des extrémités. Paris: Rignoux. Trans by T. Barlow, Collected Monographs, Vol 121, London: New Sydenham Society
12. Putnam JJ (1880) A series of cases of paraesthesia, mainly of the hands, of periodical recurrence, and possibly of vaso-motor origin. Arch Med (NY) 4:147–162
13. Ormerod JA (1883) On a peculiar numbness and paresis of the hands. St Barts Hosp Rep 19:17–26
14. Keen WW (1907) The symptomatology, diagnosis and surgical treatment of cervical ribs. Am J Med Sci 133:2:193
15. Pfeffer GB, Gelberman RH, Boyes JH, Rydevik B (1988) The history of carpal tunnel syndrome. J Hand Surg 13B:28–34
16. Sargent P (1921) Lesions of the brachial plexus associated with rudimentary ribs. Brain 44:2:95–124
17. Kinnier Wilson SA (1913) Some points in the symptomatology of cervical ribs with especial reference to muscular wasting. Proceedings of the Royal Society of Medicine 6:133–138
18. Walsh FMR, Jackson H, Wyburn-Mason R (1944) On some pressure effects associated with cervical and with rudimentary and "normal" first ribs, and the factors entering into their causation. Brain 67:3:141–177
19. Behrman S (1945) Acroparaesthesia. Proc R Soc Med 38:600–601
20. Hunt JR (1910) Occupation neuritis of the thenar branch of the median nerve: (a well defined type of neural atrophy of the hand). Trans Am Neurol Assoc 35:184

21. Moersch FP (1938) Median thenar neuritis. Proc Staff Meet Mayo Clin 13:220–222
22. Marie P, Foix C (1913) Atrophie isolée de l'éminence thénar d'origine névritique. Rôle du ligament annulaire antérieur du carpe dans la pathogénie de la lésion. Revue Neurol 26:647–649
23. Learmonth JR (1933) The principle of decompression in the treatment of certain diseases of peripheral nerves. Surg Clin North Am 13:905–913, Aug.
24. Zabriskie EG, Hare CC, Masselink RJ (1935) Hypertrophic arthritis of cervical vertebrae with thenar muscular atrophy occurring in three sisters. Bulletin of the Neurological Institute of New York 4:207
25. Wartenberg R (1939) Partial thenar atrophy. Archives of neurology and psychiatry 42:3:373
26. Zachary RB (1945) Thenar palsy due to compression of the median nerve in the carpal tunnel. Surgery, Gynecology, and Obstetrics 81:213–217
27. Cannon BW, Love JG (1946) Tardy median palsy; median neuritis; median thenar neuritis amenable to surgery. Surgery 20:210–216
28. Brain WR, Wright AD, Wilkinson M (1947) Spontaneous compression of both median nerves in the carpal tunnel: six cases treated surgically. Lancet 1:277–282
29. Harris HA (1947) Compression of median nerve in carpal tunnel (letter to the editor). Lancet 1:387
30. Phalen GS, Gardner WJ, La Londe AA (1950) Neuropathy of the median nerve due to compression beneath the transverse carpal ligament. J Bone Joint Surg 32A:109–112
31. Phalen GS, Kendrick JI (1957) Compression neuropathy of the median nerve in the carpal tunnel. JAMA 164:524–530
32. Phalen GS (1981) The birth of a syndrome, or carpal tunnel revisited (editorial). J Hand Surg 6:109–110
33. Kremer M, Gilliatt RW, Golding JSR, Wilson TG (1953) Acroparaesthesiae in the carpal-tunnel syndrome. Lancet 2:590–595
34. Woltman MW (1941) Neuritis associated with acromegaly. Archives of neurology and Psychiatry 680–682
35. Denny-Brown D, Brenner C (1944) Paralysis of nerve induced by direct pressure and by tourniquet. Archives Neurol Psychiatry 51(1):1–26
36. Poore GV (1873) On a case of writer's cramp, and subsequent general spasm of the right arm, treated by the joint use of the continuous galvanic current and the rhythmical exercise of the affected muscles. Practitioner 9:129–137
37. Stevens JC, Sun S, Beard CM, et al. (1988) Carpal tunnel syndrome in Rochester, Minnesota, 1961 to 1980. Neurology 38:134–138
38. Atroshi I, Gummesson C, Johnsson R, et al. (1999) Prevalence of carpal tunnel syndrome in a general population. JAMA 282(2):153–158
39. Atroshi I, Johnsson R, Ornstein E (1997) Endoscopic carpal tunnel release: Prospective assessment of 255 consecutive cases. J Hand Surg 22B(1):42–47
40. Amadio PC (1995) The first carpal tunnel release? J Hand Surg (British and European Vol.) 20B:I:40–41
41. Simpson JA (1956) Electrical signs in the diagnosis of carpal tunnel and related syndromes. J Neurol Neurosurg Psychiatry 19:275–280
42. Stevens JC (1987) AAEE minimonograph #26: the electrodiagnosis of carpal tunnel syndrome. Muscle Nerve 10:99–113
43. Amadio PC (1987) Carpal tunnel syndrome, pyridoxine, and the work place. J Hand Surg 12A:875–880
44. Foster JB (1960) Hydrocortisone and the carpal-tunnel syndrome. Lancet 1:454–456
45. Rempel, Evanoff B, Amadio PC, et al. (1998) Consensus criteria for the classification of carpal tunnel syndrome in epidemiologic studies. Am J Public Health 88(10):1447–1451
46. Grundberg AB (1983) Carpal tunnel decompression in spite of normal electromyography. J Hand Surg 8A(3):348–349

2 Anatomy of the Carpal Tunnel

P. Yugueros, R.A. Berger

The carpal tunnel is an inelastic fibro-osseous tunnel defined by the carpal bones and the flexor retinaculum. The osseous components of the carpal tunnel form an arch, defined by four bony prominences – proximally by pisiform and tubercle of scaphoid and distally by hook of the hamate and tubercle of trapezium. Superficially the palmaris longus tendon passes anterior to the flexor retinaculum to become continuous with the palmar fascia. Deep to the palmar fascia, a thick ligamentous band forms the superficial border of the carpal tunnel, also referred to as the transverse carpal ligament. The flexor retinaculum and the transverse carpal ligament are considered by some authors synonymous terms [1–3]. The anatomic zone of the flexor retinaculum extends from the distal radius to the proximal metaphysis of the third metacarpal. It is firmly attached to the hook of the hamate and pisiform bones on the ulnar (medial) side of the carpal tunnel and the tubercle of the trapezium and distal pole of the scaphoid on the radial (lateral) side of the carpal tunnel. The flexor retinaculum may be divided into three distinct components. The proximal portion is a direct continuation of the deep antebrachial fascia. Distally, the transverse carpal ligament represents the central portion of the flexor retinaculum. Most distally is an aponeurosis between the thenar and hypothenar muscles [4] (Fig. 2.1).

Although the carpal tunnel appears to be in open communication with the flexor compartment of the forearm proximally and the midpalmar space of the hand distally, it behaves like a closed compartment and maintains its own tissue fluid pressure levels [5]. Longitudinally the carpal tunnel is narrowest 2–2.5 cm distal to its most proximal margin (approximately at the hook of the hamate) with a mean width of 20 mm, expanding to a mean width of 25 mm at its proximal and distal margins. The transverse carpal ligament is thickest at the level of its attachment to the hook of the hamate and the tubercle of the trapezium, which is also the most narrow region of the carpal tunnel.

The radial side of the flexor retinaculum splits to form a separate tunnel for the tendon of the flexor carpi radialis muscle, forming in essence a superficial and deep layer of the retinaculum (Fig. 2.2). This tunnel is directly continuous with the fibro-osseous tunnel for

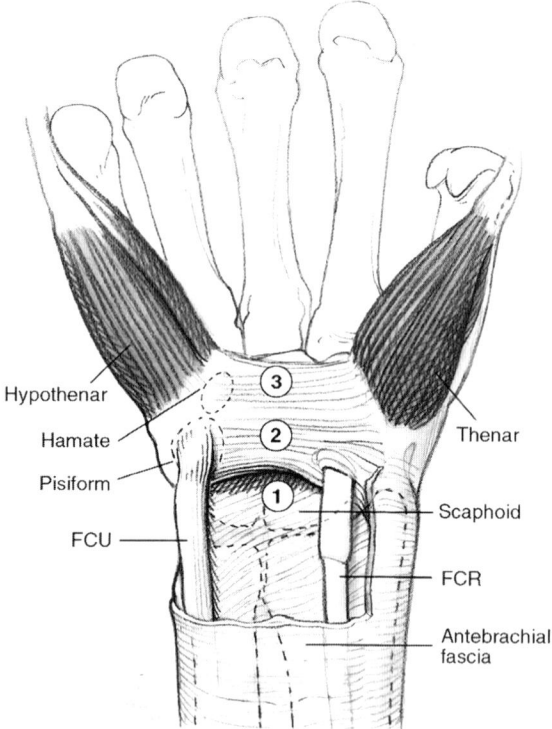

Fig. 2.1. The anterior (palmar) anatomy of the carpal tunnel. (1) demonstrates the exposed proximal entrance into the carpal tunnel between the tendons of flexor carpi ulnaris (FCU) and flexor carpi radialis (FCR). The thickest region of the flexor retinaculum is shown as (2), but it continues distally to the level of the carpometacarpal joints as a thinner structure (2)

the flexor carpi radialis tendon that forms anterior to the distal pole of the scaphoid and continues distally dorsal to the trapezial ridge.

The principle contents of the carpal tunnel are the median nerve, typically accompanied by the highly variable arteria mediana, and nine extrinsic flexor tendons. The median nerve is composed of branches from the C5 through T1 spinal cord nerve roots. It travels distally in the forearm between the flexor digitorum superficialis and profundus muscle bellies, often within the deep epimysium of the flexor digitorum superficialis. In the distal forearm, the median nerve becomes more superficial, coursing between the tendons of flex-

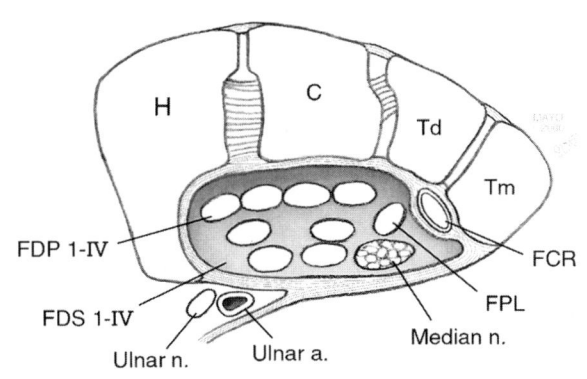

Fig. 2.2. The transverse anatomy of the carpal tunnel, through the level of the distal carpal row. H, hamate; C, capitate; Td, trapezoid; Tm, trapezium; FDP I-IV, tendons of flexor digitorum profundi; FDS I-IV, tendons of flexor digitorum superficialis; FPL, tendon of flexor pollicis longus; n, nerve; a, artery. Note that the tendon of flexor carpi radialis (FCR) is in a separate compartment

or digitorum superficialis ulnarly and flexor carpi radialis radially, dorsal or dorsoradial to the palmaris longus tendon. Approximately 5 cm proximal to the wrist crease, hence proximal to the cephalad margin of the carpal tunnel, the palmar cutaneous branch of the median nerve diverges. It parallels the median nerve for 1.6–2.5 cm and then courses separately under the antebrachial fascia between the tendons of palmaris longus and flexor carpi radialis [6, 7]. The palmar cutaneous branch of the median nerve then pierces the deep antebrachial fascia, becoming superficial to the flexor retinaculum, approximately 0.8 cm proximal to the wrist crease. It then divides into one radial and one or multiple ulnar branches which innervate the palmar skin of the proximal hand. After exiting the carpal tunnel the median nerve divides into six terminal branches. The recurrent motor branch supplies afferent innervation to the thenar muscles (flexor pollicis brevis, abductor pollicis brevis, and opponens pollicis). There are three proper digital nerves, including the radial and ulnar proper digital nerves to the thumb and the radial proper digital nerve to the index finger. These may emerge from the median nerve as a common digital nerve. Finally, two common digital nerves emerge from the median nerve. The second common digital nerve divides to form the ulnar proper digital nerve of the index finger and the radial proper digital nerve for the long finger, and the third common digital nerve divides to form the ulnar proper digital nerve for the long finger and the radial proper digital nerve for the ring finger. The first lumbrical muscle is innervated by motor branches that originate from the radial proper digital nerve to the index finger; the second lumbrical muscle is innervated by motor branches that originate from the second common digital nerve.

The point of departure of the recurrent motor branch from the median nerve may vary in its relation with the distal edge of the transverse carpal ligament. This reported variability may in fact be due to variations in the perceived distal extent of the transverse carpal ligament. Frequently (46%) the recurrent motor branch passes in a retrograde fashion into the thenar musculature, following a pattern which is labeled extraligamentous (Fig. 2.3). Less frequently (31%) the recurrent motor branch diverges from the median nerve deep to the transverse carpal ligament, within the confines of the carpal tunnel, and passes around the distal edge of the transverse carpal ligament to enter the thenar musculature, following a pattern which is called subligamentous. Least frequently (23%) the recurrent motor branch diverges from the median nerve within the limits of the carpal tunnel and appears to perforate the ligament in its course to the thenar musculature, thereby called transligamentous [8]. The fascicles ultimately destined for the recurrent motor branch have been found in 60% of dissections to arise from the extreme radial aspect of the median nerve, in 22% from the central-anterior aspect, and in the remaining 18% between the extreme radial-anterior and the central aspect of the median nerve. In 56% of reported dissections, the recurrent motor branch of the median nerve passes through a separate fascial tunnel immediately prior to entering the thenar muscles. There is no unique correlation between the presence of the distal tunnel and the motor branch orientation in the median nerve [9]. It is possible that the significant variation in the location of the motor branch of the median nerve

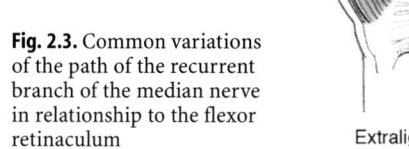

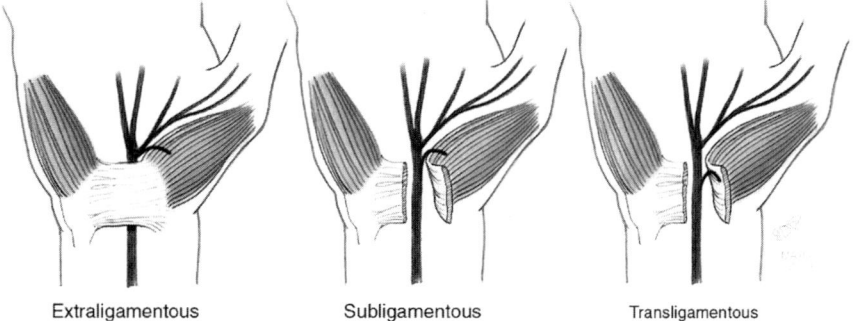

Fig. 2.3. Common variations of the path of the recurrent branch of the median nerve in relationship to the flexor retinaculum

Extraligamentous Subligamentous Transligamentous

with respect to the other fascicles may predispose to thenar muscle wasting in compression syndromes with unequal distribution of demyelination and degeneration between fascicles.

The muscles of the nine extrinsic flexor tendons which traverse the carpal tunnel originate from the medial epicondyle of the humerus and the anterior aspect of the radius, ulna, and interosseous membrane. The musculotendinous junctions are found proximal to the proximal edge of the carpal tunnel. The flexor pollicis longus muscle is the most radial structure of the group discussed here; it originates from the radius and the interosseous membrane and emerges between the superficial and deep heads of the flexor pollicis brevis muscle where it inserts into the proximal phalanx of the thumb. The flexor digitorum superficialis muscle originates from the medial epicondyle of the distal humerus and the coronoid process and proximal diaphysis of the radius, divides into four independent muscle bellies in the mid-forearm, and passes through the carpal tunnel only as deep as the flexor retinaculum into the middle phalanges of the index, long ring, and small fingers. Within the carpal tunnel, the tendons of the flexor digitorum superficialis muscle to the long and ring fingers are central and anterior relative to the index and small finger tendons. The flexor digitorum profundus muscle originates from the proximal two thirds of the ulna and the interosseous membrane. The radial half of the muscle forms the flexor digitorum profundus to the index finger and the ulnar half of the muscle forms the profundus tendons to the long, ring, and small fingers. All four tendons insert separately into the distal phalanges of the fingers. These four tendons pass through the carpal tunnel at the most dorsal aspect, dorsal to the tendons of the flexor digitorum superficialis muscle. The lumbrical muscles originate from the tendons of the flexor digitorum profundus beyond the level of the carpal tunnel.

The tendons are surrounded by mesodermal tissue, which provides vincular blood supply to the tendons as well as extratendinous lubrication and nutrition. It is composed of a continuous layer of mesoderm, forming invaginated loops around the individual tendons. The source of the blood supply to the tendinous vincula is the anterior interosseous artery. Usually there is an ulnar bursa that surrounds the superficial and deep flexors of the fingers and a separate radial bursa that surrounds the flexor pollicis longus [10].

Just above this layer of mesodermal tissue is the fibrous layer of the anterior wrist joint capsule. This capsule is composed largely of ligaments passing across the anterior surfaces of the radiocarpal, midcarpal, and carpometacarpal joints. The anterior wrist joint capsule is continuous with the periosteum of the carpal bones and the transverse carpal ligament.

References

1. Gray H, Clemente CD (1985) Anatomy of the human body. 13th ed, Lea & Febiger, Philadelphia. pp 531, 542, 551
2. Spinner M (1984) Kaplan's functional and surgical anatomy of the hand. 3rd ed JB Lippincott, Philadelphia, pp 261–263
3. Hoppenfeld S, deBoer P (1984) Surgical exposures in orthopaedics: the anatomic approach. JB Lippincott, Philadelphia, pp 162–165
4. Cobb TK, Dalley BK, Posterato RH (1993) Anatomy of the flexor retinaculum. J Hand Surg. 18:91–99
5. Steinberg DR, Szabo RM (1996) Anatomy of the median nerve at the wrist – Open carpal tunnel release – Classic. Hand Clinics 12:259–269
6. Bezerra AJ, Carvalho VC, Nucci A (1986) An anatomical study of the palmar cutaneous branch of the median nerve. Surg Radiol Anat 8:183–188
7. Taleisnik J (1973) The palmar cutaneous branch of the median nerve and the approach to the carpal tunnel. An anatomical study. J Bone Joint Surg 55A:1212–1217
8. Poisel S (1974) Ursprung und verlauf des r.muscularis des nervus digitalis palmaris communis I (N. medianus). Chir Praxis 18:471–474
9. Mackinnon S, Dellon AL (1988) Anatomic investigations of nerves at the wrist: I. Orientation of the motor fascicle of the median nerve in the carpal tunnel. Ann Plast Surg 21:32–35

Normal Anatomy and Variations of the Median Nerve in the Carpal Tunnel

H.-M. Schmidt

Carpal Tunnel

The carpal tunnel is the pathway between the flexor compartment of the forearm and the midpalmar space of the hand. Containing the median nerve and all the finger and thumb flexor tendons, they converge adjacent to the carpal tunnel and then diverge distally into the deeper palm. Also, it is a commonly used approach to the carpal bones and the joint compartments of the wrist. Variations in the volume of its contents may be possible. In cases of abnormal narrowing of the carpal tunnel as well as during motions in the wrist joints, there are changes of tunnel volume and pressure. The osseous walls are not completely rigid because the carpal bones shift against one another during the motions between forearm and hand [36]. Aberrant muscles like palmaris profundus, lumbricalis, and/or muscles bellies can also narrow the tunnel volume as well as an abnormal course of the superficial branch of the radial artery [11, 18, 29].

With flexion of the radiocarpal joint, the proximal opening of the carpal tunnel widens by about 20 % in contrast to the neutral position of the wrist [2]. In maximum extension the lunate bone shifts towards the interior. Also the distal end of the capitate bone protrudes into the carpal tunnel. The narrowing of the tunnel follows consequently. The pressure within the carpal tunnel increases under dependency of both flexion and extension and with active grip [3, 9, 15, 24, 27, 38, 44]. Also a high mean pressure within the carpal tunnel was recorded in full supination of the forearm and 90° metacarpophalangeal flexion [35].

Restriction of space and heightening of pressure in the carpal tunnel impairs the conductivity of the median nerve, not only by mechanical pressure but also by interruption of blood flow within the epineurium. An increase of pressure associated with carpal tunnel syndrome shows no influence on median nerve kinetics or kinematics in maximum wrist positions [4].

Flexor Retinaculum

The flexor retinaculum is a transverse-oriented strong ligament that contributes to maintenance of the transverse carpal arch. The main function is to serve as a flexor pulley at the wrist preventing bow-stringing of the flexor tendons. Distally oriented fibers of the forearm fascia passes into the palmar carpal ligament superficially and the flexor retinaculum deeply. The retinaculum extends between the radial and ulnar carpal eminences as a strong fibrous structure. The proximal boundary is located at the level of the proximal row of the carpal bones. The slightly curved distal rim projects over the bases of the second to fifth metacarpal bones. The mean width of the flexor retinaculum is 22 mm, slightly increasing from the radial to the ulnar side. The mean length of the flexor retinaculum proximally, as well as distally, is 26 mm. In its middle portion the fiber tract is strongest with a mean thickness of 1.6 mm. Proximally and distally the retinaculum is approximately 0.6 mm thick.

In the transition zone from the forearm to the hand, superficial reinforcements of the antebrachial fascia form the palmar carpal ligament. The fibers extend between the tendon of the flexor carpi ulnaris muscle and the ulnar border of the palmaris longus tendon. It can be divided into superficial weaker and deep stronger layers. In some cases the deep transverse fibers can compress the median nerve. The palmar carpal ligament blends with the flexor retinaculum radial to the tendon of the palmaris longus muscle.

Arteries of the flexor retinaculum form a superficial palmar and a deep dorsal vascular network [46] (Fig. 3.1). The superficial layers are supplied by branches dividing at right angles from the ulnar artery. These branches form anastomoses with short branches of the radial artery to supply the retinaculum at the origin of the thenar muscles. The dorsal surface of the retinaculum is supplied by branches of the superficial palmar arch.

Decompression of the median nerve is performed by cutting the flexor retinaculum adjacent to the hook of hamate. In addition to providing optimal protection of the branches of the median nerve, this exposure pre-

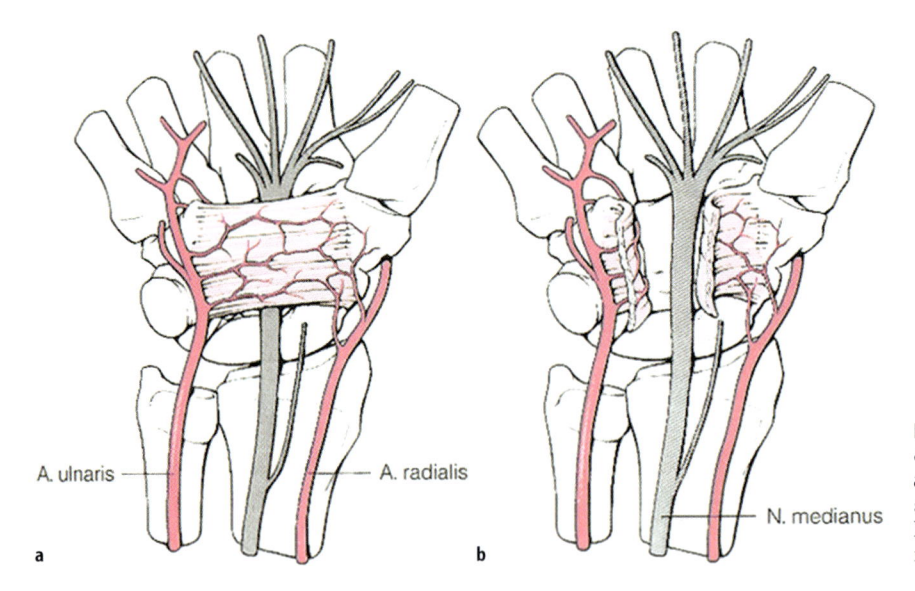

Fig. 3.1. a,b Vascularization of the flexor retinaculum. **a** Palmar surface. **b** Dorsal surface. *FR*, flexor retinaculum; *UA*, ulnar artery; *RA*, radial artery

serves a protective roof for the nerve. Nevertheless, scarring of the median nerve after open decompression very often leads to chronic pain symptoms. Loss of the sliding mobility of the nerve during wrist movements due to scar adhesions causes wound pain and reduced grip strength. Vascularized hypothenar fat flaps produce cushioning of the median nerve, restoring the sliding pathway to reduce wound tenderness [8, 10, 14, 32, 39].

The palmar cutaneous branch of the median nerve and the variable ramifications of the median and ulnar nerves are best preserved with the opening technique [21, 40]. Regularly the branch arises from the radial side of the median nerve 84 57–110 mm proximal to the wrist crease [22]. Covered by a tunnel-like fascial sheath, the nerve travels distally together with the median nerve adjacent to the tendon of the flexor carpi radialis. Ensheathed 38 mm proximal of the wrist crease, the palmar cutaneous branch of the median nerve passes dorsal to the palmar carpal ligament to the undersurface of the palmar aponeurosis. Division of the terminal endings of the branch reveal firstly smaller branches to the palmar skin overlying the palmaris longus insertion into the palmar aponeurosis. Secondly, weak radial-oriented branches reach the thenar fascia and thirdly, stronger ulnar-oriented branches traverse to a fiber complex at the radial margin of the "loge de Guyon" [12]. In some cases the palmar cutaneous branch of the median nerve passes through the palmaris longus tendon 12 mm proximal to its insertion into the palmar aponeurosis [7]. Naff and coauthors [22] reported the course of the palmar cutaneous branch of the median nerve within the tendon sheath of the flexor carpi radialis.

Measurements of the length and width of the flexor retinaculum correspond well with the dimensions of

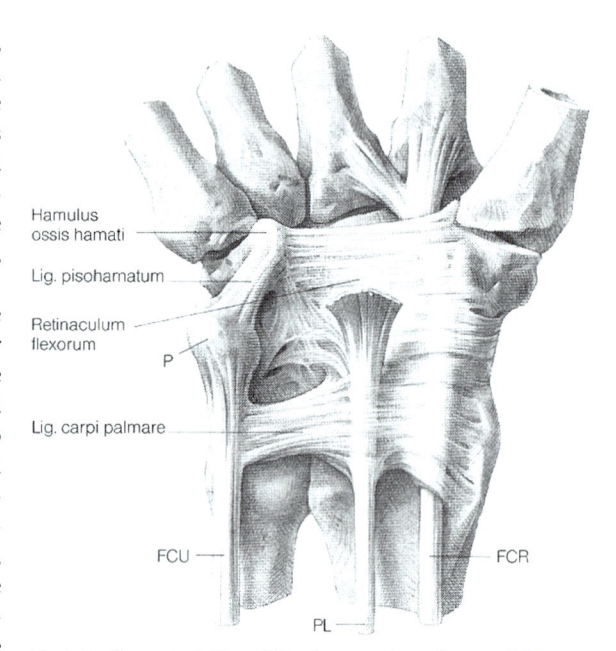

Fig. 3.2. Characteristics of the flexor retinaculum and the carpal tunnel. Length: proximal and distal 26 (21–30) mm. Width: ulnar 22 (16–27) mm; middle 22 (16–26) mm; radial 21 (18–26) mm. *FCU*, tendon of flexor carpi ulnaris; *PL*, tendon of palmaris longus; *FCR*, tendon of flexor carpi radialis; *FR*, flexor retinaculum; *PCL*, palmar carpal ligament

the carpal tunnel (Fig. 3.2). The greatest depth of the canal, approximately 12 mm, lies in the middle of the proximal opening at the level of the lunate bone. At the radial and ulnar borders of the tunnel entrance, the depth values of the canal are markedly smaller (Fig. 3.3).

The narrowest segment of the carpal tunnel, approximately 10 mm wide, is located at the level of the palmar-oriented prominence of the capitate bone

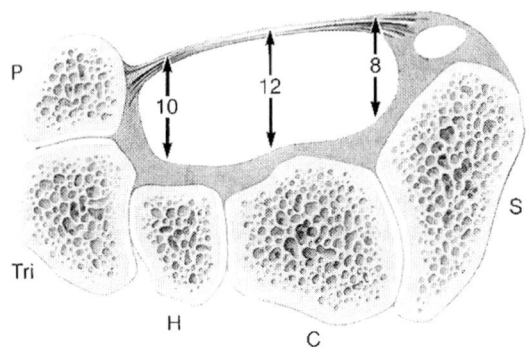

Fig. 3.3. Depth of the proximal carpal tunnel measured from the palmar side of the flexor retinaculum, and thickness of the flexor retinaculum. Thickness of the flexor retinaculum: proximal 0.6 (0.2–0.8) mm; middle 0.9 (0.4–1.6) mm; distal 0.6 (0.2–1.0) mm. Depth of the proximal carpal tunnel: radial 8 mm; middle 12 mm; ulnar 10 mm. *P*, pisiform; *Tri*, triquetrum; *H*, hamate; *C*, capitate; *S*, scaphoid

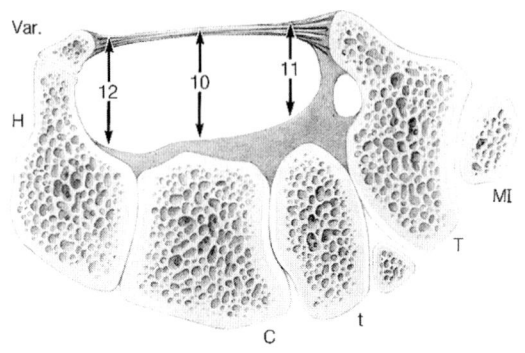

Fig. 3.4. Depth of the distal carpal tunnel measured from the palmar side of the flexor retinaculum. Depth: radial 11 mm; middle 10 mm; ulnar 12 mm. *MI*, first metacarpal; *T*, trapezium; *t*, trapezoid; *C*, capitate; *H*, hamate; *Var*, accessory hamate bone

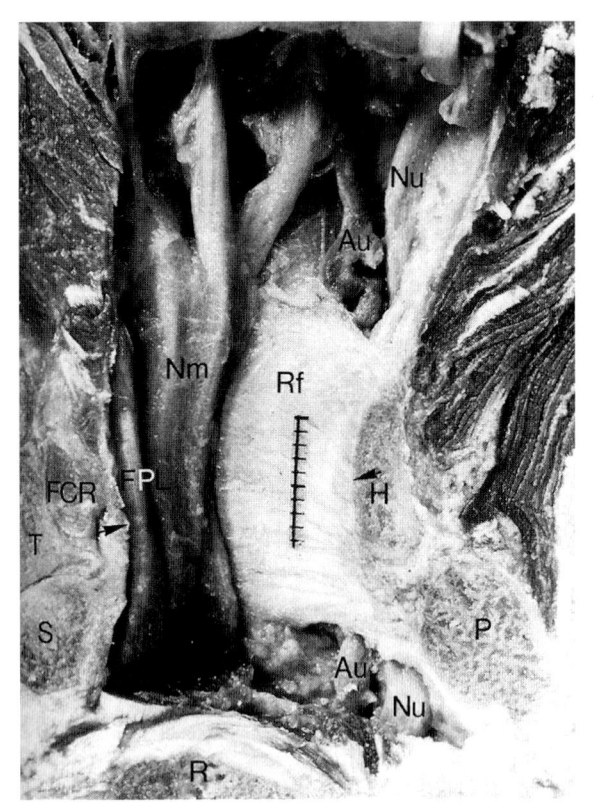

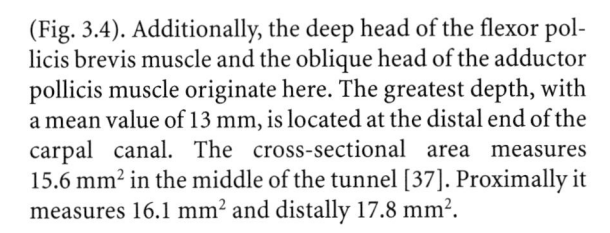

Fig. 3.5. Transverse section at the roof of the carpal tunnel. A rule is shown on the dorsal side of the flexor retinaculum (*Rf*). All flexor tendons are cut and removed distally. *Arrows* mark the "waist" of the carpal tunnel. Notice the furrows on the dorsal side of the median nerve (*Nm*). They represent indentations caused by laterally located flexor tendons. *FPL*, tendon of the flexor pollicis longus; *FCR*, tendon of the flexor carpi radialis; *T*, trapezium; *S*, scaphoid; *R*, radius; *P*, pisiform; *H*, hook of hamate; *Au*, ulnar artery; *Nu*, ulnar nerve

(Fig. 3.4). Additionally, the deep head of the flexor pollicis brevis muscle and the oblique head of the adductor pollicis muscle originate here. The greatest depth, with a mean value of 13 mm, is located at the distal end of the carpal canal. The cross-sectional area measures 15.6 mm^2 in the middle of the tunnel [37]. Proximally it measures 16.1 mm^2 and distally 17.8 mm^2.

Median Nerve

With a mean width of 6 mm, the median nerve enters the carpal canal dorsal to the flexor retinaculum. In the distal direction the width increases continuously. At the middle of the tunnel it is 6.1 mm, and at the end 7.7 mm. In thickness the median nerve decreases gradually from 2.1 mm proximally to 1.9 mm distally. Toward the palmar space of the hand the median nerve becomes more and more flattened. Throughout its course in the tunnel, the nerve shows furrow-like indentations on its dorsal surface. These are caused by intimate contact with the flexor tendons (Fig. 3.5). The number of fascicles varies from 13 proximally to approximately 35 distally [6]. At the midpoint of the distal carpal tunnel, the motor fascicle, forming the thenar branch distally, is located in the radial-palmar region of the cross-sectional area in 60% of persons, in a central position in 22%, and in a position one third of the distance between the radial and ulnar sides in 18% [20] (Fig. 3.6).

The position and course of the median nerve within the carpal tunnel shows some variations. Without curving, the nerve passes dorsal to the flexor retinaculum to the palm in two thirds of cases. Within these groups with percentages representing total cases, the nerve is shifted to the radial side of the carpal tunnel in 43.3%. Below the middle of the flexor retinaculum it is found in 21.7%, and it is shifted to the ulnar side in

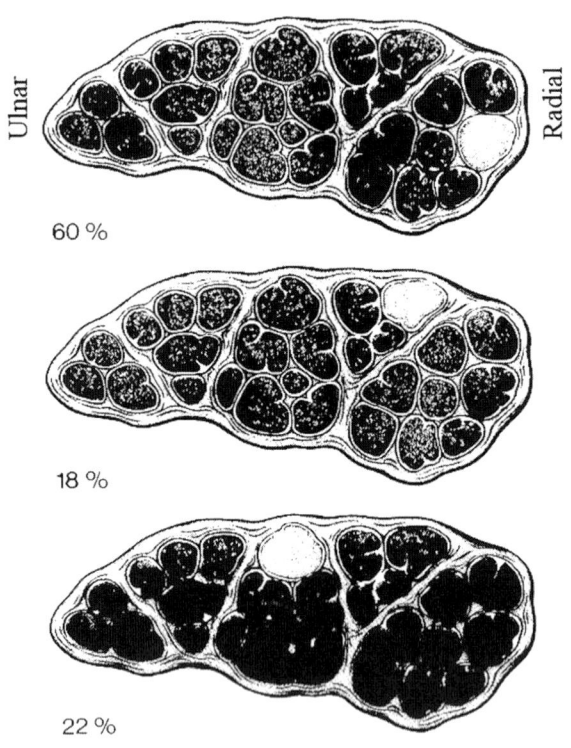

Fig. 3.6. a–c Distribution of motor fascicle orientations about the median nerve in the distal carpal tunnel. **a** 60% (radial). **b** 18% (one third of the distance between the radial and ulnar sides). **c** 22% (central position). (Adapted from [20] with permission.)

1.7%. In one third of cases the nerve curves, diverging to either the radial (21.6%) or ulnar sides (11.7%) [37] (Fig. 3.7).

In 5% of cases the median nerve lies deeply in the carpal tunnel, covered by the tendons of the finger flexors [41]. In wrist extension the median nerve is located between the flexor retinaculum and the tendons of the long finger flexor digitorum superficialis muscle [47]. In wrist flexion, however, the nerve either is flattened by pressure against the flexor retinaculum or becomes interposed between flexor tendons, most commonly the flexor digitorum superficialis II or the flexor pollicis longus. In other cases the median nerve passes between the long finger flexor digitorum superficialis or the ring finger flexor digitorum superficialis. In palmar flexion the median nerve, flexor tendons, and flexor retinaculum are thus closer to each other than in the neutral position. The space between these structures increases in wrist extension.

In the carpal tunnel, the median nerve has remarkable passive excursions. Investigations made by Nakamichi and Tachibana [23] sonographically reveal a mean nerve sliding of 2.1 mm in a transverse direction. Longitudinal excursions of the median nerve during wrist motions vary between 19.6 mm in extension and 10.4 mm in flexion [43]. A sheath-like structure with a space between the layers is closed proximally and distally. A parietal layer of loose connective tissue surrounds the median nerve [34] (Fig. 3.8).

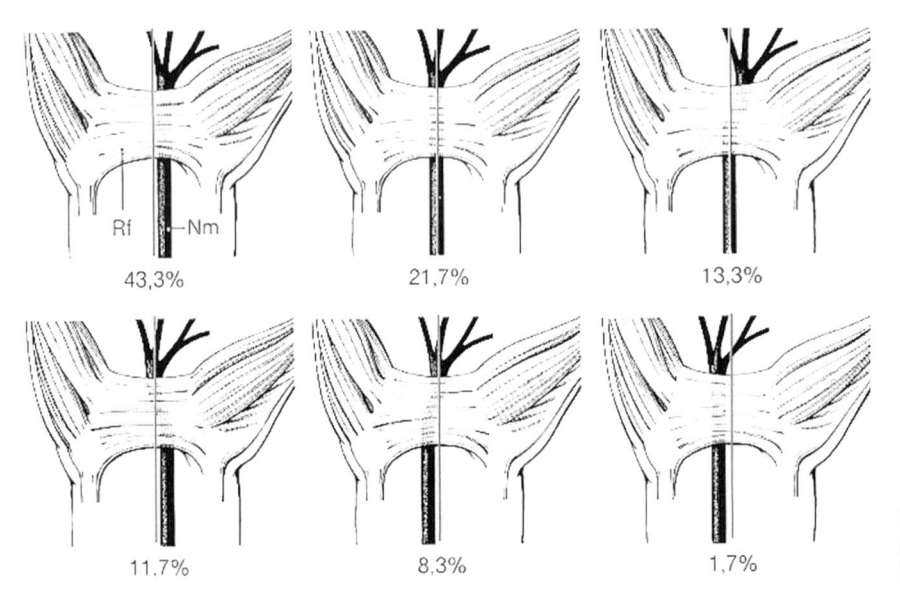

Fig. 3.7. Variations in the course of the median nerve (*Nm*). *Rf*, flexor retinaculum

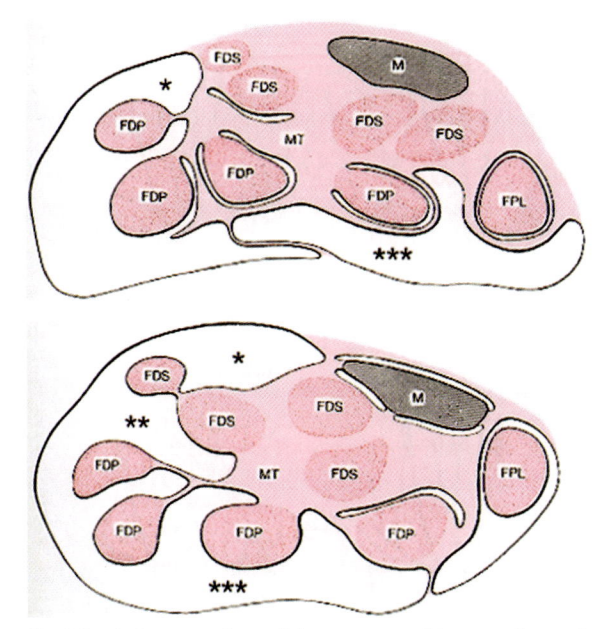

Fig. 3.8. a,b Cross-sections of the contents of the carpal tunnel with widened pretendinous (*), intertendinous (**), and retrotendinous (***) recesses. **a** Proximal carpal tunnel. **b** Distal carpal tunnel. Notice the gliding spaces of the median nerve. *M*, median nerve; *FDS*, tendons of the flexor digitorum superficialis; *FDP*, tendons of the flexor digitorum profundus; *FPL*, tendons of the flexor pollicis longus; *MT*, mesotendineum

Median Nerve Branches

At the distal end of the carpal canal the median nerve regularly divides in its terminal branches. Inside the tunnel there are a great many variations. They have been classified by Lanz [19] into four groups. The first group includes variations of the course of the thenar branch. In some cases, these branches leave the nerve within the carpal canal. They take off beneath the flexor retinaculum and then bend around it. Some of them may even perforate the retinaculum. With regard to the relation between the thenar branch and the flexor retinaculum, Poisel [33] described three subtypes: 46% of thenar branches were extraligamentous, 31% were subligamentous, and 23% were transligamentous (Fig. 3.9). In comprehensive studies Tountas and coauthors [42], Olave and coauthors [28], and Kozin [17] found the same basic subtypes as Poisel [33], but they noted different frequencies. In 80%–90% of cases an extraligamentous thenar branch was found. This may have been due to the use of different dissection techniques. The transligamentous course is of great clinical importance because of the possibility of compression within the retinacular fibers [13, 31].

The second group includes accessory branches of the median nerve in the distal area of the carpal tunnel. This variation was found in 7.2% of cases. It consists of true duplications of the thenar branch and additionally thin sensory branches, which leave the palmar or ulnar side of the main trunk of the nerve (Fig. 3.10).

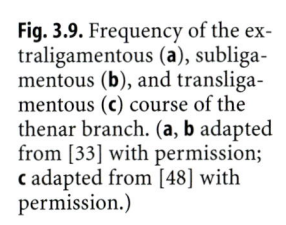

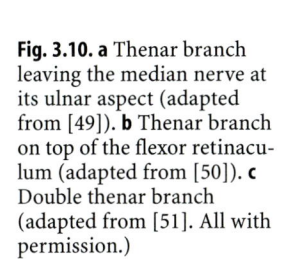

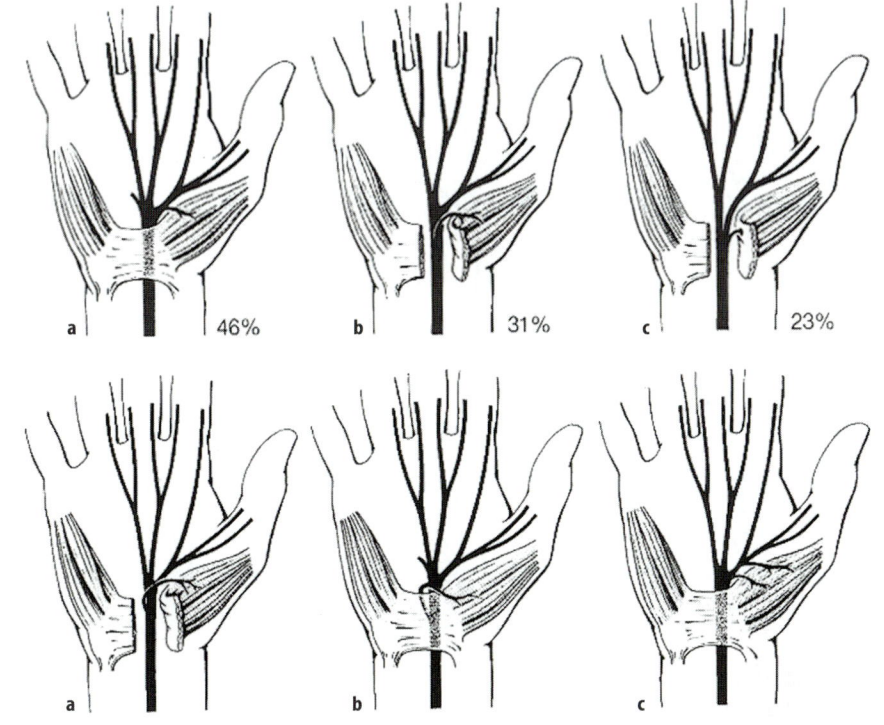

Fig. 3.9. Frequency of the extraligamentous (**a**), subligamentous (**b**), and transligamentous (**c**) course of the thenar branch. (**a, b** adapted from [33] with permission; **c** adapted from [48] with permission.)

Fig. 3.10. a Thenar branch leaving the median nerve at its ulnar aspect (adapted from [49]). **b** Thenar branch on top of the flexor retinaculum (adapted from [50]). **c** Double thenar branch (adapted from [51]. All with permission.)

In 2.8% of cases, a variation (group III) was found consisting of a high division of the median nerve at the level of the forearm (Fig. 3.11). In some cases, it is associated with a median artery [16]. Accessory lumbrical muscles have been noted passing through the bifid nerve as well. In some cases the nerve trunk may be divided into two equal-sized nerves [26]. In other cases there may be a predominance of either part, radial or ulnar. A high division of the median nerve in which the radial part passes through a separate compartment of the carpal tunnel was described by Amadio [1].

In group IV there are accessory branches of the median nerve leaving the main trunk proximal to the carpal tunnel. This variation was seen in 1.6% of cases (Fig. 3.12). Perforations of the flexor retinaculum occurred at variable levels, joining a branch or the median nerve distally [19, 25].

Most of the branches leave the median nerve radially or on its palmar side. At surgery, the nerve is approached more from the ulnar side to minimize risk of lesion to the typical branches. Landmarks to verify the point of origin of the thenar branch: *the midpoint of a line drawn between the tubercle of the scaphoid and the distal end of the flexion crease of the thumb metacarpophalangeal joint.*

The median nerve receives vascular branches from the radial, ulnar, and median arteries, and also from the superficial palmar arch within its course in the carpal canal [5, 45]. They reach the nerve from the radial or ulnar sides or they invade the interfascicular spaces

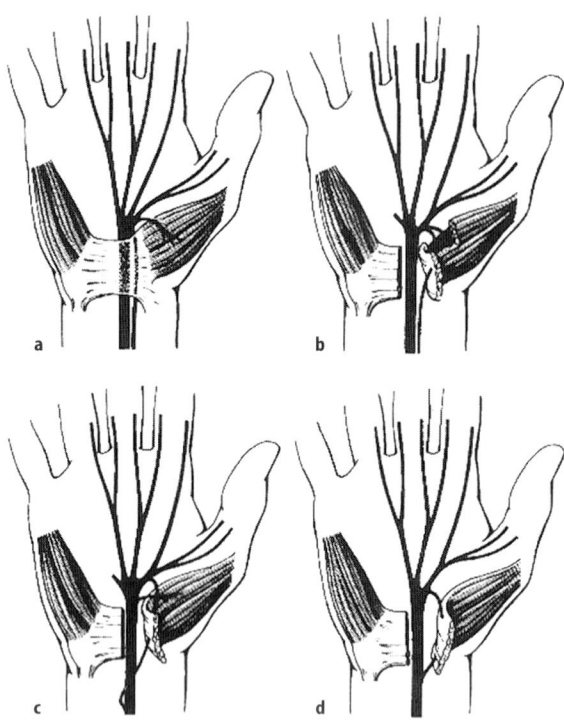

Fig. 3.12. a Accessory branch proximal to the carpal tunnel (adapted from [25]). **b** Accessory branch proximal to the carpal tunnel, perforating the flexor retinaculum (adapted from [51]). **c** Accessory branch proximal to the carpal tunnel from the ulnar aspect of the median nerve (adapted from [19]). **d** Accessory branch proximal to the carpal tunnel, running directly into the thenar muscles (adapted from [56], all with permission)

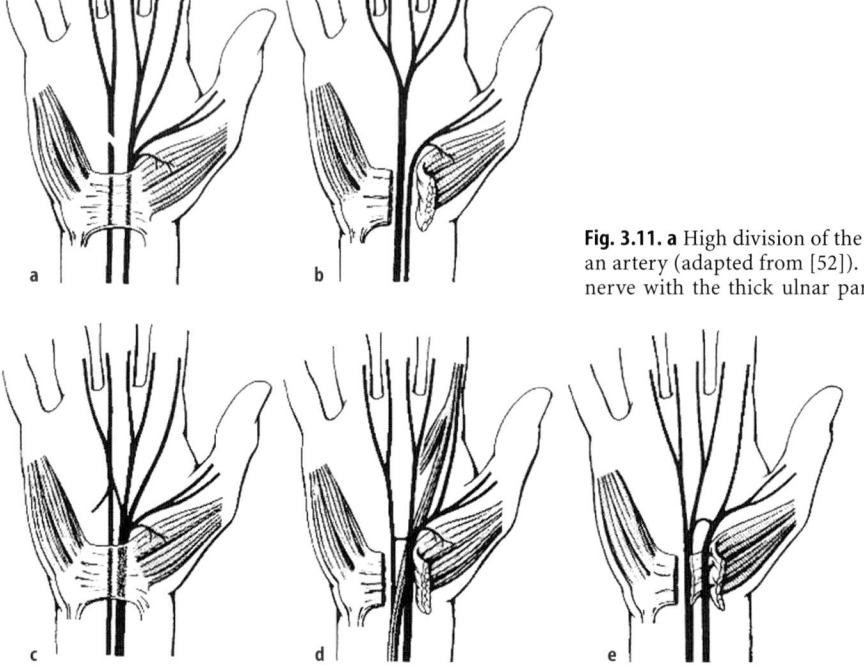

Fig. 3.11. a High division of the median nerve with the median artery (adapted from [52]). **b** High division of the median nerve with the thick ulnar part (adapted from [53]). **c** High division of the median nerve with the thin ulnar part (adapted from [54]). **d** High division of the median nerve with the accessory lumbrical muscle between the two branches (adapted from [55]). **e** High division of the median nerve in which the radial half passes through a separate compartment, sending off three motor branches to the thenar muscles (adapted from [1], all with permission.)

directly from the palmar side (Fig. 3.13). The dorsal side of the nerve is free of vessel entry. Vascular anastomoses between the mesotendineum of the flexor tendons of the carpal tunnel and the sheaths of the nerve were never seen.

Acknowledgements. The illustrations in this chapter were drawn by Gerhard Kohnle and are reprinted from Schmidt, H.-M. and U. Lanz, Chirurgische Anatomie der Hand (2003), with permission of G. Thieme Verlag, Stuttgart, Germany.

References

1. Amadio PC (1987) Bifid median nerve with double compartment within the transverse carpal canal. J Hand Surg 12 A: 366–368
2. Bade H, Reuber M, Koebke J (1994) Topologie des Karpaltunnels bei dynamischer Belastung des Handgelenks. Handchir Mikrochir Plast Chir 26: 175–181
3. Bauman TD, Gelberman RH, Mubarak SJ, Garfin SR (1981) The acute carpal tunnel syndrome. Clin Orthop 156: 151–156
4. Bay BK, Sharkey NA, Szabo RM (1997) Displacement and strain of the median nerve at the wrist. J Hand Surg 22 A: 621–627
5. Blunt MJ (1959) The vascular anatomy of the median nerve in the forearm and hand. J Anat 93: 15–22
6. Bonnel F, Mailhe P, Allieu Y, Rabischong P (1981) The general anatomy and endoneural fascicular arrangement of the median nerve at the wrist. Anat Clin 2: 201–207
7. Dowdy PA, Richards RS, Mac Farlane RM (1994) The palmar cutaneous branch of the median nerve and the palmaris longus tendon: a cadaveric study. J Hand Surg 19 A: 199–202
8. Frank U, Giunta R, Krimmer H, Lanz U (1999) Neueinbettung des N. medianus nach Vernarbung im Karpalkanal mit der Hypothenar – Fettgewebslappenplastik. Handchir Mikrochir Plast Chir 31: 317–322
9. Gelberman RH, Hergenroeder PT, Hargens AR et al. (1981) The carpal tunnel syndrome. J Bone Jt Surg 63 A: 380–383
10. Giunta R, Frank U, Lanz U (1998) The hypothenar fat – pad flap for reconstructive repair after scarring of the median nerve at the wrist joint. Ann Chir Main 17: 107–112
11. Goto S, Kojima T (1993) An anomalous muscle with an independent muscle belly associated with carpal tunnel syndrome. Handchir mikrochir Plast Chir 25: 72–74
12. Henkel – Kopleck A, Schmidt HM (2001) Zur Architektur des palmaren Faserkomplexes zwischen Palmaraponeurose und Retinaculum flexorum. Handchir Mikrochir Plast Chir 33:294–298
13. Johnson RK, Shrewsbury MM (1970) Anatomical course of the thenar branch of the median nerve – usually in a separate tunnel through the transverse carpal ligament. J Bone Jt Surg 52 A: 269–273
14. Jones SM, Stuart PR, Stothard J (1997) Open carpal tunnel release. Does a vascularized hypothenar fat pad reduce wound tenderness ? J Hand Surg 22 B: 758–760
15. Keir PJ, Wells RP, Ranney DA, Lavery W (1997) The effects of tendon load and posture on carpal tunnel pressure. J Hand Surg 22 A: 628–634
16. Kornberg M, Aulicino PL, Du Puy TE (1983) Bifid median nerve with three thenar branches. J Hand Surg 8: 553–584

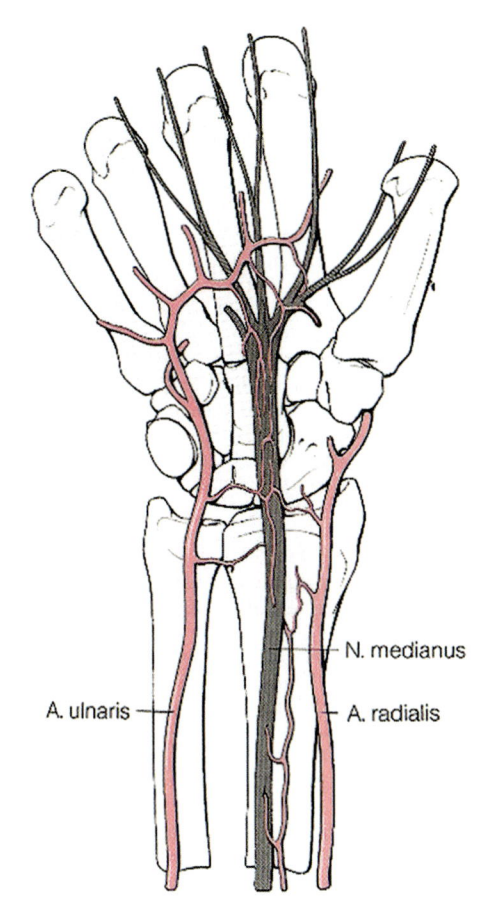

Fig. 3.13. Arterial blood supply of the median nerve. *UA*, ulnar artery; *RA*, radial artery (adapted from [5], with permission)

17. Kozin SH (1998) The anatomy of the recurrent branch of the median nerve. J Hand Surg 23 A: 852–858
18. Lange H (1997) Carpal tunnel syndrome caused by the palmaris profundus muscle. Case report. J Hand Surg. 22 B: 758–760
19. Lanz U (1977) Anatomical variations of the median nerve in the carpal tunnel. J Hand Surg 2: 44–53
20. Mackinnon SE, Dellon AL (1988) Anatomic investigations of nerves at the wrist: I. Orientation of the motor fascicle of the median nerve in the carpal tunnel. Ann Plast Surg 21: 32–35
21. Mannerfelt L, Oetker R (1986) Die chirurgische Bedeutung des Ramus palmaris n. mediani. In: Buck – Gramcko D, Nigst H (eds): Bibliothek für Handchirurgie: Nervenkompressionssyndrome an der oberen Extremität. Stuttgart, Hippokrates, pp 71–78.
22. Naff N, Dellon AL, Mackinnon SE (1993) The anatomical course of the palmar cutaneous branch of the median nerve, including a description of its own unique tunnel. J Hand Surg 18 B: 316–317
23. Nakamichi K, Tachibana S (1992) Transverse sliding of the median nerve beneath the flexor retinaculum. J Hand Surg 17 B: 213–216
24. Netscher D, Mosharrafa A, Lee M et al. (1997) Tranverse carpal ligament: its effect on flexor tendon excursion, morphologic changes of the carpal canal, and on pinch and grip strengths after open carpal tunnel release. Plast Reconstr Surg 100: 636–642

25. Ogden JA (1972) An unusual branch of the median nerve. J Bone Jt Surg 54 A: 1779–1781
26. Ogino T, Ohno K (1991) A case of bipartite median nerve at the wrist. J Hand Surg 16 B: 96–97
27. Okutso I, Ninomiya S, Hamanaka I et al. (1989) Measurement of pressure in the carpal canal before and after endoscopic management of carpal tunnel syndrome. J Bone Jt Surg 71 A: 679–683
28. Olave E, Prates JC, Gabrielli C, Pardi P (1996) Morphometric studies of the muscular branch of the median nerve. J Anat 189: 445–449
29. Olave E, Prates JC, Gabrielli C et al. (1996) Abnormal course of the superficial palmar branch of the radial artery. Surg Radiol Anat 18: 151–153
30. Olave E, Prates JC, Gabrielli, C, Pardi P (1997) Median artery and superficial palmar branch of the radial artery in the carpal tunnel. Scand J Plast Reconstr Surg 31: 13–16
31. Pfeiffer KM, Nigst H (1973) Ungewöhnliche Befunde bei der Carpaltunneloperation. Handchirurgie 5: 99–103
32. Plancher KD, Idler RS, Lourie GM, Strickland JW (1996) Recalcitrant carpal tunnel. The hypothenar fat pad flap. Hand Clin 12: 337–349
33. Poisel S (1974) Ursprung und Verlauf des Ramus muscularis des N. digitalis palmaris communis I (N. medianus). Chir Prax 18: 471–474
34. Rath T, Millesi H (1990) Das Gleitgewebe des N. medianus im Karpaltunnel. Handchirurgie 22: 203–205
35. Rempel D, Bach JM, Gordon L, So Y (1998) Effects of forearm pronation/supination on carpal tunnel pressure. J Hand Surg 23 A: 38–42
36. Robbins H (1963) Anatomical study of the median nerve in the carpal tunnel and etiologies of the carpal tunnel syndrome. J Bone Jt Surg 45 A: 953–966
37. Schmidt HM, Moser T, Lucas D (1987) Klinisch–anatomische Untersuchungen des Karpaltunnels der menschlichen Hand. Handchirurgie 9: 145–152
38. Seradke H, Jia YC, Owens W (1995) In vivo measurement of carpal tunnel pressure in the functioning hand. J Hand Surg 20 A: 855–859
39. Strickland JW, Idler RS, Lourie GM, Plancher KD (1996) The hypothenar fat pad flap for management of recalcitrant carpal tunnel syndrome. J. Hand Surg 21 A: 840–848
40. Taleisnik J (1973) The palmar cutaneous branch of the median nerve and the approach to the carpal tunnel. J Bone Jt Surg 55 A: 1212–1217
41. Tillmann B, Gretenkord K (1981) Verlauf des N. medianus im Canalis carpi. Morphol Med 1: 61–69
42. Tountas CP, Bihrle DM, Mac Donald CJ, Bergman RA (1987) Variations of the median nerve in the carpal canal. J Hand Surg 12 A: 708–712
43. Wright TW, Glowczewskie F, Wheeler D et al. (1996) Excursion and strain of the median nerve. J Bone JT Surg 78 A: 1897–1903
44. Yoshioka S, Okuda Y, Tamai K et al. (1993) Changes in the carpal tunnel shape during wrist motion. MRI evaluation of normal volunteers. J Hand Surg 18 B: 620–623
45. Zbrodowski A, Buchs JB (1983) Blood supply of the median nerve in the carpal tunnel. The Hand 15: 310–316
46. Zbrodowski A, Gajisin S (1988) The blood supply of the flexor retinaculum. J Hand Surg 13 B: 35–39
47. Zeiss J, Skie M, Ebraheim N, Jackson WT (1989) Anatomic relations between the median nerve and flexor tendons in the carpal tunnel: MR evaluation in normal volunteers. AJR 153: 533–536
48. Papathanassiou BT (1968) A variant of the motor branch of the median nerve in the hand. J Bone Jt Surg 50 B: 156
49. Entin MA (1968) Carpal tunnel syndrome and its variants. Surg Clin North Am 48: 1097
50. Mannerfelt L, Hybinette CH (1972) Important anomaly of the thenar motor branch of the median nerve. Bull Hosp Jt Dis Orthop Inst 33: 15
51. Lanz U (1975) Variationen des Nervus medianus im Bereich des Karpaltunnels. Handchirurgie 7: 159
52. Eiken O, Carstam N, Eddeland A (1971) Anomalous distal branching of the median nerve. Scand J Plast Reconstr Surg 5: 149
53. Kessler I (1969) Unusual distribution of the median nerve at the wrist. Clin Orthop 67: 124
54. Winkelman NZ, Spinner M (1973) A variant high sensory branch of the median nerve to the third web space. Bull Hosp Jt Dis Orthop Inst 34: 161
55. Schultz RJ, Endler PM, Huddleston HD (1973) Anomalous median nerve and an anomalous muscle belly of the first lumbrical associated with carpal tunnel syndrome. J Bone Jt surg 55 A: 1744
56. Linburg RM Albright JA (1970) An anomalous branch of the median nerve. J Bone Jt Surg 52 A: 182

Etiopathogenesis

R. Luchetti

Introduction

The primary cause of carpal tunnel syndrome is caused by median nerve compression inside the carpal canal. This compression is verified by phenomenon linked to an increase in internal carpal canal pressure.

Each canal has a fixed capacity; therefore, each condition that provokes an expansion of the inside of the canal will directly increase the internal pressure and consequently compress the median nerve. Anomalous contents within the canal and the position of its internal structures can decrease the available canal space. These anomalous contents are represented by edema, inflammation, hemorrhage deposits of pathologic substances such as calcium uric, and/or conditions of amyloidosis, etc.

There is a proportionally greater increase in intracanal pressure in canals that are smaller due to a congenital condition or various abnormal development.

A pre-existing pathology, such as a polyneuropathy or a more proximal compression of the same nerve, increases the possibility of compressive median nerve damage.

The greater part of CTS is not caused by systemic disease or anomalies. The most common systemic causes are diabetes mellitus, rheumatoid arthritis, and hypothyroidism. CTS can also appear during pregnancy or from hormonal alteration pathologies. Acromegaly and other collagen diseases rarely are the cause for CTS onset.

In some cases, CTS is secondary to a traumatic wrist accident or fracture. In these instances CTS has a sudden onset.

CTS can be isolated or associated with other pathologies such as De Quervain syndrome, Motta disease (trigger finger), Raynaud phenomenon, epicondylitis, or shoulder pathologies.

The medical literature reports various studies in which the incidence of CTS has various causes [1–5]. In each statistical documentation, the total of patients with identifiable causes represent only a part of an entire series. The major part of CTS causes remains unknown: this condition is termed idiopathic.

Idiopathic Forms

When the cause of CTS is not clear it is defined as idiopathic. These forms are the most frequently occurring. If a careful evaluation is performed the majority of the causes, in these cases, can be classified and are moved into another category or can be associated with other pathologies.

The idiopathic forms frequently show up as "aspecific tenovaginitis:" these alterations have not been completely demonstrated. Fuchs et al. [6], and Kerr et al. [7] have demonstrated that inflammatory cells are rarely found in the flexor tendon canals but often edema is present.

CT scans have demonstrated that the dimension of the carpal canal in idiopathic CTS patients is reduced. [8]. Idiopathic CTS can also be due to a congenital reduction in the carpal canal's shape and width.

CTS prevalently develops in patients between the age of 40–50 years. The syndrome develops quite easily when there is an increase in the sheath (edema) thickness or in occasions where there is a reduction in the carpal canal's dimensions. Actually, in cases of idiopathic CTS, there is usually another explanation as to the cause of its onset. The type and amount of work one performs can greatly influence the appearance of this syndrome. CTS more frequently occurs in the subject's dominant hand, which also happens to be the hand that works the most. Various wrist flexion and extension movements provoke an increase in pressure with repetitive phases of median nerve compression. It has been demonstrated that internal canal pressure varies with the variation of wrist position [9–16]. When the nerve is under tension it bends and rests against the canal's borders thus provoking this type of compression phenomenon.

Since this syndrome does not occur in everyone who does the same type of work, it can be hypothesized that it manifests itself only in those who already have reduced carpal canal dimensions.

Secondary Form

All the tissue that is contained in the carpal canal can become diseased and afflict the median nerve thus provoking a secondary compression. The surrounding structures and those not contained in the canal can also become diseased and invade the canal, causing the same consequences on the median nerve. The same nerve can be involved in a metabolic pathology and can be greatly susceptible to compressive phenomenon. Another secondary form that should not be forgotten is the possible presence of a median nerve tumor.

Aspecific Tenovaginitis of the Flexor Tendons

It is more appropriate to define this pathology as a thickening of the flexor tendon sheath. The pathologic proliferation of the sheath causes edema and water retention which, in the carpal canal, leads to a secondary CTS which can have either a slow or rapid onset. This cause has been demonstrated to be the basis of acute CTS forms. Patients affected by this form can demonstrate a contemporaneous onset or late and slow onset associated with other phenomenon such as trigger finger or De Quervain syndrome.

Rheumatoid Arthritis and Other Collagen Diseases

Rheumatoid arthritis is one of the causes that constantly produces a tenovaginitis and consequently CTS. Unfortunately, this disease also provokes tendon injuries that complicate the patient's medical story.

One should remember that other pathologies that cause synovial inflammation and edema can cause compression of the median nerve and the onset of CTS, for example: scleroderma, lupus, etc. In 3%–6% of patients afflicted with Sjögren syndrome, there is an associated CTS [17]. Winkelmann et al. [18] reported five cases of CTS that presented with cutaneous alterations of the connective tissue such as: fasciitis, discoid lupus, panniculus lupus. These manifestations can improve with specific medical therapy. A similar CTS form associated with fasciitis and polyarthritis can be hiding an ovarian carcinoma [19]. Other cases that have been reported to have an association with CTS are dermatomyositis, polymyositis, multicentric reticulocystitis, and lymphoma [20].

Arthritis

CTS is often associated with degenerative articular pathologies such as arthritis of the trapezio-metacarpal joint [21]. It has also been associated with scaphoid pseudoarthrosis [22].

Familiar Neuropathy

This syndrome has a familiar predisposition to compressive paralysis that afflicts people who develop acute compressive peripheral nerve injuries [23]. The nerves which are more frequently afflicted are: peroneal, radial, median, and ulnar. A slight nerve compression usually provokes the paresis and nerve compression and often the patient has even forgotten the cause of the initial event. This form often imitates a CTS idiopathic form. However, if one does perform a neurophysiologic study, a focal slowing down of nerve conduction will be found in both nerves and even in the nonsymptomatic side. The idiopathic form rarely occurs. Gray et al. [24] have published a study in which the idiopathic form has a dominant expression.

Mucopolysaccharidosis is one of these forms. Unfortunately, it is not easily diagnosed since the symptoms are quite atypical and there is a lack of night-time paresthesia along with scarce clinical symptoms.

Another rare form is familiar hypertrophic neuropathy (Dejerine-Sottas syndrome) [25].

Polyneuropathy

It is common knowledge that the patients with polyneuropathies are more susceptible to nerve compressions [26]. Frequently, the patient who is afflicted with diabetes mellitus, presents with a clear form of CTS that is a consequence of a median nerve compression in the carpal canal, associated with sensory disturbances of the upper extremities due to the polyneuropathy.

Guillain-Barré also has an association with CTS, but this is not a constant rule [27]. This also holds true for alcohol-induced neuropathies where the feet are the extremities that are afflicted first and later on the hands. But the symptoms are not typical for a clearly diagnosable CTS. In these cases the hands show an overall reduced sensibility and it is not isolated only to the median nerve distribution [28].

Rheumatic Polymyalgia

This disease process involves all the connective tissue and afflicts muscle and tendons with the formation of vascular granulomas. The involvement of these structures causes the appearance of CTS presumably from a granular tenosynovitis that has not yet completely expressed itself.

Vascular Disease

Median artery thrombosis is a cause of CTS in an acute phase. Another form of CTS, which is not yet completely clear, but appears in patients who are afflicted by chronic renal insufficiency, is when they develop a persistent arterio-venous fistula in or around the carpal tunnel and this eventually leads to a vascular breakdown [25].

Gout

Gout can cause an acute form of CTS, as well as a late onset form [29]. In 2,705 CTS cases only three cases had gout. Whereas of ten patients with gout, who prevalently had it in their hands, four had CTS [30]. The patients with typical gout had tophus gout in the flexor tendons inside the carpal canal [31]. Surgery is the treatment of choice for symptom resolution; however, it must be kept in mind that the surgical scar should be carefully watched and treated since these patients' scars tend to take a longer time to heal [32].

Amyloidosis

Amyloid deposits can cause compression of the peripheral nerves at various levels. Amyloidosis can be divided into various forms: primitive, secondary, familiar, and finally malignant paraproteinemia [33]. Patients that are afflicted with primitive amyloidosis develop nerve compressions at various levels but do not develop CTS in this phase of the disease. Instead, in familiar amyloidosis there is a strong association with CTS and with other symptoms that involve various organs and parts of the body [34]. Surgical treatment resolves the symptoms but there is a strong possibility of long-term reoccurrence.

One must remember that CTS is inserted in the context of amyloid polyneuropathies and therefore its incidence will always be inferior to the polyneuropathy itself [35].

Vitamin Deficiency

Folkers et al. [36] has published many studies regarding the relationship between CTS and a lack of pyridoxine. Strangely enough, there also exists a correlation between the appearance of CTS and an increase in the assumption of pyridoxine [37, 38].

Pregnancy and Breastfeeding

It is not quite clear as to why CTS appears during pregnancy and during breastfeeding. The symptoms begin and progress during pregnancy without reason. The third trimester is typically the moment in which the symptoms appear [39, 40]. It seems that it is due to an increase in the level of hormones that cause tissue edema and an increase in associated weight during this phase. On this basis, one would assume that once the woman has given birth the symptoms should disappear, but we have seen that this is not always true and in many cases the symptoms persist or increase after delivery [25].

CTS can even manifest itself during breastfeeding. Often it is associated with De Quervain syndrome. Research on the effect of prolactin in this sense has not lead us to any conclusions [41].

Endocrine Diseases

Edema and acromegaly are two diseases that can cause CTS. They are not very frequently occurring but clinical disturbances from CTS can be their first signs and will eventually lead the patient to seek specialized help. It has been seen that by specifically treating acromegaly, its pathological symptoms improve [42].

Diabetes mellitus is a very commonly occurring systemic disease that also is associated with the presence of CTS. Median nerve compression is only one of its many complications [43]. In these patients, the median nerve, as in their other peripheral nerves, is already involved by a polyneuropathy and is more easily subject to compression. The median nerve has to be decompressed in these cases [44].

Thyroid diseases such as hypothyroidism and hyperthyroidism can cause CTS. In hypothyroidism, the swelling of the tissue inside the carpal canal causes the syndrome. CTS can be the first sign of hypothyroidism [45]. Rarely does a hypothyroidism cause a generalized polyneuropathy [46]. The substitute medical therapy will improve the clinical symptoms. CTS that is due to hyperthyroidism is quite rare, but also, in these cases, medical treatment can improve the clinical symptoms [47]. In hyperthyroidism the increase of metabolic requests sends the median nerve in the carpal canal in crisis.

Infections

CTS can appear whenever there are any form of carpal canal infection complications that are caused by a variety of pathogenic agents. These infections can stem and/or spread from the hand or forearm. It should be remembered that this can occur in the granuloma form of tuberculosis, the form associated with leprosy (where the median nerve is less involved than the ulnar nerve), from *Borrelia* and aspecific infective agents. For the most part, the onset is acute and its progression is described in the following specific paragraphs.

Other Conditions That Occupy Carpal Canal Space

Pathological tumors that increase internal carpal canal volume cause a secondary median nerve compression. These tumors can arise from the internal structure of the carpal canal or from the flexor tendons, such as giant cell tumors that come from the sheath or from the nearby structures of the skeletal floor. Articular cysts can be listed among these culprits [48], in addition to: lipoma, hemangioma, and capitate osteoid osteoma in the endocanal [49].

CTS also appears in conditions caused by flexor tendon muscle surface anomalies [50–52] or the lumbrical muscles being inserted too proximal to the carpal canal [53]. Repetitive wrist and finger movements can cause median nerve compression and a secondary CTS. Diagnostic verification is based on isolating the cause but unfortunately, this occasionally occurs in the majority of these cases.

With the advent of endoscopic surgical techniques, a series of more precise exams can be performed before proceeding with a surgical treatment. When there is doubt as to the CTS primary cause, it is better to request an x-ray and rule out if there are calcifications, or to order an ultrasound to rule out soft tissue neoformations. These exams can be accompanied by even more sophisticated exams such as a CAT scan or a MRI.

The surgical treatment foresees, besides decompression, the removal of masses that invade the canal and can provoke the compression.

Carpal Canal Stenosis

Even in these conditions complementary exams such as CT scan, MRI, and ultrasound can be useful for making a more appropriate evaluation. Some authors have hypothesized that the smaller the canal, the higher the chance the patient has of developing CTS. This hypothesis is very subjective and has been confirmed by some and ruled out by others (see Chap. 10).

Carpal Canal Deformity

Bony anomalies can reduce the cross-section area of the carpal canal. CTS can develop as a late onset sequel due to a wrist deformity caused by a carpal bone or radial fracture or other wrist traumas [54]. Altissimi et al. [55], reported an incidence of CTS in 31% of patients following a Colles fracture. In some cases the symptoms resolved spontaneously, in others, a surgical treatment was required. The treatment included a broad decompression with a wrist-palm surgical access [56].

Congenital anomalies that cause CTS include scaphoid hypoplasia with radial dysplasia, radial bone anomalies that tend to project towards the canal, carpal bone anterior subluxation, such as Madelung's disease [57], or patients who present with osteopetrosis.

Obesity

Obesity is considered to also be one of the many causes for the onset of CTS [58]. Up until now, there has not been a scientific study to uphold a direct association between obesity and CTS. They have been associated, but it has not been determined that obesity can cause CTS directly.

Hand Edema

Various studies have demonstrated that hand edema can provoke the onset of CTS. Primary or secondary lymphedema due to mastectomy [59, 60], hand edema secondary to heart surgery [61], hand edema after an insect bite [62], are all considered possible causes for the onset of CTS.

Acute Form

CTS can be divided into an acute and chronic form on the basis of how it presents itself. The acute form occurs after a traumatic event such as a wrist fracture [2, 54, 63–66] or a carpal bone subluxation [67], crush injury, high velocity strain or repetitive hard manual labor, burn [68], or infection.

In traumatic forms (wrist fracture), CTS can even have a late onset [54]. A particularly severe form of CTS occurs in forearm and wrist crush injuries. The transverse carpal ligament must be urgently sectioned and a forearm fasciotomy should be performed [69]. Rarely does the acute form of CTS appear after a surgery where plates, screws, or tendon prosthesis have been inserted [65, 70]. CTS has been known to occur in an acute form after a Dupuytren palmar fasciotomy.

The acute form of CTS can appear even during and following wrist immobilization especially when the patient is immobilized in a plaster cast in the Cotton-Loder position in order to reduce and maintain a distal radius epiphysis fracture. Kongsholm and Olerud [71] have demonstrated a pressure increment in the carpal canal following a Colles wrist fracture, whether the wrist was positioned in either flexion or a resting neutral position. They also found that the canal pressure increased following an anesthetic infiltration at the fracture site in the attempt to reduce the fracture using a local anesthetic due to the invasion of the anesthetic liquid in the carpal canal [71].

Gelberman et al. [11] have demonstrated that there is a close association between the presence of elevated carpal canal pressure in fractured wrists that have been immobilized in flexion. In these cases the pressure is higher in respect to control groups. The acute form can occur following a medical treatment using anticoagulants [72, 73] or oral contraceptive medicine. Often, there is not a correlation between pharmaceuticals and CTS, but acute symptom onset can follow a spontaneous hemorrhage in cases of coagulopathy [74]. Rheumatoid arthritis can cause the acute onset of CTS due to acute flexor tendon tenovaginitis. The onset of acute CTS occurring from either an acute suppurative or

Table 4.1 Acute CTS causes

Wrist fractures and dislocations
Hematoma
Infections
Rheumatoid arthritis
Repetitive and intensive manual work

nonsuppurative tenovaginitis (Table 4.1). Any type of infection can cause an acute median nerve compression: an example is the appearance of an acute form of CTS in association with gonococcal tenovaginitis [75].

In addition, the rare forms of median artery thrombosis [65] should be mentioned, as well as the secondary forms due to tumors such as acute and chronic leukemia [76]. The rarest form of acute CTS can also be caused by a poisonous snake bite [77].

Particular Forms

One must remember that even if the median nerve is suffering due to a continual injury at the level of the forearm, it can still undergo a secondary compression at the carpal canal level and will demonstrate all the typical CTS symptoms. The surgical treatment usually reveals a neuroma at the forearm that should not be manipulated and a median nerve compression inside the carpal canal that should only undergo a decompression [78, 79].

Chapter 13 will discuss the truly particular forms of CTS.

Genetic Forms

The appearance of CTS in children, or adults of the same family, has brought up the supposition that there could also be a form of CTS that is genetically linked. Danta [80] reported a form of CTS that has an autosomal dominant transmission. During surgery of these cases, an abnormal thickening of the ligament has been found and sometimes there is also the presence of clinical symptoms such as trigger finger, as has been described and associated with Weil-Marchesani syndrome [81, 82]. In some cases CTS is the initial form of a hereditary neuropathy with multiple nerve compressions [36].

Mucopolysaccharidosis is a form that is associated with CTS and has already been described in the paragraph regarding familiar neuropathies There are other diseases that fall into this same category, for instance, Leri's disease [83].

Children's Forms

These are forms that do not fall into the genetic, familiar or metabolic categories. However, their cause has not been determined and their common factor is that there is an early incidence of onset in relationship to the patient's age [84, 85]. The clinical and intraoperative aspect absolutely do not differ from the previously mentioned forms and the treatment follows the same principles as the others.

Summary of CTS Causes

- Idiopathic
- Secondary
- Carpal canal stenosis (deformity congenital or acquired)
- Collagen and autoimmune diseases (tenovaginitis, rheumatoid arthritis, scleroderma, rheumatic polymyalgia, LES, gout, chondrocalcinosis, others)
- Endocrinopathy (diabetes mellitus, thyroid diseases, estrogen, progesterone, gonadotropin, growth hormone)
- Amyloidosis
- Polyneuropathy
- Infection
- Carpal canal anomaly (cysts, tumors, muscles anomalies, median artery persistence)
- Obesity
- Primary and secondary hand edema
- Acute form (fracture, crushing hand injury, hemorrhage, burn, median artery thrombosis, infection, pregnancy)
- Congenital diseases (mucopolysaccharidosis, mucolipidosis)
- Children's forms
- Consequential forms occurring from pharmaceuticals (oral contraceptives, anticoagulants, lack of vitamin B6 or excessive intake of B6, etc.)
- Others

References

1. Yamaguchi DM, Lipscomb PR, Soule EH (1965) Carpal Tunnel Syndrome. Minn Med 48 22–33
2. Phalen GS (1966) The carpal-tunnel syndrome. J Bone Joint Surg 48A 211–228
3. Cseuz KA, Thomas JE, Lambert EH et al. (1966) Long-term results of operation for carpal tunnel syndrome. Mayo Clin Proc 41: 232–241
4. Maxwell JA, Reckling FW, Kelly CR (1973) Carpal tunnel syndrome: a review of cases treated surgically. J Kansas Med Soc 74: 190–193
5. Hybbinette CH, Mannerfelt L (1975) The carpal tunnel syndrome. Acta Orthop Scand. 46: 610–620
6. Fuchs PC, Nathan PA, Myers LD (1991) Synovial histology in carpal tunnel syndrome. J Hand Surg 16A: 753–758
7. Kerr CD, Sybert DR, Albarracin NS (1992) An analysis of the flexor synovium in idiopathic carpal tunnel syndrome: report of 625 cases. J Hand Surg 17A: 1028–1030
8. Dekel S, Papaioannou T, Rushworth G (1980) Idiopathic carpal tunnel syndrome caused by carpal stenosis. Br Med J 280: 1297–1299

9. Gelberman RH, Hergenroeder PT, Hargens AR et al. (1981) The carpal tunnel syndrome. A study of carpal canal pressures. J Bone Joint Surg 63A, 380–383
10. Werner CO, Elmquist D, Ohlin P (1983) Pressure and nerve lesion in the carpal tunnel. Acta Orthop Scand 54, 312–316
11. Gelberman RH, Szabo RM, Motensen WW (1984) Carpal tunnel pressure and wrist position in patients with Colles' fractures. J Trauma 24, 747–749
12. Szabo RM, Gelberman RH (1987) The pathophysiology of nerve entrapment syndromes. J Hand Surg 12A, 880–884
13. Luchetti R, Schoenhuber R, DeCicco G et al. (1989) Carpal-tunnel pressure. Acta Orthop Scand 60 (4), 397–399
14. Rempel D, Manojlovic R, Levisohn DG et al. (1994) The effect of wearing a flexible wrist splint on carpal tunnel pressure during repetitive hand activity. J Hand Surg 19A, 106–110
15. Weiss ND, Gordon L, Bloom T et al. (1995) Position of the wrist associated with the lowest carpal-tunnel pressure: implication for splinting design. J Bone Joint Surg 77-A, 11, 1695–1699
16. Luchetti R, Schoenhuber R, Nathan P (1998) Correlation of segmental carpal tunnel pressures with changes in hand and wrist positions in patients with carpal tunnel syndrome and controls. J Hand Surg 23B: 5: 598–602
17. Binder A, Snaith ML, Isenberg D (1988) Sjogren's syndrome: a study of its neurological complications. Br J Rheumatol 27: 275–280
18. Winkelmann RK, connolly SM, Doyle JA (1982) Carpal tunnel syndrome in cutaneous connective tissue disease: generalized morphea, lichen sclerossus, fasciitis, discoid lupus erythematosus, and lupus panniculitis. J Am Acad Dermatol 7: 94–99
19. Medsger TA, Dixon JA, Garwood VF (1982) Palmar fasciitis and polyarthritis associated with ovarian carcinoma. Ann Intern Med 96: 424–431
20. Quinones CA, Perry HO, Rushton JG (1966) Carpal tunnel syndrome in dermatomyositis and scleroderma. Arch Dermatol 94: 20–25
21. Florack TM, Miller RJ, Pellegrini VD et al. (1992) The prevalence of carpal tunnel syndrome in patients with basal joint arthritis of the thumb. J Hand Surg 17A: 624–630
22. Leviet B, Ebelin M, Meriaux JL, Vilain R (1984) Syndrome du canal carpien et pseudoarthrose du scaphoide. Rev Chir Orthop 70: 79–81
23. Dubi J, Regli F, Bischoff A (1979) Recurrent familial neuropathy with liability to pressure palsies. J Neurol 220: 43
24. Gray RG, Poppo MJ, Gottlieb NL (1979) Primary familial bilateral carpal tunnel syndrome. Ann Intern Med 91: 37
25. Dawson DM, Hallett M, Millender LH (1983) Entrapment neuropathies. Boston, Little Brown Co.
26. Potts F, Shahani BT, Young RR (1980) Study of the coincidence of carpal tunnel syndrome and generalized peripheral neuropathy. Musce Nerve 3: 440
27. Lambert EH, Mulder DW (1964) Nerve conduction in the Guillain-Berrè syndrome. Electroencephalogr Clin Neurophysiol 17: 86
28. Victor-Torras M, Garcia AF, Barriero-Tella P et al. (1985) Manifestation of scheie mucopolysaccharidosis I: carpal tunnel syndrome in childhood. Case report. Arch Neurobiol (Madr) 48: 113–123
29. Champion D (1969) Gouty tenosynovitis and the carpal tunnel syndrome. Med J Aust 1: 1030–1032
30. Moore JR, Weiland AJ (1985) Gouty tenosynovitis. J Hand Surg 10A: 291–295
31. Akizuki S, Matsui T (1984) Entrapment neuropathy caused by tophaceous gout. J Hand Surg 9B: 331–332
32. Lainga J, Waslen GD, Penney CJ (1986) Tophaceous gout presenting with bilateral hand contractures and carpal tunnel syndrome (letter). J Rheumatol 13: 230–231
33. Cohen AS, Benson MD (1975) Amyloid neuropathy. In PJ Dyck, PK Thomas, Lambert EH (Eds), Peripheral Neuropathy. Philadelphia: Saunders.
34. Thomas PK (1975) Genetic factors in amyloidosis. J Med Genet 12: 317–326
35. Kyle RA, Bayrd ED (1975) Amyloidosis: review of 236 cases. Medicine 54: 271
36. Folkers K, Ellis J, Watanabe T (1978) Biochemical evidence for a deficiency of vitamin B6 in the carpal tunnel syndrome based on a crossover clinical study. Proc Nat Acad Sci USA 75: 3410
37. Schaumberg H, Kaplan J, Windebank A et al. (1983) Sensory neuropathy from pyridoxine abuse. New England J Med 309 (8): 445–448
38. Amadio P (1987) Carpal tunnel syndrome, pyridoxine, and the work place. J Hand Surg 12A: 875–880
39. Gould JS, Wissinger HA (1978) Carpal tunnel syndrome in pregnancy. South Med J 71: 144–154
40. Wand JS (1990) Carpal tunnel syndrome in pregnancy and lactation. J Hand Surg 15B: 93–95
41. Rossi E, Sighinolfi E, Bortolotti P et al. (1984) Nocturnal prolactin secretion in carpal tunnel syndrome. Ital J Neurol Sci 5: 405–408
42. Nabarro JD (1987) Acromegaly. Clin Endocrinol (Oxf) 26: 481–512
43. Brown MJ, Asbury AK (1984) Diabetic neuropathy Ann Neurol 15: 2–12
44. Dellon AL (1992) Treatment of symptomatic diabetic neuropathy by surgical decompression of multiple peripheral nerves. Plast Reconstr Surg 89: 689–697
45. Golding DN (1970) Hypothyroidism presenting with musculoskeletal symptoms. Ann Rheum Dis 29: 10–14
46. Fincham RW, Cape CA (1968) Neuropathy in mixedema. A study of sensory nerve conduction in the upper extremities. Arch Neurol 19: 464–466
47. Beard L, Kumar A, Estep HL (1985) Bilateral carpal tunnel syndrome caused by Graves' disease. Arch Intern Med 145: 345–346
48. Jensen TT (1990) Isolated compression of the motor branch of the median nerve by a ganglion. Case Report. Scand J Plast Reconstr Hand Surg 24: 171
49. Herndon JH, Eaton RG, Littler JW (1974) Carpal tunnel syndrome: an unusual presentation of osteoma osteoide of the capitate. J Bone Joint Surg. 56A: 1715
50. Hayes CW (1974) Anomalous flexor digitorum sublimis with incipient carpal tunnel syndrome. Plast Reconstr Surg 53: 479
51. Smith RJ (1971) Anomalous muscle belly of flexor digitorum sublimis causing carpal tunnel syndrome. J Bone Joint Surg 53A: 1215
52. Aghasi MK, Rzetelny V Axer A (1980) The flexor digitorum superficialis as a cause of bilateral carpal tunnel syndrome and trigger wrist. J Bone Joint Surg 62A: 134
53. Jabaley ME (1978) Personal observations on the role of the lumbrical muscle in carpal tunnel syndrome. J Hand Surg 3: 82
54. Abbott LC, Saunders JB deCM (1933) Injuries of the median nerve in fractures of the lower end of the radius. Surg Gynecol Obstet 57: 507–516
55. Altissimi M, Antenucci R, Fiacca C, Mancini GB (1986) Long-term results of conservative treatment of fractures of the distal radius. Clin Orthop 206: 202–210
56. Lewis MH (1978) Median nerve decompression after Colles's fracture. JBJS 60B:195–196
57. Luchetti R, Mingione A, Monteleone M, Cristiani G (1988) Carpal tunnel syndrome in Madelung's deformity. JHS 13B: 19–22

58. Nathan PA, Keniston RC, Myers LD, Meadows KD (1992) Obesity as a rsk factor for slowing of sensory conduction of the median nerve in industry. A cross-sectional and longitudinal study involving 429 workers. JOM 34: 379–383
59. Ganel A, Engel J, Sela M, Brooks M (1979) Nerve entrapments associated with postmastectomy lymphedema. Cancer 44: 2254–2259
60. Smith WK, Giddins GEB (1999) Lymphoedema and hand surgery. J Hand Surg 24B: 138
61. Arnold AG (1977) The carpal tunnel syndrome in congestive cardiac failure. Postgrad Med J 53: 623–624
62. Lazaro III L (1972) Carpal-tunnel syndrome from an insect sting. A case report. J Bone Joint Surg. 54A: 1095–1096
63. Seddon H (1975) Surgical disorders of the peripheral nerves, 2nd ed Edinburgh, Churchill Livingstone
64. Watson-Jones R (1976) Fractures and joint injuries, 5th ed, ed Wilson JN, vol 2, pag 755, Edinburgh, Churchill Livingstone
65. Bauman T, Gelberman RH, Mubarak SJ, Garfin S (1981) The acute carpal tunnel syndrome. Clin Orthop Rel Res 156, 151–156
66. McCarroll HR (1984) Nerve injuries associated with wrist trauma. Orthop Clin North Am 15: 279–287
67. Rawlings ID (1981) The management of dislocations of the carpal tunnel lunate. Injury 12: 319–330
68. Adamson JE, Srouji SJ, Horton CE, Mladick RA (1971) The acute carpal tunnel syndrome. Plast Reconstr Surg 47: 332–336
69. Askin G, Finley R, Parenti J et al. (1986) High-energy roller injuries to the upper extremity. J Trauma 26: 1127–1131
70. DeLuca FN, Cowen NJ (1975) Median-nerve compression complicating a tendon graft prothesis. J Bone Joint Surg 57A: 553
71. Kongsholm J, Olerud G (1986) Carpal tunnel pressure in the acute phase after colles' fracture. Arch Orthop Trauma Surg 105: 183–186
72. Hartwell SW, Kurtay M (1966) Carpal tunnel compression caused by hematoma associated with anticoagulant therapy. Cleveland Clin 33; 127–129
73. Copeland J, Wells HG Jr, Puckett CL (1989) Acute carpal tunnel syndrome in a patient taking coumadin. J Trauma 29: 131–132
74. Case DB (1967) An acute carpal tunnel syndrome in a haemophiliac. BrJ Clin Pract 21: 254–255
75. DeHertogh D, Ritland D, Green R (1988) Carpal tunnel syndrome due to gonococcal tenosynovitis. Orthopedics 11: 199–200
76. Kilpatrick T, Leyden M, Sullivan J et al. (1985) Acute median nerve compression by haemorrhage from acute myelomonocytic leukaemia. Med J Aust 142: 51–52
77. Schweitzer G, Lewis JS (1981) Puff adder bite – an unusual cause of bilateral carpal tunnel syndrome. A case report. S Afr Med J 60: 714–715
78. McGrath MH, Polayes IM (1979) Posttarumatic median neuroma: a cause of carpal tunnel syndrome. Ann Plast Surg 3: 227–230
79. Martinelli P, Poppi M, Gaist G et al. (1985) Posttraumatic neuroma of the median nerve: a cause of carpal tunnel syndrome. Eur Neurol 24: 13–15
80. Danta G (1975) Familial carpal tunnel syndrome with onset in childhood. J Neurol Neurosurg Psychiatry 38: 350
81. Dellon AL, Trojak JE, Rochman GM (1984) Median nerve compression in Weill-Marchesani syndrome. Plast Reconstr Surg 74: 127–130
82. Panciera P, Panciera C (1996) Sindrome del tunnel carpale bilaterale in bambino con sindrome di Weil-Marchesani. Riv Chir Riab Mano Arto Sup 33 : 61–63
83. Watson-Jones R (1949) Leri's pleonosteosis, carpal tunnel compression of the median nerves and Morton's metatarsalgia. J Bone Joint Surg 31B: 560–571
84. Miner ME, Schimke RN (1975) Carpal tunnel syndrome in pediatric mucopolysaccharidoses: report of four cases. J Neurosurg. 43: 102
85. Sainio K, Merikanto L, Larsen TA (1987) Carpal tunnel syndrome in childhood. Dev Med Child Neurol 29: 794–797

5 The Pathophysiology of Median Nerve Compression

R. Luchetti

Introduction

Chronic nerve compression is the result of different trauma mechanisms such as traction, friction, and repetitive compression.

Nerves are static structures, when the articulation or limb moves the nerve must adapt and glide a few millimeters [1] along its course. Nerves pass through various narrow anatomical canals extending from the vertebral foramen to the most distal part of the limb, These canals do not represent fixed points, therefore, the nerve must freely glide inside them. Their fixed point is where they emerge from the vertebral foramen and from the surrounding collateral areas with respective final terminations (muscular or sensitive branches, etc). Even a minor amount of localized and surrounding tissue edema can interfere with passive nerve (gliding) movements. During limb movement, a nerve that is not very mobile will be stretched, thus causing its ulterior damage such as irritation, edema and or microinjuries that cause the consequential formation of scar adhesions. Scar tissue causes increased localized pressure and reduces nerve gliding, thus leading to a permanent nerve compression. This type of compression is often called "nerve entrapment."

The anatomical basis for the development of this type of injury can be from osteo-fibrotic canals; for example, the carpal tunnel, cubital tunnel, and the intervertebral foramen, but also from incongruous "sharp" fascial borders along with muscle contractions, (as in the case of the Fröhse arch for the posterior interosseous nerve or the proximal part of the flexor carpi ulnaris for the ulnar nerve). There are various factors that can contribute to the development of a nerve compression or stretching at this level, such as posture and nonphysiologic movements, repetitive muscle contraction or even an increase or decrease in structure volume within the canal (Fig. 5.1).

In order to better understand the physiopathological mechanism of nerve compression injuries, one must have a thorough knowledge of both the anatomical and nerve physiology of the structures that are involved. It is essential that one knows even the microanatomy of the specific nerve since each nerve is contained in different tissue structures and each one responds to compressive forces in an individual manner depending on its make-up and the physiopathological event that is taking place. One must remember that compression nerve injuries are not only a *mechanical* problem. The precocious signs and symptoms which the patient initially reports are often the result of intraneural structural alterations, prevalently affecting the nerve's microcirculation due to tissue pressure, and occurs before the first sign of structural damage has occurred to the nerve fiber.

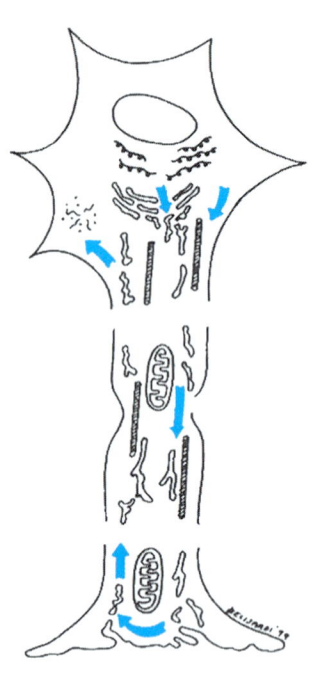

Fig. 5.1. Schematic drawing of neuronal axon flow

Anatomy Notes

The Neuron

The neuron is made up of a cellular body and its processes: dendrites and axons. It is a highly specialized cell. The cellular body of the motor neuron is situated in the anterior horn of the spinal cord, while the sensory neurons are located in the spinal root ganglions. Together, they branch out into the periphery. Those branches that come from the motor cells are called axons, and from sensitive branch ramifications, (dendrites). The production of essential substances for maintaining the vitality of the neuron is concentrated in the cellular body and the distal part of the axons, (synapses included), are structurally and functionally dependent on connections with the cellular body. Requirements for intracellular transport inside the neuron-*axonal transport* is very high. By means of axonal transport the substances produced in the cell body are transported to the outskirts along the axons, stopping at different levels: this type of transport is called *antegrade axonal transport*. The material transported is comprised of protein, vesicular membranes, neurotransmitters, lipids, mitochondria, and RNA (Table 5.1). There are five known types of antegrade axonal transport [2]. The type of axonal transport is divided into two groups based on transport velocity: slow or fast. The *slow transport* (0.1 – 30 mm/day) involves cytoskeletal elements (microtubule and neurofilament subunits) and axo-plasma elements of microtrabecular matrix (ex. actin) (Table 5.2). *Fast transport* (20 – 400 mm/day) regards the major part of small vesicular organs and both membranous and soluble material (Table 5.3).

Axonal transport is bidirectional. The materials that come from the axonal terminations are transported towards the cell body; this movement is *retrograde axonal transport* (Table 5.4) and the velocity of this type of transport is variable. A transport velocity of about 300 mm/day actually exists, (slightly less than the fast antegrade transport) and a slow transport of 3 – 8 mm/day. Part of the transported material is made up of recycled material that originally had been transported in an antegrade direction. The extracellular material is prevalently coming from the nerve endings or from the nerve fiber section zone which has the goal of reaching the cell body in order to give it information concerning the axon state and its endings, the sheath and nerve fiber protection system, as well as the target cells. This information system has a *trophic effect* role on the cell body. Scientific data exists which confirms the true validity of these target cells that transport their information via retrograde axonal flow. A characteristic aspect is a type of cell body alteration called *chromatolysis*, which can follow the axonal nerve fiber sectioning. Peripheral nerve compression produced a similar cell body alteration as well. It has been suggested that in such situations the loss of retrograde transport material can cause initial signs of cell body modification, demonstrating chemical and metabolic substance release that blocks the retrograde axonal transport thus provoking the same effects on the cell body. A cell body alteration of this kind can cause the neuron to die (dying back) [3]. By knowing the interactions that take place between the cell body, its endings and the cell alarm system, which works by means of bidirectional transport, one can understand the fundamental importance of understanding the pathophysiology of nerve compression injury. It is also important to consider this complex (cell body-axon-cell alarm system) as a single structure (neuron unit) so that one can understand why a peripheral nerve compression can induce functional alterations at a central level.

Table 5.1. Anterograde axonal transport

Proteins
Membrane
Vessels
Neurotransmitters
Lipids
Mitochondria
RNA

Table 5.2. Slow anterograde axonal transport

Cytoskeletal elements
Microtubules and neurofilaments
Axoplasm

Table 5.3. Fast anterograde axonal transport

Vesicles
Mitochondrial and proteins
Membrane material
Microtubules

Table 5.4. Retrograde axonal transport (fast and slow flow)

Recycled materials
Extracellular materials from:
Nerve terminals
Targets
Schwann cell

The Nerve Trunk

The peripheral nerve is a composite tissue where nerve fibers are positioned extremely close together in order to form a fasciculus. The nerve fibers can be divided based on their dimension and myelin sheath, which represents the way in which they function (Table 5.5).

The various nerve trunk components have the goal of maintaining continuity, nutrition, and fiber protection. The intraneural microvascular system, which is well developed, is the basis for supplying continual energy, which is necessary in maintaining nerve impulse conduction and axonal transport.

Some fasciculus are surrounded by a perineurium that makes up the laminated sheath (in layers) and is of considerable mechanical strength. The perineurium represents a barrier for the diffusion of various external substances, such as ferritin and exogenous proteins. The perineurium contributes to the chemical iso-

Table 5.5 Typology and function of the nerve fibers

Group	Diameter (u)	Conduction Velocity (m/s)	Function
A	2.5–22	15–100	Myelinated afferent and efferent somatic fibers (sensory and motor fibers)
B	3	3–15	Myelinic autonomic preganglial fibers (visceral)
C	0.2–1.5	0.3–1.6	Unmyelinated afferent somatic and postganglial efferent autonomic fibers (pain, pilomotor, sudomotor, and vasomotor)

lation of the nerve fiber from its surrounding tissue, creating an ionic intrafascicular sheath. Internally, the nerve fibers are packed together in fascicles by another type of connective tissue that is called *endoneurium*. This tissue is composed of fibroblasts and collagen fibrils. The cutaneous nerve's endoneurium seems to have a greater number of deeply positioned collagen fibrils that can count on their protection from the surrounding structures. This greater collagen richness reflects its need for protection from the more superficial part of the nerve fibers (Fig. 5.2).

The fascicles are immersed in a connective tissue called the epineurium that contains a large amount of intraneural vascular structures. The epineurium represents a lax and soft connective tissue that wraps itself around and protects the fascicles. The quantity of epineural and perineural connective tissue varies in different levels, nerves, and individuals. Usually, the nerve contains more epineurium where it passes over the articulation and this helps to minimize the compressive effect, friction and traction that occurs during articular movement. The epineurium is denser superficially, and forms a sheath around the nerve separating it from its surrounding structures.

Intraneural Microvascular System

The peripheral nerves are vascularized structures [4] with a well-developed microvascular system comprised of the epineurium, perineurium, and endoneurium. The vessels have an interconnecting system between the various tissue layers. Transmission of impulses, such as axonal transport, require a continual energy supply that is driven by the intraneural microvascular system and this system seems to have a great reserve and compensatory capacity in relationship to the damage of nearby vascular structures. The vessels in the epineurium are set up in a longitudinal direction. The vessels are present in all tissue layers, both superficial and profound and between the fascicles. The epineural vessels form an anastomosis with the perineural vascular plexus whose vessels also run in a longitudinal direction and branch into various perineurium strata (Fig. 5.3). The perineural anastomosis vessels pass through perineural layers in a very characteristic way, oblique, and towards the endoneural strata (Figs. 5.4, 5.5). This oblique perineural vessel passage makes up a

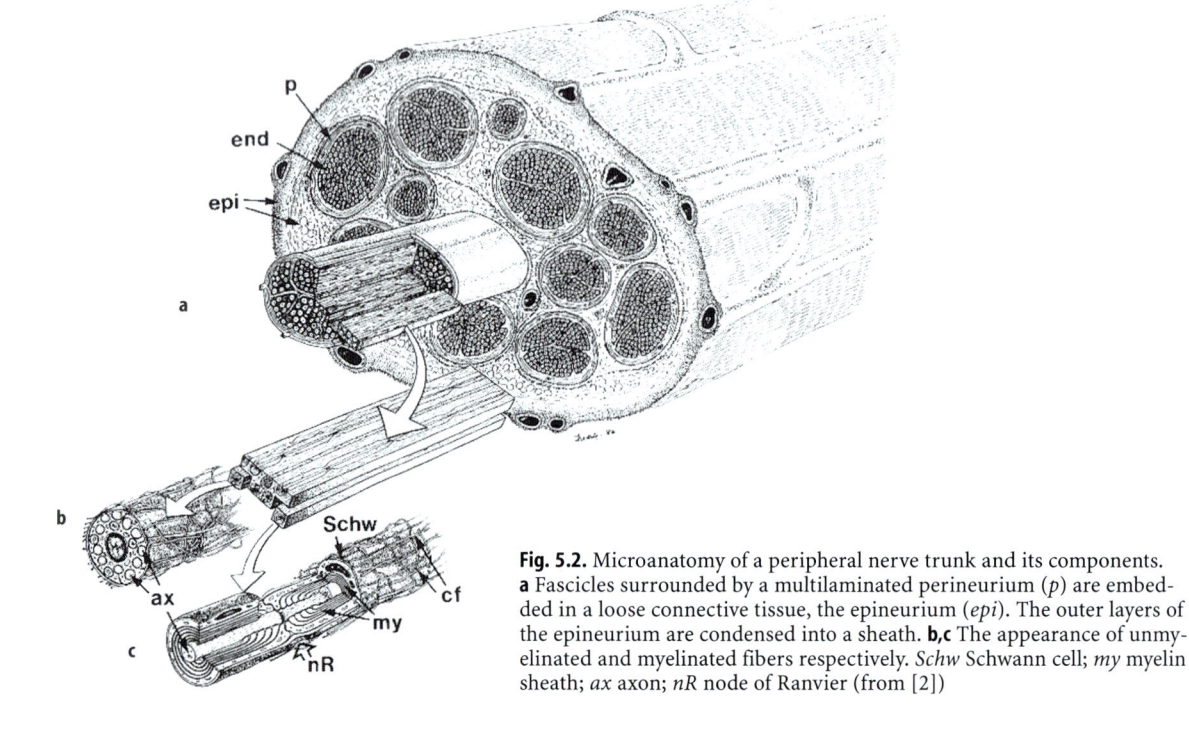

Fig. 5.2. Microanatomy of a peripheral nerve trunk and its components. **a** Fascicles surrounded by a multilaminated perineurium (*p*) are embedded in a loose connective tissue, the epineurium (*epi*). The outer layers of the epineurium are condensed into a sheath. **b,c** The appearance of unmyelinated and myelinated fibers respectively. *Schw* Schwann cell; *my* myelin sheath; *ax* axon; *nR* node of Ranvier (from [2])

5 The Pathophysiology of Median Nerve Compression

Fig. 5.3. Intraneural vascularization. Vessels are abundant in all layers of the nerve, forming a pattern of longitudinally oriented vessels. Extrinsic vessels (*exv*) are, via regional feeding vessels (*rv*), supporting vascular plexa in superficial and deep layers of the epineurium (*epi*), perineurium (*p*) and endoneurium (*end*). Note the oblique course of vessels penetrating the perineurium (*arrows*) and the intrafascicular "double loop formations" (*) (from [2])

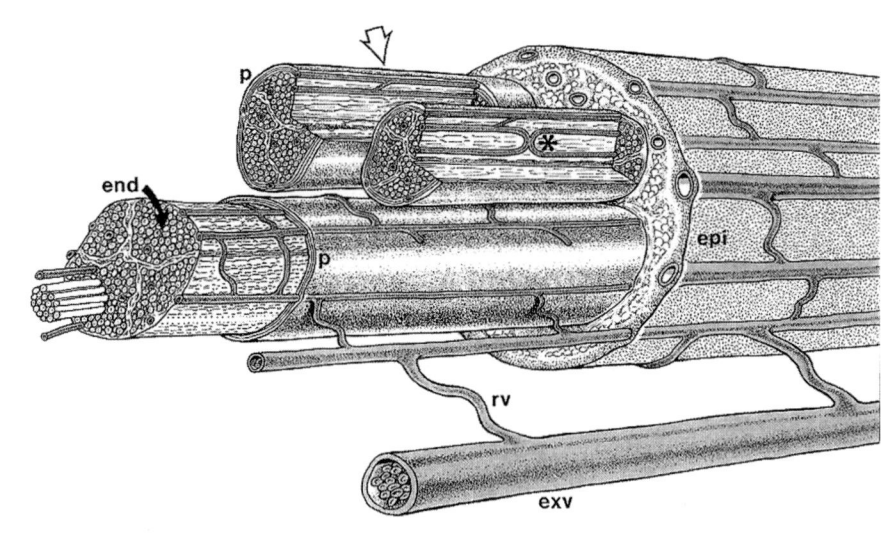

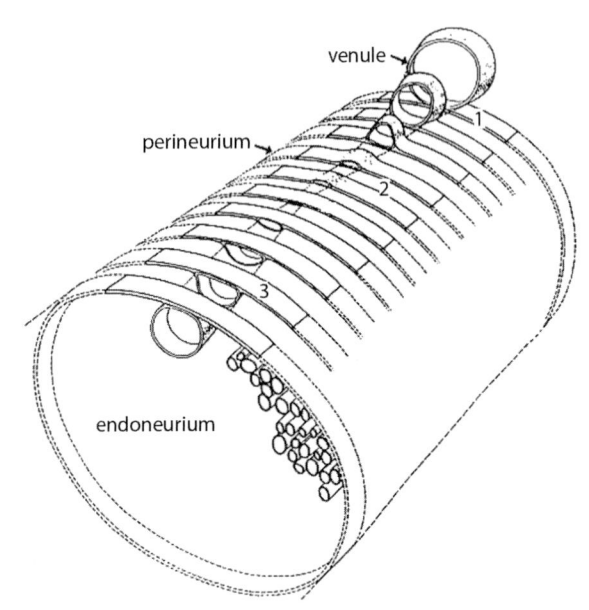

Fig. 5.4. Serial transverse sections of rat sciatic nerve fascicles showing a venule traversing the perineurium (*left*) and drawing of all sequential sections (from [2])

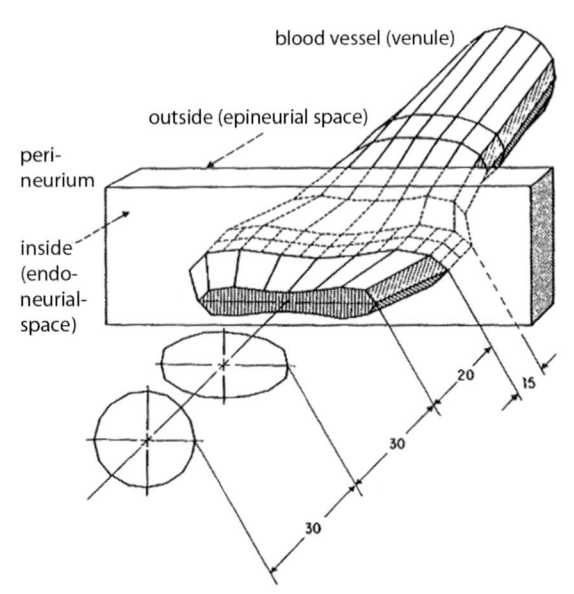

Fig. 5.5. Three-dimensional computer analysis of deformation of cylindrical blood vessel as it passes through the perineurium of an edematous fascicle. Tissue properties are well defined and believed to represent pathophysiological values present in edematous neuropathies. Endoneurial fluid pressure 6 mm Hg. The perspective of the drawing is from inside to endoneurium (from [2])

sort of valve mechanism at the point where the vessels are subject to obliteration in situations where there could be an increase in intrafascicular fluid pressure. An endoneural microvascular network exists at a intrafascicular level and is made up of not only capillaries but also arterioles and venules. The endoneural vascular bed is present in the entire length of the fascicles. Due to numerous anastomoses in all directions the endoneural capillary circuit is not really influenced by nerve trunk movements and because of the perineural barrier function, the endoneural blood flow is surprisingly well protected by eventual excessive intraneural dissection, like that which can occur during an internal neurolysis.

Blood-Nerve Barrier

The fascicles and their contents can be considered to be an extension of the central nervous system (CNS) towards its periphery. The perineurium is considered to be an extension of the pia mater of the CNS. Only some structural and functional characteristics of the CNS vessels have been found in the peripheral nervous system. The barrier of certain substances that circulate in the CNS blood (blood-brain barrier) is present and is called "blood-nerve barrier" [5]. The permeability of intraneural vessels to proteins that are in its microcirculation has been demonstrated by using fluoroscopy and radioactive tracers. Certain substances can easily pass through the vessels endothelium of the epineurium, while others are unable to pass or can only pass through in a reduced manner through the *endothelium* of the *endoneural* vessels. The structural basis for this barrier effect is derived from the narrowing of the endothelial cell junctions. The rheumato-nervous barrier is an essential element for maintaining endoneural homeostasis.

Nerve Fibers

Nerve fibers can be subdivided into myelinated or nonmyelinated types (Table 5.1). Schwann cells exist in both types and they wrap themselves around the nerve fiber (axon). The relationship between the Schwann cell and the axons is fundamentally different between the myelinated and nonmyelinated fibers. In the nonmyelinated fibers, the Schwann cell can wrap itself around more than one fiber, while in the myelinated, each axon is associated with only one Schwann cell for each level. The Schwann cell membrane wraps itself in a spiral manner around the axon, thus producing a alternating strata of lipids and proteins which make up the myelin sheath. Schwann cells unite with the myelinated fibers one after another at the Ranvier nodes junction. At this exact point, the cellular processes allow for an exchange between intra- and extracellular ions; this process oversees the statuary propagation of impulses from one node to another. Obviously, the conduction of impulses is different between fibers that are covered in a thick myelin sheath, and those that are scarcely covered, resulting in a much slower response propagation.

Pathophysiology

The Effect of Compression on the Nerve Fiber

The severity of a nerve injury that has been induced by an acute and or chronic compression is based on the duration of the compressive trauma. The onset, as is the nerve's recovery, can be variable and reflects the basic pathophysiology of the injury. The nerve fibers demonstrate their susceptibility to the compression in variable ways in relationship to their caliber, fascicular location, as well as the fascicles location within the nerve trunk [6]. The larger fibers are more susceptible to ischemia and compression in respect to the finer fibers, and the fibers that are located in the fascicle's periphery suffer more in respect to those that are more centrally located. Similarly, the nerve fibers that are located in the more superficial fascicles are injured more than those which are more central. Furthermore, the nerve trunk's constitution, at the site of compression, is an important factor in determining the extent of nerve compression damage: the larger fascicles that are contained in a small quantity of epineural tissue are more vulnerable to numerous compressions, rather than the little fascicles that are arranged and immersed in a large quantity of epineural tissue [2].

The physiopathologic basis of acute and chronic compression are controversial: both ischemic and mechanical factors have been proposed as the primary causes of the functional defect. The problem is difficult to address since all the compressive forces, by definition, include ischemic factors secondary to the obliteration of nerve microvessels. Generally, a moderate or slight compression that results in a functional compromise which is immediately reversible and consequential to the compression demonstrates direct finding of microvascular insufficiency, whereas, mechanical factors that provoke a focal myelin damage can make up etiologic factors of primary importance in injuries that require, above all, a longer recovery time.

The Compression Effect on Microvascular Intraneural Structures

The local compression effect has been experimentally studied on animals using various miniature compression models (Figs. 5.6, 5.7). Rydevik [7, 8], found in his intraoperative microscopic study that external compression of 20–30 mm Hg induces a slower epineurium venule flow. If the compressive pressure increases, the endoneurium capillary flow also is reduced. At a pressure of 80 mm Hg a complete intraneural flow stasis occurs in only the compressed nerve segment (ischemia) (Table 5.6). Rydevik's results have been recently reconfirmed by other authors.

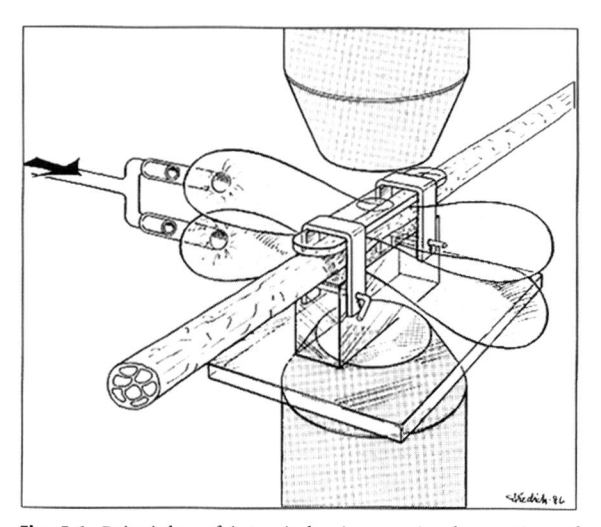

Fig. 5.6. Principles of intravital microscopic observation of intraneural microcirculation in rabbit tibial nerve under compression. The nerve is compressed by two transparent cuffs inflated to desired pressure (from [2])

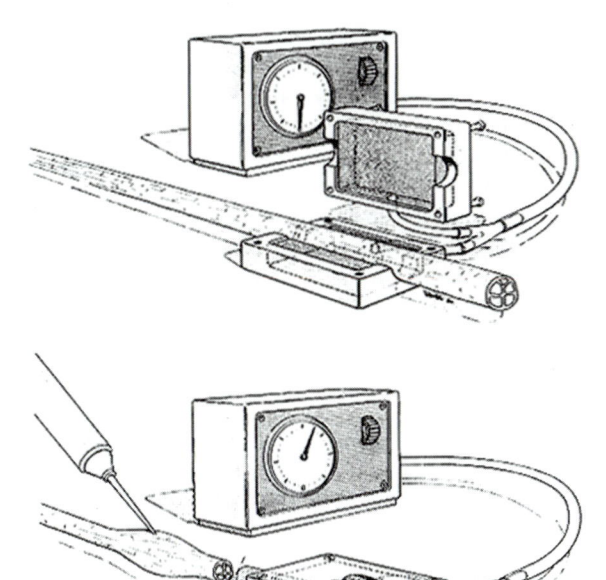

Fig. 5.7. Graded compression of the nerve by a miniature cuff, used for studies of vascular permeability and axonal transport (from [2])

Table 5.6. Effect of pressure on intraneural microvascular flow

Pressure (mmHg)	Effect
20–22	Reduction of epineurial venous flow
40–50	Reduction of capillary flow
80	Complete stasis

[8]

Axonal Transport and Nerve Compression

In 1948, Weiss and Hiscoe [9] reported that nerve constriction indicates swelling and fluid accumulation in the area that lies proximal to the site of injury. They uphold that this is due to an obstruction effect on the axoplasm inside the nerve fiber. In theory, one can believe that compression interferes with the axonal transport in a direct and mechanical or secondary manner by means of intraneural vessel obliteration with consequent anoxia. In experimental studies [10, 11], where the nerve has been compressed at a local level by using a pneumatic tourniquet, it has been demonstrated that even limited compression can inhibit axonal transport. Fast axonal transport, studied by means of tracer protein transport, remains normal up until a 20 mmHg pressure is reached for 2 h; if the duration is increased (8 h), an accumulation of material is seen proximal to the site of compression. A pressure of 30 mmHg for 2 h will cause a partial or complete inhibition. A blockage of fast axonal transport is reversible within 24 h only if

Table 5.7. Effect of pressure on fast anterograde axonal transport

Pressure (mmHg)	Duration (hours)	Effect
20	2	Absent
20	8	Block proximal to site of compression
30	2	Partial or complete block
50	2	Reversible block in 24 h
200	2	Reversible block in 3 days
400	2	Reversible block in 7 days

[11, 43, 46]

Table 5.8. Effect of pressure on slow anterograde axonal transport

Pressure (mmHg)	Duration (hours)	Effect
20	8	Absent
30	8	Protein accumulation

[46]

Table 5.9. Effect of pressure on retrograde axonal transport

Pressure (mmHg)	Duration (hours)	Effect
20–30	8	Axonal transport inhibition
200	8	Axonal transport block

[43, 46] Dahlin et al. 1984, Dahlin and McLean 1986

it does not exceed a compression of more 50 mmHg. The transport blockage is reversible only after 3 days, if 200 mmHg of pressure has been applied for only 2 h and within 7 days after 400 mmHg of pressure has been applied for 2 h (Table 5.7). In another experimental study, it has been demonstrated that if axonal transport metabolic injury already exists, for example, in rats with diabetes induced by streptozotocin, the fast axonal transport is significantly involved with respect to a control group. This indicates that nerves of diabetic animals are more susceptible to compression with respect to the nerves of healthy animals.

Slow axonal transport has been studied by Dahlin and McLean [12] (Table 5.8). A compression of 20 mmHg that is applied for more than 8 h does not cause an accumulation of material that is transported by a slow flow, whereas a pressure of 30 mmHg applied for 8 h is always followed by significant fluid accumulation but not all of the proteins that have been transported by the slow flow.

These results indicate that even the lowest compression pressure can interfere with either the slow or fast axonal flow. Even low pressures are, however, of interest since similar pressures have been found in the carpal canal in patients that are afflicted with CTS. The same low pressures can even involve retrograde axonal transport (Table 5.9). In an animal experimental study, it

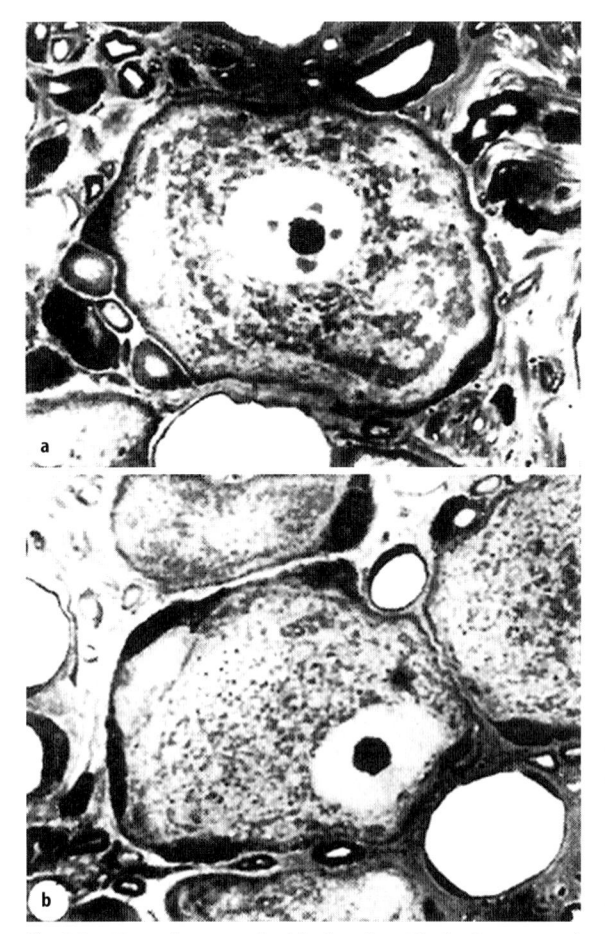

Fig. 5.8. a Normal nerve cell with abundant Nissl substance and central nucleus. The cell is from a ganglion where the vagus has not been subjected to any trauma. **B** Nerve cell with dispersed Nissl substance (chromatolysis) and peripheral displacement of nucleus. The cell is taken from a ganglion where vagus nerve was compressed at 30 mmHg for 2 h at 1 week before evaluation of morphology (methylene blue and Azur II: × 1000) (from [2])

was demonstrated that 20–30 mm Hg of pressure that is applied for 8 h induces retrograde axonal transport inhibition. Compression of 200 mmHg for 8 h induces a greater inhibition to this type of flow. Dahlin observed the neuron cell body's morphology to be modified after an application of low pressure compression of the respective nerve fibers. At a pressure of 30 mm Hg one can observe a volume and nuclear density increase, nucleus eccentricity, and dispersion of Nissl substance (chromatolysis) up to 7 days after compression (Fig. 5.8). This type of cell body behavior is well known and occurs only after a severe crush or nerve dissection injury.

Pressure Effect on Nerve Fibers

Compression of a nerve trunk can cause damage by means of direct pressure or associated tangent forces with the redistribution of tissue from the compressed and noncompressed area. Different experimental studies have demonstrated that this tissue redistribution is often not measurable by using compression instruments and it is damaging for the injured fibers, while a pressure that is more uniformly applied to the nerve causes minor fiber damage Interesting studies have been performed with regard to nerve compression that has occurred from the application of external compression instruments. In this situation the nerve is not directly compressed along all the surface application of the tourniquet but prevalently at the border level where the tangent forces are maximal. In an experimental study on monkeys, it has been demonstrated that the Rainer nodes move towards the noncompressed part of the nerve. The paranodal myelin is relocated from a part of the node and folds into the other. This change in position occurs both in the proximal and distal part of the compressive tourniquet and is followed by a segmental demyelinization and a successive conduction blockage, reversible after weeks or months. The focal demyelinization that is observed [13–15] is believed to be a direct consequence of mechanical pressure provoked by the compressive tourniquet. Powell and Myers [16] demonstrated local Schwann cell necrosis appears before focal demyelinization occurs. The necrosis can be provoked by a local ischemic effect since this physiopathological mechanism is the most probable one for successive paranodal demyelinization.

Intraneural Edema from Compression

Compression with consequential total and subtotal ischemia can produce damage to all the intraneural tissue including the Schwann cells, nerve fibers, and the intraneural microvessels. A microvascular injury can be associated with an increase in membrane permeability to proteins, while long-lasting ischemic periods can be followed by intraneural edema as soon as the blood flow has been reestablished [17–20]. This local swelling, called "nonreflux phenomenon" [21, 22, 23] or "closed compartment syndrome," is a phenomenon which is well known and occurs in the muscle tissue following severe ischemic nerve and muscle injury. The effect this phenomenon has on the nerves is quite critical and can cause a functional barrier in the perineurium stratum [24].

The intrafascicular vessels are particularly resistant to ischemia. Complete ischemia that lasts 6 h can be followed by a complete microvascular recovery with or without thrombosis. This phenomenon can be in relation to a local release of plasminogen-activating factors from the endothelium of endoneural blood vessels undergoing prolonged periods of ischemia, for example, 8 h or more, an intense endoneural edema associated with a "nonreflux phenomenon." Animal experiments have demonstrated that this type of endoneural edema

Table 5.10. Effect of pressure on intraneural edema

Pressure (mmHg)	Duration (hours)	Effect
50	2	Epineurial edema
200–400	2	Endoneurial edema (at compression borders)
200	6	Endoneurial edema (at central segment)

[43, 46]

Table 5.11. Effect of intraneural edema on the microvascular flow

Pressure (mmHg)	Duration (hours)	Effect
80	2	Immediate flow recovery
400	2	Partial or absent recovery

[8]

is followed by irreversible damage to the nerve's function.

When a nerve undergoes a local compression, one should take into account the width and length of the tourniquet that is being applied, as well as the pressure duration since the distribution of intrafascicular edema, once the tourniquet is deflated, since the damage provoked is based on these factors. Modifications of intraneural microvascular permeability have been experimentally studied at different compression levels (50–200–400 mmHg) by using a miniature tourniquet that is applied around the nerve (Table 5.10). Compression of 50 mmHg for 2 h induces an edema that remains strictly in the epineurium. The edema does not reach the endoneurium due to the barrier effect of the perineural stratum. Pressure of 200–400 mmHg for 2 h demonstrated a significant amount of microvascular damage to the compressed segment's margins. This was indicated by the venous leakage of infused tracer material. Consequently, an intense amount of endoneural edema was found at the compression margins, while it was not present in the center of the compressed segment. Compression at 200 mmHg for 2 h or 400 mmHg for 15 min was followed by endoneurial edema in only some of the fascicles at the compression margins, but instead a longer compression duration produced the appearance of edema in all the fascicles. If the pressure was 200 mmHg and was applied for 4 h or 6 h, the edema was evident even in the compressed segment's center. The data demonstrates that compression dimensions and duration play a very important role in determining intraneural edema, and that vascular injuries are more evident at the compressed zone's margins. Nerve fiber injuries occur at margin levels and this phenomenon is called a "margin effect."

Rydevik's experiments [7, 8] have demonstrated that 80 mmHg of pressure applied for 2 h caused an immediate microvascular recovery; however, nerves that were compressed at 400 mmHg, for the same time period, did not demonstrate or demonstrated only a partial recovery of the compressed segment's microcirculation, even after 7 days had passed (Table 5.11). This "nonreflux phenomenon" is based on a massive amount of intraneural edema in the compressed nerve segment, associated with a direct mechanical injury of the intraneural microvessels at the compressive margin level – together impeding reperfusion of the compressed segment.

Lundborg [2] and also Powell and Myers [16], have studied the effect of interneural edema that appears in the nerves following local compression from minipneumatic tourniquets. Normally the internal tissue pressure of the fascicles is slightly positive (2.0 +/– 1.0 cm H_2O) [25, 26]. The tissue pressure is evaluated by using a micropipette after applied compression from 1 to 24 h, while contemporaneously the nerve fiber, its ultrastructure, and endoneural contents are histologically evaluated for a period of time up until 28 days after the compression release. One can observe an increase in endoneural edema and tissue fluid pressure up to 4 times per hour after compression removal of 80 mmHg, for 4 h up until 3 times after compression at 30 mmHg for 8 h (Table 5.12). It has even been possible to register a similar pressure value 24 h after surgery and endoneural edema was still present even after 28 days from the time of compression application. Microscopic studies revealed pathologic alterations of the subperineural fibers with demyelinization even in nerves that had undergone a pressure of only 10 mmHg. The Schwann cells demonstrate, after undergoing a compression of 80 mmHg for only 2 h, swelling and cytoplasmic disintegration for a period of up to 28 days from the time of treatment.

The increase in tissue fluid pressure runs parallel with an increase in endoneural edema, which is essential when one understands either acute or chronic nerve compression pathophysiology. The constant increase of endoneural tissue fluid pressure can cause nerve fiber damage and modifications in the endoneural fluid's electrolytic composition thus causing nerve conduction damage. The increase in endoneural fluid pressure interferes with the endoneural capillary microcirculation, therefore, total endoneural capillary

Table 5.12. Effect of pressure on the endoneurial edema

Pressure (mmHg)	Duration (hours)	Effect
80	4	8.5
30	8	6.0

[16]

collapse does not occur. A pressure of endoneural fluid three times its norm has been seen and is associated with a significant reduction in the nerve's blood flow. Endoneural edema increases the difficulty of obtaining diffusion of oxygen between the capillaries and the axons, leading to an endoneural hypoxia phenomenon. Hypoxia can affect different parts of the endoneural space and extends itself in a very variable manner. In galactose neuropathies, an endoneural edema with increased endoneural fluid pressure occurs and the oxygen tension in the subperineurium and nerve fascicle centers is significantly low. The endoneural edema can not leak out from the endoneural space, thus a diffusion barrier exists and the endoneural space pressure remains high for a long period of time. Endoneural edema is subject to a fibrotic transformation due to an invasion of fibroblasts, and consequently an intraneural scar that once formed is irreversible.

Ischemia Versus Compression – Clinical Experiments

Lewis [27] created a special instrument for exerting a pressure of 60–70 mm Hg on human radial and median nerves. He found that this compression was sufficient to block nerve conduction and he arrived at the conclusion that the block depended on an intraneural microvessel occlusion. Various other experiments have theoretically come to the same conclusion excluding mechanical factors. An experiment of Lundborg [28] put an end to this dilemma. The experiment consisted of applying controlled pressure to median nerves in human subjects. This experiment utilized a pressure gauge (wick catheter) in order to register the continual pressure inside the carpal canal near the median nerve (Figs. 5.9, 5.10). The hands of voluntary subjects underwent an external compression at the carpal canal level (near the palm) by using a specifically made instrument. In this way the applied pressure could be controlled and monitored over time, even inside the canal and near the median nerve. Contemporaneously, motor and sensory nerve conduction was controlled using a battery of specific tests that registered clinical symptoms and the appearance of motor or sensory deficits. A pressure of 30 mm Hg caused the onset of the first neurophysiological modifications associated with sensory symptoms (paresthesia). A complete sensory and motor nerve conduction block (VCS and VCM) appeared, but only after an endo-canal pressure of about 40–50 mm Hg or greater was reached. In these cases the VCS was the first to demonstrate a slowing down in its sensory potential amplitude after 25–50 min from external compression application. Instead, motor potentials followed the same course but with a latency of 10–30 min (Table 5.13). These experiments demonstrate that the critical pressure level for microvessels that causes their obliteration with consequent ischemia and total nerve conduction block is around 40–50 mm Hg.

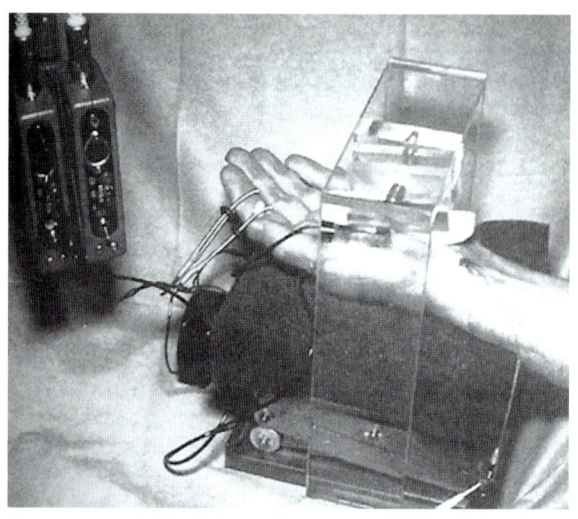

Fig. 5.9. Experimental device for applying external pressure to the carpal canal of human volunteers. A Wick catheter was introduced into the carpal canal to monitor local tissue pressure. Localized pressure was applied to the carpal tunnel by raising the lower platform towards the fixed roof of the compression device (from [2])

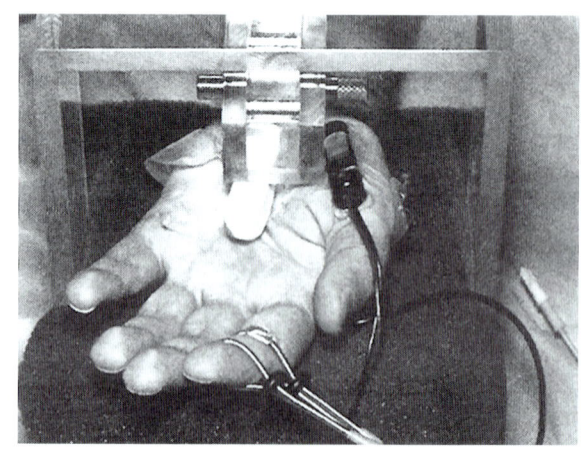

Fig. 5.10. Close-up of model in **Fig. 5.9**, showing surface electrodes for motor and sensory fiber recordings and mould used for applying localized pressure to the carpal canal (from [2])

Table 5.13. Effect of pressure on the median nerve conduction velocity at wrist

Pressure (mmHg)	Duration (min)	Effect
30		Slowing of NCV + paresthesia
40–50		SCV and MCV block
40–50	20–50	SAP absence
40–50	35–80	MUP absence

[28]

The evidence that it was the ischemia and not the mechanical effect of compression by itself determining the damage of the nerve fiber was demonstrated in a subsequent experiment. After having applied an external compression to the wrist, which causes the disappearance of the median nerve's VCS, a tourniquet is applied to the upper arm and pumped up to a pressure that is superior to the patient's systolic pressure; once this pressure is reached the local pressure that has been applied to the wrist is removed. Even though the direct local pressure applied to the nerve has been removed, its sensory nerve conduction does not return until the upper arm tourniquet is removed: at this point both motor and sensory function returns immediately.

The significant importance of ischemia has been demonstrated in successive hypertension patients. In these subjects, sensory conduction is blocked at 60–70 mmHg, and at a pressure threshold of 20 mmHg higher with respect to the above-mentioned 40–50 mmHg, thus demonstrating that is sufficient to cause a sensory conduction block in patients with normal tension [29, 30].

Chronic Nerve Compression

The signs and symptoms in a chronic nerve compression are the combined effect of persistent compression and the nerve's subsequent inflammatory reaction causing a direct mechanical injury to the nerve fibers. Repetitive compression, lengthening, stretching, and friction are factors that contribute to an increase in vascular permeability, chronic edema, and endoneural fibrous tissue formation. Myelin damage and axonal degeneration are results of defective microvascular flow and repetitive trauma on the nerve fibers. The importance of mechanical factors has been emphasized by experiments performed by Ochoa [13–15] and Gilliat [31], while the significance of microvascular insufficiency has been upheld by other authors [2, 7, 8, 32, 33].

Various experimental models have been studied in order to evaluate the pathophysiology and pathologic anatomy of chronic nerve compression injuries. It has been possible to follow a study on spontaneous injuries in an animal species (guinea pigs) that during development encounters spontaneous median nerve compression at the carpal canal level. The natural development of this compressive syndrome has been quite useful for the study of chronic compressive nerve pathologies. A detailed study has been done by examining its histologic and ultrastructure aspects. The typical injuries are called "tadpole lesion" [2]. This type of injury has been found in human median nerves at the wrist and in ulnar nerves at the elbow, as well as in the lateral femoralcutaneous nerve of the thigh associated with paresthetic pain.

The injuries have also been experimentally induced by directly applying a structure on the nerve in order to produce a constriction. A silicone tube of an adequate diameter and thickness was applied to the sciatic nerve of rats by Mackinnon [34], so that it would produce a chronic irritation, epineural and perineural fibrosis until deterioration of the blood-nerve barrier was reached and consequent injury to the large nerve fibers. Similar experiments were reproduced by Horiuchi and Nemoto [35, 36] that induced long-duration-controlled compression to the sciatic nerves' of dogs by using metal clips. A compression of 30 mmHg provoked a flattening of the nerve, while immediately proximal and distal to the nerve compression an intraneural edema and swelling appeared.

Seiler's [37] experiment is quite interesting regarding a double chronic crushing to the nerve. Four months after tibial nerve compression to a rat by means of a silicone tube, a second compression (using the same mechanism) was applied more distally. The neurophysiologic study that was done 4 months later

Fig. 5.11. Experimental "double crush model" as designed by Nemoto. Sciatic nerves of adult dogs were compressed by a special spring-clip device inducing a pressure of about 30 mmHg. Group 1: one clip was applied to the sciatic nerve 3 cm distal to the sciatic tuberculum. Group 2: two clips applied simultaneously 2 cm apart. Group 3: two clips applied at the same sites as in group 2 but the second applied 3 weeks after the first (from [2])

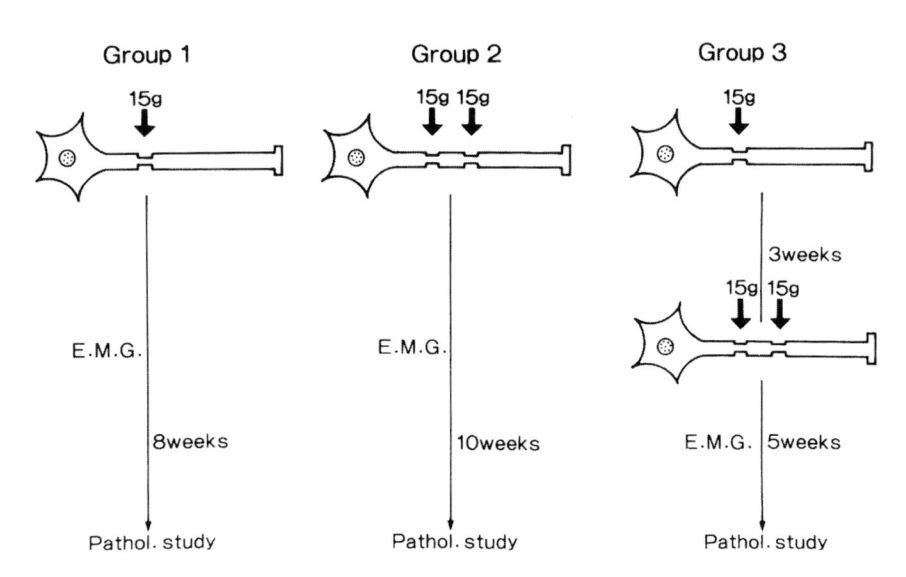

showed a significant decrease in motor velocity conduction time in comparison to a group who only underwent a single compression.

Nemoto [36] has also conducted an experiment that confirms the existence of a double level of compression by using metal clips which induce a chronic compression when applied with a pressure of about 30 mm Hg at two different levels along dogs' sciatic nerves. Ten weeks after applying these compressive forces to the nerve, Nemoto demonstrated that the proximal compression increased the vulnerability of the nerve's distal part and lead to a successive compression (Fig. 5.11).

Stages of Compressive Nerve Injuries

Theoretical and Clinical Considerations

The susceptibility of nerve fibers to compression varies in relationship to their caliber and intrafascicular topography, for which each compressive nerve injury represents a *mixed injury,* with the extent of injury on the various nerve fiber populations. In addition, it has been seen that the stages of nerve compression should be defined based on the nature of the functional injury and the type of functional recovery, as well as on the anatomical-pathologic picture of various nerve trunk tissue components.

Metabolic Conduction Block

The term, metabolic conduction block (physiologic) refers to a local lack of oxygen based on a circulatory arrest, with inhibition to impulse transmission in structurally intact parts of the nerve fibers. This type of block can be induced by a weak local compression, for example, peroneal compression, as occurs when one leg is crossed over the other. In this situation, the foot falls asleep, but the block is immediately reversible when the pressure is removed. Another condition is when a tourniquet is applied to the upper arm with a pressure which is superior to the patient's arteriole systolic pressure. Local ischemia is induced by the tourniquet's pressure and an alteration in sensory and motor conduction occurs due to the nerve being compressed, but the conduction is immediately recovered when the tourniquet is removed. The time required for this functional recovery to occur is in relation to the duration of the ischemia and intraneural edema that occurs secondary to endothelial anoxia contributing to the increase in recovery time. The time limit for ischemia that then transfers itself into a metabolic block in an irreversible nerve injury is 6–8 h.

Neuroapraxia

Neuroapraxia refers to another type of nerve conduction block in which the continuity of axons is maintained without a degenerative onset, but conduction through the compression site recovers only after some weeks or months. This term was introduced by Seddon [38, 39]. This type of injury is thought to correspond to an acute phenomenon, with local damage to the myelin at the Rainer nodes, as has been described by Denny-Brown and Brenner [40] and Ochoa [15]. The block persists until the myelin injury has healed. This is a process that usually takes some weeks to months. As Seddon [38] has originally observed, the neuroapraxia presents itself as a motor paralysis saving only the sensitive and sympathetic nerve fibers.

"Saturday night paralysis" of the radial nerve, that occurs after a humeral fracture, represents a typical example of a neuroapraxic injury. In this case, there is a complete paralysis of radially innervated muscles that are distal to the compression site, but the sensitive fibers are not involved. Sometimes the compression is more intense or occurs in patients that have pre-existing metabolic pathologies. Therefore, the way in which it expresses itself clinically is not of the typical nature, but instead, also demonstrates a sensitive paresthesia associated with the motor one. The axonal continuity is maintained; the radially innervated muscles can be activated by a stimulus that is applied distal to the compression. Usually, there is a functional recovery after some weeks or months from the time of initial injury and it coincides with a remodeling of the myelin sheath. If there is no evident recovery after 4 months one can conclude that the local healing processes (bone callus fracture entrapments) have impeded the injury repair or the injury was so significant that it lead to the nerve's Wallerian degeneration.

A nerve compression due to the application of a compressive tourniquet is another classic example of a neuroapraxia injury. It has been reported in the scientific literature that its functional damage varies on the basis of simple sensibility disturbances and a paralysis of all three principal upper extremity nerves. Even the tourniquet application time can be quite variable from 15 min to 2 and one half hours. The frequency of this pathology has been estimated to be 1/5,000. These results make it clear that nerve injuries are not proportional to the limb's ischemic time. The tourniquet's manometer registers calibration errors in a great number of cases. The pressure that results right below the tourniquet or around its borders, which has induced the nerve structures compression injury, actually varies from 350 to 1,200 mm Hg.

Sunderland [41] has introduced a more detailed classification for nerve injuries based on anatomical landmarks (types I–V). In this neuroapraxia classification, type I refers to a local myelin injury to intact nerve fibers, without Wallerian degeneration.

Axonotmesis

Axonotmesis implies the loss of local axon continuity but the endoneural tubes remain intact. The injury corresponds to an advanced compression or excessive traction that causes an interruption in axonal continuity, therefore inducing axonal degeneration. The endoneural tubes are spared and the functional recovery reflects the time required by the axons to regenerate in the original endoneural tubes until they reach a peripheral target. Axon growth is guided by the original tubes; the prognosis is good regarding regeneration. Surgery will not be required, but it is not easy to define the real entity of the pathology and peripheral nerve injury; as mentioned above, they are mixed and frequently a surgical decompression treatment is associated with an internal neurolysis.

Neurotmesis

Neurotmesis signifies axon continuity loss and whichever nerve trunk element has been affected, including the endoneural covering, the perineurium and the epineurium. According to Seddon's [38] original classifications, neurotmesis is a term that is used to describe the nerve state that has been completely sectioned or is totally damaged from fibrosis and no longer can obtain spontaneous recovery. Sunderland [41] has divided this type of injury into three subgroups (types III – V). Type III includes nerves which have lost their axon continuity of the endoneural tubes while the perineurium is still intact. In this situation, the continuity and orientation of the endoneural tubes is lost and the injury is often associated with a intrafascicular fibrosis. Type IV includes nerves which have lost the continuity of the perineurium with maintenance of the endoneurium; while type V includes the loss of continuity of the entire nerve trunk. Neurotmesis requires a surgical treatment in order to regain complete functional recovery.

Conclusion

It is easy to understand that both chronic and acute nerve injuries are complex to treat. The interference with the intraneural microcirculation, the axonal transport, and the impulse transmission can form a clinical basis for the presentation of symptoms and clinical signs, both in the initial phase, as well as in the advanced phases of nerve compression. The term "nerve compression injury" from a physiopathologic point of view, is not correct and does not indicate that the intraneural inflammatory reaction has been caused by a friction mechanism and/or overstretching, both which play essential roles as etiologic factors.

The various stages of CTS that have been proposed try to demonstrate the involvement of both etiologic factors, as well as physiopathological ones. The initial stage of CTS is characterized by night-time paresthesia and is based on night-time intraneural microvascular insufficiency due to an increase in night-time tissue pressure in the carpal canal. The incremental increase in tissue fluid pressure reflects the exclusion of the muscle pump, the redistribution of body fluid in the horizontal position, and palmar flexion of the wrist. One should not forget that in addition to night-time vascular pressure reduction, which is linked to the circadian rhythm, there is also the reduction of perfusion pressure inside the carpal canal. The symptoms are based on the nerve's local metabolic disorganization, resulting in a deprivation of oxygen secondary to intraneural microcirculation involvement. The symptoms are reversible when the wrist position, the muscle pump, and the body posture normalize themselves or when the transverse carpal ligament is sectioned.

In more advanced CTS cases, edema is persistent first in the epineurium and then in the endoneurium. Constant microcirculation involvement and an increase in tissue fluid pressure maintain the patient's symptoms, but decompression can still be reversible if it occurs contemporaneously with the recovery of interneural flow and the edema is then drained from the area. Focal injury of the nerve fiber components occurs in this stage with injury to the myelin sheath caused by pressure and secondary nerve ischemia. Neuroapraxic injuries require quite a long time to recuperate and fiber function can return to normal only after many months from the time of decompression.

A long-enduring edema can be invaded by fibroblasts and transform itself into fibrosis. In this situation, some of the fibers can be involved only by a metabolic phenomenon and others by demyelinization with greater damage (neuroapraxia) while others can end up with axonal degeneration (axonotmesis). Nerve decompression can be followed by a very variable time frame for functional recovery and depends on the severity of the injury. Sometimes a timely functional recovery can occur: the recovery of certain functions can be rapid (due to metabolic damage) while other recovery is much more slow (months or years). In some cases, functional recovery does not occur since there is a interneural scar, in addition to axonal degeneration (permanent functional damage).

Double Level Compression (Double Crush)

It is known that an increase of CTS occurs in patients suffering from cervico-brachialgia. Upton and McComas [42] proposed the theory of a double level compression (double crush). This implies that the successive nerve trunk compression can have a cumulative effect causing the distal part of the proximally compressed nerve to be susceptible to compression. Current knowledge of the influence of compression on axonal transport makes this theory very convincing. Probably even clinical nerve compression features at more than one level find an explanation in physiopathologic terms. The anterograde axonal transport produces sufficient material for the axons, as well as for their terminations, and naturally, whatever condition that interferes with the axonal transport can interfere, for example, with the membrane composition in the distal part of the axon itself. An axon membrane defect can indicate a resistance defect to external compression forces in relation to the healthy membrane.

Dahlin's studies [43] on the effect of low compression in relation to retrograde axonal transport suggest that modifications which the membrane undergoes is of great importance. The amount of pressure which is similar to that which has been registered in the CTS patient's carpal tunnel demonstrated a retrograde axonal transport block and the onset of morphological modifications in the nerve cell bodies inside the ganglion. The response of the cell bodies is probably an expression of the loss of neurotrophic factors that have been synthesized by the Schwann cells or by the target tissue. A cell body that is damaged is not able to adequately control the anterograde axonal transport and the proximal part of the axon can therefore suffer from lack of material. In this way, a distal nerve compression can theoretically be the cause for a proximal compression injury of the same nerve, making up the so-called inverted double crush syndrome. Carroll [44] and Hurst [45] have pointed out that it is possible to explain why, when following a simple surgical decompression of the carpal tunnel, sometimes more proximally located typical compression symptoms are activated.

Finally, it should be remembered that there is a high possibility that a nerve compression occurs in nerves which are already afflicted with a metabolic pathology or a polyneuropathy. This is the case in diabetic patients that manifest median nerve compression at the wrist. The "double crush" concept is identical, the only difference is that the proximal compression does not exist but nerve suffering continues from a pre-existing metabolic pathology. Dahlin et al. [46] have conducted specific studies regarding this topic.

References

1. McLellan DL, Swash M (1976) Longitudinal sliding of the median nerve during movement of the upper limb. J Neurol Neurosurg Psychiatry 39: 566–570
2. Lundborg G (1988) Nerve Injury and Repair. Churchill Livingstone Edinburgh
3. Dahlin LB, Nordborg C, Lundborg G (1987) Morphological changes in nerve cell bodies induced by experimental graded nerve compression. Exp Neurol 95: 611
4. Lundborg G (1979) The intrinsic vascularization of human peripheral nerves: Structural and functional aspect. J Hand Surg 4: 34
5. Shanthaveerappa TR, Bourne GH (1963) The perineural epithelium. Nature and significance. Nature (Lond) 199: 577
6. Sunderland S (1976) The nerve lesion in the carpal tunnel syndrome. J Neurol Neurosurg Psychiatry 39: 615
7. Rydevik B, Lundborg G (1977) Permeability of intraneural microvessels and perineurium following acute, graded experimental nerve compression. Scand J Plast Reconstr Surg 11: 179
8. Rydevik B, Lundborg G, Bagge U (1981) Effects of graded compression on intraneural blood flow. An in vivo study on rabbit tibial nerve. J Hand Surg 6: 3
9. Weiss P, Hiscoe HB (1948) Experiments on the mechanism of nerve growth. J Exp Zoology 107: 315–395
10. Lundborg G, Nordborg C, Rydevik B, Olsson Y (1973) The effect of ischemia on the permeability of the perineurium to protein tracers in rabbit tibial nerve. Acta Neurol Scand 49: 287
11. Rydevik B, McLean WG, Sjostrand J, Lundborg G (1980) Blockage of axonal transport induced by acute, graded compression of the rabbit vagus nerve. J Neurol Neurosurg Psychiatry 43: 690
12. Dahlin LB, McLean WG (1986) Effects of graded experimental compression on slow and fast axonal transport in rabbit vagus nerve. J Neurol Sci 72: 19
13. Ochoa J (1980) Nerve fiber pathology in acute and chronic compression. In GE Omer, M Spinner (Eds): Management of peripheral nerve problems. Philadelphia, WB Saunders Co, pp 487.
14. Ochoa J, Marotte L (1973) The nature of the nerve lesion caused by chronic entrapment in the guinea-pig. J Neurol Sci 19: 491
15. Ochoa J, Fowler TJ, Gilliatt RW (1972) Anatomical changes in peripheral nerves compressed by a pneumatic tourniquet. J Anat 113: 433
16. Powell HC, Myers RR (1986) Pathology of experimental nerve compression. Lab Invest 55: 91
17. Myers RR, Powell HC (1981) Endoneurial fluid pressure in peripheral neuropathies. In AR Hargens (Ed): Tissue Fluid Pressure and Composition. Baltimore, Williams and Wilkins, pp 193.
18. Myers RR, Powell HC, Costello ML et al. (1978) Endoneurial fluid pressure: direct measurement with micropipettes. Brain Res, 148: 510
19. Myers RR, Costello ML, Powell HC (1979) Increased endoneurial fluid pressure in galactose neuropathy. Muscle & Nerve 2: 299
20. Myers RR, Heckman HM, Powell HC (1983) Endoneurial fluid is hypertonic. Results of microanalysis and its significance in neuropathy. J Neuropathol Exp Neurol 42: 217
21. Matsen FA (1980) Compartmental Syndromes. New York, Grune and Stratton
22. Mubarak SJ, Hargens AR (1981) Compartment syndromes and Volkmann's contracture. Phladelphia, WB Saunders Co
23. Hargens AR, Akeson WH, Mubarak SJ et al. (1978) Fluid balance within the canine anterolateral compartment and its relationship to compartment syndromes. J Bone Joint Surg 60A: 499–505
24. Lundborg G, Myers R, Powell H (1983) Nerve compression injury and increased endoneurial fluid pressure: a "miniature compartment syndrome." J Neurol Neurosurg Psychiatry 46: 1119

25. Low PA, Dyck PJ (1977) Increased endoneurial fluid pressure in experimental lead neuropathy. Nature (Lond) 269: 427
26. Low PA, Marchand G, Knox F, Dyck PJ (1977) Measurement of endoneurial fluid pressure with polyethylene matrix capsules. Brain Res 122: 373
27. Lewis T, Pickering GW, Rothschild P (1931) Centripetal paralysis arising out of arrested bloodflow to the limb, including notes on a form of tingling. Heart 16: 1–32
28. Lundborg G, Gelberman RH, Minteer-Convery M et al. (1982) Median nerve compression in the carpal tunnel. Functional response to experimentally induced controlled pressure. J Hand Surg 7: 252
29. Gelberman RH, Szabo RM, Williamson RV et al. (1983) Tissue pressure threshold for peripheral nerve viability. Clin Orthop 178: 285
30. Szabo RM, Gelberman RH, Williamson RV, Hargens AR (1983) Effects of increased systemic blood pressure on the tissue fluid pressure threshold of peripheral nerve. J Orthop Res 1: 172
31. Gilliatt RW (1981) Physical injury to peripheral nerves. Physiologic and electrodiagnostic aspect. Mayo Clin Proc 56: 361
32. Lundborg G (1970) Ischemic nerve injury. Experimental studies on intraneural microvascular pathophysiology and nerve function in a limb sujected to temporary circulatory arrest. Scand J Plast Reconstr Surg, Suppl 6
33. Lundborg G (1975) Structure and function of the intraneural microvessels as related to trauma, edema formation, and nerve function. J Bone Joint Surg 57A: 938
34. MacKinnon S, Dellon AL, Hudson AR, Hunter DA (1984) Chronic nerve compression – an experimental model in the rat. Ann Plast Surg 13: 112
35. Horiuchi Y (1983) Experimental study on peripheral nerve lesions. Compression neuropathy. J Jap Orthop Assoc 57: 789
36. Nemoto K (1983) An experimental study on the vulnerability of the peripheral nerve. J Jpn Orthop Ass 57: 1773
37. Seiler WA, Schlegel R, MacKinnon S, Dellon AL (1983) Double crush syndrome: experimental model in the rat. Surg Forum 34: 596
38. Seddon HJ (1943) Three types of nerves injury. Brain 66: 237
39. Seddon HJ (1972) Surgical disorder of the peripheral nerves. London, Churchill Livingstone, pp 34.
40. Denny-Brown D, Brenner C (1944) Paralysis of nerve induced by direct pressure and by tourniquet. Arch Neurol Psychiatry 51: 1
41. Sunderland S (1978) Nerves and nerve injuries. London, Churchill Livingstone
42. Upton AR, McComas AJ (1973) The double crush in the nerve entrapment syndromes. Lancet 2: 359
43. Dahlin LB, Rydevik B, McLean WG, Sjostrand J (1984) Changes in fast axonal transport during experimental nerve compression at low pressures. Exp Neurol 84: 29
44. Carroll RE, Hurst LC (1982) The relationship of thoracic outlet syndrome and carpal tunnel syndrome. Clin Orthop 164: 149
45. Hurst LC, Weissberg D, Carroll RE (1985) The relationship of double crush to carpal tunnel syndrome (an analysis of 1,000 cases of carpal tunnel syndrome). J Hand Surg 10B: 202
46. Dahlin LB, Meiri KF, McLean WG et al. (1986) Effects of nerve compression on fast axonal transport in streptozotocin-induced diabetes mellitus. An experimental study in the sciatic nerve of rats. Diabetol 29: 181

6 Ischemia-Reperfusion Injury as a Common Etiology of "Idiopathic" Carpal Tunnel Syndrome: Biochemical and Immunohistochemical Evidence

A.E. Freeland, M.A. Tucci, V. Sud

Disclaimer: No benefits in any form have been received or will be received from a commercial party related directly or indirectly to the subject of this chapter.

Introduction

Carpal tunnel syndrome (CTS) is a frequent source of pain, impairment, and disability. Decompression of the carpal canal is currently the most common operation currently performed by hand surgeons and has attained almost epidemic proportions [17]. There are approximately 450,000 carpal tunnel releases (CTR) performed annually in the USA at a medical cost in excess of two billion dollars annually [39]. Medical costs, lost wages, and lost industrial performance are staggering.

In many cases, the onset of CTS is insidious and progressive. In these instances, the etiology has proven illusive and consequently labeled as "idiopathic" [20]. These patients fulfill the following criteria: (1) typical signs and symptoms of CTS [29, 37]; (2) no significant past medical history (no history of trauma, diabetes mellitus, crystalline arthropathy, metabolic disease, endocrine imbalance, inflammatory arthritis, or other related systemic disease) [39]; (3) documented abnormalities in the preoperative electrodiagnostic studies [14]; (4) normal standard wrist x-rays; and (5) no evident structural cause of compression of the median nerve intraoperatively other than hyperplasia, edema, and fibroplasia of the flexor tenosynovium. A cohort of similar patients exists that do not develop abnormal electrophysiologic changes [26]. Manual workers, especially women, have been severely afflicted. Repetitive forceful motion has often been implicated.

A growing body of evidence indicates that the common final pathway for the development of carpal tunnel syndrome is increased interstitial fluid pressure within the carpal canal and the median nerve, owing to microcirculatory venous stasis within a confined space [20, 25, 47, 50]. Experimental studies suggest that the changes in carpal tunnel syndrome follow a dose response curve in relation to the amount and duration of the interstitial fluid pressure and may be reversible up to a point, with physical therapy or surgical decompression [26]. Numerous intrinsic, extrinsic, or "idiopathic" factors may individually or collectively cause or contribute to this increased pressure [20]. Anatomic, pathophysiologic, biochemical, and histologic components of CTS integrate to explain and characterize this phenomenon.

Anatomic Factors

The carpal tunnel may function as a confining space [4]. Patients developing carpal tunnel syndrome tend to have smaller than normal carpal canals [7, 15, 40]. The ratio of the contents of the carpal tunnel to its volume diminishes as the wrist becomes smaller [6]. This may explain in part the increased prevalence of carpal tunnel syndrome seen in women as compared to men. Normal, and especially hypertrophic, lumbrical muscles that may develop particularly in manual workers, further diminish carpal tunnel volume with finger flexion [5]. Anomalous muscles may similarly cause encroachment within the carpal canal.

Pathophysiologic Factors

The cross-sectional area of the carpal tunnel diminishes with progressive wrist flexion or extension, while interstitial pressure increases [10, 13, 20, 56]. Repetitive forceful gripping and wrist motion may increase carpal canal pressure [2, 52, 54]. Externally applied pressure or vibration to the palm of the hand increases carpal tunnel pressure [22]. These forms of mechanical pressure may lead to venous stasis in the carpal canal, which in turn may lead to endothelial cell ischemia at the capillary level. Increased capillary permeability and fluid extravasation into the carpal canal follow. Persistent edema and increased interstitial pressure eventually lead to decreased axonal transport and intraneural blood flow followed by fibroblastic activity and scar formation in and about the nerve [24–27, 38].

Meyer reported that degenerative changes in ischemic loose connective tissue with ample access to fluid perpetuated additional swelling because of the altered tissue glycosaminoglycan and hyaluronan content. He noted that the tendency of loose connective tissue to expand under normal conditions is countered by collagen and microfibrillar networks restraint of expansion of hyaluronan. During periods of ischemia and reperfusion, there is a negative interstitial fluid pressure, suggesting that the tensile forces exerted on the tenosynovium are reduced, thus augmenting the diffusion of fluid into the tenosynovium. Sud et al. confirmed that fluid diffusion occurs at a faster rate and in higher volume in the tenosynovium harvested from "idiopathic" carpal tunnel patients than in that harvested from normal tenosynovium [49].

Progressive tenosynovial edema tends to compress the structures within the carpal canal. While the tendons within the carpal tunnel are firm and resistant to ischemic changes, the median nerve is soft, pliable, and vulnerable to pressure. Similar concurrent primary ischemia, edema, and fibrosis may occur in the connective tissue components of the median nerve. The ischemia and edema produced by this phenomenon promotes fibroplasias, causing destruction and replacement of the normal epineurium with scar tissue. Extraneural and, later, intraneural median nerve blood flow, axonal transport, and conductivity are progressively compromised in relation to the magnitude and duration of interstitial fluid pressure elevation [27, 38, 47, 48, 50]. Nerve deformity (flattening and hourglass deformity) and axonal damage may occur. Nerve excursion is decreased [26].

Biochemical Factors

An expanding body of evidence supports the contention that ischemic and oxidative cellular damage and biochemical changes mediate the occurrence of "idiopathic" carpal tunnel syndrome.

Reactive Oxygen Intermediates (ROIs)

Experimental and clinical evidence now suggests that ROIs are bioactive molecules in both physiological and pathological conditions [41]. The production of aldehyde compounds such as malondialdehyde (MDA) at very low and nontoxic concentrations has been shown to modulate and affect several cell functions including signal transduction, gene expression, and cell proliferation.

Intermittent local ischemia and reperfusion during periods of recovery can cause oxidative cellular and tissue injuries [51, 55]. Reactive oxygen intermediates (ROI) and other pro-oxidant agents elicit in vivo and in vitro oxidative decomposition of omega-3 and omega-6 polyunsaturated fatty acids of membrane phospholipids (i.e., lipid peroxidation). This leads to the formation of a complex mixture of aldehyde end products, including malondialdehyde (MDA), 4-hydroxy-2,3-nonenal (HNE), and other 4-hydroxy-2, 3-alkenals (HAKs) of different chain length. These aldehyde molecules are the ultimate mediators of the toxic cellular effects elicited by oxidative stress. With continued oxidative stress, the human body's normal antioxidant defensive system becomes overwhelmed and cellular injury ensues. Myelinated nerves, being a rich source of lipids, are a predominant target for free radical-mediated lipid peroxidation and they are more severely affected by compression than are nonmyelinated fibers [27, 38].

MDA in excessive quantities has long been recognized as a reliable marker in cellular reperfusion damage caused by lipid peroxidation. ROI damage has been reported in rat peripheral nerve injuries following acute compression [45]. Serum and tenosynovial MDA levels from carpal tunnel patients are elevated in comparison with control tissue [11] (Tables 6.1, 6.2, Figs. 6.1, 6.2).

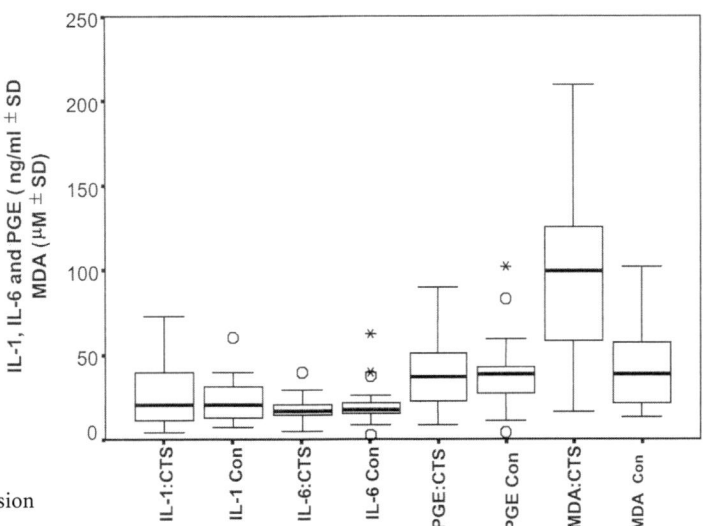

Fig. 6.1. Results of serum analysis in control and "idiopathic" carpal tunnel patients (with permission from [11])

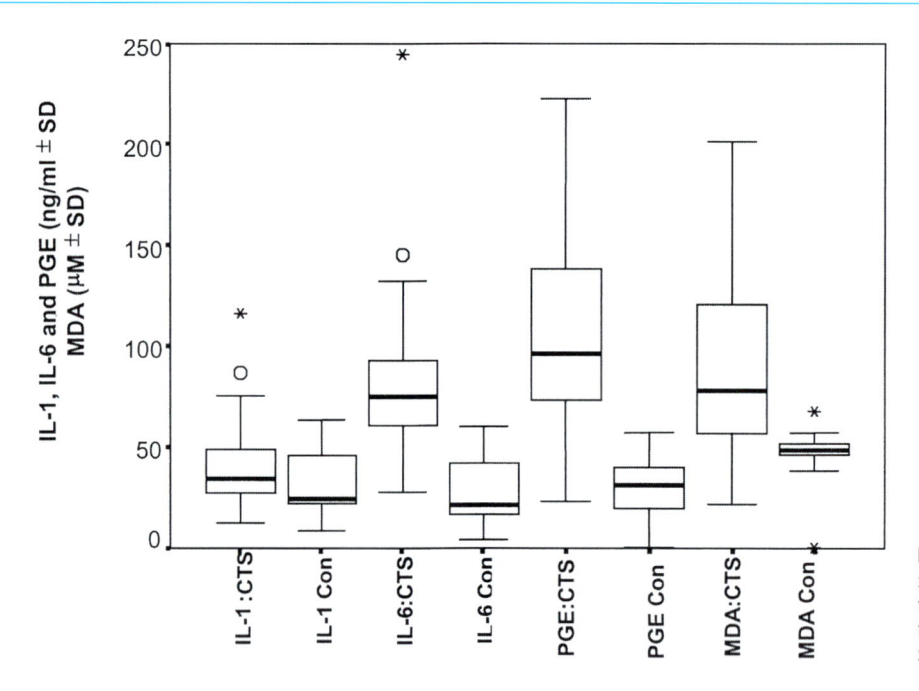

Fig. 6.2. Results of flexor tenosynovial analysis in control and "idiopathic" carpal tunnel patients (with permission from [11])

Table 6.1. Serum analysis quartiles and Mann-Whitney p values for comparing CTS patients and controls

Response	CTS†	Controls	p values
IL-1	20 (11, 40)	20 (13, 33)	0.84
IL-6	17 (14, 21)	17 (15, 21)	0.55
PGE	37 (23, 52)	38 (27, 45)	0.73
MDA	99 (58, 127)	39 (19, 63)	≤0.001

† Median (25th, 75th percentiles)

Table 6.2. Tenosynovium analysis quartiles and Mann-Whitney p values for comparing CTS patients and controls

Response	CTS*	Controls	p values
IL-1	34 (27, 52)	24 (21, 52)	0.26
IL-6	75 (59, 95)	21 (14, 48)	≤0.001
PGE	96 (71, 139)	31 (18, 41)	≤0.001
MDA	78 (57, 123)	48 (45, 53)	≤0.001

* Median (25th, 75th percentiles)

Prostaglandin E$_2$

Cellular ischemia and injury initiate the metabolism of arachidonic acid into cyclooxygenase products such as prostaglandin E$_2$. Prostaglandin E$_2$ is a potent vasodilator known to increase the sensitivity of nerve endings to chemical and mechanical stimuli and thus may contribute to the pain experienced by CTS patients [18, 42]. Recent studies by Berg et al. have shown that prostaglandin (PGE) may cause an increased negativity of interstitial fluid pressure creating a rapid rise in edema formation, contributing to impaired tissue function [1].

The quantity of PGE$_2$ in the tenosynovium of CTS patients has been reported as nearly four times that of controls ($p<0.001$) [11]. In contrast, there is no reported difference in the serum level of PGE$_2$ in these two groups (Tables 6.1, 6.2, Figs. 6.1, 6.2). This disparity in regional versus systemic prostaglandin production may be explained by the fact that these compounds are sustained locally, but are rapidly metabolized systemically.

Cytokines

Many different cell types can produce cytokines both intrinsically and as a result of stimulation with various agents. Cytokines are powerful mediators of cellular homeostasis and may act systemically as hormones after local production [8].

Interleukin-6 (IL-6)

IL-6 stimulates the production of acute phase proteins and was initially described in terms of its activities in the immune system and as a component of inflammatory processes. IL-6 is now known to be a multifunctional cytokine that is produced by and acts upon many cell types, e.g., fibroblasts and neurons and has pleiotropic effect, including modulation of cellular proliferation, differentiation, and maturation; wound healing; angiogenesis; cellular motility; pain sensitivity; certain carcinoma cell lines; and other cellular metabolic activities [3, 36, 42].

IL-6 plays an essential role in the development, differentiation, regeneration, and degeneration of neurons in the peripheral and central nervous system, but is normally undetectable [21, 34]. Cellular damage created by synovial and neural ischemia can also contribute to the production of cytokines [30]. IL-6 is responsible for changes in neuronal peptides that are associated with constriction-type nerve injuries [35]. Chronic compression of the nerve in animal models produces substantial detectable IL-6 in some motor and sensory neurons and neural connective tissue.

IL-6 induces the proliferation of synovial fibroblasts in the presence of soluble IL-6 receptors [32]. Serum levels of IL-6 are not statistically different between CTS patients and controls, although tenosynovial levels of IL-6 were three times higher in the carpal tunnel group ($p<.001$) [11]. (Tables 6.1, 6.2, Figs. 6.1, 6.2) These data suggest that IL-6 may play a local role in the pathophysiologic process of carpal tunnel syndrome.

Interleukin-1 (IL-1)

IL-1 is produced primarily by macrophages and is associated with the activation of T-cells as well as with induction of growth factors and inflammatory mediators [9]. Serum and flexor tenosynovial analyses have shown no difference in the levels of IL-1 between CTS patients and controls [11]. (Tables 6.1, 6.2, Figs. 6.1, 6.2)

Histologic Factors

Most cases of idiopathic CTS have in common an obvious cloudy white, nontransparent, fibrous hypertrophy of the synovium of the flexor tendons [12]. Biochemical changes are consistent with the clinical and histopathological picture seen in most "idiopathic" carpal tunnel patients. Histologic studies of the tenosynovium from "idiopathic" carpal tunnel patients have revealed it to be typical of connective tissue undergoing degeneration under repeated mechanical stress [19, 46]. There are relatively few inflammatory cells [12, 19, 23, 46]. "Idiopathic" carpal tunnel syndrome appears an "-osis" rather than an "-itis."

All of the steps of the mechanism for this fibrosis have not been elucidated, but increased levels of free oxygen radicals, PGE_2, and IL-6 probably contribute to this phenomenon. Each of these substances has been associated with stimulating tissue fibrogenesis [18, 30, 44]. Hematoxylin and eosin staining of the tenosynovium of "idiopathic" carpal tunnel patients has recently reconfirmed the earlier observations of noninflammatory edema and hyperplasia of the flexor tenosynovium along with angiogenesis [11] (Fig. 6.3a, b).

Angiogenesis is a multistep process in which many growth factors and cytokines have essential roles. Two types of angiogenesis-promoting agents have been characterized: (1) those that indirectly stimulate angiogenesis [e.g., tumor necrosis factor (TNF-α and transforming growth factor beta (TGFβ], and (2) those that act as direct angiogenic factors, [e.g., acidic and basic fibroblast growth factors (aFGF and bFGF), vascular endothelial growth factor (VEGF), and more recently IL-6].

Immunohistochemical staining clearly shows the presence of IL-6 in the endothelial cells around the newly formed vessels in the synovium of "idiopathic" carpal tunnel patients as compared to the synovium of control patients (Fig. 6.4a, b). When this tissue was stained for IL-1 and IL-6 by immunohistochemical techniques, the increased IL-6 production was localized to the perivascular regions of the synovial tissue, suggesting that one site of IL-6 production or activity is in the endothelial cells that have been damaged by tissue ischemia. Ischemic connective tissue components of the nerve may also secrete elevated levels of MDA, PGE_2, and IL-6, but this has not yet been proven.

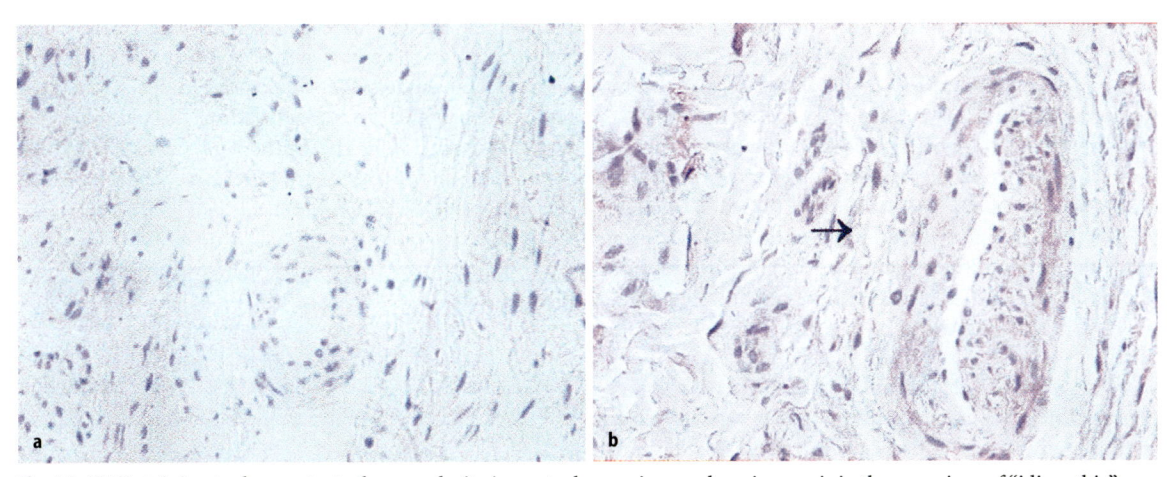

Fig. 6.3. H&E staining to demonstrate the vascularity in control synovium and angiogenesis in the synovium of "idiopathic" carpal tunnel patients (with permission from [11])

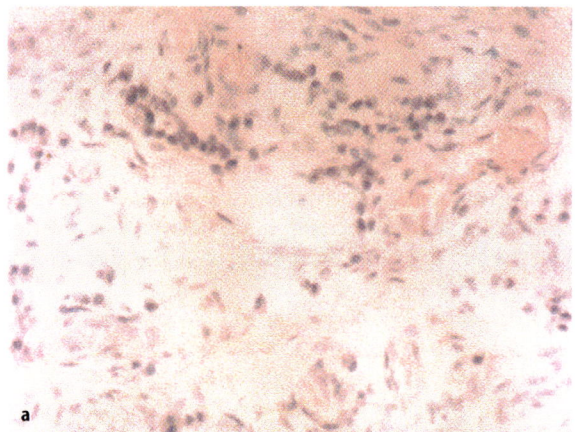

Fig. 6.4. Immunohistochemical staining to demonstrate the difference in IL-6 concentration in control tenosynovium and the tenosynovium from "idiopathic" carpal tunnel patients (250×) (with permission from [11])

Discussion

CTS is the most frequently encountered peripheral compressive neuropathy [39]. Classically, this condition was found to occur predominantly in middle-aged females and manifested itself initially with nocturnal pain and paresthesias along the sensory distribution of the median nerve [29, 43]. Over the last decade, there has been a dramatic change in the patient population. Young industrial workers of either sex, whose work involves repetitive motion, are now presenting with the signs and symptoms of carpal tunnel syndrome. These patients comprise a large subset of the group of afflictions popularly known as "cumulative trauma disorders" [17, 28].

In the "cumulative trauma disorder" population, CTS symptoms may not always be substantiated by objective findings and frequently persist despite well-established treatment methods [16, 26]. This has led many hand surgeons to argue that the majority of these patients are frauds or conscious malingerers. No data exist to support this concept, however, and the estimated incidence of true fraud is less than 5% [33]. Whether this exponential increase in the prevalence of CTS is owing to psychosocioeconomic issues or physiologic processes has been the subject of much debate [17, 28]. What is generally agreed upon is that despite a greater understanding of the effects of compression on nerves, very little has been known about the pathophysiologic mechanisms in idiopathic CTS until recently [20].

Discussion of the pathophysiology of compressive neuropathies begins by understanding the ischemic changes within the nerve caused by mechanical compression. These disturbances in intraneural blood and oxygen flow in first the perineural, and later the intraneural, regions of the nerve lead to irregularities in axonal transport and fibrosis of the nerve tissue itself. The result is abnormal impulse generation, progressive conduction delay, and eventually axonal damage [24–27, 38, 47, 48, 50]. Clinically this presents as pain, paresthesias, decreased sensation, and weakness [29, 43].

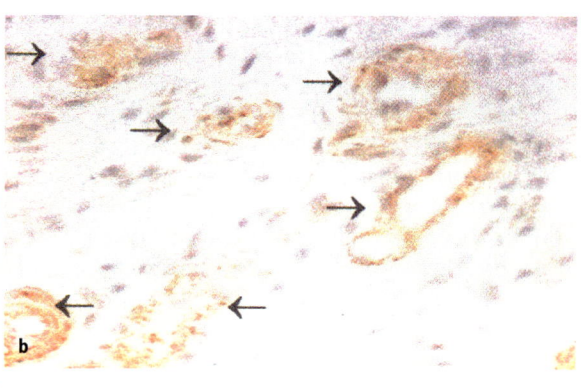

Intermittent reperfusion of cellular tissue during periods of recovery from ischemia prior to and immediately after carpal tunnel release produces free oxygen radicals. Alternating compression and perfusion may occur, particularly in repetitive function cumulative trauma disorders. With continued oxidative stress the human body's normal antioxidant defensive system becomes overwhelmed and cellular injury ensues. There may be a secondary neurogenic response as well. Tissue injury and responses may occur in both the tenosynovium and the median nerve.

Data indicates that biochemical mediators that include free oxygen radicals, PGE_2, and IL-6 may ultimately be involved in the pathophysiology of idiopathic CTS. Currently, it is not known how these various biologic factors influence each other to produce the tenosynovial hyperplasia that may cause, contribute to, or perpetuate compression of the median nerve in the carpal tunnel, but the data suggest an interrelationship that produces a vicious cycle of events resulting in pathological destruction of the tissue. This link may prove to be critical in understanding the pathogenesis associated with both the initial and persistent symptoms seen in untreated, nonoperatively treated, and surgically treated CTS patients.

References

1. Berg A, Ekwall AK, Rubin K et al. (1998) Effect of PGE1, PGI2, and PGF2 alpha analogs on collagen gel compaction in vitro and interstitial pressure in vivo. Am J Physiol 274: 663–671
2. Braun RM, Davidson K, Doehr MA (1989) Provocative testing in the diagnosis of dynamic carpal tunnel syndrome. J Hand Surg 14A: 195–197

3. Castell JV, Gomez-Lechon MJ, Hirano DM et al. (1987) Recombinant human interleukin-6 (IL-6/BSF-2/HSF) regulates the synthesis of acute phase protein in human hepatocytes. FEBS Letter 232: 347–349
4. Cobb TK, Dalley BK, Posteraro RH, Lewis RL (1992) The carpal tunnel as a compartment: An anatomic perspective. Orthop Rev 21: 451–453
5. Cobb TK, An K-N, Cooney WP, Berger RA (1994) Lumbrical muscle incursion into the carpal tunnel during finger flexion. J Hand Surg 19A: 434–438
6. Cobb TK, Bond JR, Cooney WP, Metcalf BJ (1997) Assessment of the ratio of carpal tunnel contents to carpal tunnel volume in patients with carpal tunnel syndrome. J Hand Surg 22A: 635–639
7. Dekel S, Papaioannou T, Rushworth G (1980) Idiopathic carpal tunnel syndrome caused by carpal stenosis. Br Med J [Clin Res]; 280: 1297–1301
8. DiGiovine FS, Mee JB, Duff GW (1996) Immunoregulatory cytokines. In: Henderson BH (ed) Therapeutic modulation of cytokines. CRC Press, New York, pp 37–65
9. Dinarello CA Interleukin-1 and its biologically related cytokines (1989) In: Dixon FJ (ed) Advances in immunology. Academic Press, San Diego, pp 153–159
10. Ditmars Jr DM, Houin HP (1986) Carpal tunnel syndrome. Hand Clin 2: 525–532
11. Freeland AE, Tucci MA, Barbieri RA et al. (2002) Biochemical evaluation of serum and flexor tenosynovium in carpal tunnel syndrome. Microsurgery 22: 378–385
12. Fuchs PC, Nathan PA, Myers LD (1991) Synovial histology in carpal tunnel syndrome. J Hand Surg 16A: 753–758
13. Gelberman RH, Hergenroeder PT, Hargens AR et al. (1981) The carpal tunnel syndrome. A study of carpal tunnel pressures. J Bone Joint Surg 63A: 380–383
14. Gelberman RH, Pfeffer GB, Galbraith RT et al. (1987) Results of treatment of severe carpal tunnel syndrome without internal neurolysis of the median nerve. J Bone Joint Surg 69A: 896–903
15. Gelmers HJ (1981) Primary carpal tunnel stenosis as a cause of entrapment of the median nerve. Acta Neurochir 55:317–320
16. Hadler NM (1990) Cumulative trauma disorders: An iatrogenic concept. J Occup Med 32: 28–41
17. Hadler NM (1997) Repetitive upper extremity motions in the workplace are not hazardous. J Hand Surg 22A: 19–29
18. Hall AK, Behrman HR (1982) Prostaglandin: Biosynthesis, metabolism and mechanism of cellular action. In: Lee JB (ed) Prostaglandin Elsevier, New York, pp 1–38
19. Kerr CD, Sybert DR, Albarracin NS (1992) An analysis of the flexor synovium in idiopathic carpal tunnel syndrome: Report of 625 cases. J Hand Surg 17A: 1028–1030
20. Kerwin G, Williams CS, Seiler JG (1996) The pathophysiology of carpal tunnel syndrome. Hand Clin 12: 243–251
21. Kiefer R, Lindholm D, Kreutzberg GW (1993) Interleukin-6 and transforming growth factor-beta 1 mRNAs are induced in rat facial nucleus following motor neuron axonotomy. Eur J Neurosci 5: 775–781
22. Lin R, Lin E, Engle J, Bobis JJ (1983) Histomechanical aspects of carpal tunnel syndrome. Hand 15: 395–399
23. Lluch AL (1992) Thickening of the synovial flexor tendons: Cause or consequence of carpal tunnel syndrome? J Hand Surg 17B: 209–212
24. Lundborg G, Myers R, Powell H (1983) Nerve compression injury and increased endoneural fluid pressure: A miniature compartment syndrome. J Neurol Neurosurg Psychiatry 46: 1119–1124
25. Lundborg G, Dahlin LB (1996) Anatomy, function, and pathophysiology of peripheral nerves and nerve compression. Hand Clin 12: 185–193
26. Mackinnon SE. (2002) Pathophysiology of nerve compression. Hand Clin 18: 231–241
27. Mackinnon SE, Dellon AL, Hudson AR, Hunter DA (1984) Chronic nerve compression – an experimental model in the rat. Ann Plast Surg 13: 112–120
28. MacKinnon SE, Novak CB (1997) Repetitive strain in the workplace. J Hand Surg 22A: 2–18
29. Mackinnon SE, Novak CB, Landau WM (2000) Clinical diagnosis of carpal tunnel syndrome. JAMA 284: 1924–1926
30. Meager A (1986) Introduction to cytokines and their physiology. In: Henderson BH (ed) Therapeutic modulation of cytokines. CRC Press, New York, pp 3–36
31. Meyer FA (1983) Macromolecular basis of globular protein exclusion and of swelling pressure in loose connective tissue (umbilical cord). (1983) Biochim Biophys Acta 22:388–399
32. Mihara M, Moriya Y, Kishimoto T, Ohsugi Y (1995) Interleukin-6 (IL-6) induces the proliferation of synovial fibroblastic cells in the presence of soluble IL-6 receptors. Brit J Rheum 34: 321–325
33. Millender LH, Conlon M (1996) An approach to work-related disorders of the upper extremity. JAAOS 4: 134–142
34. Murphy PG, Grondin J, Altares M, Richardson PM (1995) Induction of interleukin-6 in axonomized sensory neurons. J Neurosci 15: 5130–5138
35. Murphy PG, Ramer MS, Borthwick L et al. (1999) Endogenous interleukin-6 contributes to hypersensitivity to cutaneous stimuli and changes neuropeptides associated with chronic nerve constriction in mice. Eur J Neurosci. 11: 2243–2253
36. Nijsten NWN, DeGroot ER, Ten Duis HJ et al. (1987) Serum levels of interleukin 6 and acute phase responses. Lancet 17: 921–923
37. North ER, Kaul MP (1996) Compression neuropathies: Median. In: Peimer CA (ed) Surgery of the hand and upper extremity. McGraw-Hill, New York, pp 1307–1336
38. O'Brien JP, Mackinnon SE, MacLean AP et al. (1987) A model of chronic nerve compression in the rat. Ann Plast Surg 19: 430–435
39. Palmer DH, Hanrahan LP (1995) Social and economic costs of carpal tunnel surgery. AAOS Instructional Course Lectures 44: 167–172
40. Papaioannou T, Rushworth G, Atar D, Cekel S (1992) Carpal canal stenosis in men with idiopathic carpal tunnel syndrome. Clin Orthop 285:210–213
41. Parola RG, Dianzani MU (1999) 4-hydroxy-2,3 alkenals as molecular mediators of oxidative stress in the pathogenesis of liver necrosis. Int J Mol Med 4: 425–432
42. Pettipher ER (1996) Cytokines in inflammation: An overview. In: Henderson BH (ed) Therapeutic modulation of cytokines. CRC Press, New York, pp 67–80
43. Phalen GS (1966) The carpal tunnel syndrome: Seventeen years' experience in diagnosis and treatment of six hundred fifty-four hands. J Bone Joint Surg 48A: 211–228
44. Poli G, Parola M (1997) Oxidative damage and fibrogenesis. Free Radical Biol Med 22: 287–305
45. Ress AM, Babovic, Angel MF et al. (1995) Free radical damage in acute nerve compression. Ann Plast Surg 34: 388–395
46. Schuind F, Ventura M, Pastels JL (1990) Idiopathic carpal tunnel syndrome: Histologic study of flexor tendon synovium. J Hand Surg 15A: 497–503
47. Seiler JG, Milek MA, Carpenter GK, Swiontkowski MF (1989) Intraoperative assessment of median nerve blood flow during carpal tunnel release with laser Doppler flowmetry. J Hand Surg 14A: 986–991
48. Slater RR, Bynum DK (1993) Diagnosis and treatment of carpal tunnel syndrome. Orthop Rev 22: 1095–1105

49. Sud V, Tucci MA, Freeland AE et al. (2002) Absorptive properties of synovium harvested from the carpal tunnel. Microsurgery 22: 316–319
50. Sunderland S (1976) The nerve lesion in the carpal tunnel syndrome. J Neurol Neurosurg Psychiatry 39: 615–626
51. Suzuki YJ, Forman HJ, Sevanian A (1997) Oxidants as stimulators of signal transduction. Free Radical Biol Med 22: 269–285
52. Szabo RM, Chidgey LK (1989) Stress carpal tunnel pressures in patients with carpal tunnel syndrome and normal patients. J Hand Surg 14: 624–627
53. Szabo RM, Gelberman RH (1997) The pathophysiology of nerve entrapment syndromes. J Hand Surg 12A: 880–884
54. Szabo RM, Madison M (1992) Carpal tunnel syndrome. Orthop Clin North Am 23: 103–109
55. Yagi K. (1987) Lipid peroxides and human diseases. Chemistry & Physics of Lipids 45: 337–351
56. Yoshioka S, Okuda Y, Tamai K, Koda Y (1993) Changes in carpal tunnel shape during wrist joint motion: MRI evaluation of normal volunteers. J Hand Surg 18B: 620–623

Carpal Canal Pressure Measurements: Literature Review and Clinical Implications

R. Luchetti, R. Schoenhuber

Initial Studies

The first evaluative reviews regarding the use of a measurement system for determining carpal tunnel pressure was introduced by Brain et al. in 1947 [1]. The second evaluative review appeared in the medical literature 10 years later and was published by Tanzer [2]. Sophisticated and nondangerous instrumentation was not available at that time in order to measure actual carpal tunnel pressure in live subjects. Both authors used rudimentary methods (Foley no. 14 catheter connected to a manometer) and measured cadavers' carpal tunnel pressure by studying the pressure measurements obtained when the wrist was placed in various postures: flexion and above all extension. In Brain's studies, wrist extension pressure was three times that obtained in flexion (Table 7.1). These same results were then reconfirmed by Tanzer, who further demonstrated that the carpal pressure was higher in the more proximal part of the carpal canal, with the wrist flexed, rather than extended, whereas, the pressure was higher in the distal part of the canal only when the wrist was extended. Based on anatomo-surgical landmarks, where the median nerve widens immediately proximally to the proximal carpal canal margins, both Brain and Tanzer concluded that "...the wrist produces more abnormal symptoms when flexed in respect to when it is extended, even if the experimental studies have demonstrated that *an increase in carpal pressure occurs in wrist extension*."

About 20 years later, Smith et al. [3], substituted the median nerve in the carpal canals of cadaver with a plastic cylindrical tube that was filled with water and connected to a pressure measurement transducer, demonstrating that during wrist extension the pressure in the carpal canal underwent an overall increase. This study is of particular importance since it demonstrated that the second and third flexor tendons contributed to an increase in median nerve compression when the wrist was flexed. It has been proposed, based on these findings, that the Phalen test be modified: this "sensibility maneuver" that is a part of the test, foresees that the patient performs a three-finger pinch using the thumb, second, and third fingers with the wrist flexed in a Phalen position for 1–2 min.

Clinical Studies

Bauman et al. in 1981 [4], performed the first study that was done on live subjects that presented with acute symptoms for median nerve compression at the wrist level (Table 7.2). Baumann used a wick catheter to demonstrate the importance of CTS canal pressure during its acute phase, after a wrist fracture.

Clinical implications such as an acute increase in carpal canal pressure had already been hypothesized Abbott et al. in 1933 [5]. Abbott demonstrated that liquid (Berlin blue and Lipiodol) injected into the median nerve sheath, accumulated at the proximal part of the canal if the wrist was positioned in maximum flexion. He upheld that this liquid block was due to an increase in pressure under the ligament and was provoked by the position of wrist flexion. He took these findings one step further and discussed the risk of plaster casting a wrist in a Cotton-Loder position (wrist flexed) after a distal epiphysis radial fractures since it most likely could cause a median nerve injury due to a significant increase in pressure below the proximal border of the flexor retinaculum provoking compression. Some years later, other studies appeared in the medical literature regarding intracanal pressure in fractured wrists. Two interesting studies were done by Kongsholm and Olerud [6] and Mack et al. [7] regarding carpal canal pressure behavior after a Colles type wrist fracture. Both studies found that the canal pressure was truly high with the wrist in a rest position, reaching as much as

Table 7.1. Studies performed on cadavers

Authors	Year	Wrist position		
		Rest mm H$_2$O	Flexion mm H$_2$O	Extension mm H$_2$O
Brain et al.	1947	/	100	300
Tanzer	1959	/	High (proximal site)	Very high (proximal and distal)
Smith	1977	/	77	96

Table 7.2 Clinical studies of carpal tunnel pressure measurement performed on CTS patients and controls

		CTS patients				Controls		
		Wrist				Wrist		
Authors	Year	Rest	Flexion	Extension	Method	Rest	Flexion	Extension
Abbott	1933	Perfusion	Block	Block	Liquid injection	/	/	/
Bauman	1981	34	75	80	Wick catheter	2	42	43
Gelberman	1981	32	94	110	Wick catheter	3	31	30
Werner	1983	31	105	113	Slit catheter	/	/	/
Gelberman	1984	18	27	85	Wick catheter	/	/	/
Chaise	1984	25	90	100	Constant infusion	6	30	30
Kongsholm	1986	36	60	/	Wick catheter	6	15	/
Gellmann	1988	12	95	160	Wick catheter	8	42	200
Luchetti	1989	21	/	/	Constant infusion	13	/	/
Szabo	1989	5	37	50	Slit catheter	5	16	26
Rojviroj	1990	12	27	33	Slit catheter	4	9	13
Seradge	1995	44	98	119	Constant infusion	24	80	101
Luchetti	1998	14	60	84	Camino catheter	8	44	48

36 mmHg and 52 mmHg in some studies. The carpal canal is not anatomically localized to the level of a distal radius wrist fracture [8, 9] (Figs. 7.1, 7.2); the mechanism of the increase in pressure was not quite clear and was thought to be due to hemorrhaging or tissue edema that occurred within the carpal canal [6]. The introduction of an anesthetic liquid into the fracture site produced an increase in carpal canal pressure. Mack et al. [7], by using the appropriate pressure measurement system [4], confirmed the possibility of distinguishing acute median nerve compression by the contusion of the nerve itself after undergoing a trauma. In cases where the nerve was damaged from trauma, the endocanal pressure was not elevated. Sometimes, two phenomena coexist.

Gelberman et al. [10] utilized wick catheters to demonstrate that the endocanal pressure was higher in idiopathic CTS patients than in normal subjects. In neutral rest wrist postures, the average pressure that is registered in the patients' carpal canal is 32 mmHg. When the wrist is flexed to 90° the pressure reaches a value of 94 mmHg, but is 110 mmHg when the wrist is extended. This last data has not been well considered but it does reflect the results of the previous experimental studies. In a successive study, conducted by Gelberman et al. [11], it has been demonstrated that even with only 20° of wrist extension the carpal canal pressure has the tendency to be higher than that in the same degrees of wrist flexion. The pressure was measured at 40° of wrist flexion, but was not compared to the same degrees of

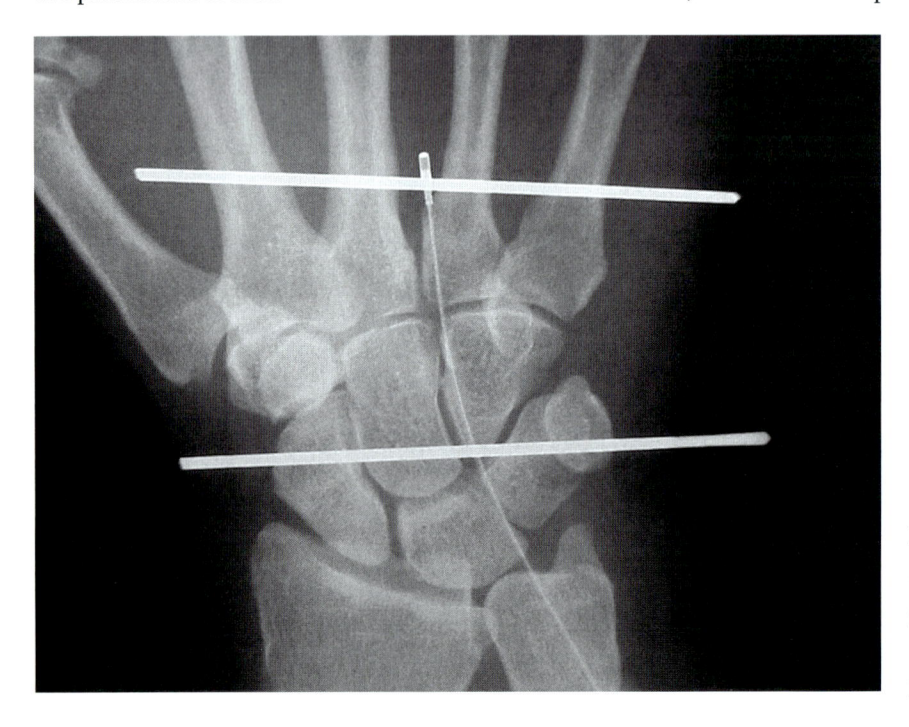

Fig. 7.1. AP view of x-ray of left wrist showing catheter into the carpal canal. Two K-wires were used as markers of proximal and distal borders of the carpal tunnel in comparison with the carpal bones

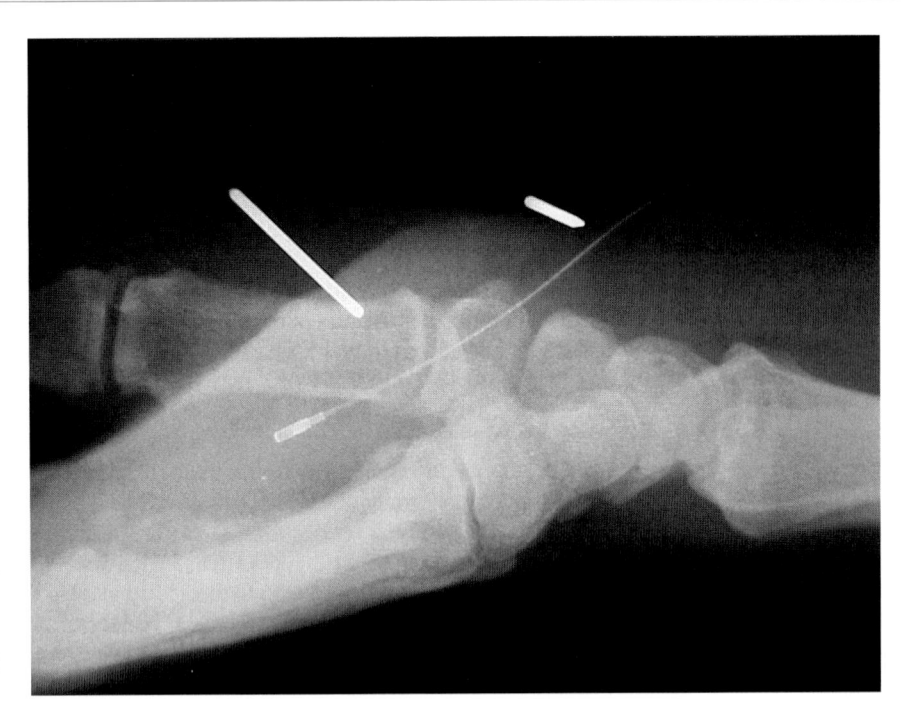

Fig. 7.2. Lateral view of x-ray of left wrist showing catheter into the carpal canal. The two K-wires used as superficial markers of proximal and distal borders of the carpal tunnel demonstrate the deep position of the catheter under the flexor retinaculum of the carpal canal

wrist extension. Therefore, the goal of this study was to verify the danger of a wrist flexion position on the median nerve when maintained in a plaster cast after reduction. The conclusion of this study was to ascertain that conservative treatment of a Colles fracture by reduction and immobilization in a plaster cast, in a position of wrist flexion and ulnar deviation (Cotton-Loder position), had the capacity to cause a compressive neuropathy of the median nerve at this level.

In successive years, other authors confirmed the presence of high carpal canal pressure in CTS patients. Werner et al. in 1983 [12] utilized continuous infusion techniques, obtaining similar results to that of Gelberman; the average resting pressure was 31 mmHg and increased to 105 mmHg with passive wrist extension, while reaching 75 mmHg in flexion. Carpal canal pressure modifications have also been evaluated when the fingers were either extended or flexed. With the fingers flexed and the wrist extended, the pressure reached a value of 113 mmHg, whereas, when the wrist was flexed the pressure rose to 60 mmHg.

Lundborg et al. [13, 14] have contributed very interesting studies on carpal canal pressure fluctuations in human volunteer patients. The studies demonstrated that there was a direct correlation between an increase in carpal canal pressure, nerve dysfunction, and clinical symptoms [13]. Even in this study, a wick catheter was used to measure carpal canal pressure. A pressure of 30 mmHg measured in the carpal canal was defined as pathologic, or better yet, "critical pressure level." This pressure level has the capacity to damage the median nerve over time, and is considered chronic (see Chap. 4 entitled Etiopathogenesis, Chap. 5 entitled Pathophysiology). A year later, Lundborg et al. [14] coined the term "miniature compartment syndrome" which defined the median nerve as having a similar behavior to that of a muscle compartment if under chronic compression. This data was supported by previous studies done by Low and Dyck [15] and Myers et al. [16], which demonstrated the perineurium "barrier" function.

Other alternative studies regarding carpal canal pressure determined that the internal pressure level is not always critical and does not always reach the values that have been reported by other authors, sufficient to damage nerve function. Luchetti et al. [17], used a constant infusion technique and were able to demonstrate that the average low pressure was 26 mmHg with respect to those reported in healthy subjects. These results were similar to those revealed by Szabo and Gelberman [18] and Rojviroj et al. [19], although different methods were used to obtain the carpal canal pressure data. It has been postulated that even in cases in which the intracanal pressure was lower than 30 mmHg and even if the pressure around the median nerve did not reach critical levels, it could produce an increase in intraneural pressure that could become higher over time [14–16].

Gellman et al. [20] evaluated carpal canal pressure behavior in paraplegic patients that suffered and those that did not suffer from CTS. The pressure was always higher in wrist extension than in any other wrist position.

Dynamic Evaluation

Dynamic studies have been used to evaluate carpal canal pressure behavior when the wrist and hand are placed under effort and to evaluate recovery time. Szabo and Gelberman [18] have followed these trials using a "slit catheter," an evaluation system without constant infusion, but due to the tip's shape it is less likely to occlude. This type of catheter is very useful for evaluating muscle compartment pressure under effort for both short and medium time periods. The intracanal pressure study in CTS patients has been based on a subdivision of three groups in relation to the severity of their pathology: initial, intermediate, and advanced stages, considering the clinical aspects and the electromyography. These patients, together with a control group, underwent repetitive wrist movements. The method was called "stress test." During the effort trial and in the recovery phase (return to a low pressure), the pressure was significantly higher in patients that were effected by CTS in the initial and intermediate phases with respect to the control group. This confirms that the carpal canal pressure had the same behavior as the muscle compartment. Instead, in the advanced cases, the pressure was not different than that of the control group. These findings confirm that the carpal canal should be considered a "functionally" closed compartment. Even if at rest the pressure was inferior to 30 mm Hg, the use of this test is valid for selecting those patients at risk for developing an occupational (CTS).

Parallel studies on nerve function have demonstrated that after a "stress test," CTS patients demonstrate positive clinical finding and negative conventional neurophysiological results. These findings demonstrate that there is a discrepancy in the sensibility of performing only a neurophysiological evaluation [18, 21]. This is an important finding that needs to be taken into consideration when determining which patients are at risk or are affected by CTS.

Centimetric Evaluation of Endocanal Pressure

The centimetric pressure measurement method in the carpal canal was first proposed by Luchetti et al. [17] by using both constant and continual infusion techniques (Figs. 7.3–7.6). The aim of this method was to verify the greatest level of nerve compression through distinguishing maximum pressure levels in the carpal canal and correlate them with previous neurophysiologic studies [22–24]. The resulting pressure was significantly higher in CTS patients with respect to control subjects, with the highest pressure level registered at about 2.5–3.5 cm distal to the wrist crease, corresponding to the area that lies just before or on the same level as the distal border of the carpal canal. However, the greatest pressure level was located in the carpal canal's distal area, while the pressure entity diminished as soon as the catheter was within reach of the proximal or distal canal aperture. When graphing out the pressure measurements taken from the areas inside the canal moving in a proximal-to-distal direction, the graph takes on a bell-shape curve. These findings correlate to those already documented by Cobb et al. [25] who demonstrated that the carpal canal is an open canal (Fig. 7.7).

Probably this phenomenon can be explained by the canal's form, which is narrow at its distal aspect and has already been demonstrated in anatomical studies [26] or by studies done using CAT or MRI scans [27–32]. The median nerve follows the anatomical conformation of the carpal canal deeper in an antero-posterior

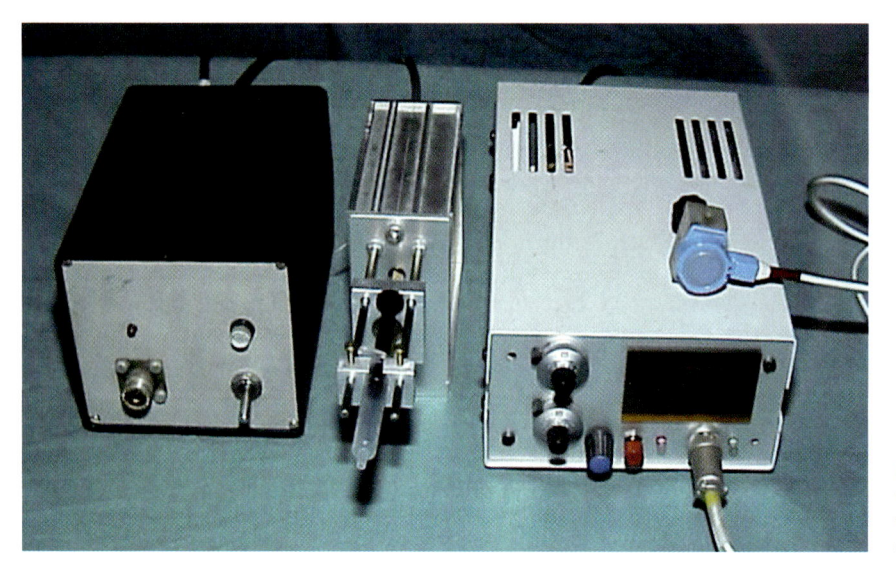

Fig. 7.3. Experimental device to measure the pressure into the carpal canal by using constant infusion technique

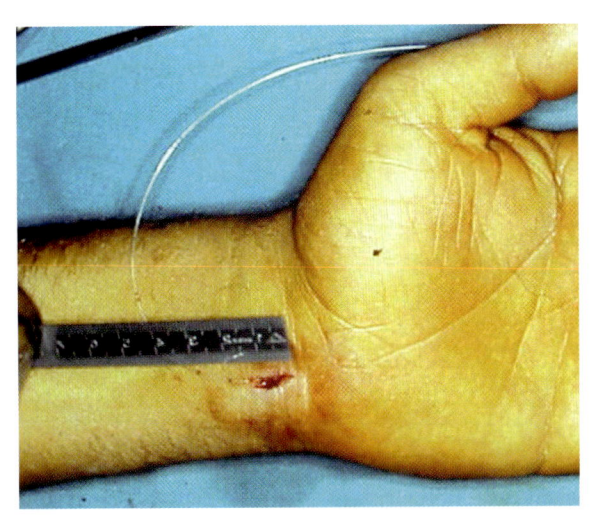

Fig. 7.4. Catheter introduced into the carpal canal through a wrist short incision proximally to the distal wrist crease in order to measure the pressure

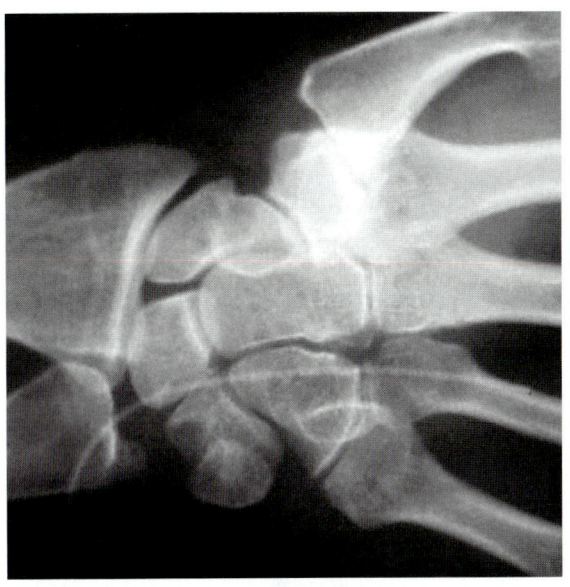

Fig. 7.5. X-ray of the wrist of the patient in Fig. 7.4 showing position of the catheter into the carpal canal

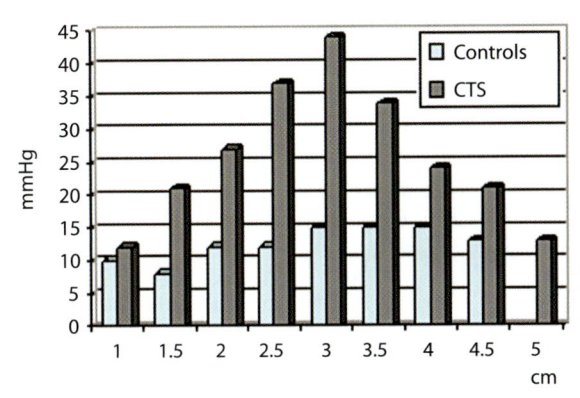

Fig. 7.6. Segmental evaluation of the carpal canal pressure. 0 cm corresponds to the distal wrist crease

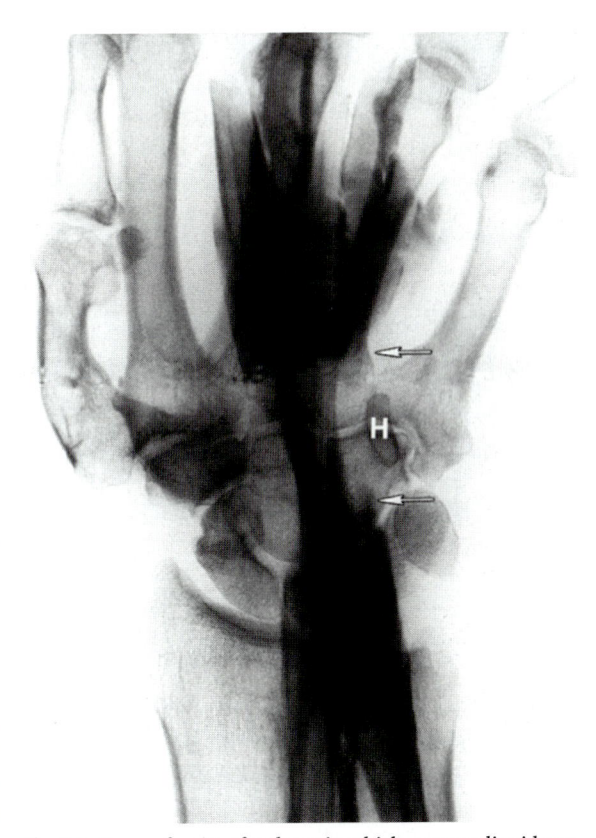

Fig. 7.7. X-ray of wrist of cadaver in which contrast liquid was introduced into the flexor tendons compartment proximal to the carpal canal. Contrast liquid depicts size, shape, dimension, and position of the carpal canal in comparison with the wrist carpal bones. *White arrows* show the proximal and distal level of the carpal canal. *H*: hook of hamate (Reproduced with permission from [25])

and proximal-distal sense with respect to the palmar cutaneous surface (Fig. 7.8). Therefore, the tract from the palm to the wrist is not straight and the nerve undergoes a slight angulation during wrist flexion and extension movements with successive compression. The depth of the canal influences the neuroelectric registration during neurophysiologic studies.

The neurophysiologic studies of Kimura [22], Brown and Yates [33], Luchetti et al. [23], and Nathan et al. [24] conducted on the median nerve at the wrist level using centimetric techniques (Figs. 7.9, 7.10) have confirmed that the nerve dysfunction is localized, with greater frequency, in the distal part of the canal, corresponding to the pressure results. If the carpal canal was actually closed or "functionally closed" we should observe a constant pressure level like that which occurs in muscle compartments of limbs [34, 35].

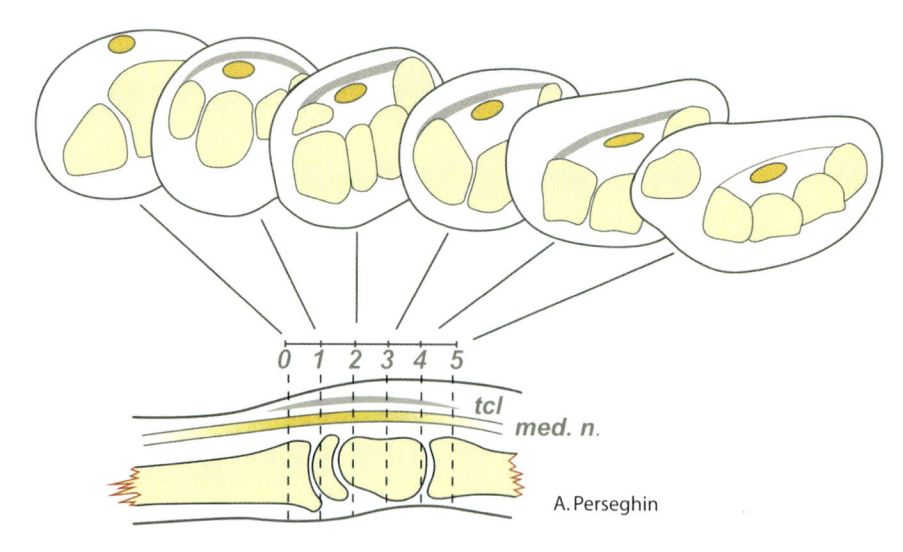

Fig. 7.8. Serial transverse sections of the wrist at the level of the carpal canal (from 0 to 5 cm) demonstrating the position of median nerve (*med.n.*) under the transverse carpal ligament (*tcl*)

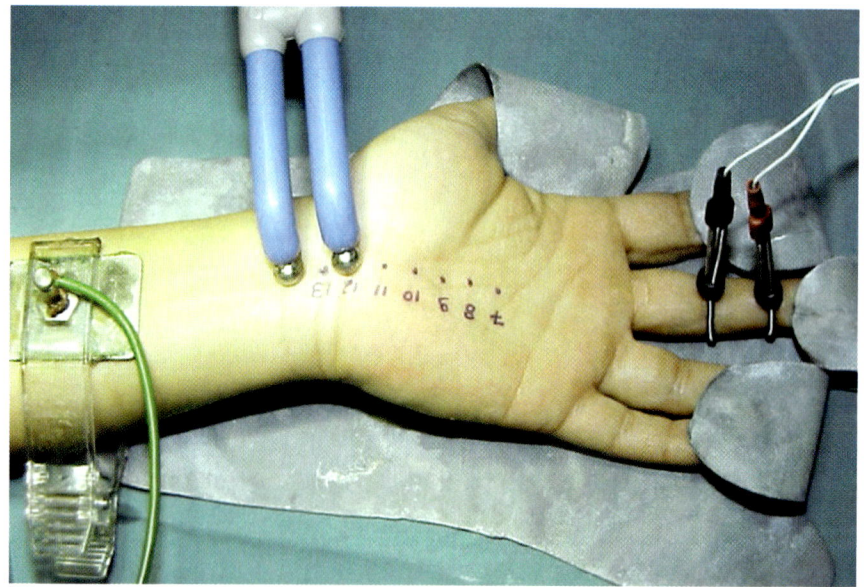

Fig. 7.9. Electrophysiological study of median nerve conduction through the carpal canal. Segmental electrical stimulation of the median nerve at the wrist is performed according to the inching technique (Kimura test): 0 cm level corresponds to the distal wrist crease

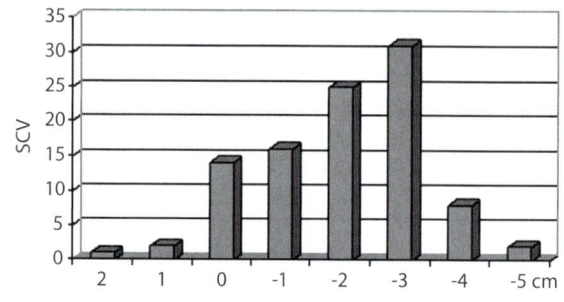

Fig. 7.10. Median nerve SCV at wrist by using the inching technique. 0 cm corresponds to the distal wrist crease

Further evolution of these studies is represented by comparative evaluation studies between internal canal pressure levels and intraoperative neurophysiologic evaluation of the median nerve at the wrist using centimetric techniques [36]. The pressure is prevalently increased at the level of the distal canal and in this same position, the median nerve's sensitive conduction velocity is slowed down. Overall, the comparison does not reach statistically significant values. Unfortunately, the evaluation method is not correct, containing two noncomparative variables. In addition, the neuroelectric study was done intraoperatively, on an already decompressed nerve, while the pressure evaluation was done preoperatively when the transverse carpal ligament still had its integrity and the nerve was still compressed. However, this study has supplied useful information about the immediate neuroelectric behavior of the median nerve as soon as it has been decompressed [37, 38]. A portion of the patients, who had the initial stages of severity, according to Lundborg, had an evident immediate recovery in sensitive conduction velocity as soon as the decompression was performed.

Endocanalar Pressure, Wrist Posturing Splints Used During Activities of Daily Living

Some authors have taken into account the various wrist positions and how they effect intracarpal pressure [10]. They have focused their studies on the development of functional wrist splints. These splints are usually integrated into the standard conservative CTS treatment protocol and the wrist is placed in a rest position. One should not forget that a prolonged immobilized wrist already afflicted by CTS can easily develop clinical symptoms.

Prefabricated wrist splints tend to position the wrist at 20° of extension. This position has been defined as a "functional wrist position" [39]. However, it has also been demonstrated that when the wrist is placed in extension there is a greater amount of intracanal pressure than when placed in flexion [10].

Luchetti et al. [40] conducted a study on CTS patients demonstrating that the application of a nighttime splint, which positioned the wrist at 20° of extension, increased intracanal pressure but did not produce results that were greater than those subjects who were not splinted, and in neither group did the results reach significant statistics. In the same study, it was found that the intracanal night-time pressure showed a slow increase and was higher than that which was measured at 6:00 in the morning. In a successive study, Weiss et al. [41] confirmed that by maintaining the wrist in slight extension (functional position) it was not adequate to reduce intracanal pressure. In addition, it has been demonstrated that by positioning the wrist in slight ulnar deviation, intracanal pressure is greater than that in radial deviation. This data should be utilized for fabricating wrist splints that can unintentionally cause an increase in carpal canal pressure.

With regard to the relationship between wrist angulation and intracanal pressure, Rempel et al. [42] demonstrated the effect of prono-supination and the use of splints. In their study, lower canal pressure was obtained when the wrist was at 45° of pronation. The wrist splint did not cause an increase in intracanal pressure as had been previously demonstrated in a study conducted by Luchetti et al. [40]. The same group [43] completed a follow-up study on carpal canal pressure when the fingers were placed at 0°, 45°, and 90° and in relationship to variable wrist postures (flexion-extension and radial /ulnar deviation). Even in this study, the pressure was higher when the wrist was in extension than when flexed. The pressure was also higher when the MFs were in a position of 0° with respect to 45° and 90° in all degrees of ulnar and radial deviation and wrist extension. These results are very important for understanding the effect of certain work activities that place specific pressure on the carpal tunnel and lead to CTS. In order to reduce the occurrence of manual-work-induced CTS, one must consider the findings from these studies and modify specific instruments and hand postures that provoke CTS. These findings also should be considered when indicating the type of wrist splint that should be specifically fabricated for individual patient wear, in order to reduce the effect of intracanal pressure. There are also many other interesting studies that one can find in the medical literature regarding wrist posture, functional manual activities and intracanal pressure.

Seradge et al. [44] used a continual infusion method and demonstrated that intracanal pressure was always significantly higher in CTS patients with respect to control subjects both at rest and during active maximum flexion or extension of the wrist. The study was conducted in typical work conditions in which the subject was asked to grasp and maintain an object in hand, perform isolated finger flexion against resistance, and make a closed fist. The pressure of the forearm flexor compartment was contemporaneously evaluated and the results were inferior with respect to the intracanal pressure in both the patients and control subjects. Even in the study conducted by Szabo and Gelberman [18], a rebound effect was not found, possibly due to the improper use of the catheter. They do not use a wick catheter in their studies and therefore they can be unreliable due to the obstruction of the catheter's point, which was found in a series of preliminary studies. It is better to use a catheter with three lateral holes, as has been proposed in the study by Luchetti et al. [17]. These conclusions should raise considerations regarding their eventual clinical applications: reduction of specific activities that require repetitive grasping, and/or wrist flexion and extension, sustaining heavy objects with the hands, isolated resistance of single digits (such as three-point pinch and typing). Short interruptions of repetitive wrist and hand manual labor should be suggested to the patient so they do not incur a constant increase in canal pressure. The recent proposal of a new fiber optic catheter [45, 46] (Fig. 7.11), with the possibility to directly register the pressure at the same point of its application (inching technique), has avoided the problems that are linked to the preceding measurement methods: occlusion, fragility, instability, and scarce rapidity of measurement. Luchetti et al. [47] repeated the same pressure centimetric studies along the median nerve tract within the carpal canal both at rest (wrist extension functional position of 15°) (Fig. 7.12), as well as passive wrist flexion and extension of 45° (Figs. 7.13, 7.14) in CTS patients and control subjects. When measuring the pressure during grasping activities, the wrist was placed in the same position parameters. The results obtained, and compared with the previous findings, indicated that the pressure was higher in the CTS patients than in the control subjects, higher in wrist extension than in flexion, but in patients with the wrist in

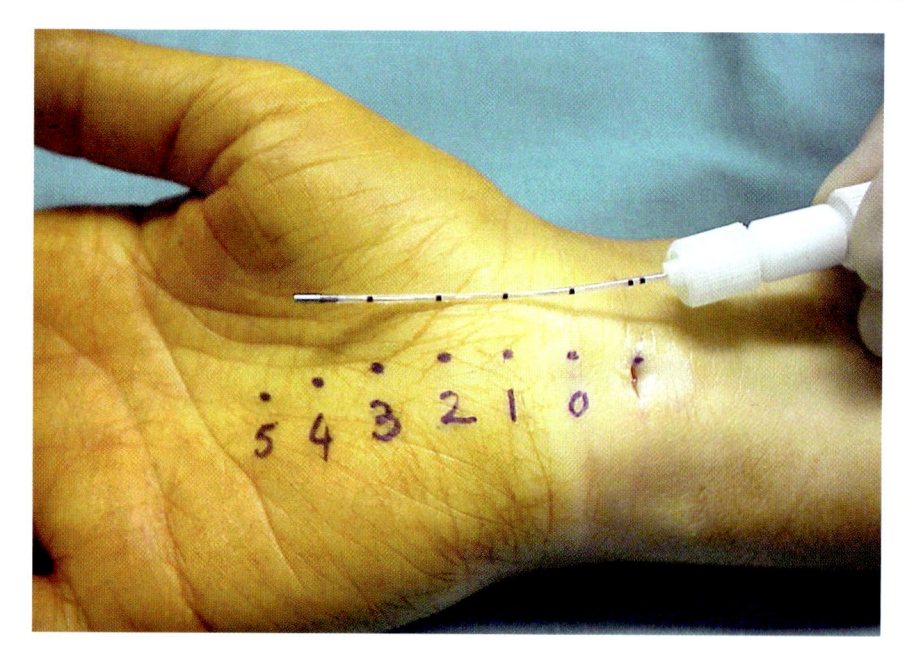

Fig. 7.11. Same patient as Fig. 7.9. Camino catheter for pressure measurement ready to be introduced into the carpal canal. Markers on the catheter ensure measuring the pressure along the canal at the same skin markers of the electrophysiological study: the 0 cm level corresponds to the distal wrist crease

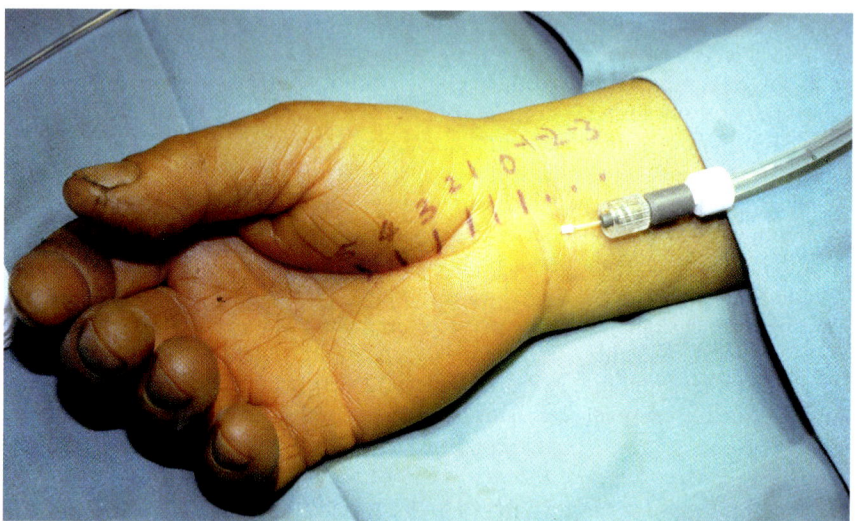

Fig. 7.12. Camino catheter introduced into the carpal canal starting 1 cm before the distal wrist crease

a rest position, rarely did the canal pressure values reach a critical level of 30 mm Hg, for each segment of the intracanal centimetric evaluation. With respect to other previous studies, the following has been found: (1) an elevated pressure registered at the central segment level and not in the carpal canal's distal tract; (2) a greater pressure with the wrist extended instead of in flexion, when the hand grasps; (3) an elevated pressure located distal to the carpal canal in both patients and control subjects and only in the wrist rest position.

The results of another scientific study that made a comparison between pressure values and median nerve latent sensitive fiber values inside the carpal canal in healthy subjects and those with CTS will be completed and published shortly. Thus far, the data obtained in relationship to the behavior of the canal pressure in CTS patients and in control subjects is reported in Fig. 7.15. It has been found that the CTS patients have a higher pressure value than the control subjects and their pressure increases in proportion to the severity of their disease. Finally, inside the canal, a pressure distribution has been distinguished and can be traced out as the shape of a bell curve with greater pressure points in the central segment and with the tendency to move towards the distal margin (revealed in advanced disease cases).

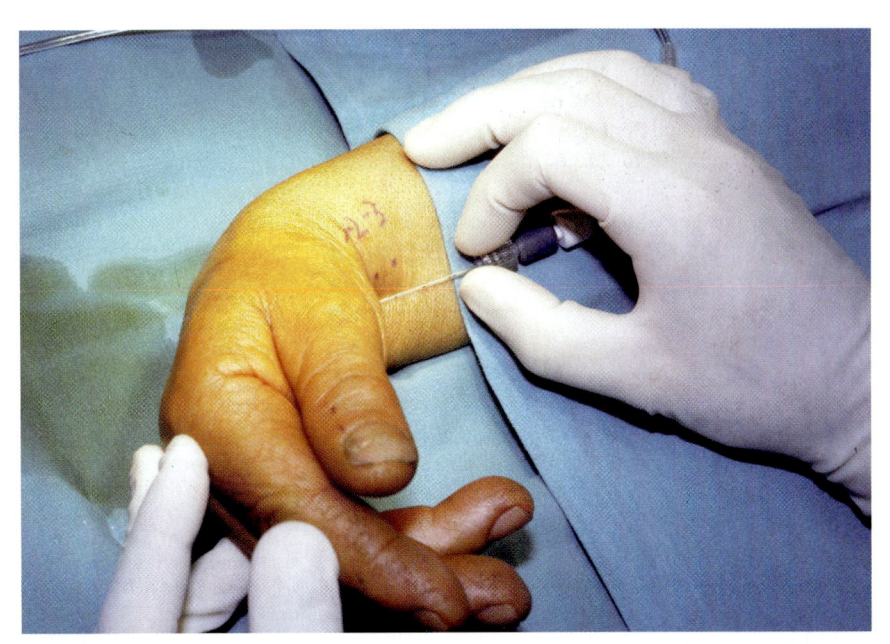

7 Carpal Canal Pressure Measurements: Literature Review and Clinical Implications

Fig. 7.13. Pressure measurement in the carpal canal performed during wrist flexion

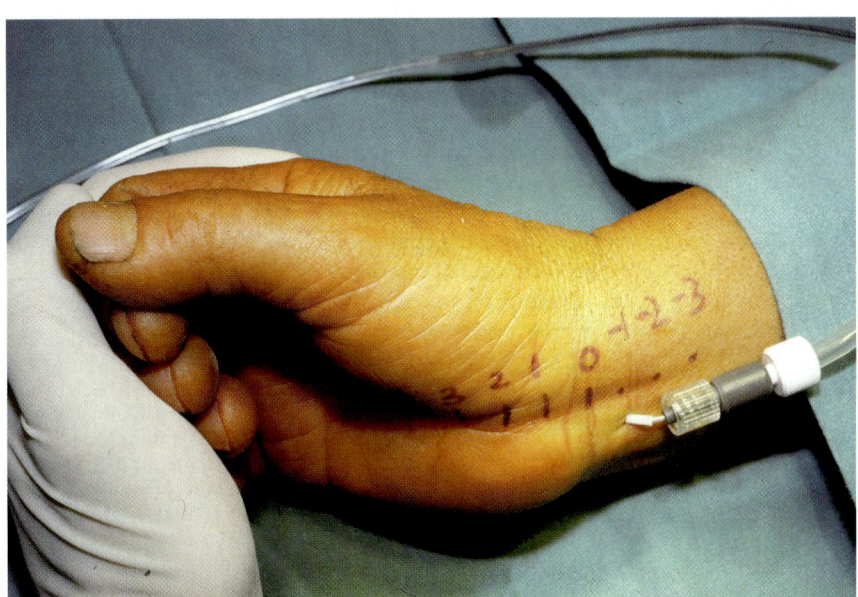

Fig. 7.14. Pressure measurement in the carpal canal performed during wrist extension

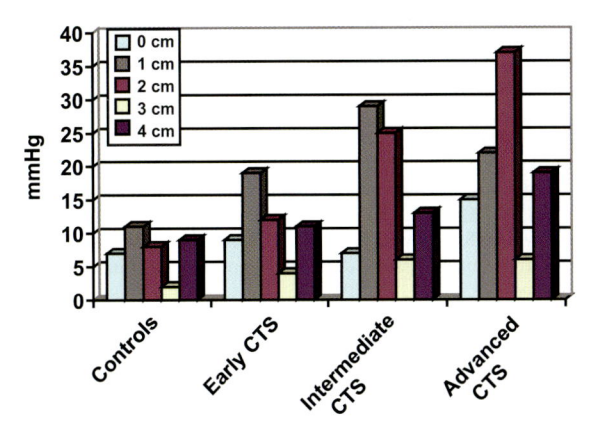

Fig. 7.15. Carpal canal pressure: segmental study

Conclusion

This brief historical review on the measuring of carpal canal pressure, besides confirming the pathophysiologic basis of this disease process, also establishes:

1. Literature results that are in accordance with an average carpal canal pressure which is higher in CTS patients with respect to control subjects [10, 13, 14], even if critical values of 30 mmHg [17–19, 44] are not reached.
2. The pressure is higher during wrist extension than flexion [10, 11, 20, 40, 47].

3. The progressive pressure that increases with wrist extension can be controlled by using a wrist extension splint which limits the wrist to 20° of extension so that a functional posture is obtained during activities of daily living but without exaggerated extension [40–42].
4. Pressure studies during wrist flexion extension movements [43, 47], prono-supination [42], and radial ulnar deviation [41, 43], supply useful parameters that can be applied when modifying work instruments.
5. The pressure is higher in the distal [23] or central-distal canal corresponding to the area where neuroelectric damage has occurred [22–24, 33].
6. The carpal canal is not a closed or functionally closed compartment, since it has been demonstrated that when tracing pressure areas a bell shaped curve is formed [17, 25]. The findings of an elevated pressure located more distally in the carpal canal (palm) is just another confirmation of this finding. It seems to be correlated to a hypothesis based on the insertion of the lumbrical palm muscles inside the canal [9, 48].
7. Various instrumentation exists for measuring the intracanal pressure by means of continual infusion [17] or blocked [18] to the most recently developed instrumentation that uses a catheter fiber optic method [47]. All these pressure evaluation instruments have confirmed, and are in accordance with, findings that the highest intracanal pressure is found in CTS patients with respect to control subjects. Canal pressure during grasping maneuvers show pressure values that are significantly superior to those obtained when the hand and wrist are in a rest position with prolonged functional recovery time after completing an effort [18, 44].
8. The pressure is abnormally elevated in acute conditions following an external compression or a wrist fracture [4, 6, 7, 11, 13, 14, 20].
9. Surgical treatment is the only solution for normal pressure recovery inside the carpal canal; endoscopic treatment has proved to be quite valid [49, 50] demonstrating normal pressure return immediately after the transverse carpal ligament is sectioned with a contemporaneous reduction in clinical symptoms.

Clinical Implications

Carpal canal pressure measurements can not be used as a routine diagnostic exam for determining if one is afflicted with CTS. This method of measurement is used for scientific means, as has been carefully described in the previous paragraphs. It has its useful indications in cases of acute posttrauma, where there is a doubt as to if there is a "direct nerve injury from trauma or an indirect trauma relative to an increase in endocanal pressure." Bauman et al. [4], Kongsholm and Olerud [6], and Mack et al. [7] have published and confirmed that in crush injuries, with direct median nerve trauma, there is a nearly normal endocanal pressure; but in secondary CTS cases there is an excessive increase in intracanal pressure.

References

1. Brain WR, Wright AD, Wilkinson M (1947) Spontaneous compression of both median nerves in the carpal tunnel. Six cases treated surgically. Lancet 1, 277–282
2. Tanzer R (1959) The carpal tunnel syndrome. A clinical and anatomical study. J Bone Joint Surg 41A, 626–634
3. Smith EM, Sonstegard DA, Anderson WH Jr (1977) Carpal tunnel syndrome: contribution of flexor tendons. Arch Phys Med Rehab 58, 379–385
4. Bauman T, Gelberman RH, Mubarak SJ, Garfin S (1981) The acute carpal tunnel syndrome. Clin Orthop Rel Res 156, 151–156
5. Abbott LC, Saunders JB DeC M (1933) Injuries of the median nerve in fractures of the lower end of the radius. Surg Gynec Obstet 57, 507–516
6. Kongsholm J, Olerud C (1986) Carpal tunnel pressure in the acute phase after Colles' fracture. Arch Orthop Trauma Surg 105, 183–186
7. Mack GR, McPherson SA, Lutz RB (1994) Acute median neuropathy after wrist trauma. The role of emergent carpal tunnel release. Clin Orthop Rel Res 300, 141–146
8. Cobb TK, Dalley BK, Posteraro RH, Lewis RC (1993) Anatomy of the flexor retinaculum. J Hand Surg 18A, 91–99
9. Cobb TK, An KN, Cooney WP, Berger RA (1994) Lumbrical muscle incursion into the carpal tunnel during finger flexion. J Hand Surg 19B (4), 434–438
10. Gelberman RH, Hergenroeder PT, Hargens AR et al. (1981) The carpal tunnel syndrome. A study of carpal canal pressures. J Bone Joint Surg 63A, 380–383
11. Gelberman RH, Szabo RM, Motensen WW (1984) Carpal tunnel pressure and wrist position in patients with Colles' fractures. J Trauma 24, 747–749
12. Werner CO, Elmquist D, Ohlin P (1983) Pressure and nerve lesion in the carpal tunnel. Acta Orthop Scand 54, 312–316
13. Lundborg GN, Gelberman RH, Minteer-Convery MA et al. (1982) Median nerve compression in the carpal tunnel. Functional response to experimentally induced controlled pressure. J Hand Surg 7, 252–255
14. Lundborg GN, Myers R, Powell H (1983) Nerve compression injury and increased endoneurial fluid pressure: a "miniature compartment syndrome." J Neurol Neurosurg Psychiat 46, 1119–1124
15. Low RA, Dyck PJ (1977) Increased endoneurial fluid pressure in experimental lead neuropathy. Nature 269, 427–428
16. Myers RR, Powell HC, Costello MC et al. (1978) Endoneurial fluid pressure: direct measurement with micropipettes. Brain Res 148, 510–515
17. Luchetti R, Schoenhuber R, DeCicco G et al. (1989) Carpal-tunnel pressure. Acta Orthop Scand 60 (4), 397–399
18. Szabo RM, Gelberman RH (1987) The pathophysiology of nerve entrapment syndromes. J Hand Surg 12A, 880–884
19. Rojviroj S, Sirichativapee W, Kowsuwon W et al. (1990) Pressure in the carpal tunnel. A comparison between pa-

tients with carpal tunnel syndrome and normal subjects. J Bone Joint Surg 72B, 516–518
20. Gellman H, Chandler DR, Petrasek J et al. (1988) Carpal tunnel syndrome in paraplegic patients. J Bone Joint Surg 70A; 517–519
21. Read RL (1991) Stress testing in nerve compression. Hand Clin 7 (3), 521–526
22. Kimura J (1979) The carpal tunnel syndrome. Localization of conduction abnormalities within the distal segment of the median nerve. Brain 102: 619–635
23. Luchetti R, Schoenhuber R, Landi A (1988) Localized nerve damage recorded intraoperatively in carpal tunnel syndrome. Electromyogr Clin Neurophysiol 28, 379–383
24. Nathan PA, Srinivasan H, Doyle LS, Meadows KD (1990) Location of impaired sensory conduction of the median nerve in carpal tunnel syndrome. J Hand Surg 15B: 89–92
25. Cobb TK, Dalley BK, Posteraro RH, Lewis RC (1992) The carpal tunnel as a compartment. An anatomic perspective. Orthop Rev 21 (4) 451–453
26. Robbins H (1963) Anatomical study of the median nerve in the carpal tunnel and etiologies of the carpal-tunnel syndrome. J Bone Joint Surg 45A, 953–966
27. Zucker-Pinchoff B, Hermann G, Srinivasan R (1981) Computed tomography of the carpal tunnel: a radioanatomical study. J of CAT 5 (4), 525–528
28. Bleecker ML, Bohleen M, Moreland R, Tipton A (1985) Carpal tunnel syndrome: role of carpal canal size. Neurology 35, 1599–1604
29. Middleton WD, Kneeland JB, Kellman GM et al. (1987) MR imaging of the carpal tunnel: normal anatomy and preliminar findings in the carpal tunnel syndrome. AJR 148, 307–316
30. Mesgarzadeh M, Schneck CD, Bonakdarpour A, Mitra A, Conaway D (1989) Carpal tunnel: MR Imaging. Part II. Carpal tunnel syndrome. Radiology 171, 749–754
31. Zeiss J, Skie M, Ebraheim N, Jackson WT (1989) Anatomic relations between the median nerve and flexor tendons in the carpal tunnel: MR evaluation in normal volunteers. AJR 153, 533–536
32. Cobb TK, Dalley BK, Posteraro RH, Lewis RC (1992a) Establishment of carpal contents / canal ratio by means of magnetic resonance imaging. J Hand Surg 17A, 843–849
33. Brown WF, Yates SK (1982) Percutaneous localization of conduction abnormalities in human entrapment neuropathies. Canadian J Neurol Sci 14; 391–400
34. Hargens A, Romine J, Sipe J et al. (1979) Peripheral nerve conduction block by high muscle compartment pressure. J Bone Joint Surg 61A, 192–200
35. Hargens AR (1989) Measurement of tissue fluid pressure as related to nerve compression syndromes. In Szabo RM, ed. Nerve compression syndromes. Diagnosis and treatment. Slack, 41–65
36. Luchetti R, Schoenhuber R, Alfarano M et al. (1990a) Carpal tunnel syndrome: correlations between pressure measurement and intraoperative electrophysiological nerve study. Muscle & Nerve 13, 1164–1168
37. Luchetti R, Schoenhuber R, Landi A (1988a) Assessment of sensory nerve conduction in carpal tunnel syndrome before, during and after operation. J Hand Surg 13B, 386–390
38. Luchetti R, Schoenhuber R, Alfarano M et al. (1991) Neurophysiological assessment of the early phases of carpal tunnel syndrome with the inching technique before and during operation. J Hand Surg 16B (4), 415–419
39. Baxter-Petralia PL (1990) Therapist's management of carpal tunnel syndrome. In: Hunter JM, Schneider LH, Makkin EJ, Callahan AD (eds): Rehabilitation of the hand: surgery and therapy. St Louis, CV Mosby, 640–646
40. Luchetti R, Schoenhuber R, Alfarano M et al. (1994) Serial overnight recordings of intracarpal canal pressure in carpal tunnel syndrome patients with and without splinting. J Hand Surg 19B 35–37
41. Weiss ND, Gordon L, Bloom T et al. (1995) Position of the wrist associated with the lowest carpal-tunnel pressure: implication for splinting design. J Bone Joint Surg 77-A, 11, 1695–1699
42. Rempel D, Manojlovic R, Levisohn DG et al. (1994) The effect of wearing a flexible wrist splint on carpal tunnel pressure during repetitive hand activity. J Hand Surg 19A, 106–110
43. Keir PJ, Bach JM, Rempel DM (1998) Effects of finger posture on carpal tunnel pressure during wrist motion. J Hand Surg 23A: 1004–1009
44. Seradge H, Jia Yi-C, Owens W (1995) In vivo measurement of carpal tunnel pressure in the functioning hand. J Hand Surg 20A: 855–859
45. Ostrup RC, Luerssen TG, Marshall LF, Zornow MH (1987) Continuous monitoring of the intracranial pressure with a miniature fiberoptic device. J Neurosurg 67, 206–209
46. Crenshaw AG, Styf JR, Mubarak SJ, Hargens AR (1990) A new "transducer-tipped" fiber optic catheter for measuring intramuscular pressures. J Orthop Res 8 (3), 464–468
47. Luchetti R, Schoenhuber R, Nathan P (1998) Correlation of segmental carpal tunnel pressures with changes in hand and wrist positions in patients with carpal tunnel syndrome and controls. J Hand Surg 23B: 5: 598–602
48. Yii NW, Elliot D (1994) A study of the dynamic relationship of the lumbrical muscles and the carpal tunnel. J Hand Surg 19B, (4), 439–443
49. Okutsu I, Ninomiya, S, Hamanaka I et al. (1989) Measurement of pressure in the carpal tunnel before and after endoscopic management of carpal tunnel syndrome. J Hand Surg 71A: 679–683
50. Hamanaka I, Okutsu I, Shimizu K et al. (1995) Evaluation of carpal tunnel pressure in carpal tunnel syndrome. J Hand Surg 20A; 848–854

Part II

Diagnosis

Clinical Diagnosis

M. Ceruso, R. Angeloni, G. Lauri, G. Checcucci

Diagnosis of carpal tunnel syndrome is substantially clinical. The most common subjective symptom is "nocturnal acroparesthesia," consisting of a painful tingling sensation which may even disturb sleep. Paresthesias are generally resolved by changing the position of the upper limb, by shaking or massaging it, or letting it hang down. Many patients also report relief after immersing their hand in cold water. Paresthesias may even occur during the day and are often triggered by certain positions or activities such as the act of sewing, driving, holding the phone or a book while reading. During a first look, a high percentage of patients are not able to describe on which fingers paresthesia occurs; they thus relate it to the whole hand and often, to the back of the hand as well as to the palmar surface. When asked to be more precise or, after performing some semeiotic maneuvers aimed at reproducing symptomatology, they adequately describe spreading of the disorder to the three radial fingers and to the radial side of the fourth finger. They furthermore recognize induced paresthesia as "overlapping" the spontaneous one, albeit of a lesser entity [1]. Moreover, sensitivity disorders are frequently related to only one finger, generally the middle finger or the thumb, or to both middle fingers. Often, the pain radiates out to the forearm or to the shoulder. Some patients refer that pain in these sites is dominant or is the only pain they experience. Also, as previously stated, following provocation maneuvers, they recognize that the pain is like the spontaneous symptom.

At times, paresthesia is reported as a sensation of insufficient blood supply to the fingers. Generally, this is a subjective perception of the symptom and must be distinguished from those rare pathologic conditions which involve objective symptoms of altered digital vascularization. Lastly, the patients commonly lament reduced manual dexterity because they frequently drop small objects which they cannot hold. This can be attributed to reduced sensitivity or to a weakened ability to the opposing grasp between the thumb and the long fingers.

Diagnosis based exclusively on electromyographic tests should be discouraged [2]. The incidence of false negatives, in fact, is statistically significant and data reported in the literature ranges between 8% and 12%. On the other hand, the instrumental sensitivity of electromyography may register subclinical conduction alterations which do not require surgical treatment (false positives) [3, 8].

The study of the patient's medical history is important in order to establish differential diagnosis and to plan possible treatment when the described symptomatology proves to be secondary to other pathologic conditions, and must thus be included in the sphere of more complex syndromes.

The carpal tunnel syndrome more frequently affects females and is concomitant to alterations in the estrogenic-progestogen hormonal balance. Nonetheless, it can also be observed in males and at all ages. In unusual cases, it is necessary to ascertain possible previous traumas of the wrist or proximal traumas along the path of the nerve or its roots. Concomitant diseases, whether current or previous, should also be taken into account since they may explain the onset of symptoms and may require priority treatment and not only local treatment for wrist compression (for example, endocrine diseases or metabolic diseases such as diabetes or thyroid disorders; major rheumatologic diseases, chronic renal failure).

Manual work may also influence the onset of CTS. Use of vibrating hand tools, activities carried out with the wrist mainly in the flexed position, inadequate training for heavy physical activities all increase the chances of onset of the carpal tunnel syndrome. Hobbies and sports activities may also be responsible for the onset of this disease. In these cases, interruption or changing the way these activities are performed may even lead to complete resolution of the disease.

Objective testing is based on provocation tests and on the evaluation of motor and sensitivity deficits which may be present in the territory of median nerve distal distribution.

Phalen attributed importance to Tinel's classic test [3, 4] and described the wrist flexion test. The Tinel sign (Fig. 8.1) involves percussion over the median nerve along its pathway from the forearm to the wrist in the proximal distal direction. It is positive when paresthesias are elicited in the territory of nerve distribu-

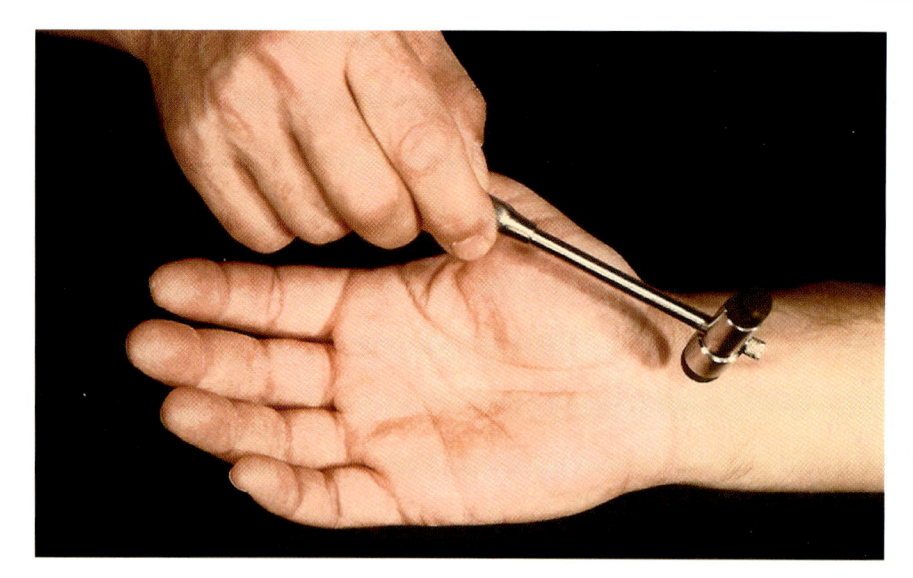

Fig. 8.1. Tinel's sign is performed applying repeated digital percussion over the median nerve in a proximo-distal direction

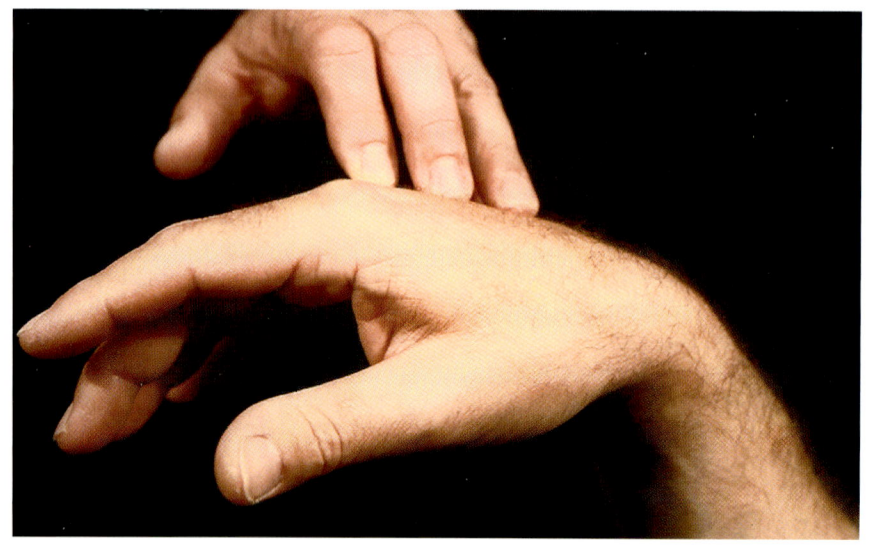

Fig. 8.2. Phalen's test is a provocation test done through maximal wrist flexion maintained for approximately 60 s. This increases pressure on the median nerve

tion. The Tinel sign, however, is diagnostically valid in a percentage between 58% and 67% of the cases of patients whose electromyographic tests are positive; in 20% of the cases, instead, Tinel's sign may be positive in the absence of compression disease [5]. Kuschner et al. [6] therefore concluded that the Tinel sign, alone, is not sufficient to establish a diagnosis of CTS.

Another important test is Phalen's test. This is done by holding the wrist in maximal flexion for several seconds: if a sensation of numbness as well as paresthesia on the first three fingers occurs within 60 s, it is considered diagnostic (Fig. 8.2). Phalen believed that this was due to compression of the nerve between the proximal edge of the transverse ligament and the adjacent flexor tendons. It has been demonstrated that Phalen's test is positive in 66%–88% of the patients with CTS, even if it can be positive in almost 20% of normal patients. A positive response obtained by combining Phalen's and Tinel's test is diagnostically important insofar as it identifies close to 90% of positive patients with CTS [7, 9].

Analogous to the wrist flexion test is the compression test of the median nerve, described by Durkan [5]. This test is considered specific for the diagnosis of CTS; it involves evaluating the onset of paresthesia in the territory of median nerve distribution when the physician applies pressure with his thumb at the level of the carpal tunnel for approximately 30 s (Fig. 8.3). Durkan reports that this test is positive in 87% of patients with CTS. For Williams [10] this test is positive in 100% of patients. While the flexion test may be positive in a certain percentage of normal patients (10%), it is, in any case, one of the tests that should normally be performed in order to objectively evaluate CTS; it can replace Phalen's test in those cases in which flexion of the wrist cannot be achieved because of concomitant diseases.

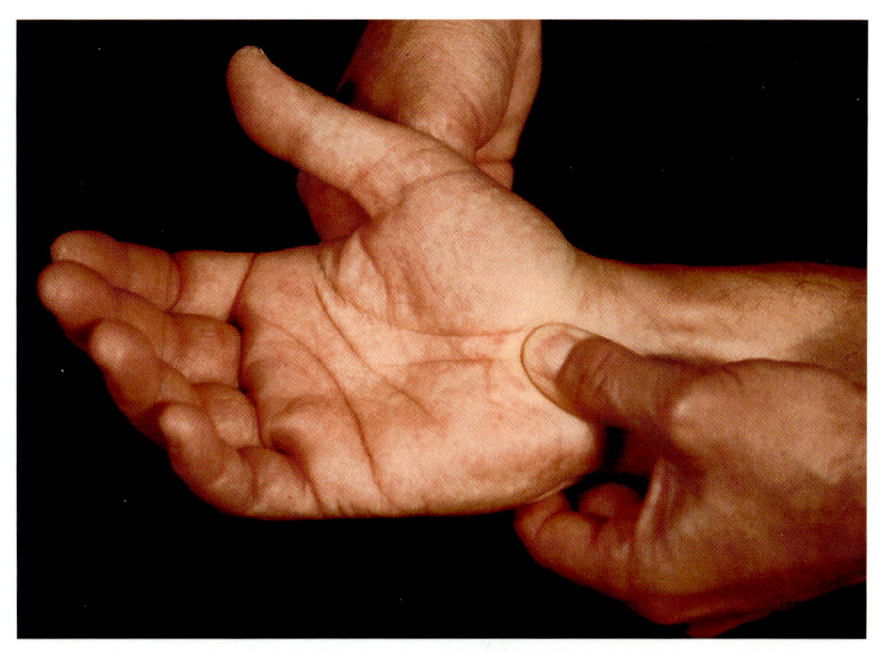

Fig. 8.3. The compression test, as described by Durkan, is considered positive when patient symptoms are reproduced applying a direct digital pressure for approximately 30 s

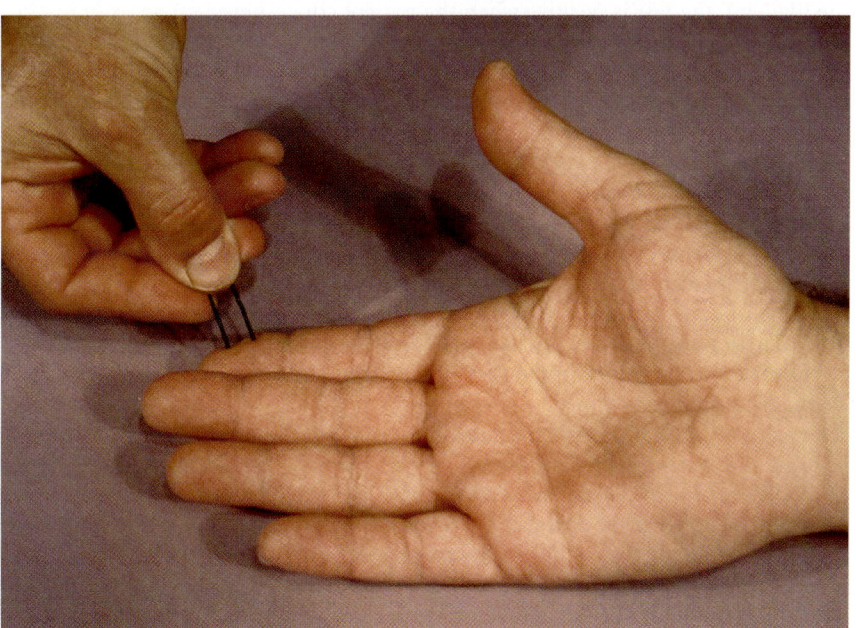

Fig. 8.4. Abnormal two-point discrimination is evaluated using the Weber's test

The tourniquet test described by Gilliat and Wilson in 1953 [11] proved to be scarcely useful in diagnosing CTS.

Measurement of the pressure inside the carpal canal [12] was the object of accurate studies aimed at demonstrating correlation between intercarpal pressure variations and the onset of the carpal tunnel syndrome [12].

Bedeschi (1986) underscored the significance of palpation in revealing increased local tension in the anterior region of the wrist. This finding seems to be correlated to an increased carpal tunnel pressure [13].

Tests aimed at evaluating sensitivity are divided into two major groups: innervation density tests and threshold tests.

Weber's test two-point discrimination test [14–15] is the best-known test for innervation density; it is generally normal in mild or moderate cases of CTS (Fig. 8.4).

The most widely used test is Van Frey's pressure test with Semmes-Weinstein monofilaments. This test involves perpendicular application on the finger tips of monofilaments with different thicknesses; the amount of pressure applied is just enough to obtain flexion of

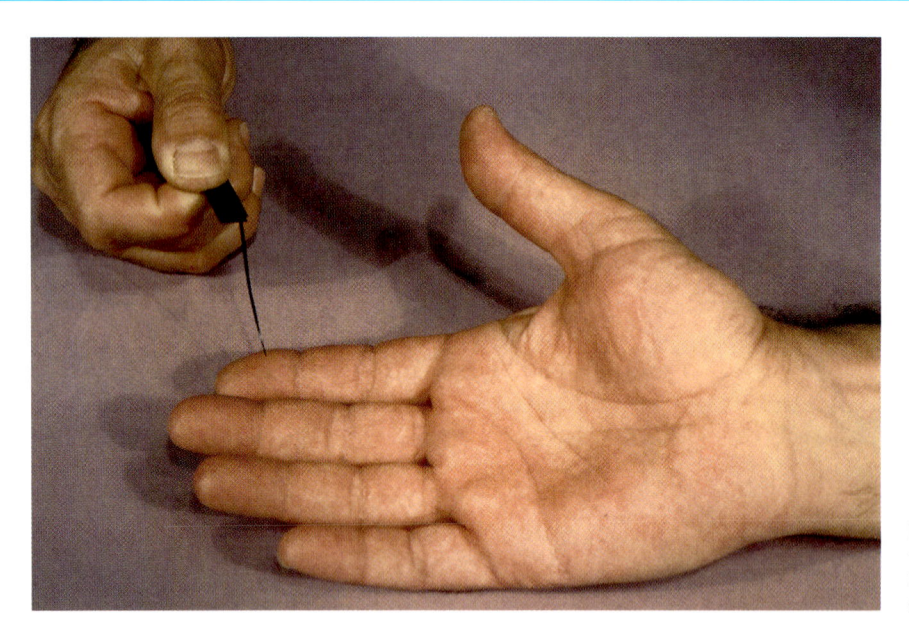

Fig. 8.5. Von Frey's pressure test is performed using the Semmes-Weinstein monofilament set

the filament: the test is positive when the patient correctly identifies the stimulated finger (Fig. 8.5). During a study carried out on a series of patients with CTS, Van Frey's test proved to be significant in 52% of the cases while Weber's two-point discrimination test was significant only in 30% of the cases.

Another threshold test is the vibration test described by Szabo et al. [16]. Nonetheless, just as the ability to discriminate between two points deteriorates with age, so does the perception of vibrations, regardless of the presence of compression of the median nerve in the wrist. These tests, therefore, are less valid in older patients since the variations in the threshold value with ageing have not been defined.

Sensitivity evaluation tests must prove to be altered only in the territory of distribution of the median nerve. Therefore, if extension of hypo-anesthesia to the palm is present, the involvement of the sensitive palmar branch (originating proximally to the transverse ligament) should be suspected and further differential diagnostic evaluations should be undertaken.

In some cases (medical-legal evaluations or insurance evaluations), it may be necessary to verify "subjective control" exercised by the patients in provocation tests and in tests undertaken to evaluate sensitivity, since the reliability of these test is based on the answer provided to the physician. For this purpose, Ames [17] described the evaluation test carried out when the wrist is in a neutral position. After performing Phalen's test, the patient is asked to form a fist and to place the metacarpal heads against each other for 1 min, while keeping the wrist extended. The test is considered positive (therefore, the patient is considered unreliable) if the onset of typical paresthesias is reported.

Clinical diagnosis of the carpal tunnel syndrome is based on an examination of the muscles of the thenar prominences; in normal anatomical conditions, they are innervated by the motor branch of the median nerve which arises from the nerve where it emerges from the carpal canal.

The muscle function which is the easiest to test is that of the thumb's short abductor muscle. The patient is asked to place the first finger perpendicular to the palm and to resist pressure exercised, directly in adducted direction, on the distal phalanx (Fig. 8.6). Correct execution of the requested movement and the force applied to counter resist is evaluated by comparing it to the other hand. It should be noted that even with a weak short abductor, the requested movement can still be done, albeit in an altered manner. The first digital ray, in fact, may be abducted with APL which is innervated from the radial nerve, and can be brought toward the palm with the long flexor which is innervated by the median nerve proximally to the carpal tunnel. The position of the thumb in these circumstances is, at any rate, easily recognizable in light of inevitable flexion of IP and since the patient can never position his thumb at 90° from the palm's surface.

The opponens pollicis muscle is tested by asking the patient to join the tip of his thumb to the tip of the fifth finger. While the clinician tries to open this position, the patient is asked to resist. Actually, in this case, all the thenar muscles are contracted and the opponens pollicis muscle alone cannot be evaluated.

Likewise, evaluation of the thumb's short flexor muscle is scarcely significant. The latter in fact is made up of two heads of which only one is innervated by the median nerve. Furthermore, according to a statistically significant incidence, both heads may be dependent on the innervations of the ulnar nerve.

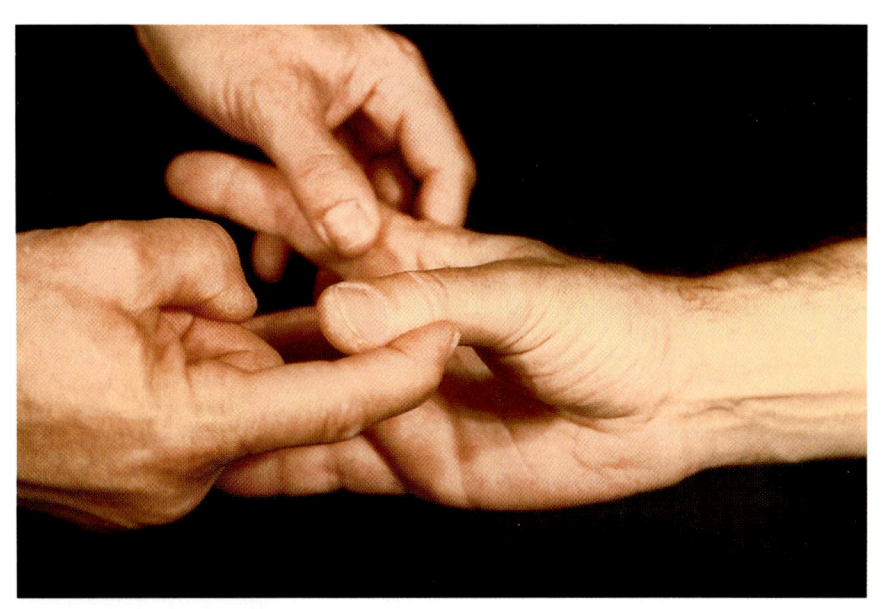

Fig. 8.6. Abductor Pollicis Brevis is tested asking the patient to place his thumb perpendicular to the palm and to resist the pressure which is applied by the examiner

Table 8.1. Significance of clinical tests

Clinical test	Significance
Phalen	Acceptable (+ Tinel)
Tinel	Acceptable (+ Phalen)
Carpal compression	Acceptable (+ Tinel)
Tourniquet	Not significant
APL Hypotrophy	Acceptable, if present
Weber	Acceptable, varying significance
Van Frey	Acceptable, varying significance

Therefore, it is important to take into account the reliability and validity of the tests employed in the clinical examination of the patient. For the sake of exemplification, we refer to the recent synthesis [18–19] published by R.G. Marx et al., which points to the different degrees of significance achieved with the various tests comprising the objective examination. For each of these, it is necessary to understand the degree of reliability and validity in order to have a standardized reference of an essential series of signs and symptoms in order to establish a correct diagnosis (Table 8.1).

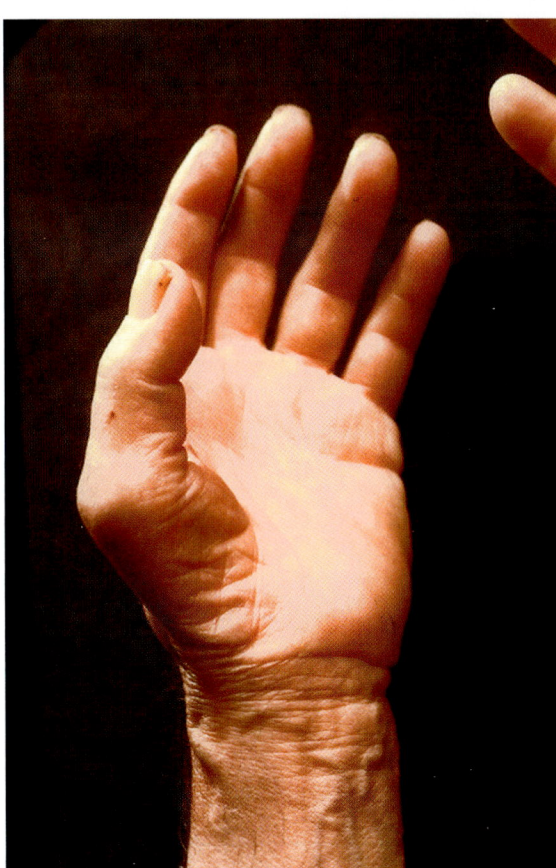

Fig. 8.7. Atrophy of the thenar muscles

Lastly, hypotrophy or atrophy of the thenar muscle must also be verified; the degree of atrophy is, in fact, proportional to nerve damage (Fig. 8.7). Atrophy is a sign of axonal lesion of the nerve while demyelinized lesions produce hyposthenia without atrophy.

References

1. Louis D (1992) The carpal tunnel syndrome in the work place. In Millender L, Louis D, Simmons B (eds), Occupational Disorders of Upper Extremity. Churchill – Livingstone, New York, Chap 12, pp 145–154
2. Louis D, Hankin F (1987) Simptomatic relief following carpal tunnel decompression with normal electroneuromyographic studies. Orthopedics 10: 434
3. Phalen G, Gardner W, LaLonde A (1950) Neuropathy of the median nerve due to compression beneath the trasverse carpal ligament. J Bone Joint Surg (Am) 32: 109

4. Phalen G (1951) Spontaneous compression of median nerve and wrist. JAMA 145: 1128
5. Durkan JA (1991) A new diagnostic test for carpal tunnel syndrome. J Bone Joint Surg 73A: 535–538
6. Kuschner SH, Ebramzadeh E, Johnson D et al. (1992) Tinel's sign and Phalen's test in carpal tunnel syndrome. Orthopaedics 15: 1297–1302
7. Seror P (1988) Phalen's test in the diagnosis of carpal tunnel syndrome. J Hand Surg (Br) 13: 383
8. Kanz JN, Larson MJ, Sabra A et al. (1992) The carpal tunnel sindrome: diagnostic utility of the history physical examination findings. Ann Intern Med 112: 321–327
9. Kanz J, Larson M, Fossel A et al. (1991) Validation of a surveillance case definition of carpal tunnel syndrome. Am J Public Health 81: 189
10. Willimas M, Mackinnon SE et al. (1992) Verification of the pressure provocative test in carpal tunnel syndrome. Ann Plast Surg. 29: 8–11
11. Gilliat RW, Wilson TG (1953) A pneumatic-tourniquet test in carpal tunnel syndrome. Lancet 2: 595–597
12. Luchetti R, Shoenhuber R, Nathan P (1988) Correlation of segmental carpal tunnel pressures with changes in hand and wrist positions in patiens with carpal tunnel syndrome and controls. J Hand Surg (Br) 23: 598–602
13. Bedeschi P (1986) Un nuovo segno clinico nella diagnosi della sindrome del tunnel carpale: la rivelazione palpatoria dell'aumento della tensione locale. Atti XII Congr. Naz. It. Ric. Chir.: 113–116
14. Borg K, Lindblum U (1988) Diagnostic value of quantitative sensory testing (QST) in carpal tunnel syndrome. Acta Neural Scand 7: 537
15. Dellon AL, Mackinnon SE, Crosby PM (1995) Reliability of two-point discrimination measurements. J Hand Surg (Am) 9: 104
16. Szabo RM, Gelberman RH, Willimson R et al. (1984) Vibration sensory testing in acute peripheral nerve compression. J Hand Surg (Am) 9: 104
17. Ames EL (1994) Wrist neutral test. In: Kasdan M, Amadio P, Bowers W, ed Mosby, Technical tips for hand surgery. St. Louis, pp 162–163
18. Marx RG, Hudak PL, Bombardier C et al. (1998) The riability of physical examination for carpal tunnel syndrome. J Hand Surg 23B: 499–502
19. Marx GR, Bombardier C, Wright JG (1999) What do we know about the reliability and validity of physical examination tests used to examine the upper extremity? J Hand Surg (Am) 22:185–193

Neurophysiological Assessment of Carpal Tunnel Syndrome

R. Schoenhuber, L. Capone, R. Gentile, R. Pentore

Introduction

In recent years decompression of the median nerve has become one of the most frequently performed surgical procedures, even if only 30–40 years ago carpal tunnel syndrome (CTS) was hardly recognized by most physicians. The frequent complaint of tingling in the hand and pain in the arm had been variously interpreted over the years [1] and various treatments had been proposed according to the underlying theory. The widespread availability of neurophysiological techniques in the 1970s and 1980s allowed the recognition of CTS as the most frequent cause of hand paresthesias and has made this diagnosis quite popular among physicians and patients. Initially, a neurophysiological confirmation of the clinical diagnosis was considered mandatory; today many operations are made without a prior nerve conduction study and many surgeons, neurologists, and general physicians think that nerve conduction studies are an expensive option which could be avoided.

For them, numbness und tingling with median nerve distribution which causes nocturnal awakening and improves by flicking the hand are sufficient for the diagnosis of CTS, but this can hardly be considered the gold standard and the association with successful decompression make this definition circular. Clinical neurophysiologists continue to stress the high sensitivity of their techniques, while epidemiologists and clinical methodologists insist on the opposite. It seems, therefore, worthwhile to put the problem of neurophysiological diagnosis of CTS, the most frequent referral diagnosis in many laboratories, in a wider context and consider the place of clinical neurophysiology in today's clinical medicine from a historical point of view and within the framework of health services organizations.

Soon after WWII, in the 1950s, when cheap surplus material from the armies became available it was used in a few European physiology laboratories for signal amplification and recording from nervous tissue. A few years later this equipment had been commercialized, initially by British and Danish companies. Quite early it became evident that the main value of the technique was in its high time and spatial resolution, easing, among other things, the localization of nerve compression and defining its physiopathology, severity, and time course. The diffusion of expertise in the field of clinical neurophysiology paralleled the interest in the peripheral nervous system. In those years, the different pathologies were identified and a model for focal nerve lesions developed; at the same time the application of the same recording setup was used in the clinic for diagnostic purposes.

While for most peripheral nervous diseases the result of the clinical neurophysiological examination was interesting but most often not followed by a change in clinical behavior, for nerve entrapments the surgeon relied more and more on the topographical diagnosis made by the electromyographer. Soon the role of the clinical neurophysiologist was recognized by other health care professionals. In several places, where EMG had already established its value, it became current practice that the primary care physician sent their patient to the EMG lab with the explicit request of suspected CTS, while earlier patients with similar symptoms were considered suffering from cervical radiculopathy.

With greater availability of EMG laboratories, the referring physician (typically the primary care physician, the orthopedic surgeon, or the physiatrist) now chooses among several professionals using several different criteria to evaluate the advantage of an examination. Different stakeholders rate the utility of a neurophysiological consultation differently: for the practitioner and the patient as well, diagnostic accuracy is the most important aspect, which in turn depends on the applied technique and clinical interpretation reflected by a clearly written, structured report which depends heavily on the experience and training of staff. Other criteria are more and more becoming important for the patients themselves: the availability of the examination, which means a short waiting list, cost and reimbursement issues such as coverage by one's insurance or a reasonable fee, but also other factors influencing patient acceptance of the examination, such as accessibility, friendly staff, and a nice ambience.

The Neurophysiological Examination

The goals of an electrodiagnostic examination are basically to localize the lesion; to show the involvement of motor, sensory fibers, or both; to define the physiologic basis (axon loss, demyelination) and the severity of the lesion (degree of axonal loss, the continuity of axons), as well as the time course of the lesion (evidence of reinnervation or of ongoing axonal loss). The main objective of the neurophysiological assessment of a patient with supposed CTS is to confirm the clinical suspicion of median nerve compression at wrist suggested by history and clinical examination. Sensory and motor nerve conduction velocity of the median nerve and other nerve segments with the needle electromyographic examination of one or several muscles allows the diagnosis of other diseases often associated with CTS such as radiculopathies, plexopathies, and others not evidenced by clinical examination alone. In the preoperative work-up of a CTS patient the neurophysiological examination allows quantification of the severity and the type of nerve lesion; moreover, it can be of some value in litigation should the intervention be less than satisfactory for the patient.

Simpson in 1958 [2] first showed a focal slowing of median motor nerve conduction at wrist in CTS patients, showing the clinical applicability of neurophysiological methods in the diagnosis of entrapment neuropathies. The same year Gilliat and Sears [3] introduced sensory conduction into the diagnosis of CTS. More and more tests have been suggested in the following years and have shown to increase the sensitivity for slighter forms of entrapment (Table 9.1).

Table 9.1. Neurophysiological tests for the diagnosis of CTS

Median nerve sensory conduction studies
Finger-wrist conduction
Palm-wrist conduction
Serial palmar stimulation (inching)
Ipsilateral comparison
   Median-ulnar (ring finger)
   Median-radial (thumb)
   Amplitude comparison
   Distal proximal (hand-forearm)

Median nerve motor conduction studies
Distal motor latency
Residual motor latency
Recording from lumbricals
Palmar stimulation
Serial palmar stimulation (inching)
Forearm motor conduction velocity

Electromyography
Evidence of axonal damage
Neuronal discharges

Median Nerve Sensory Conduction Studies

Several methods have been proposed for recording sensory potential from the median nerve, and their use differs widely among laboratories. Direct comparison between results is difficult even if each laboratory uses standard techniques. Particular care should be taken to maintain constant stimulating and recording parameters, such as interelectrode distance and temperature, which should be higher than 34 °C [4]. With the antidromic stimulation technique, the sensory action potential (SAP) is elicited by median nerve stimulation at palm and wrist and recorded by ring electrodes positioned proximally on each finger. With orthodromic stimulation the SAP is recorded at wrist or even more proximally (elbow, axilla, Erb's point) by stimulating each median innervated finger. Surface or needle electrodes can be used for recording and stimulation of sensory nerve fibers. The latency of the negative peak of the SAP depends on the distance from the stimulating electrodes

Even if differences have been shown between orthodromic and antidromic stimulation, in their practical application the two techniques are equivalent. The latency at the beginning of the SAP reflects the velocity of the fastest conducting sensory nerve fibers. In many laboratories, however, because of its higher reproducibility the positive or negative peak latency is used. Sensory conduction can be reported as sensory latency, maintaining the distance between stimulating and recording electrodes constant or as sensory conduction velocity along the measured segment, when the distance between stimulating and recording electrodes is divided by the latency. The amplitude of the SAP can be measure from the negative to the positive peak or from baseline to the negative peak. Since the amplitude of SAP is in the microvolt range, averaging several successive potentials is necessary to reduce the background noise and obtain a reliable SAP. Amplitudes of antidromic potentials are higher that those obtained by orthodromic stimulation, as are those obtained by needle cording compared to surface recording.

Normative values differ among laboratories and each laboratory should standardize its own technique for collecting its own normative values. According to Stevens [5] sensory peak latency obtained at the index finger by antidromic stimulation should have a latency of ≤ 3.5 ms and an amplitude of ≥ 25 µV.

For orthodromic stimulation peak sensory latency is ≤ 4.0 ms [3]. Median nerve sensory conduction velocity between finger and wrist in a normal population is 67.5 ± 4.7 ms, from wrist to elbow 67.7 ± 4.4 ms [4].

It was clear from the beginning of clinical neurophysiology that in CTS sensory nerve conduction studies are more frequently affected than motor nerve conduction studies. Melvin in 1973 [6] found a latency increase in the finger wrist tract in 88 % of his CTS patients. Conduction time within and across the carpal tunnel can be calculated by stimulating the median nerve at wrist and at mid-palm and recording from a median innervated finger or by stimulating the finger or palm and recording at wrist or more proximally [7]: with both techniques similar sensory latency values are obtained. All digital sensory branches are usually affected in CTS, but sensory conduction of the third and fourth finger seems more often affected than the second [8]. However, the SAP of the fourth finger is often absent either because both its digital branches originate from the ulnar nerve, or because the sensory fibers for the fourth finger within the median nerve are located in a position which make them more susceptible to compression within the carpal tunnel [9]. In 1979, Kimura [10] introduced serial sensory conduction velocity obtained by orthodromic stimulation at a 1-cm interval (inching) along the median nerve from palm to wrist. The mean difference between successive stimulation segments was 0.2 ms/cm proximal from the tunnel, but increased (>0.5 ms/cm) immediately distally to the carpal ligament and became again normal in the more distal part, suggesting a focal slowing underneath the carpal ligament. In at least half of the patients with CTS, a more diffuse slowing along the entire palm-to-wrist segment was present. With the same technique, a difference of ≥ 0.4 ms/cm in 81 % and ≥ 0.5 ms/cm in 54 % CTS patients was found [11].

Comparison Methods: Sensory Median to Ulnar and Median to Radial Nerve Fibers

The high diffusion of comparison tests in the diagnostic approach to patients with suspected CTS depends on their supposed higher sensitivity and specificity, particularly in less advanced stages of CTS. An method previously often used in many laboratories is the comparison of SAP amplitudes recorded from both hands. Another possible comparison is between median and ulnar or median and radial nerve SAP, which allows minimization of the effects of variability due to age and temperature which reduce the test's sensitivity.

Usually the median nerve sensory latency from the second finger and the ulnar sensory latency of the fifth finger differs < 0.4 ms [12]. The comparison of median and ulnar fourth finger sensory potential latencies is the most sensitive test for CTS, particularly if a sensory potential with a double negative peak, one (earlier) from the ulnar and another (later) from the median nerve is present, as found in 78 % of affected hands [13].

By first finger stimulation one can record a SAP from the median nerve at wrist and from the superficial sensory branch of the radial nerve where it crosses the tendon of the extensor longus pollicis muscle along the lateral margin of the radius. To compare directly the latencies, the distances between recording and stimulating electrode pairs must be the same [14] or nerve velocities must be calculated to allow for distance differences. For antidromic recording, ring finger electrodes on the first finger are used and both median and radial nerves are stimulated at a 10-cm distance [15]. In unaffected hands, latency difference is < 0.5 ms [14, 15].

Median Nerve Motor Conduction Studies

For median nerve motor, nerve conduction velocity is usually measured by surface electrodes from the thenar eminence. The active electrode is positioned on the motor point of the abductor pollicis brevis muscle, about two thirds proximally on the line from the metacarpo-phalangeal joint to the carpo-metacarpal joint of the first finger. From this position the electrode records potentials from several muscles beyond the abductor pollicis brevis, namely the opponens pollicis, flexor brevis, and adductor pollicis, but also the first interosseus dorsalis muscle.

The reference electrode is best put on the metacarpo-phalangeal joint of the thumb. Stimulating sites are typically at wrist, medially to the tendon of flexor carpi radialis muscle, at the elbow in the antecubital space medially to the biceps tendon, in the axilla, or in the supraclavicular space.

The distal motor latency (DML) from the first deflection of the compound motor action potential (CMAP) obtained by wrist stimulation, its amplitude, and shape are considered. The same criteria are used for all potentials obtained from more proximal stimulation. The distance between the stimulation point at the wrist and the recording electrode should be measured and kept constant during the whole examination. Stimulus intensity should be increased up to the maximal CMAP amplitude reflecting stimulation of the whole population of motor nerve fibers. By supramaximal stimulation of the median nerve at wrist, sometimes also ulnar nerve fiber could be stimulated: a CMAP of the thenar muscles with an initial positive deflection suggests a volume-conducted contribution from ulnar innervated muscles, which could be avoided by reducing stimulus strength or by slightly moving stimulus electrodes in a radial direction. If the median nerve CMAP at wrist is greater than by stimulating at the elbow, there could be again a volume-conducted contribution from ulnar or an innervation anomaly in the forearm.

In a few, most severe cases, in order to measure accurately the DML, needle electrodes should be put in the abductor pollicis brevis muscle.

Normative values of the DML of the median nerve depend on the length of the stimulated segment, and therefore on the distance between stimulating and recording electrodes. At a 7 cm distance LMD should be < 4.7 ms [5], and at a 4 cm distance < 4.4 ms [4]. In CTS, LMD is increased in about 51 % of cases [5].

Several tests have been proposed to increase the sensitivity of motor conduction velocity. Residual motor latency tries to correct DML by comparing it to forearm velocity [16]. Recording simultaneously from the second lumbrical muscle and the abductor pollicis muscle, the latency difference should not be higher than 0.4 ms [17]. Usually nerve conduction blockages or slowing are quite easily localized to the compressed segment. With stimulation at palm a normal conduction can be shown distally [10]. There are some patients in which median nerve conduction velocity is slowed also more proximally, suggesting a more marked compression with fiber loss, usually associated with a reduced CMAP. An anatomical variant of the median nerve is the Martin-Gruber anastomosis in which fibers originating from the median nerve in the antecubital space cross over to the ulnar nerve following the anterior interosseous nerve. These fibers cross the wrist with the ulnar nerve and innervate the thenar, hypothenar, and interossei muscles. An increased DML of median nerve without the corresponding increase of proximal latencies causes an erroneous calculation of conduction velocity, which seems to be increased. In extreme cases, the DML is higher than the proximal latency! In some patients with an increased DML there is also an increase of the minimum F-wave latency obtained from thenar muscles [18]. The increased minimum median nerve F-wave latency with normal distal motor and sensory latencies does not allow differentiation of a CTS from a proximal median neuropathy or brachial plexopathy; in these cases, the study of other nerve segments enables the diagnosis of a polyneuropathy.

Needle Electromyography

The usefulness of needle electromyography (EMG) in the diagnosis of CTS is still a matter of discussion. EMG documents the most severe cases, those which clinically show an atrophy of thenar muscles and where sensory loss appears. In less severe cases, which claim only sensory symptoms, it is very often completely normal. Most often the abductor pollicis brevis muscle is tested and spontaneous activity (fibrillation potentials and positive sharp waves) are searched for, as well as the recruitment pattern (frequency, amplitude, and duration of motor unit potentials). The probability of finding alteration with needle EMG increases with an increased DML [19]. Axonal nerve damage findings, both acute and chronic, are important for prognosis and for recovery following surgical decompression.

In cases where EMG shows neurogenic signs in the abductor pollicis brevis, it is suggested to examine another muscle innervated by the same root, but by another nerve, such as the abductor digiti minimi or the first dorsal interosseous nerve, in order to exclude a concomitant C8-Th1 radiculopathy. The examination of more proximal median innervated muscles such as the pronator quadratus or the pronator teres allow the diagnosis of a more proximal entrapment. It should be noticed that patients presenting with symptoms indicative of CTS can have a completely different diagnosis at neurophysiological examination. A proximal median neuropathy with entrapment at the level of the pronator teres muscle or at Struthers' ligament can show a nerve conduction similar to that seen in CTS, with a small median CMAP, absent or small median SAP, and a reduced motor and sensory conduction velocity in the forearm. Usually, in these cases there is not an increased distal latency, as is usually found in CTS. One should always remember that even if CTS is the most frequent cause of hand pain, it is not the only one. Only the needle EMG examination allows us to confirm the diagnosis of proximal median neuropathy, with denervation signs in at least one median innervated muscle above the wrist.

Other less common but nevertheless possible causes are cervical radiculopathies and even less frequently plexopathies or syringomyelia. The coexistence of cervical radiculopathy and CTS known as double crash syndrome has been described in 1973 by Upton and McComas, who suggested a proximal lesion at root level which would reduce the resilience of the median nerve at wrist, making it more susceptible to compression by the transverse ligament.

Also, a C6 root compression might simulate CTS; sometimes both these lesions coexist. Quite often the differential diagnosis based only on history or clinical examination is difficult. At needle EMG in 6 % – 14 % of CTS patients, signs of cervical root involvement can be found [21]. The importance of this diagnosis of a coexisting radiculopathy is important, since surgical decompression at wrist will leave the more proximal root lesion unaffected and therefore the operation might fail.

In cases in which conduction velocity studies do not show any slowing or blockage, needle EMG looks for other causes of arm pain or tingling. For patients with a diffuse nerve involvement in the sense of a polyneuropathy differential diagnosis is difficult, but can have therapeutically important consequences

In patients suffering from diabetes, renal failure, or with other polyneuropathies, their nerves are more susceptible to mechanical damage such as in an entrapment. It is therefore important to thoroughly examine a patient in which distal latencies also of the legs are recorded, as well as needle recording from distal and more proximal muscles in order to completely assess the extent of nerve damage. Patients with brachial plexus lesions or syringomyelia are also more prone to have more distal nerve entrapments. While nerve conduction studies can show the presence of this kind of pathology, needle EMG define the severity.

Conclusions

Over the last decades the increasing availability of neurophysiological examination has made the diagnosis of CTS better known to health care professionals and also to the general public. The widespread use of nerve conduction studies has confirmed CTS as the most frequent cause of hand numbness and tingling and arm pain. Most often the examination confirms the clinical suspicion, but in some rarer cases it results in a different diagnosis, or in more causes of the presenting symptoms. In these cases the surgeon might reconsider his therapeutic indication.

The real value of the neurophysiological examination for CTS is challenged today by the more critical and more cost-conscious individuals. No routine examination can, so far, demonstrate the increased tendency of a damaged nerve to spontaneously discharge and so give rise to paresthesia in the early phase of nerve compression. All of the above-described techniques can only define even the slightest delay of conduction or block of the faster nerve fibers, but not the initial phenomenon of increased excitability and ectopic impulse generation [22, 23]. In patients with an initial CTS, in its still irritative stage, the neurophysiological examination will be normal and only over time, if the patient worsens, will follow-up studies become diagnostic for CTS.

Moreover, as with every examination and test, there is also the risk of abnormal results in the absence of clinical symptoms. This is, of course, not the case for patients with symptoms sent for evaluation, but recent epidemiological surveys in occupational medicine show the relatively high prevalence of false positives [24]. When a patient is sent for a consultation, the clinical neurophysiologist should examine the patient, confirm or exclude the suspected diagnosis, and suggest alternatives [25]. An approach which uses standardized protocols (Table 9.2) and clearly definite criteria of abnormality (Table 9.3) makes the process easier and more efficient [26, 27].

As long as the diagnostic yield of imaging methods is not defined and direct pressure measurements within the carpal are still potentially dangerous, the methods of clinical neurophysiology provide the best available diagnostic tool. The hand surgeon will always be best advised to use his judgment based on history and examination, considering the report of the clinical neurophysiologist as one of the elements needed for clinical decision making. For this it is important to know the indications, as well as the limits of neurophysiological techniques.

Table 9.2. Protocol proposed for the neurophysiological diagnosis of CTS

Sensory nerve conduction
Orthodromic stimulation with surface electrodes at palm and on every finger at 12 cm from wrist on the first phalanx, recording with surface electrodes from wrist. Absolute sensory latencies measured from the negative peak, comparison of median and ulnar ring finger latencies, in doubt compare with the unaffected hand.

Motor nerve conduction
Median nerve stimulation at wrist and in the antecubital space, recording with surface electrodes from the APB muscle, measurement of the distance with the arm extended, calculation of conduction velocity. Amplitude of both potentials and DML are considered.
Ulnar nerve stimulation at wrist and above elbow, recording with surface electrodes from ADQ muscle, measurement of the distance with the arm slightly flexed, calculation of conduction velocity. Amplitude of both potentials and DML are considered.

Needle electromyography
M. abductor pollicis brevis (median)
M. abductor digiti quinti (ulnar) (optional and should be examined only if the abductor pollicis is affected)
M. extensor digitorum communis and brachioradialis (radial) (optional and should be examined only if the abductor pollicis is affected)

Table 9.3. Diagnostic criteria for carpal tunnel syndrome

Evidence of sensory nerve fiber compression
Absent or delayed motor nerve SAP (>3.4 ms)
Increased median-to-ulnar latency difference of the fourth finger SAP (≥ 0.5 ms)

Evidence of motor nerve fiber compression
Increased distal motor latency (>4.2 ms)
Denervation signs in the abductor pollicis brevis muscle

References

1. Lishman WA, Russel WR (1961) The brachial neuropathies. Lancet 2:941–947
2. Simpson JA (1958) Electrical sign in the diagnosis of carpal tunnel and related syndromes. J Neurol Neurosurg Psychiatry 19: 275–280
3. Gilliat RW, Sears TA (1958) Sensory nerve action potentials in patients with peripheral nerve lesions. J Neurol Neurosurg Psychiatry 19: 109–119
4. Kimura J (1989) Electrodiagnosis in disease of nerve and muscle: principles and Practice (second edition) Philadelphia, FA Davis Company pp 501–505
5. Stevens JC (1997) AAEE minimonograph #26: the electrodiagnosis of carpal tunnel syndrome. Muscle Nerve 20: 1477–1486
6. Melvin JL, Schuchmann JA, Lanese RR (1973) Diagnostic specificity of motor and sensory nerve conduction variables

in the carpal tunnel syndrome. Arch Phys Med Rehabil 54: 69–74
7. Mills KR (1985) Orthodromic sensory action potentials from palmar stimulation in the diagnosis of carpal tunnel syndrome. J Neurol Neurosurg Psychiatry 48: 250–255
8. Cioni R, Passero S, Paradiso C, Giannini F, Battistini N, Rushworth G (1989) Diagnostic specificity of sensory and motor nerve conduction variables in early detection of carpal tunnel syndrome. J Neurol 236: 208–213
9. Tackmann W, Kaeser HE, Magun HG (1981) Comparison of orthodromic and antidromic sensory nerve conduction velocity measurements in the carpal tunnel syndrome. J Neurol 224: 257–266
10. Kimura J (1979) The carpal tunnel syndrome: localization of conduction abnormalities within the distal segment of the median nerve. Brain 102: 619–635
11. Nathan PA, Meadows KD, Doyle LS (1988) Sensory segmental latency values of the median nerve for a population of normal individuals. Arch Phys Med Rehabil 69: 499–501
12. Felsenthal G (1977) Median and ulnar distal motor and sensory latencies in the same normal subject. Arch Phys Med Rehabil 58: 297–302
13. Uncini A, Lange DJ, Solomon M, Soliven B, Meer J, Lovelace RE (1989) Ring finger testing in carpal tunnel syndrome: a comparative study of diagnostic utility. Muscle Nerve 12: 735–741
14. Carroll GJ (1987) Comparison of median and radial nerve sensory latencies in the electrophysiological diagnosis of carpal tunnel syndrome. Electroencephalogr Clin Neurophysiol 68: 101–106
15. Johnson EW, Sipski M, Lammertse T (1987) Median and radial sensory latencies to digit I: normal values and usefulness in carpal tunnel syndrome- Arch Phys Med Rehabil 68: 140–141 and 388
16. Kraft GH Halvorson GA (1983) Median nerve residual latency: normal values and use in diagnosis of carpal tunnel syndrome. Arch Phys Med Rehabil 64: 221–226
17. Logigian EL, Busis NA, Berger AR et al. (1987) Lombrical sparing in carpal tunnel syndrome: anatomic, physiologic, and diagnostic implications. Neurology 37: 1499–1505
18. Kimura J (1983) F-wave determination in nerve conduction studies. Adv neurol 39: 961–975
19. Kimura I, Ayyar DR (1985) The carpal tunnel sindrome: electrophysiological aspect of 639 symptomatic extremities. Electromyogr Clin Neurophysiol 25: 151–164
20. Upton AR, Mc Comas AJ (1973) The double crush in nerve entrapment syndromes. Lancet 2: 359–362
21. Kuntzer T (1994) Carpal tunnel syndrome in 100 patients: sensitivity, specificity of multi-neurophysiological procedures and estimation of axonal loss of motor sensory and sympathetic nerve fibers. J Neurol Sci 127: 221–229
22. Gilliat RW (1980) Paresthesiae. In: Abnormal nerve and muscle as impulse generators, Culp WJ, Ochoa JL (eds.) New York, Oxford University Press pp 477–489
23. Ochoa JL, Torbjörk HE (1980) Paraesthesias from ectopic impulse generation in human sensory nerves. Brain 103: 835–853
24. Atroshi I, Gummesson, Johnsson R, Ornstein E (2003) Diagnostic properties of nerve conduction tests in population-based carpal tunnel syndrome. BMC Muscoskeletal Disorders 4: 9 http://www.biomedcentral.com/1471–2474/4/9
25. Smith BE (2003) What good is EMG to the patient and practitioner? Seminars in Neurology 23: 335–342
26. Jablecki CK, Andary MT, Floeter MK, Miller RG, Quartly CA Vennix MJ, Wilson JR (2002) Practice parameter: Electrodiagnostic studies in carpal tunnel syndrome. Neurology 58: 1589–1592
27. Hermann DN, Logigian EL (2002) Electrodiagnostic approach to the patient with suspected mononeuropathy of the upper extremity. Neurol Clin N Am 20: 451–478
28. Rosenbaum R (1999) carpal tunnel syndrome and the myth of the Eldorado. Muscle Nerve 22: 1165–1167

Diagnostic Imaging

E. Cerofolini

Diagnostic imaging has always had a minor role in the diagnosis of carpal tunnel syndrome (CTS), which is based mostly upon clinical findings and nerve conduction studies. Both conventional radiography [1] and computed tomography [2–4] have not been widely used because the information provided is of little use. More recently, high resolution magnetic resonance [5–8] and high frequency ultrasound [9–12] have been able to demonstrate median nerve compression along with the detection of space-occupying lesions within the carpal tunnel and flexor tendon pathology. Sliding of the median nerve during dynamic studies with flexion of the fingers can also be evaluated. MR and US can also be employed in the diagnosis of post-operative conditions and surgical complications.

Magnetic Resonance

MR images have an intrinsic high contrast resolution showing different signal intensity for tendons, tendon sheaths, nerves, muscles, fat, bone, and vessels: this makes MRI an ideal tool to visualize the carpal tunnel contents. In order to obtain high quality images of the wrist, a dedicated surface coil should be employed; the phased array surface coils allow faster acquisition times which can be traded off for higher resolution, allowing a better depiction of anatomical details. The patient can be positioned in different ways inside the magnet depending on the configuration of the surface coils employed: prone with the arm extended over the head or more comfortably supine with the arm resting along the body. In this position, however, the wrist is at the periphery of magnetic field, causing some signal loss and inhomogeneities. Spin-echo T1-weighted and T2-weighted sequences along with gradient echo sequences are usually employed. Suppression of fat signal is sometimes used to enhance contrast between fluids and surrounding tissues. MR allows the acquisition of scans along any direction of the space and also volume acquisition, which can be subsequently be postprocessed and reconstructed. Axial scans are the most useful for the depiction of carpal tunnel anatomy (Fig. 10.1). The flexor tendons are imaged in cross sections and show very low signal intensity due to the absence of moving protons. In the axial plane they appear as small, dark, oval structures devoid of signal. The flexor pollicis longus (FPL) tendon appears as a structure separated from the other flexor tendons even if contained within the carpal tunnel; it runs deep to the median nerve in the proximal sections while it moves radially in the most distal ones. The four superficial flexor tendons (SF) are visualized as separate structures; at times the fifth superficial and deep tendons are close together and not clearly separable on the MR images. The second superficial flexor tendon is located next to the median nerve. The four deep flexor tendons (DF) are usually visualized as individual structures but at times they can appear as a whole with no definite separation among them. The median nerve displays a higher signal intensity than the tendons, similar to muscle. The median nerve usually lies close to the flexor retinaculum, which has a lower signal intensity. In the proximal carpal tunnel, at the level of the pisiform, the average median nerve cross sections diameters are 2 mm (thickness) by 4 mm (width); distally, at the level of the hook of the hamate, the nerve has a more flat shape (2 mm thick by 5 mm wide). The flexor retinacu-

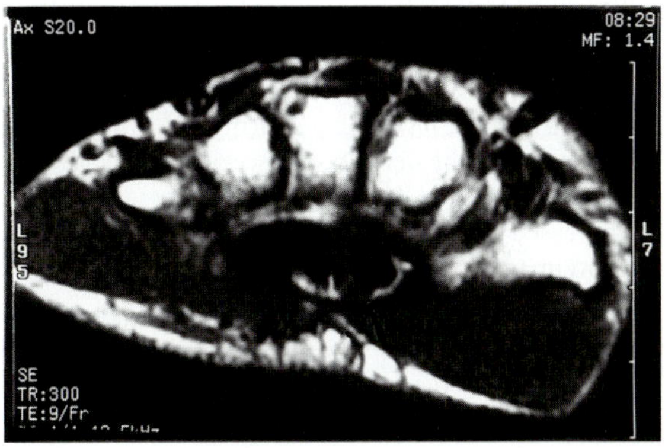

Fig. 10.1. MR T1-weighted axial scan. Normal anatomy. The carpal tunnel is delimited ventrally by the flexor retinaculum, a fibrous structure with low signal intensity (*arrow*) and by the carpal bones dorsally. The median nerve is seen as a intermediate signal intensity (similar to muscle) structure close to the retinaculum (*curved arrow*). The flexor tendons have a very low signal intensity and they are individually visualized

lum appears as a fibrous, low intensity, linear structure delimiting the volar side of the carpal tunnel; the distal insertions upon the hook of the hamate and the trapezium, where the retinaculum is thicker, are constantly visualized, while the proximal ones upon the pisiform and scaphoid are less often identified. The high intensity signal fat tissue interposed among the flexor tendons provides an excellent natural contrast. The signal of vessels varies according to the kind of MR sequence being employed and can be either high or absent, but they can always be identified without the need of contrast media. In sagittal sections the median nerve can also be well visualized and its relationship with the flexor retinaculum and flexor tendons can be evaluated. Images acquired along this scan plane only rarely provide additional information to that available in the axial images. Coronal sections are less valuable since the scan plane is parallel to the structures being studied (retinaculum, median nerve and tendons) and are less frequently utilized. Some anatomic variations may cause an increase in the volume of the contents of carpal tunnel where the space is already limited, and they can be responsible for compression of the median nerve. One possible variation is a persistent median artery [13], which is a small vessel that normally obliterates after birth. Its presence in symptomatic patients can be relevant even if it's not usually the only cause of CTS. The extension of portions of lumbrical muscle within the carpal tunnel can act as a space-occupying mass and can ultimately cause or contribute to the development of the CTS [14, 15]. The lumbrical muscles can be easily identified with MR. Caution should be taken not to examine patients with the fingers flexed since they originate from the deep flexor tendons which are retracted proximally during flexion, pulling backward the lumbrical muscle that will be located within the tunnel [16]. In the presence of CTS, the following modifications can be observed in the median nerve (Figs. 10.2, 10.3):

- Diffuse or focal swelling of the nerve best discerned at the level of the pisiform
- Flattening of the nerve best discerned at the level of the hamate
- Increased signal intensity on T2-weighted spin-echo images

When enlarged proximally, the nerve may assume an oval shape sometimes defined as pseudo-neuroma (Fig. 10.3). In order to define the presence of a focal nerve enlargement, a detailed evaluation of its size on axial images at various levels from distal to proximal sections should be performed with the use of ratios of nerve size. The ratio between the cross-sectional areas of the median nerve at the pisiform and at the distal radius should be 1, while in patients with CTS it is greater than 2. Another sign of CTS is flattening at the level of the hook of the hamate due to compression by the tendons. The involved median nerve usually displays an increased signal intensity on T2-weighted images. Another sign of advanced CTS is hypotrophy and increased signal of hypothenar muscles due to denervation with fatty infiltration [17]. Inflammation of the

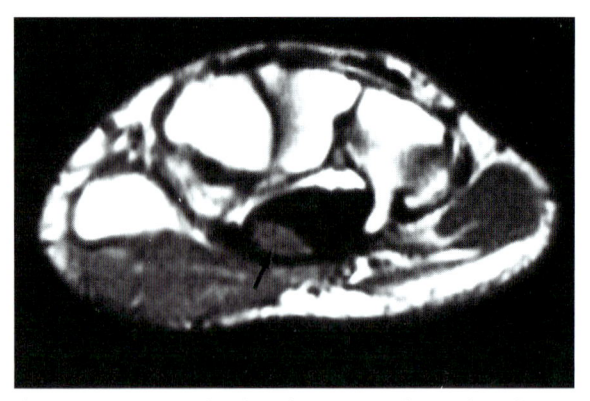

Fig. 10.2. MR T1-weighted axial scan. Carpal tunnel syndrome. The median nerve (*arrow*), compressed between the flexor retinaculum and the flexor tendons, looks quite enlarged and swelled in this advanced case of CTS

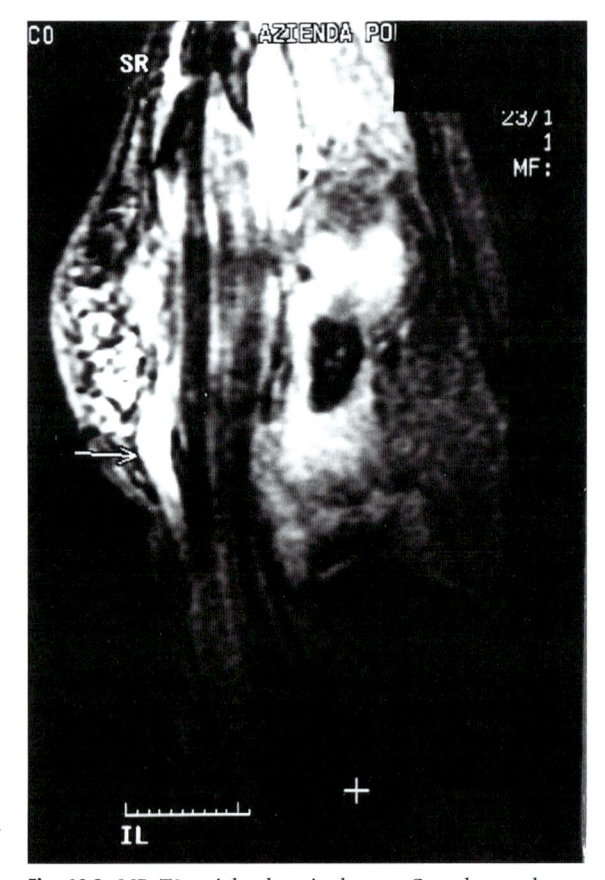

Fig. 10.3. MR T2-weighted sagittal scan. Carpal tunnel syndrome. Swelling of the median nerve at the entrance in the carpal tunnel with a nodular appearance (pseudoneuroma) and marked increase of signal intensity (*white arrow*)

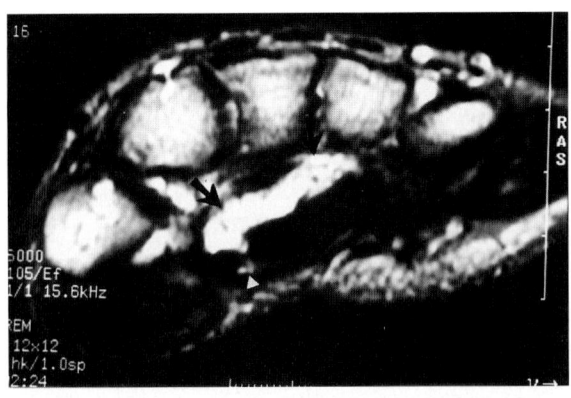

Fig. 10.4. MR T2-weighted axial scan. Carpal tunnel angioma. Between the flexor tendons and the carpal bones there's a high signal intensity space-occupying lesion (*arrows*) that turned out to be an angioma. The lesion produced an indirect compression on the median nerve that shows increased signal intensity (*white arrowhead*) due to inflammation

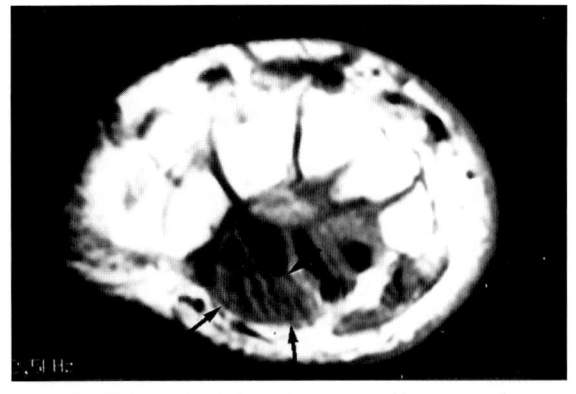

Fig. 10.5. MR T1-weighted axial scan. Lipofibromatous hamartoma. The median nerve looks extremely enlarged and infiltrated by an intermediate signal intensity tissue that causes spreading of fascicles, making them recognizable individually (*arrows*)

flexor tendon sheaths is an important cause of CTS [18] and can be seen on MR as increased thickness and signal intensity on T2-weighted images; distances among low signal intensity tendons is increased. An effusion may be present in case of bursitis. For this reason flexor retinaculum may show a palmar bowing at the level of the hamate due to increased volume of the structures within the carpal tunnel.

The use of contrast media can enhance the increased signal of tendon sheaths and the median nerve, but its use is seldom necessary. Chronic tenosynovitis is found at surgery with a relatively high incidence in some reports. This finding is less frequently detected at MR examinations probably because in less severe forms it is more easily discerned with comparative examinations such as ultrasound. Anatomical changes can be subtle [5] and be discerned only by comparing the two sides even though not infrequently both wrists are involved. All aspects described so far are signs of nerve impairment and inflammation of tendon sheaths; in the literature there are discordant data regarding their specificity and sensitivity in the diagnosis of CTS: very high according to some [19] and very low according to others [20]. Brits et al. found that the alterations of the median nerve depicted with MR can even precede the modifications of nerve conduction. Among other rare causes of CTS there are cystic ganglia [21], lipomas, angiomas (Fig. 10.4), neurinomas, and other space occupying lesions such as lipofibromatous hamartoma (Fig. 10.5) of median nerve [22].

Accumulation of fat tissue in obese patients or amyloid (either primarily or secondarily to long-term hemodialysis) can sometimes be a cause of CTS and are seen respectively as areas of high signal intensity on T1-weighted images or low signal intensity on T2-weighted images. Modifications of the bony walls of the tunnel can determine a compression upon the nerve such as in case of fractures, luxations, or hypertrophic repair tissue. There are forms of latent CTS that manifest themselves only after exercise. The corresponding MR findings have been recently described: transient swelling and increased signal of median nerve, bowing of retinaculum, and hyperintensity of tendon sheaths [23]. MRI has been employed in dynamic studies aimed at demonstrating the changes in the relationship between the nerve and the tendons during flexion of the fingers [24, 25].

Postsurgery Findings

In an MR study performed before and after surgical carpal tunnel release obtained with transverse carpal ligament resection, it has been shown that the main effect of surgery is an enlargement of the carpal canal with palmar dislocations of its content [26]. This has been attributed to the palmar sliding of the newly formed carpal ligament rather than to a real widening of the canal itself. Persistence of symptoms after surgery can be due to various causes, and among them the most common ones are incomplete resection of the ligament or the presence of perineural scar tissue [27]. Both can be evaluated with MR especially if scans prior to surgery are available for comparison. Another cause of persistence or worsening of symptoms is iatrogenic transection of median nerve [28], which can be difficult to demonstrate with MR. The presence of an amputation neuroma can eventually be seen, along with muscle atrophy secondary to denervation. An algodystrophic syndrome may complicate a successful surgical procedure; in this case MR can accurately show the presence of bone marrow edema of wrist bones.

Ultrasound Studies

With ultrasound, information similar to that obtained with MR can be obtained at a much lower cost and with much greater availability. It also easily allows a dynamic study, which is very difficult to obtain with MR. Anatomical details as well as contrast resolution are lower than with MR; the bony structures are not visualized and the ultrasound images are less attractive to the surgeons who are the ultimate users of imaging examinations. It also has to be underlined that the accuracy of ultrasound studies are strongly operator-dependent. Ultrasonographic study of carpal tunnel has to be performed with linear array transducers with frequencies as high as 17 MHz, available in some recent equipment. Color and power Doppler can be at times be useful to identify vessels within the tunnel. A stand-off pad to better focus the most superficial areas, can be used if the higher frequency probes are not available. The patient should sit comfortably in front of the operator with the palms up and moderately extended fingers. The study is performed in the transverse and longitudinal scan planes. Ultrasound allows the visualization of all the soft tissue components of carpal tunnel (tendons, median nerve, and transverse carpal ligament) while the bony structures are not evaluated.

The nine flexor tendons show a marked hyperechogenicity with a fibrillar internal architecture, and the two layers, superficial and deep, are displayed. The median nerve runs superficially with respect to the tendons; it is less echogenic than the tendons and the internal structure can be defined as fascicular since, especially with very high frequencies probes, the nerve fascicles can be identified: they appear as small echogenic dots in the transverse plane and as thin lines in the longitudinal scans [29, 30]. It is easily differentiated from the tendons of the second and third fingers that run deep to it (Fig. 10.6). In transverse sections, the nerve has an elliptical shape. Transverse carpal ligament delimitates the carpal tunnel on the palmar side; it has a quadrangular shape and it's made of fibrous tissue. On ultrasound images it appears as a slightly echogenic linear band with a thickness of 1–1.5 mm.

Ultrasonographic diagnosis of CTS depends upon the depiction of abnormalities of the anatomical structures within the CT and first of all those involving the median nerve [9, 10]. The nerve may show a swelling in the proximal carpal tunnel or right before its entrance into it (Fig. 10.7). Flattening of the nerve in the distal canal can be observed (Fig. 10.8). Enlargement of the nerve can be uniform or sometimes be so relevant as to assume a pseudotumoral appearance (so-called pseudoneuroma). Some authors [31] have found that the maximum normal cross-sectional area of the nerve at the level of the pisiform where it is greatest should not exceed 10^2 mm. Maybe easier and more reliable to eval-

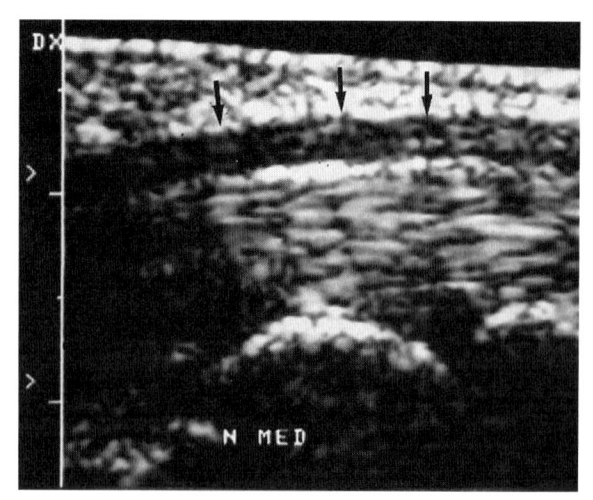

Fig. 10.6. Ultrasound longitudinal scan. The normal median nerve (*arrows*) can be easily recognized due its superficial position and the hypoechoic fascicular structure as compared to the hyperechoic fibrillar structure of flexor tendons. The thickness of the nerve is uniform

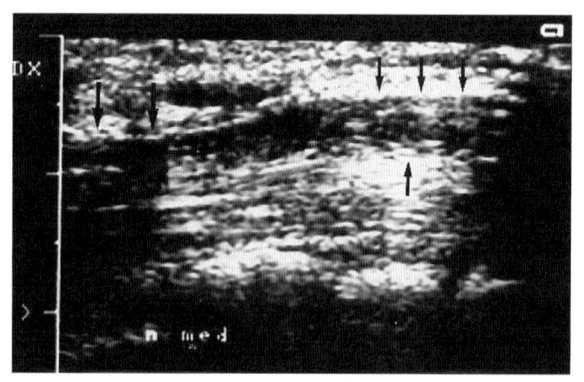

Fig. 10.7. Ultrasound longitudinal scan. Carpal tunnel syndrome. The median nerve is flattened at the level of the transverse ligament (*large arrows*) while it looks thickened and swollen proximally (*small arrows*)

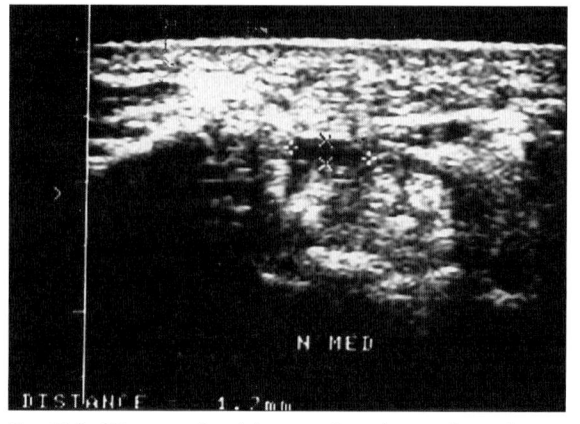

Fig. 10.8. Ultrasound axial scan. Carpal tunnel syndrome. Marked flattening of the median nerve is present at the level of its entrance in the tunnel (*markings*). The rate between the largest and smallest diameters is used to calculate the flattening index of the nerve

uate is the flattening index expressed by the rate between the largest and smallest cross-sectional diameters evaluated at the level of the distal CT: its normal value should not exceed 3 [11]. The ultrasonographic examination of the median nerve should always be completed with a dynamic evaluation during active and passive flexion of the fingers in order to evaluate the transverse and longitudinal sliding of the nerve with respect to the flexor tendons of the second and third fingers [32]. This an important pathophysiological parameter, but it is very difficult to quantify sonographically and its evaluation might lack objectivity; some authors have established for the transverse sliding a minimum value of 1.75 mm. In a recent paper [33], no decrease of longitudinal nerve sliding was found in patients with CTS as compared with control subjects, and these results suggest that local nerve strain from restricted longitudinal nerve movement does not contribute to the symptoms of idiopathic CTS. Carpal transverse ligament or flexor retinaculum abnormalities detected with ultrasound include palmar bowing and thickening(Fig. 10.9). Normally, the flexor retinaculum runs in a linear pattern but when there is CTS it may show palmar bowing due to increased volume of the contents of the CT. Palmar displacement can be determined on axial scans by measuring the distance between the top of the retinaculum and a line traced between the trapezium and the hamate: the value should not exceed 4 mm (Fig. 10.10). In advanced cases of CTS the transverse ligament may show marked thickening and decreased echogenicity.

A frequent finding in patients with CTS is the presence of tenosynovitis of flexor tendons with thickening of tendon sheaths. This can be easily detected on ultrasound studies since in this condition the single tendons are widely separated by the enlarged hypoechogenic sheaths (Fig. 10.11) and much better identified, while in normal cases they tend to merge into an indistinct echogenic structure. In cases of unilateral involvement these changes can be even better appreciated with comparative examination. In advanced cases tenosynovitis may form large masses dislocating the tendons [34]. Ultrasound is also able to detect space occupying lesions within the canal whose nature is usually benign. Cysts, lipomas, and vascular lesions, by means of color-Doppler studies, can be identified while in other cases the ultrasonographic determination of the nature of the mass is less specific. Another useful application of ultrasound is the evaluation of operated patients without improvements of symptoms. In these case the presence of scar tissue surrounding and entrapping the nerve can at times be found (Figs. 10.12, 10.13). Iatrogenic lesions of the median nerve can be recognized in the presence of amputation neuromas. The presence of a new-formed transverse ligament is also difficult to assess.

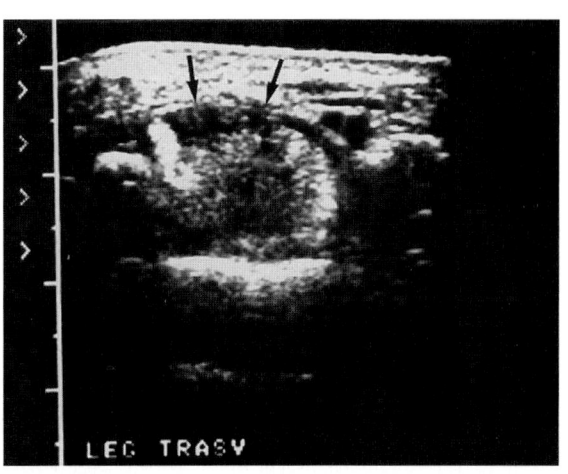

Fig. 10.9. Ultrasound longitudinal scar. Transverse ligament. In this patient with CTS the ligament is clearly depicted because it is thickened due to volar bowing

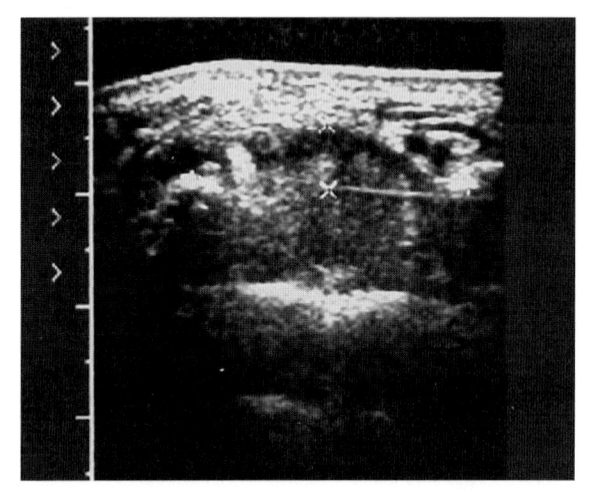

Fig. 10.10. Ultrasound axial scan. In this patient with CTS there's thickening and bowing of the transverse ligament. The line drawn between the hamate and the trapezium is used to evaluate palmar displacement

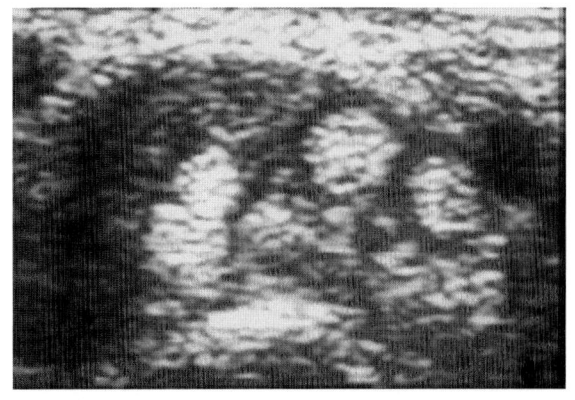

Fig. 10.11. Ultrasound axial scan. Flexor tendons tenosynovitis. The hypoechoic tissue surrounding the tendons represent the thickened tendon sheaths, allowing a better delineation of their margins

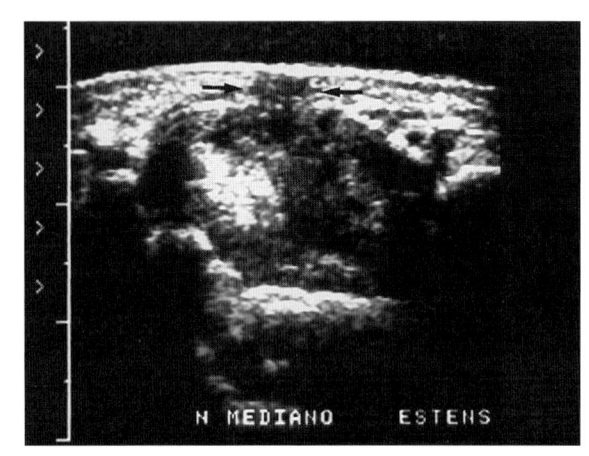

Fig. 10.12. Ultrasound axial scan. In this patient with persistence of symptoms after surgery, the hypoechoic tissue (*arrows*) represent scar formation that extends from the subcutaneous plane to the nerve surrounding it, and causing compression and reduced sliding during motion of the fingers

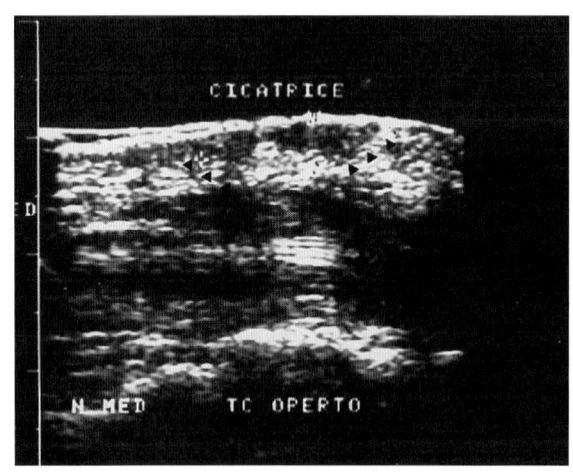

Fig. 10.13. Ultrasound longitudinal scan. Patient with persistence of symptoms after CTS release. A voluminous hypoechoic tissue scar (*head arrows*) determines compression of the median nerve. This is a typical case in which a dynamic ultrasound evaluation of the median nerve sliding is indicated to determine its fixation

References

1. Engel J, Zinneman H, Tsurh Fari J (1978) Carpal tunnel syndrome due to carpal osteophyte. Hand 10: 283–286
2. Zucker-Pinchoff B, Hermann G, Srinivasan R (1981) Computed Tomography of the carpal tunnel: a radioanatomical study. J Comput Assist Tomogr 5: 525–528
3. Bleeker ML, Bohlman M, Moreland R, Tipton A (1985) Carpal tunnel syndrome: role of carpal canal size. Neurology 35: 1599–1605
4. Jessurun W, Hillen B, Zonnenveld F et al. (1987) Anatomical relations in the carpal tunnel: a computed tomographic study. J Hand Surg 12: 64–70
5. Middleton WD, Bruce Kneeland J, Kellman GM et al. (1987) MR imaging of the carpal tunnel: normal anatomy and preliminary findings in the carpal tunnel syndrome. AJR 148: 307–313
6. Mesgarzadeh M, Schneck CD, Bonakdarpour A et al. (1989) Carpal tunnel: MR imaging. Part I: normal anatomy. Radiology 171: 749–756
7. Mesgarzadeh M, Schneck CD, Bonakdarpour A et al. (1989) Carpal tunnel: MR imaging. Part II: carpal tunnel syndrome. Radiology 171: 750–761
8. Healy C, Watson JD, Longstaff A, Cambell MJ (1990) MRI of the carpal tunnel J Hand Surg 15B: 243–251
9. Buchberger W, Schon G, Strasser K, Jungwirth W (1991) High-resolution ultrasonography of the carpal tunnel J Ultrasound Med 10: 531–539
10. Buchberger W, Judmeier W, Birbamer G et al. (1992) Carpal tunnel syndrome:diagnosis with high-resolution sonography AJR 159: 793–800
11. Chen P, Maklad N, Redwine M, Zelit D (1997) Dynamic high-resolution sonography of the carpal tunnel. AJR 168: 533–541
12. Ferrari FS (1997) L'ecografia con alta risoluzione nello studio della sindrome del tunnel carpale Rad Med 93: 336–341
13. Luyendijk W (1986) The carpal tunnel syndrome: the role of a persistent median artery Acta Neurol 79: 52–57
14. Asai M, Wong ACW, Matsunaga T, Akahoshi Y (1986) Carpal tunnel syndrome caused by aberrant lumbrical muscle associated with cistic degeneration of synovium: a case report. J Hand Surg 11A: 218–221
15. Zeiss J (1995) MR demonstration of an anomalous muscle in a patient with a coexistent carpal and ulnar tunnel syndrome Clin Imaging 109: 102–107
16. Ham SJ (1996) Changes in the carpal tunnel due to action of the flexor tendons: visualization with MRI. J Hand Surg 21: 997–1003
17. Britz GW, Haynor DR, Kunz C et al. (1995) Carpal tunnel syndrome: correlation of MRI, clinical, electrodiagnostic and intraoperative findings. Neurosurgery 37: 1097–1103
18. Radack DM, Schweitzer ME, Taras J (1997) Carpal tunnel syndrome: are the MR findings a result of population selection bias. AJR 169: 1649–1655
19. West GA (1994) MR imaging signal changes in denervated muscles after peripheral nerve injury Neurosurgery 35: 1077–1083
20. Schuind F, Ventura M, Pastels JL (1990) Idiopathic carpal tunnel syndrome: histologic study of flexor tendon synovium. J Hand Surg 15A: 497–503
21. Kerrigan JJ, Berton JM, Jaeger SH (1988) Ganglion cysts and carpal tunnel syndrome. J Hand Surg 13A: 763–770
22. Guthikonda M, Setti Rengachary S, Gregory Balko M, Van Loveren H (1994) Lipofibromatous hamartoma of thre median nerve: case report with MR imaging correlation. Neurosurgery 35: 127–131
23. Brahme SK, Hodler J, Braun RM et al. (1997) Dynamic MR imaging of carpal tunnel syndrome. Skeletal Radiol 26: 482–488
24. Zeiss J, Skie M, Ebraheim N, Jackson W (1989) Anatomic relations between the median nerve and the flexor tendons in the carpal tunnel. MR evaluation in normal volunteers. AJR 153: 533–538
25. Ham SJ, Kolman WFA, Heeres J et al. (1996) Changes in the carpal tunnel due to action of the flexor tendons: visualization with MRI. J Hand Surg 21A: 997–1002
26. Richman JA, Gelberman RH, Rydevik BJ et al. (1989) Carpal tunnel syndrome: morphological changes after release of the transverse carpal ligament. J Hand Surg 14A: 852–858
27. Murphy RX, Chernofsky MA, Osborne MA, Wolson AH (1993) MRI in the evaluation of persistent carpal tunnel syndrome. J Hand Surg 18A: 113–119
28. Silberman-Hoffman O, Touan C, Miroux F et al. (1998) Contribution of MR imaging for the diagnosis of median

nerve lesion after endoscopic carpal tunnel release. Ann Chir Main 17: 291–297
29. Fornage BD (1988) Peripheral nerves of the extremities: imaging with US. Radiology 167: 179–185
30. Silvestri E., Martinoli C et al. (1995) Echotexture of peripheral nerves: correlation between US and histologic findings and criteria to differentiate tendons. Radiology 197: 291–296
31. Rankin EA (1988) Carpal tunnel syndrome: issues and answers. J Natl Med Assoc 87: 369–373
32. Nakamichi K, Takibana S (1995) Transverse sliding of the median nerve beneath the flexor retinaculum. J Hand Surg 20B: 460–466
33. Erel E, Dilley A, Greening J et. al. (2003) Longitudinal sliding of the median nerve in patients with carpal tunnel syndrome. The Journal of Hand Surgery 28:439–443
34. Nakamichi K, Tachibana S (1993) The use of ultrasonography in detection of synovitis in carpal tunnel syndrome. J Hand Surg 18B: 176–183

11 Quantitative Assessment of Historical and Objective Findings: A New Clinical Severity Scale of CTS

F. Giannini

Introduction

The quantification of impairment is a fundamental phase in the approach to any disease. It can be considered a step of the diagnostic procedure providing better classification of severity, enabling comparison of patient groups, and supplying baseline assessment for follow-up studies and for outcome evaluation after different therapies.

Historical data (symptoms), physical examination (signs), and electrodiagnostic study are the clues for recognition and characterization of the Carpal Tunnel Syndrome (CTS) patient. The neurophysiological aspects of this syndrome have been widely studied [1, 2] and most common electrodiagnostic methods provide quantitative data per se. Some neurophysiological classifications or grading scales based on sensory and motor median nerve conduction abnormalities have also been developed [3, 4]. Although electrodiagnostic examination is considered the most accurate single test, it cannot be regarded as a diagnostic gold standard because of false negatives, about 15% of symptomatic referred cases [2], and false positives, nearly 18% in the general population [5] and asymptomatic industrial workers [6]. The combination of electrophysiological findings and symptoms has been stated to provide the most accurate diagnosis of CTS in epidemiological studies, whereas the combination of symptoms and signs provide the most diagnostic information when electrodiagnostic study is not available [7]. Accurate clinical assessment should therefore be regarded as a crucial step in medical practice. In most cases, diagnosis is based on history and subjective symptoms. Objective physical examination does not reveal any abnormality in many hands with CTS, and sensory or motor deficits can be only detected in severe cases. Many authors have focused their studies on symptoms reported by patients and signs obtained by physical examination, separately and combined, comparing them with electrophysiological abnormalities. The sensitivity/specificity and the positive/negative predictive value of most common clinical items have been widely reported.

Objective Findings

Regarding objective findings, sensory loss, thenar muscle strength, and provocative tests have been assessed quantitatively. Here will be discussed the diagnostic accuracy and utility of tests in follow-up studies (see Chap. 8 entitled Clinical Diagnosis for proper application and interpretation of these tests).

Sensibility Testing

The tests most commonly used to assess hand sensibility are the static or moving two-point discrimination test and threshold test. The static and moving two-point discrimination test evaluates innervation density of large myelinated fibers [8], the former measuring slowly adapting fiber-receptors and the latter measuring quickly adapting fiber-receptors. The results of these tests are patient-age-dependent and may be influenced by wide interobserver variability. Many factors other than CTS, such as hand edema, temperature, and presence of callus, limit specificity. No correlation between this sensibility test and median nerve conduction findings has been found. In fact, the two-point discrimination test is generally normal in mild or moderate CTS [9]. Under such conditions, nerve fiber density may be almost normal or slightly reduced and stimulus perception may be replaced by cortical mechanisms of integration, whereas sensory nerve conduction study already reveals some abnormalities. In a recent meta-analysis of the literature, the pooled positive and negative likelihood ratios (LR+ and LR–) were estimated at 1.3 and 1.0, respectively [10]. Moreover, low responsiveness to change has been found in postsurgical assessment, leading to poor reliability as an outcome measurement [11].

Similar conclusions have been drawn for vibrometry testing with tuning fork, the first method proposed for measuring the threshold of quickly adapting fiber-receptors in peripheral nerve disease [12]. The sensitivity and specificity are low (pooled LR+ 1.6 and LR– 0.8) [10] and reproducibility is insufficient (Cohen ϰ coefficient 0.40) [13]. More elaborate and expensive devices have subsequently been developed to improve accuracy in measuring and monitoring vibration threshold. Since these techniques are very time consuming, they have never become common in clinical practice.

The Semmes-Weinstein monofilament test evaluates the sensibility threshold of the same nerve fiber population and seems to be more accurate than innervation density tests for assessing sensory impairment in CTS. The sensitivity and specificity of monofilament testing in CTS diagnosis vary in the literature, mostly because of differences in methods and control populations. When tested in clinically defined patients, the sensitivity was 0.65 and specificity 0.88 [14], whereas in comparison with electrodiagnostic findings both resulted 0.59 [15]. A recent study showed sufficient specificity but very low sensitivity of the classical (liberal) test applied to the first three radial fingers. When sensory threshold was measured comparing middle to little finger (conservative test), sensitivity increased but specificity unfortunately decreased. The authors concluded that the Semmes-Weinstein monofilament testing is useless in suspected CTS [16]. Although the results of this test mprove after surgical release, no correlation with patient satisfaction has been reported [11].

Motor Testing

Motor function testing of the median nerve is quickly and easily performed and involves observing the bulk of the thenar muscles and assessing the strength of resisted thumb abduction and resisted pinching between thumb and little fingers. Hypotrophy of the thenar muscles is evaluated by comparison with the opposite side or other hand muscles, whereas weakness can be quantified on the basis of the 0–5 MRC grading scale or by using grip or pinch dynamometers. Motor deficits occur late in the course of the disease and only in severe cases of CTS, and therefore do not help in the recognition of most patients, but when present, they clearly differentiate subjects with and without CTS (LR+ 1.8 and LR– 0.5) [10]. Reproducibility of this test is poor with Cohen $\varkappa$ coefficient 0.25 [13]. Moreover, low responsiveness has been shown after surgery [11].

Provocative Testing

Provocative tests used in CTS diagnosis are based on stressing the wrist in order to induce or exacerbate symptoms (paresthesia or pain) in hand territory innervated by an impaired median nerve. Some of them, such as wrist-flexion (Phalen's test) or wrist-extension (reverse Phalen's test), median nerve percussion (Tinel's test), and compression (pressure provocation test), have become routine investigative procedures. Studies into the diagnostic accuracy of these clinical signs in comparison with electrodiagnostic findings have produced contrasting results. Sensitivity ranged from 0.10 to 0.91 and specificity from 0.33 to 0.86 for Phalen sign [10]. Similar variations have been reported for the pressure provocation test (sensitivity 0.28–0.63, specificity 0.33–0.74), Tinel test (sensitivity 0.23–0.60, specificity 0.64–0.87) [10], and reverse Phalen's test (sensitivity 0.41–0.90; specificity 0.56–1.0) [17–19]. These discrepancies may be related to clinical, methodological, and statistical factors, including referral bias, small number of patients examined, different diagnostic criteria of CTS, different characteristics of control subjects, and examination techniques. However, such wide variation is probably due to the fact that many clinical features actually depend on the severity of nerve impairment, and whether or not a sign is present could depend on the stage of CTS.

To verify this hypothesis we conducted a study on the four above-mentioned provocative tests in 179 patients with clinical and electrophysiological findings consistent with idiopathic CTS, 147 healthy control subjects, and 39 patients with polyneuropathy of different types [20]. The diagnostic accuracy of each test, alone and in combination, is summarized in Table 11.1. None of the conventional tests reached sufficient diagnostic accuracy, especially in distinguishing CTS from polyneuropathy. Indeed, most signs may often be evoked in peripheral nerve diseases other than CTS patients, the Tinel sign being the most frequent (44% in polyneuropathy group), as previously observed [21]. Combining the different tests did not significantly improve diagnostic accuracy, as found in other studies

Table 11.1. Diagnostic accuracy of provocative test alone or in combination (179 CTS patients)

	Compared to control group ($n=147$)				Compared to polyneuropathy group ($n=39$)		
	Sensitivity	Specificity	PPV	NPV	Specificity	PPV	NPV
Phalen sign	0.59	0.93	0.91	0.65	0.72	0.90	0.27
Wrist extension	0.55	0.96	0.94	0.63	0.82	0.93	0.26
Pressure provocation test	0.42	0.99	0.97	0.58	0.95	0.97	0.26
Tinel sign	0.41	0.90	0.83	0.56	0.56	0.81	0.17
One positive sign in a pair[a]	0.64–0.73	0.84–0.95	0.84–0.94	0.67–0.73	0.49–0.77	0.86–0.93	0.24–0.35
Both positive signs in a pair[a]	0.20–0.41	0.97–1.00	0.95–1.0	0.50–0.57	0.77–1.00	0.93–1.00	0.32–0.51
Any signs	0.83	0.84	0.87	0.80	0.47	0.76	0.37

[a] Values are minimum and maximum of the six possible pairs of signs; PPV, positive predictive value; NPV, negative predictive value (reprinted from [20] with permission from Elsevier)

Table 11.2. Sensitivity of the four provocative tests in relation to the clinical and electrophysiological severity of CTS

	Phalen	Wrist extension	Pressure	Tinel
Hi-Ob Scale				
Stage 1 ($n=46$)	0.63	0.56	0.26	0.37
Stage 2 ($n=63$)	0.73	0.57	0.54	0.46
Stage 3 ($n=42$)	0.55	0.68	0.52	0.45
Stage 4 ($n=18$)	0.33	0.39	0.44	0.44
Stage 5 ($n=10$)	0.10	0.10	0	0.10
P	0.0004	0.014	0.0015	0.25
Neurophysiological classes				
Stage 1 "MIN" ($n=25$)	0.72	0.48	0.36	0.40
Stage 2 "MILD" ($n=16$)	0.44	0.56	0.37	0.44
Stage 3 "MOD" ($n=94$)	0.65	0.60	0.43	0.40
Stage 4 "SEV" ($n=34$)	0.53	0.59	0.62	0.53
Stage 5 "EXT" ($n=10$)	0.10	0.10	0	0.10
P	0.0046	0.046	0.010	0.20

(reprinted from [20] with permission from Elsevier)

[17, 22, 23]. Sensitivity was also calculated according to a historical-objective severity scale (see below, "A New Clinical Scale: Validation of the Measurement") and a five-point neurophysiological classification [3]. Table 11.2 shows a significant decreasing trend of sensitivity with increasing clinical and neurophysiological severity. Although it would be reasonable to expect a correlation between abnormal tests findings and the clinical and electrophysiological severity of CTS, none of the previous studies addressed this aspect. The ability of many conventional provocative tests to induce positive sensory symptoms, such as paresthesia and pain, by means of increasing intracarpal tunnel pressure, probably weakens in the course of the disease because of progressive axonal loss. Our data clearly demonstrated that the sensitivity of provocation tests depends on the severity of the CTS, in the sense that the prevalence of abnormal findings is significantly less in advanced clinical and electrophysiological stages of the disease.

In conclusion, traditional provocative tests have limited value in distinguishing patients with and without CTS and are not useful in follow-up studies because positivity generally persists after surgery.

Historical Findings

A common opinion in clinical practice is that major clues for the diagnosis of CTS are to be found in the patient's history.

Hand Diagram

The first attempt to standardize historical data is the hand diagram, adapted from that used in the evaluation of back pain and proposed by Katz et al. in 1990 [23, 24].

Before physical and electrodiagnostic examination, patients are asked to shade the areas and quality of their symptoms on a hand diagram. The rating system is based on the anatomic allocation of pain/paresthesia or reduced sensation and leads to four hand diagram patterns of increasing diagnostic certainty: "classic," symptoms in at least two of digits 1, 2, or 3, palm and dorsum of hand excluded; "probable," same distribution with palmar symptoms allowed unless confined to the ulnar aspect; "possible," symptoms in at least one of digits 1, 2, or 3; "unlikely," no symptoms in same digits. The diagnostic sensitivity and specificity of "classic" or "probable" hand diagrams in selected populations are 0.64 and 0.73 with LR+ 2.4 and LR– 0.5, respectively [23]. When administered in an unselected population, these patterns have lower absolute diagnostic values (0.50), but are confirmed to be better positive predictors than Tinel sign, Phalen sign, sensory loss, and nocturnal symptoms [24]. It is therefore very unlikely that a patient with a "classic" or "probable" pattern does not have CTS. In order to assess hand diagrams as a predictor of surgical outcome, a subsequent study classified the symptoms into three groups, dividing the hand into six anatomical regions, and compared the results with a symptom/function, self-administered questionnaire and the SF-36 mental health subscale, before and six months after surgery [25]. Several distinct symptom patterns were associated with the three prominent outcomes and the hand diagram may be able to preoperatively identify worse or less satisfying outcomes, as in patients receiving Workers' Compensation. Nevertheless, the method used for statistically meaningful quantification of the diagram is too complex and lacks practical utility for assessment of symptom severity in follow-up studies.

Self-Administered Questionnaires

Besides conventional physical or instrumental assessments of objective impairment, the methodology of outcome studies requires standardized and reliable measures of patients' main subjective concerns. In the CTS, as in several other conditions, patients mainly seek relief of symptoms and functional improvement. In other words, outcome evaluation of any treatment cannot dismiss the patient's point of view ("patient-oriented" evaluation). For this purpose, generic measurements of health-related quality of life, such as the Nottingham Health Profile (NHF) [26] and the Medical Outcome Survey Short Form-36 (SF-36) [27], and anatomical region-specific outcome instruments, such as the Disabilities of the Arm, Shoulder and Hand (DASH) self-administered questionnaire [28], were employed in patients with CTS [29–31]. Moreover, some disease-specific questionnaires, such as the Boston Carpal Tunnel Questionnaire (BCTQ) [32] and others subsequently modified [33–35], were developed for the assessment of clinical severity and therapeutic outcome. Chapter 50, Outcomes Assessment Protocols, of the current book extensively deals with this fundamental issue.

A New Clinical Scale: Validation of the Measurement

Using severity scores based only on patient-oriented items in the above questionnaires, symptoms and functions are generally summarized by one or two scores that do not, however, characterize the main clinical feature of each patient. This aim may be achieved by a clinical classification that incorporates both the patient's and the physician's point of view. For instance, a patient (usually young) often complains of severe symptoms but physical examination fails to reveal abnormalities, whereas another patient (usually elderly) may show severe sensory and motor deficits, even complete thenar muscle atrophy, but only complain of mild symptoms. If patients underestimate their functional impairment, BCTQ scores will be lower than that of patients with a less severe degree of the disease. A simple and reliable means of assessing symptoms and signs together was still lacking in the literature until we proposed a new clinical Historical-Objective (Hi-Ob) scale [36]. The scale is a modified version of a previously reported scale [37]. It was not designed for a proper diagnostic purpose but to classify clinical severity of CTS patients and has been used in broad Italian multicenter studies (see Chap. 51, "Carpal Tunnel Syndrome: Multicenter Studies With Multiperspective Assessment: Results of the Italian CTS Study Group") [38–41].

Among data obtained from clinical history and physical examination (required for independent diagnosis of CTS), we have selected the following findings to create the Hi-Ob grading scale: (A) any kind of paresthesia in the hand (numbness, tingling, burning etc.) with regard to its temporal onset and duration, (B) sensory function in hand territory innervated by the median nerve, (C) motor function of median-innervated muscles of the hand, (D) trophism of the thenar eminence and (E) pain, reported as dull or aching discomfort in the hand, forearm, or upper arm. The Hi-Ob scale therefore consists of two figures. The first is a ordinal scale (Hi-Ob) of increasing severity, determined by symptoms and objective findings (A–D), namely:

Stage 0: No symptoms suggesting CTS
Stage 1: Only nocturnal paresthesia
Stage 2: Diurnal paresthesia
Stage 3: Sensory deficit
Stage 4: Hypotrophy and/or motor deficit of median-innervated thenar muscles
Stage 5: Complete atrophy or paralysis of median-innervated thenar muscles

The second figure regards the presence or absence of pain (item E), a dichotomous categorical score obtained from a forced-choice answer (yes or no) of the patient. In other words, an associated mark was defined. The final score is a number (stage) with or without the pain variable (PAIN). For example, a case with nocturnal and diurnal paresthesia as well as pain, is scored "2P," a case with sensory but nonmotor deficit, without pain is scored "3." The scale is therefore "mixed," the score PAIN being a single patient-oriented item. There are certain practical recommendations for correctly applying the Hi-Ob scale:

0: After critical analysis of reported symptoms, assign "0" only if no symptoms were present in the previous two weeks.
1: Assign "1" regardless of which and how many median-innervated fingers have the symptom; assign "1" even in the case of paresthesia on awakening, if disappearance is rapid.
2: See first line above; assign "2" even in the case of transient diurnal symptoms after repetitive movements or prolonged postures.
3: Use cotton wool to compare sensation of the palmar aspect of the second and third vs. fifth finger; assign "3" for hypoesthesia or sensory lack of one or both median-innervated fingers; the test may also be done by other commonly used methods of sensory evaluation, such as Semmes-Weinstein monofilament or two-point discrimination test.
4: Assign "4" when there is selective hypotrophy of thenar muscles compared to other hand muscles, or weakness evaluated by resistance to thumb abduction at right angle to the palm.
5: Assign "5" for muscle atrophy defined as concavity of thenar eminence with respect to the plane of palm or paralysis defined as inability to abduct thumb ventrally from palm.

PAIN: Assign "P" if pain was present in the previous 2 weeks.

The items of the scale were suggested by personal clinical experience, by the studies mentioned above, and by AAN recommendations [1] and appear "appropriate to the task" and internally consistent. Indeed, the progression of the score from subjective sensory symptoms to severe motor impairment is in line with the pathological basis of the disease and reflects different stages in the development of the median nerve lesion inside the carpal tunnel [42]. In this respect, the earlier degree, due to increase in intrafascicular pressure, is characterized by hyperexcitability and spontaneous discharge of some sensory fibers, causing episodes of paresthesia and/or pain, often distributed in a patchy manner over the median field, but with no clinical sensory loss. In the next stage, endoneural edema causes structural changes and conduction block in more vul-

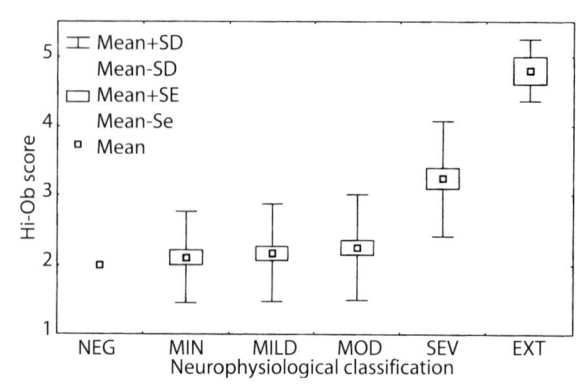

Fig. 11.1. Relationship between neurophysiological picture and clinical scale (reprinted from [36] with permission from Elsevier)

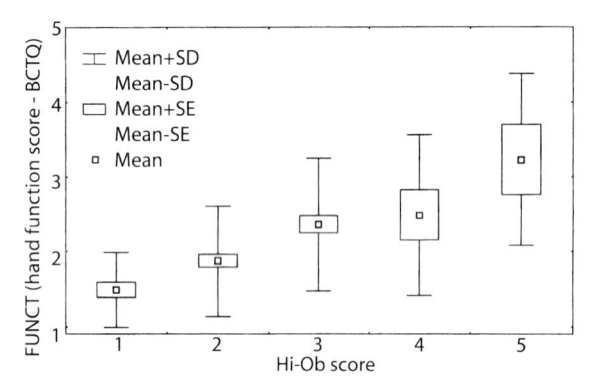

Fig. 11.2. Relationship between clinical scale and hand function (reprinted from [36] with permission from Elsevier)

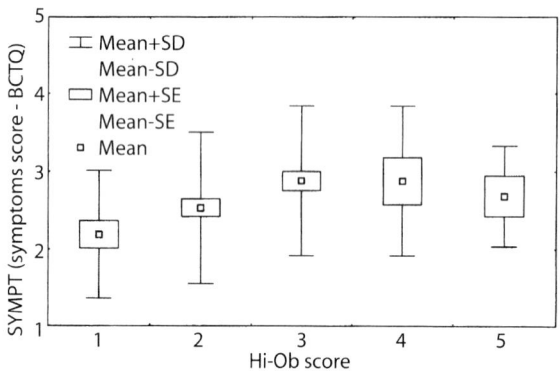

Fig. 11.3. Relationship between clinical scale and symptoms (reprinted from [36] with permission from Elsevier)

nerable nerve fibers, first inducing sensory deficit and later weakness of thenar muscles. In the final stage, very few thinner fibers survive inside fibrotic fascicules: sensation is lacking and the thenar muscles become paralyzed and wasted.

In order to validate this scale we studied 168 consecutive idiopathic CTS hands through a multiperspective assessment using validated neurophysiological and patient-oriented measurements of CTS severity. The results obtained with the Hi-Ob scale were compared with 11-item "symptom" scores (SYMPT) and 8-item "functional" scores (FUNCT) of the BCTQ [32]. They were also compared with a previously described nominal six-point neurophysiological classification (NEGATIVE, MINIMAL, MILD, MODERATE, SEVERE, AND EXTREME), based on the degree of motor and sensory (conventional, segmental, or comparative) conduction impairment of the median nerve, according to a protocol inspired by AAN and AAEM recommendations [3]. Correlation analysis showed that the Hi-Ob scale was positively related to duration of symptoms with high statistical significance ($p<0.001$, $r=0.36$). A highly significant positive relationship was also observed between Hi-Ob score and neurophysiological classes ($p<0.001$, $r=0.42$) (Fig. 11.1). Only two hands, one with Hi-Ob score 2 and the other with Hi-Ob score 2P, had normal electrophysiological findings in all tests (NEG). A significant linear correlation was observed between Hi-Ob score and FUNCT ($p<0.001$, $r=0.41$) (Fig. 11.2). Although a significant relationship was observed between Hi-Ob and SYMPT ($p<0.005$, $r=0.23$), we noticed that patients with Hi-Ob score 5 had a milder symptom picture than patients with minor clinical impairment (Hi-Ob score 4 and 3) (Fig. 11.3).

The second dichotomous categorical score was used to define two groups of hands. Statistical analysis of these two groups of hands showed that PAIN (64% of hands) is not significantly related to age and duration of symptoms but was significantly related to Hi-Ob stages, SYMPT, and FUNCT scores ($p<0.001$), and neurophysiological classification ($p<0.02$). PAIN was more frequent in MOD and SEV groups of neurophysiological classification and in stages 2, 3, and 4 of Hi-Ob classification, being less frequent in earlier and more advanced cases. The Hi-Ob scale was designed to evaluate the subjective item "pain" as a separate category since not all patients complain of pain but, when reported, this symptom has great influence on the severity of the clinical picture. Indeed, pain is often the key symptom for surgical evaluation in clinical practice. Another reason is that pain often appeared to be quite unrelated to the other clinical features of CTS.

This study showed that our mixed scale covers all types and degrees of the disease. In fact, it allowed us to reliably assess most CTS hands without a history of objective motor-sensory impairment. It also enabled assessment of severe CTS by objective measurement at physical examination.

The analysis of reproducibility of the proposed scale was performed according to the Snedecor and Cochrane methods. Four independent observers, blind to the electrodiagnostic results, assessed 50 consecutive patients to evaluate interobserver error. The observers also scored Hi-Ob scale twice at an interval of at least 2 days to evaluate the intraobserver error. Paired comparison between observer scores showed high interobserver reliability and intraobserver reproducibility (Cohen ϰ coefficient >0.75).

To confirm interobserver reproducibility and to test the responsiveness of the Hi-Ob scale to changes in clinical status, we prospectively studied a consecutive series of 254 hands (219 patients) with idiopathic CTS, referred for surgical decompression [43]. The same multiperspective protocol was applied before and 6 months after surgery. Interobserver variability was evaluated by comparing stages assigned by the neurophysiologist and by the neurosurgeon before surgery. The percentage of assignments to the same severity stage by the two observers was 78% with a Cohen κ coefficient 0.69 (95% CI: 0.62–0.76), indicating high statistical agreement.

The responsiveness of the scale was tested by comparing the neurophysiologist's stages before the operation and 6 months later, using a nonparametric test for paired data (sign test). A significant improvement in severity score was observed in the whole statistical sample ($p<0.001$). With regard to pain, all patients referred for surgery had a positive item (P+) by virtue of patient selection criteria. After the operation, pain persisted in only 19 hands (7%). Surgery led to improvement of the mean BCTQ score and the mean neurophysiological score, confirming the relationship between pre- and postoperative values of these parameters, as reported in other studies [44, 45]. The presurgical relation between Hi-Ob stage and BCTQ or neurophysiological classification also persisted after the operation ($p<0.001$). Absence of symptoms (stage 0) was achieved by almost all subjects initially in Hi-Ob stages 1 and 2. Thirty percent of hands in stage 3 were also symptom-free and without sensory deficit after decompression. Hands in higher stages (4 and 5), with motor deficit and/or wasting of muscles, rarely changed stage. This may reflect the relations between clinical symptoms and physiopathological events underlying CTS, characterized by severe axonal loss in advanced phases of the disease. Nevertheless, pain disappeared in most patients in stages 4 and 5. These results as a whole indicated that the Hi-Ob scale very reliably reflects clinical events in CTS, and is coherent with other validated measures. Inter- and intraobserver testing confirmed that the scale gives highly reproducible results. This may be due to the clear terminology and simple methods used in stage definition, facilitating scoring. The Hi-Ob scale also proved to be responsive to changes in clinical status after surgical decompression and sufficiently descriptive of clinical improvement.

Conclusions

On the basis of the literature reviewed and the above remarks, we conclude that no single clinical item has sufficient predictive value for CTS. An accurate clinical diagnosis of CTS can only be obtained by complete historical interview and careful physical examination, including recognition of a wide range of symptoms and signs. Among various standardized tools, the hand symptom diagram ("classic" or "probable" patterns) may be of some diagnostic utility as screening of symptomatic patients and, in combination with electrophysiological tests, seems to have the best predictive value for defining cases of CTS. However, the hand diagram is unable to quantify the severity of clinical impairment and seems to be not useful for follow-up studies.

For this purpose, the most widely used instrument is the BCTQ, the first specific patient-oriented score proposed for CTS. Its internal consistency, validity, and reproducibility have been demonstrated and its sensitivity to clinical change has been confirmed by many studies.

Besides patient-oriented evaluation, the Historical-Objective scale proposed by us proves to be a reliable, reproducible, and responsive measurement, able to characterize and quantify clinical severity of patients "from a physician's point of view."

Together with the BCTQ and neurophysiological classification, the Historical-Objective scale was recently proposed as a standardized protocol of outcome evaluation for surgical release of CTS, useful for routine clinical management and for scientific purposes [46].

References

1. AAN, AAEM, AAPMR (1993) Practice parameter for electrodiagnostic studies in carpal tunnel syndrome: summary statement. Muscle Nerve 16:1390–1393
2. AAN, AAEM, AAPMR (2002) Practice parameter: Electrodiagnostic studies in carpal tunnel syndrome. Muscle Nerve 25:918–922
3. Padua L, Lo Monaco M, Gregori B, Valente EM, Padua R, Tonali P (1997) Neurophysiological classification and sensitivity in 500 carpal tunnel syndrome hands. Acta Neurol Scand 96:211–217
4. Bland JDP (2000) A neurophysiological grading scale for carpal tunnel syndrome. Muscle Nerve 23:1280–1283
5. Atroshi I, Gummesson C, Johnsson R et al. (1999) Prevalence of carpal tunnel syndrome in a general population. JAMA 282:153–158
6. Nathan PA, Takigawa K, Keniston RC et al. (1994) Slowing of sensory conduction of the median nerve and carpal tunnel syndrome in Japanese and American industrial workers. J Hand Surg [Br] 19:30–34
7. Rempel D, Evanoff B, Amadio PC et al. (1998) Consensus criteria for the classification of carpal tunnel syndrome in epidemiologic studies. Am J Public Health 88:1447–1451
8. Moberg E (1958) Objective methods for determining the functional value of sensibility in the hand. J Bone Joint Surg 40:454–476

9. Marlowe ES, Francis JB, Berkowitz AR (1999) Correlation between two-point discrimination and median nerve sensory response. Muscle Nerve 22:1196–1200
10. D'Arcy CA, McGee S (2000) Does this patient have carpal tunnel syndrome? JAMA 283:3110–3117
11. Katz JN, Gelberman RH, Wright EA et al. (1994) Responsiveness of self-reported and objective measures of disease severity in carpal tunnel syndrome. Med Care 32:1127–1133
12. Dellon AL (1980) Clinical use of vibratory stimuli to evaluate peripheral nerve injury and compression neuropathy. Plast Reconstr Surg 65:466–476
13. Marx RG, Hudak PL, Bombardier C et al. (1998) The reliability of physical examination for carpal tunnel syndrome. J Hand Surg [Br] 23:499–502
14. Szabo RM, Slater RR, Farver TB et al. (1999) The value of diagnostic testing in carpal tunnel syndrome. J Hand Surg [Am] 24:704–714
15. Buch-Jaeger N, Foucher G (1994) Correlation of clinical signs with nerve conduction tests in the diagnosis of carpal tunnel syndrome. J Hand Surg [Br] 19:720–724
16. Pagel KJ, Kaul MP, Dryden JD (2002) Lack of utility of Semmes-Weinstein monofilament testing in suspected carpal tunnel syndrome. Am J Phys Med Rehabil 81:597–600
17. de Krom MCTF, Knipschild PG, Kester ADM, Spaans F (1990). Efficacy of provocative tests for diagnosis of carpal tunnel syndrome. Lancet 335:393–395
18. Werner RA, Bir C, Armstrong TJ (1994) Reverse Phalen's maneuver as an aid in diagnosing carpal tunnel syndrome. Arch Phys Med Rehabil 75:783–786
19. LaBan MM, Friedman NA, Zemenick GA (1986) "Tethered" median nerve stress test in chronic carpal tunnel syndrome. Arch Phys Med Rehabil 67:803–804
20. Mondelli M, Passero S, Giannini F (2001) Provocative tests in different stages of carpal tunnel syndrome. Clin Neurol Neurosurg 103:178–181
21. Jabre JF, Dillard JW, Salzsieder BT et al. (1995) The use of multiple Tinel's sign in identification of patients with peripheral neuropathy. Electromyogr Clin Neurophysiol 35:131–136
22. Gellman H, Gelberman RH, Mae Tan A, Botte MJ (1986) Carpal tunnel syndrome. An evaluation of the provocative diagnostic tests. J Bone Joint Surg 68:735–737
23. Katz JN, Larson MG, Sabra A et al. (1990) The carpal tunnel syndrome: diagnostic utility of the history and physical examination findings. Ann Int Med 112:321–327
24. Katz JN and Stirrat CR (1990) A self-administered hand diagram for the diagnosis of carpal tunnel syndrome. J Hand Surg 15A:360–363
25. Bessette L, Keller RB, Lew RA et al. (1997) Prognostic value of a hand symptom diagram in surgery for carpal tunnel syndrome. J Rheumatol 24:726–734
26. Hunt SM, McEwen J, McKenna SP (1986) Measuring health status. Croon Helm, Beckenham
27. Ware JE, Snow KK, Kosinski M, Gandek B (1993) SF-36 Health Survey: manual and interpretation guide. New England Medical Center, Health Institute, Boston
28. Hudak PL, Amadio PC, Bombardier C, and the Upper Extremity Collaborative Group (UECG) (1996) Development of an upper extremity outcome measure: the DASH (disabilities of the arm, shoulder and hand) [corrected]. Am J Ind Med 29:602–608
29. Vaile JH, Mathers DM, Ramos-Remus C, Russel A (1999) Generic health instruments do not comprehensively capture patient perceived improvement in patients with carpal tunnel syndrome. J Rheumatol 26:1163–1166
30. Gummesson C, Atroshi I, Ekdahl C (2003) The disabilities of the arm, shoulder and hand (DASH) outcome questionnaire: longitudinal construct validity and measuring self-rated health change after surgery. BMC Musculoskeletal Disorders 4:11, http://www.biomedical.com/1471–2474/4/11
31. Gay RE, Amadio PC, Johnson JC (2003) Comparative responsiveness of the disabilities of the arm, shoulder, and hand, the carpal tunnel questionnaire, and the SF-36 to clinical change after carpal tunnel release. J Hand Surg [Am] 28:250–254
32. Levine DW, Simmons B, Koris MJ et al. (1993) A self-administered questionnaire for the assessment of severity of symptoms and functional status in carpal tunnel syndrome. J Bone Joint Surg 75A:1585–1592
33. Herskovitz S, Berger AR, Lipton RB (1995) Low-dose, short-term oral prednisone in the treatment of carpal tunnel syndrome. Neurology 45:1923–1925
34. You H, Simmons Z, Freivaldos A et al. (1999) Relationship between clinical symptom severity scales and nerve conduction measures in carpal tunnel syndrome. Muscle Nerve 22:497–501
35. Bland JDP (2000) The value of the history in the diagnosis of carpal tunnel syndrome. J Hand Surg [Br] 25:445–450
36. Giannini F, Cioni R, Mondelli M et al. (2002) A new clinical scale of carpal tunnel syndrome: validation of the measurement and clinical-neurophysiological assessment. Clin Neurophysiol 113: 71–77
37. Giannini F, Passero S, Cioni R et al. (1991) Electrophysiologic evaluation of local steroid injection in carpal tunnel syndrome. Arch Phys Med Rehabil 72:738–742
38. Padua L, Padua R, Lo Monaco M et al. (1999) Multiperspective assessment of carpal tunnel syndrome: a multicenter study. Italian CTS Study Group. Neurology 53:1654–1659
39. Padua L, Padua R, Aprile I, Tonali P (1999) Italian multicentre study of carpal tunnel syndrome. Differences in the clinical and neurophysiological features between male and female patients. J Hand Surg [Br] 24:579–582
40. Padua L, Padua R, Aprile I et al. Italian CTS Study Group (2001) Multiperspective follow-up of untreated carpal tunnel syndrome: a multicenter study. Neurology 56:1459–1466
41. Padua L, Aprile I, Caliandro P et al. Italian Carpal Tunnel Syndrome Study Group (2002) Carpal tunnel syndrome in pregnancy: multiperspective follow-up of untreated cases. 59:1643–1646
42. Sunderland S (1991) Nerve injuries and their repair. A critical neurology appraisal. Churchill Livingstone, London
43. Mondelli M, Ginanneschi F, Rossi S et al. (2002) Inter-observer reproducibility and responsiveness of a clinical severity scale in surgically treated carpal tunnel syndrome. Acta Neurol Scand 106:263–268
44. Mondelli M, Reale F, Sicurelli F, Padua L (2000) Relationship between the self-administered Boston Questionnaire and electrophysiological findings in follow-up of surgically-treated carpal tunnel syndrome. J Hand Surg [Br] 25:128–134
45. Padua L, Lo Monaco M, Padua R et al. (1995) Carpal tunnel syndrome: neurophysiological results of surgery based on preoperative electrodiagnostic testing. J Hand Surg [Br] 22:599–601
46. Reale F, Ginanneschi F, Sicurelli F, Mondelli M (2003) Protocol of outcome evaluation for surgical release of carpal tunnel syndrome. Neurosurgery 53:343–351

Differential Diagnosis of Carpal Tunnel Syndrome

P.C. Amadio

Carpal tunnel syndrome is a common clinical condition, occurring in as much as 5% of the population [1, 2]. Although it is quite common, the differential diagnosis can be quite complex. This is because the diagnostic criteria of carpal tunnel syndrome are, to some extent, subjective.

Carpal tunnel syndrome is primarily diagnosed from a typical pattern of symptoms, including nocturnal paresthesias in the median nerve distribution, and certain specific activity-aggravated paresthesias, such as paresthesias from prolonged grip, as would occur for example in holding a book or newspaper or the steering wheel of an automobile [3]. Patients often describe shaking the hands to relieve the symptoms. Some patients describe pain radiating up the arm, even as far as the shoulder.

Sometimes patients may not be clear, either in their own minds, or in communication, with regard to the location of the symptoms, specifically to the median nerve distribution. In addition, patients may not be clear as to the nature of the symptoms, referring to the difficulty as pain, numbness, or tingling variably and perhaps not even recognizing that a physician makes a significant distinction between those three terms, while the patient may consider them relatively synonymous. Weakness, awkwardness, and lack of dexterity are all common symptoms associated with carpal tunnel syndrome, but, of course, can be associated with many other conditions [3, 4].

That being said, in many cases the diagnosis of carpal tunnel syndrome is clear cut. Patients with nocturnal paresthesias limited to the median nerve distribution, aggravated by specific symptoms, and with physical findings which localize to the median nerve at the level of the wrist, are commonly seen. In such patients, the clinician can be fairly confident as to the diagnosis.

In many other patients, the diagnosis is not so clear, because of the varying nature of the symptoms presented. Pain is the most confusing symptom. Many specific and nonspecific conditions can present with pain, carpal tunnel syndrome among them. If this is the only symptom and there are no physical findings, then a diagnosis of carpal tunnel syndrome is not particularly likely. However, the patient or clinician may believe that a diagnosis of carpal tunnel syndrome exists, because of associated circumstances, such as occupation. In such cases, it is important to establish a diagnosis by other means, such as electrodiagnostic testing [5–10].

Numbness and paresthesias are also common symptoms of carpal tunnel syndrome, but may of course be caused by other neurological and nonneurological disorders, especially when the symptoms are constant, and do not follow the characteristic pattern of aggravation at night or with activity seen in carpal tunnel syndrome [6]. These other conditions are discussed below. Again, electrodiagnostic testing is often helpful in distinguishing these conditions from carpal tunnel syndrome.

Weakness, atrophy, or loss of dexterity are also symptoms that can be associated with carpal tunnel syndrome, but which may be present in many other conditions, both neurological and nonneurological. Injuries and even congenital anomalies can be confused with carpal tunnel syndrome, when a diagnosis is based primarily on a complaint of weakness or loss of dexterity.

Useful tests to establish the diagnosis of carpal tunnel syndrome are few. The most valuable is electrodiagnostic testing [5]. Electromyography and nerve conduction studies have been well described and remain for many clinicians the gold standard diagnostic test. However, there are many false negative cases [11], in which the clinical diagnosis is extremely clear-cut but electrodiagnostic testing is normal. This is to be expected, as the electrodiagnostic tests reflect significant neurophysiological abnormalities. When findings are more mild or less chronic, electrodiagnostic changes may not be present.

There are other tests which are very useful to help to rule out a diagnosis of carpal tunnel syndrome [12]. X-rays of the wrist may show a fracture or other abnormality to explain symptoms of pain and weakness, or even occasional paresthesias. X-rays of the cervical spine may show evidence of cervical spondylosis. Laboratory studies may show evidence of abnormalities of blood sugar, inflammatory markers such as rheumatoid factor or sedimentation rate, or endocrine markers such as thyroid hormone levels, which may explain the

Table 12.1. Other neurological diagnoses that may present with a clinical picture similar to CTS

Intracranial neoplasm
Multiple sclerosis
Cervical radiculopathy
Cervical syringomyelia
Thoracic outlet syndrome
Pancoast tumor
Peripheral nerve tumor (schwannoma, hamartoma, etc.)
Idiopathic brachioplexitis (Parsonage-Turner syndrome/neuralgic amyotrophy)
Lower trunk brachial plexopathy
Pronator syndrome
Ulnar neuropathy
Radial neuropathy
Generalized neuropathy (diabetes/mononeuritis multiplex)
Churg-Strauss syndrome
Median nerve contusion

symptoms without the necessity to invoke a diagnosis of carpal tunnel syndrome [13]. In rare cases, a magnetic resonance imaging (MRI) or other tests may be useful to rule out diagnoses such as nerve tumors, particularly in the region of the brachial plexus [14].

Perhaps the most common and confusing differential diagnoses will occur when sorting out carpal tunnel syndrome from neurological disorders. There are many neurological disorders which can present with symptoms of pain, numbness, or weakness in the hands (Table 12.1). These are discussed below.

Intracranial neoplasms can sometimes present with history of numbness or tingling in the hand, weakness in the hand, or loss of coordination in the hand [6, 15–17]. Often, these findings will be associated with hyperreflexia, however, indicating that the diagnosis is more central. In addition, the pattern of weakness or hypoesthesia will typically not be in a distribution limited to that of the median nerve. Thus, a careful neurological examination, combined with appropriate imagining studies such as MRI, is the key factor in sorting out CNS neoplasia from carpal tunnel syndrome.

Multiple sclerosis can be superficially confused with carpal tunnel syndrome, but can be readily distinguished by a careful neurological evaluation, since the diagnosis of multiple sclerosis requires, as its name suggests, multiple events and multiple sites of pathology, none of which would be typical for carpal tunnel syndrome. Other CNS disorders, such as amyotrophic lateral sclerosis or Charcot-Marie-Tooth disease, are pure motor neuropathies, and affect distal muscles diffusely, so that all the intrinsic muscles show weakness, and not just those of the thenar eminence [4].

Cervical radiculopathy is probably the most common neurological condition which can be confused with carpal tunnel syndrome, or which may coexist with carpal tunnel syndrome. Again, careful neurological evaluation will demonstrate weakness or numbness in proximal dermatomes or myotomes, not consistent with a diagnosis of focal median neuropathy. Pain or symptoms in the neck, particularly those aggravated with neck motion or neck compression, are also useful clues. Symptoms aggravated by coughing and sneezing are much more likely to be due to cervical radiculopathy than carpal tunnel syndrome.

Cervical syringomyelia can also be confused with carpal tunnel syndrome. The characteristic patterns of numbness or weakness, however, are quite different, reflecting the cervical spine origin of the symptoms.

Brachial plexus disorders can also be confused with carpal tunnel syndrome. In thoracic outlet syndrome, the symptoms are typically in the ulnar nerve distribution, and thus can be again distinguished by a careful neurological evaluation [18]. Pancoast tumor can be confused with carpal tunnel syndrome in that symptoms may be present in the hand, but the neurological distribution will be rather different, depending on the specific location of the Pancoast tumor [19]. It would be extremely unlikely for a tumor at the lung apex to specifically affect only the fibers going to the median nerve, particularly as some of these come from the medial cord and some from the lateral cord of the brachial plexus. Similarly, postradiation neuritis of the brachial plexus can cause extremity pain, hand numbness, and hand weakness, but the pattern will not be limited to the median nerve distribution, and electrodiagnostic tests will localize to the plexus and not the wrist [14].

Idiopathic brachial plexitis, otherwise known as Parsonage-Turner syndrome or neuralgic amyotrophy, is another condition which can be confused with carpal tunnel syndrome, but the findings are typically rather different [4]. Idiopathic brachial plexitis begins typically with a prodrome of severe proximal limb pain, followed in 7–10 days by marked weakness in one or more peripheral nerves, with little numbness. The distribution is typically not specifically in the distal median nerve distribution, although more proximal branches of the median nerve, such as the anterior interosseous nerve, may be affected. Such findings, out of the distribution of the median nerve in the carpal tunnel, argue strongly against the diagnosis of carpal tunnel syndrome. In doubtful cases, electrodiagnostic testing can help sort out the pathology.

Tumors within peripheral nerves can also simulate carpal tunnel syndrome [4]. This can be particularly difficult if the tumor is within the carpal tunnel, as is often the case with lipofibromatous hamartoma of nerve [20]. The key distinction here will be a relatively long history of a mass. Unlike the swelling of the flexor synovium that one can see in carpal tunnel syndrome, the nerve tumor enlargement will not move with active finger motion. MRI is oftentimes useful in sorting out the diagnosis more specifically.

Pronator syndrome is a specific neuropathy at the median nerve, more proximal than the carpal tunnel, which may be confused with carpal tunnel syndrome [21, 22]. Here there is significant overlap with the symptoms, but in pronator syndrome there may also be weakness of the anterior interosseous nerve. Some clinicians consider that a pronator syndrome exists when the patient has all the physical findings of carpal tunnel syndrome, but also has tenderness over the pronator area. In my experience, this is more likely to be a proximal-referred tenderness of the nerve associated with carpal tunnel syndrome, and not a true pronator syndrome. In cases in which a clinician considers pronator syndrome to be present, electrodiagnostic tests should always be performed. If the tests do not confirm a more proximal level of entrapment, then the diagnosis should be considered to be carpal tunnel syndrome, and the patient treated accordingly.

Patients with ulnar or radial neuropathy can be confused with carpal tunnel syndrome, particularly when a careful neurological examination is not done [7, 15, 19, 23, 24]. Numbness or tingling in the hand can occur with either, as can hand weakness. However, the distribution will be rather different in ulnar neuropathy or radial neuropathy, than in median neuropathy. Again, in doubtful cases, electrodiagnostic testing is quite useful in establishing the correct diagnosis.

Endocrine disorders such as diabetes mellitus can be associated with a generalized neuropathy [25]. This most often affects multiple nerves in the upper and lower extremity and that becomes the key factor in differential diagnosis. In the presence of neuropathies involving multiple nerves, other diagnoses besides isolated carpal tunnel syndrome should be considered. A specific disorder, uniquely present in patients with diabetes, kidney failure, and an upper extremity vascular shunt, is ischemic monomelic neuropathy [26]. In this condition the true pathology is the result of diabetic neuropathy aggravated by a vascular steal. The hallmark is a strong distal to proximal gradient of severity of the neuropathy, with severe changes in the most distal muscles and nerve, and progressively normal findings as one goes proximally. The only effective treatment is to remove the vascular shunt (usually after successful transplantation, or a change to peritoneal dialysis).

An uncommon cause of multiple neuropathies is Churg-Strauss syndrome [4]. Patients with asthma, allergic granulomatosis, and angiitis can develop multiple peripheral neuropathies. The disease is inflammatory and is treated with anti-inflammatory medication. Surgical decompression is typically not indicated.

Trauma to the median nerve can also be confused with carpal tunnel syndrome. This can be the case, for example, in patients with distal radius fractures [27–29]. In such patients, an acute carpal tunnel syndrome can develop due to hematoma within the carpal canal. In addition, however, the median nerve can be directly contused. In the latter case, surgical decompression may not be helpful. In doubtful cases, carpal tunnel pressure testing can be done, to establish the correct diagnosis. In patients with carpal tunnel syndrome, carpal canal pressure should be elevated. In cases of median nerve contusion, the pressure would be normal.

In addition to the many neurological conditions that can be confused with carpal tunnel syndrome, there are many nonneurological diagnoses that may present with a clinical picture similar to carpal tunnel syndrome [30] (Table 12.2).

Vascular disorders can often be confused with carpal tunnel syndrome because they may cause symptoms of paresthesias, and, when more evident in the radial artery distribution, can also overlap with the median nerve distribution of carpal tunnel syndrome. Raynaud's phenomenon can be confused with carpal tunnel syndrome because it can be aggravated by similar activities but, unlike carpal tunnel syndrome, Raynaud's phenomenon will have coldness and color changes in the finger tips [31]. In doubtful cases, noninvasive vascular studies such as cold stress testing and digital plethysmography can be done to establish the correct diagnosis. Hypothenar hammer syndrome, or ulnar artery thrombosis, can also be confused with car-

Table 12.2. Nonneurological diagnoses that may present with a clinical picture similar to CTS

Vascular
Raynaud's phenomenon
Hypothenar hammer syndrome (injury to ulnar artery in hand with secondary involvement of the ulnar nerve)
Hand-arm vibration syndrome

Congenital
Thumb hypoplasia

Traumatic
Wrist sprain or ligament injury
Carpal fracture
de Quervain's syndrome
Intersection syndrome
Flexor carpi radialis tenosynovitis
Linburg's syndrome
Flexor carpi ulnaris tenosynovitis
Trigger finger.

Degenerative
Osteoarthritis

Infectious
Sporothrix
Atypical or typical mycobacterial infection

Other Inflammatory
Rheumatoid arthritis
Gout

Miscellaneous
Nonspecific hand pain

pal tunnel syndrome causing similar vascular changes, but these are more typically on the ulnar side of the hand, are often associated with injury, and again can be differentiated by the presence of abnormal vascular studies and, often, the absence of neurological changes, particularly changes in the median nerve distribution.

Hand/arm vibration syndrome is another condition which can be confused with carpal tunnel syndrome, particularly in the working population [32–34]. Those who work with vibrating tools can develop a small fiber neuropathy as well as a small vessel vasculopathy. The symptoms of paresthesias can be quite similar to those of carpal tunnel syndrome, but, in hand/arm vibration syndrome the symptoms will be present in all the fingertips not just in the median nerve distribution and will typically not be associated with nerve conduction abnormalities in the carpal tunnel itself. Again, specific physical examination and electrodiagnostic testing can be helpful, as well as a careful history eliciting the exposure to vibrating tools.

Rarely, congenital hypoplasia of the thumb, if mild, can go unrecognized into adulthood and then be confused with carpal tunnel syndrome [35]. However, in such cases, the electrodiagnostic testing will be normal and x-rays may show hypoplasia of the thumb skeleton as well.

There are many traumatic conditions that can be confused with carpal tunnel syndrome. Wrist sprain or ligament injury can produce wrist pain which could be confused with the pain of carpal tunnel syndrome but of course would not be associated with neurological abnormality. Carpal fractures may similarly be associated with activity-related symptom aggravation and may be difficult to diagnose, particularly fractures of the hook of the hamate [36]. In doubtful cases, computed tomography can be quite helpful in establishing the correct diagnosis. Any patient with a history of significant injury to the hand, or symptoms of hand pain or paresthesias which came on after a history of hand trauma, should be evaluated for the possibility of carpal fracture.

There are a number of soft tissue conditions around the hand and wrist which can also be confused with carpal tunnel syndrome, particularly by the generalist who may be evaluating a patient with hand pain. Tenderness along one of the major wrist flexors, such as the flexor carpi radialis or flexor carpi ulnaris, can be confused with carpal tunnel syndrome, in that there is pain in the wrist associated with activity, but of course in the case of tendon-related symptoms, there would be no paresthesias or numbness, and electrodiagnostic testing would be normal. A more difficult case to sort out is that of Linburg's syndrome [37]. In this syndrome, there is a connection in the distal forearm between the tendons of the flexor pollicis longus and the flexor digitorum profundus of the index finger, so that these two digits move together, rather than separately. Since there are many activities in which the index finger might extend while the thumb flexes, or vice versa, shear stress on the tendons and tenosynovium may injure the connection, cause pain, and may also irritate the median nerve. However, in Linburg's syndrome, electrodiagnostic testing will be normal, and the characteristic Linburg sign will be present, in which the symptoms are aggravated by active flexion of the thumb associated with passive extension of the index finger, or vice versa. Provocative tests for carpal tunnel syndrome will typically be normal.

Trigger fingers and trigger thumbs can also be associated with, or confused with, carpal tunnel syndrome, particularly since some patients do report numbness in the effected finger when triggering is present. However, the clinical diagnosis should be relatively easy to sort out, once the examiner palpates the tendon sheaths for triggering, and notes that provocative tests for carpal tunnel syndrome and sensibility in the median distribution are normal.

Arthritic conditions can be associated or confused with carpal tunnel syndrome, particularly scaphotrapezial arthritis [38], but also osteoarthritis of the interphalangeal joints, which can cause pain or stiffness in the fingers that the patient may describe variably as being associated with numbness. X-rays of the hand will help to establish the diagnosis of osteoarthritis, and electrodiagnostic testing would of course be normal in patients who did not also have carpal tunnel syndrome.

There are various etiologies of inflammatory synovitis within the wrist which may be relatively low grade and which may simulate carpal tunnel syndrome or may actually produce a median neuropathy after chronic exposure. Low grade infections such as those associated with sporotrichosis or atypical mycobacteria and other granulomatous infections can produce a flexor synovitis that can cause median nerve symptoms [39–41]. In some cases, the treatment for these infections can be purely medical, in others, a combination of surgical synovectomy with or without flexor retinaculum release, and antibiotic therapy may be curative.

There are also, of course, noninfectious inflammations of the flexor synovium that can cause or simulate carpal tunnel syndrome, particularly inflammation associated with rheumatoid or either sero-positive or sero-negative rheumatoid arthritis, systemic lupus erythematosus, psoriatic arthritis, or gout [42–44]. In such cases, the clinician's index of suspicion can be raised by eliciting a history of involvement of other joints, morning stiffness, and intermittent exacerbations not associated with activity. Laboratory studies are obviously quite helpful in establishing a diagnosis of inflammatory arthropathy, and should be performed when these diagnoses are considered.

The most confusing and vexing element in the differential diagnosis has been left for last. Many patients have nonspecific hand symptoms which may be described as pain, numbness, weakness, tingling, or loss of dexterity. Such patients may have symptoms aggravated by work and may be quite convinced, either because of what they have read or the encouragement of colleagues, that carpal tunnel syndrome is present. However, it is important for the clinician to insist on clear diagnostic criteria, based on physical examination, history, and laboratory testing, before establishing a diagnosis of carpal tunnel syndrome. If there is no history of aggravation with characteristic activities or at night, no evidence on clinical examination of irritability of the median nerve, if the symptoms are not limited to the median nerve distribution, and if testing of median nerve physiology shows no evidence of abnormality, then the clinician should be hesitant to establish a diagnosis of carpal tunnel syndrome. It is not necessary to provide a diagnosis simply because a patient has presented to the clinician with an ailment. Pain, unassociated with any specific pathological entity, can occur, does occur, and is often the only "diagnosis" present, particularly in young, otherwise healthy individuals. The clinician should not hesitate to enter a diagnosis of "hand pain" if that is the only thing that can be conclusively demonstrated after a thorough clinical evaluation. It may well do a disservice to the patient, to provide a diagnosis of "possible carpal tunnel syndrome" because the label implies a specific problem with a specific treatment, when such specificity is not truly supported by the clinical evidence. Indeed, once such a label is applied, it may be very difficult to dissuade the patient, their employer, their insurance company, and other clinicians, that the label is truly not justified, simply because it has been made in the past, and regardless of the evidence to support the diagnosis. Clinicians must, therefore, be quite careful and conscientious in performing a thorough differential diagnosis for carpal tunnel syndrome, and applying the label only when it is justified.

References

1. Gummesson C et al. (2003) Chronic upper extremity pain and co-occurring symptoms in a general population. Arthritis & Rheumatism 49(5): p. 697–702
2. Atroshi I et al. (1999) Prevalence of carpal tunnel syndrome in a general population.[see comment]. JAMA 282(2): p. 153–8
3. Rempel D et al. (1998) Consensus criteria for the classification of carpal tunnel syndrome in epidemiologic studies. American Journal of Public Health 88(10): p. 1447–51
4. Rosenbaum R, Ochoa J (1993) Carpal Tunnel Syndrome and Other Disorders of the Median Nerve. 1 ed. London: Butterworth. 358
5. Atroshi I et al. (2003) Diagnostic properties of nerve conduction tests in population-based carpal tunnel syndrome. BMC Musculoskeletal Disorders 4(1): p. 9
6. Corwin HM, Kasdan ML (1998) Electrodiagnostic reports of median neuropathy at the wrist. Journal of Hand Surgery – American Volume 23(1): p. 55–7
7. Haig AJ, Tzeng HM, LeBreck DB (1999) The value of electrodiagnostic consultation for patients with upper extremity nerve complaints: a prospective comparison with the history and physical examination. Archives of Physical Medicine & Rehabilitation 80(10): p. 1273–81
8. Jordan R, Carter T, Cummins C (2002) A systematic review of the utility of electrodiagnostic testing in carpal tunnel syndrome.[see comment]. British Journal of General Practice 52(481): p. 670–3
9. Jablecki CK et al. (1993) Literature review of the usefulness of nerve conduction studies and electromyography for the evaluation of patients with carpal tunnel syndrome. AAEM Quality Assurance Committee. [see comment]. Muscle & Nerve 16(12): p. 1392–414
10. Kilmer DD, Davis BA (2002) Electrodiagnosis in carpal tunnel syndrome. Hand Clinics 18(2): p. 243–55
11. Kitsis CK et al. (2002) Carpal tunnel syndrome despite negative neurophysiological studies. Acta Orthopaedica Belgica 68(2): p. 135–40
12. Spinner RJ, Bachman JW, Amadio PC (1989) The many faces of carpal tunnel syndrome. [see comment]. Mayo Clinic Proceedings 64(7): p. 829–36
13. van Dijk MA et al. (2003) Indications for requesting laboratory tests for concurrent diseases in patients with carpal tunnel syndrome: a systematic review. Clinical Chemistry 49(9): p. 1437–44
14. Hussussian CJ, Mackinnon SE (1999) Postradiation neural sheath sarcoma of the brachial plexus: a case report. Annals of Plastic Surgery 43(3): p. 313–7
15. Rhomberg M, Herczeg E, Piza-Katzer H (2002) Pitfalls in diagnosing carpal tunnel syndrome. European Journal of Pediatric Surgery 12(1): p. 67–70
16. Stabile MJ, Warfield CA (1990) Differential diagnosis of arm pain. Hospital Practice (Office Edition) 25(1): p. 55–8, 61, 64
17. Witt JC, Stevens JC (2000) Neurologic disorders masquerading as carpal tunnel syndrome: 12 cases of failed carpal tunnel release. Mayo Clinic Proceedings 75(4): p. 409–13
18. Abe M, Ichinohe K, Nishida J (1999) Diagnosis, treatment, and complications of thoracic outlet syndrome. Journal of Orthopaedic Science 4(1): p. 66–9
19. Kaufman MA (1996) Differential diagnosis and pitfalls in electrodiagnostic studies and special tests for diagnosing compressive neuropathies. Orthopedic Clinics of North America 27(2): p. 245–52
20. Amadio PC, Reiman HM, Dobyns JH (1988) Lipofibromatous hamartoma of nerve. Journal of Hand Surgery – American Volume 13(1): p. 67–75
21. Rehak DC (2001) Pronator syndrome. Clinics in Sports Medicine 20(3): p. 531–40
22. Werner CO, Rosen I, Thorngren KG (1985) Clinical and neurophysiologic characteristics of the pronator syndrome. Clinical Orthopaedics & Related Research (197): p. 231–6
23. Fisher MA, Gorelick PB (1985) Entrapment neuropathies. Differential diagnosis and management. Postgraduate Medicine 77(1): p. 160–74
24. Folberg CR, Weiss AP, Akelman E (1994) Cubital tunnel syndrome. Part I: Presentation and diagnosis. Orthopaedic Review 23(2): p. 136–44
25. Perkins BA, Olaleye D, Bril V (2002) Carpal tunnel syndrome in patients with diabetic polyneuropathy. [see comment]. Diabetes Care 25(3): p. 565–9
26. Valji K et al. (1995) Hand ischemia in patients with hemodialysis access grafts: angiographic diagnosis and treatment. Radiology 196(3): p. 697–701
27. Botte MJ, Gelberman RH (1998) Acute compartment syndrome of the forearm. Hand Clinics 14(3): p. 391–403

28. Gelberman RH, Szabo RM, Mortensen WW (1984) Carpal tunnel pressures and wrist position in patients with colles' fractures. Journal of Trauma-Injury Infection & Critical Care 24(8): p. 747–9
29. Bauman TD et al. (1981) The acute carpal tunnel syndrome. Clinical Orthopaedics & Related Research (156): p. 151–6
30. Crossman MW et al. (2001) Nonneurologic hand pain versus carpal tunnel syndrome: do psychological measures differentiate? American Journal of Physical Medicine & Rehabilitation 80(2): p. 100–7
31. Grassi W et al. (1998) Clinical diagnosis found in patients with Raynaud's phenomenon: a multicentre study. Rheumatology International 18(1): p. 17–20
32. Falkiner S (2003) Diagnosis and treatment of hand-arm vibration syndrome and its relationship to carpal tunnel syndrome. Australian Family Physician 32(7): p. 530–4
33. Miller RF et al. (1994) An epidemiologic study of carpal tunnel syndrome and hand-arm vibration syndrome in relation to vibration exposure. [see comment]. Journal of Hand Surgery – American Volume 19(1): p. 99–105
34. Pelmear PL, Taylor W (1994) Carpal tunnel syndrome and hand-arm vibration syndrome. A diagnostic enigma. Archives of Neurology 51(4): p. 416–20
35. Danner R (1983) Unilateral thenar hypoplasia. Clinical Neurology & Neurosurgery 85(2): p. 123–8
36. Bishop AT, Beckenbaugh RD (1988) Fracture of the hamate hook. Journal of Hand Surgery – American Volume 13(1): p. 135–9
37. Linburg RM, Comstock BE (1979) Anomalous tendon slips from the flexor pollicis longus to the flexor digitorum profundus. Journal of Hand Surgery – American Volume 4(1): p. 79–83
38. Crosby EB, Linscheid RL, Dobyns JH (1978) Scaphotrapezial trapezoidal arthrosis. Journal of Hand Surgery – American Volume 3(3): p. 223–34
39. Amadio PC (1998) Fungal infections of the hand. Hand Clinics 14(4): p. 605–12
40. Brutus JP et al. (2001) Atypical mycobacterial infections of the hand: report of eight cases and literature review. Chirurgie de la Main 20(4): p. 280–6
41. Hurst LC et al. (1987) Mycobacterium marinum infections of the hand. Journal of Hand Surgery – American Volume 12(3): p. 428–35
42. Cantini F et al. (1999) Remitting seronegative symmetrical synovitis with pitting oedema (RS3PE) syndrome: a prospective follow up and magnetic resonance imaging study.[see comment]. Annals of the Rheumatic Diseases 58(4): p. 230–6
43. Dennis RH, Ransome 2nd JR (1996) Giant cell arteritis presenting as a carpal tunnel syndrome. Journal of the National Medical Association 88(8): p. 524–5
44. Fitzcharles MA, Esdaile JM (1990) Atypical presentations of polymyalgia rheumatica. Arthritis & Rheumatism 33(3): p. 403–6

Carpal Tunnel Syndrome: Rare Causes

A. Landi, A. Leti Acciaro, N. Della Rosa, A. Pellacani

Carpal tunnel syndrome (CTS), in its idiopathic form, is an extremely frequent entrapment neuropathy in the clinical practice.

Several extrinsic or intrinsic processes [1–3] are involved in the etiology of such a syndrome: some of them are common whereas others are rare [4, 5]. The latter may pose particular management issues and they may require specific diagnostic, therapeutic, and rehabilitative expedients (Table 13.1).

We can differentiate between secondary compressions and intrinsic anatomic anomalies of the median nerve or extrinsic anomalies of osteo-muscular or vascular origin, such as, for instance: fractures and fracture-dislocation of the wrist bones, hematoma and post-traumatic tendon ruptures, as well as epiphyseal malformations and deformities of the wrist and carpal bones. Thesaurismotic and amyloid deposits can lead to nerve compression at the site of deposit in several connective, endocrinal, systemic, neoplastic, and metabolic disorders (especially the ones affecting the hemopoietic system). Soft tissue and bone tumors may become manifest as "space occupying" lesions, compressing the nerve inside the carpal tunnel. Last but not least, CTS in children is particularly interesting because of its peculiar aspects.

Anatomic Anomalies

Anatomic anomalies involving the bone-muscle-tendon structures of the carpal tunnel can entail median nerve compression. The short palmar muscle, which

Table 13.1. Classification of rare causes of carpal tunnel syndrome

Anatomic anomalies	Muscular anomalies
	    Muscular hypertrophies
	    Supernumerary muscles
	    Myotendinous junction variations
	Carpal bone anomalies
	    Supernumerary bones
	    Melorheostosis, osteopetrosis, etc.
	Median artery
	Median nerve anomalies

Traumatic lesions	Radius distal epiphysis fractures Carpal dislocation fractures Perilunar dislocation with volar dislocation of the semilunar Scaphoid pseudoarthrosis with FPL rupture Tendon ruptures
Malformations Congenital anomalies	Madelung's disease Macrodactyly Dejerine-Sottas disease Weill-Marchesani Leri's pleonosteosis
Focal neuropathies Connective tissue disease	Rheumatoid and psoriatic arthritis SLE Mixed connective tissue disease Eosinophilic fasciitis Systemic sclerosis Scleroderma Myxedema

Endocrine disorders	Hypersomatotropism Hypothyroidism
Infectious diseases	Hansen's disease Mycobacterium Sarcoidosis Histoplasmosis Parvovirus
Metabolic diseases and intracanalicular deposits	Gout and pseudogout Calcinosis Mucopolysaccharidosis and mucolipidosis Amyloidosis Diabetes
Tumors	Neurofibroma Lipomatous macrodystrophy Lipomas and fibrolipomas Median nerve's hemangioma Osteochondroma of the synovial sheath Villonodular pigmented tenosynovitis Ganglions Osteoid osteoma Lymphomas
Induced coagulopathies Hemopathies	Hemophilia Neoplasias

can almost totally replace a terminal tendon with a large muscular structure, represents one of the most frequent causes, as the rare forms of duplicative, digastric or hypertrophic anomalies of the *palmaris longus* muscle and the flexor digitorum superficialis muscle [6], as well as hypertrophy of the I and II lumbrical muscle. In this situation, if median nerve compression is not macroscopic, a simple section of transverse ligament may be sufficient to resolve the symptoms; if not, excision of the supernumerary or hypertrophic [7–10] muscle will be necessary.

Similarly, entrapment syndromes may arise from the presence of supernumerary carpal bones or for certain deformities which can be observed in association with hyperostosis or eburnation osteosis affecting the most superficial bone segments of the extremities, as in melorheostosis or osteopetrosis [1].

In such pathologies, a diligent clinical history and scrupulous radiologic exam play a crucial diagnostic role, especially considering the patient's young age and the limited symptomatology.

The median artery [11] may cause an acute form of CTS, with massive thrombosis of the corresponding vessel and consequent acute or chronic nerve ischemia. The median artery may also play a major role in the vascularization of the radial three fingers, especially if it is associated, as occurs in 10% of cases, with the absence of the superficial palmar arch. Resection of the obstructed segment (Fig. 13.1), according to Leriche's rules, may be sufficient to relieve the painful symptoms. Microsurgical reconstruction of the vessel is required only if it plays a major role in vascularization of the radial fingers (Allen's test).

Surgical treatment of CTS is particularly complicated when the nerve presents anatomical anomalies. Median nerve duplication [5] is one of the most frequent reasons for failure of surgical treatment, due to the position of the compression where one of the two nerve endings moves inside a deep accessory compartment, normally not decompressed by customary techniques. In such cases, in the absence of any other disorders, clinical suspicion alone of an anatomic anomaly may be of great help, and will prompt a thorough exploration of all carpal tunnel structures. Under such conditions, the use of mini-invasive and endoscopic techniques is obviously contraindicated whereas static or dynamic ultrasound sonography may prove extremely useful for preoperative diagnosis.

Traumatic Lesions

The median nerve can be directly damaged or it can suffer secondary compression in trauma affecting the wrist and carpus [12–15]. Whereas in traumatic lesions of the distal epiphysis of the radius, Colles fractures can be a relatively frequent cause of CTS. Perilunar dislocation fractures of the carpus, especially in case of complete volar dislocations of the lunate, are considered one of the rare, often unrecognized, causes. A rapid resolution of the neurological symptomatology usually follows a prompt diagnosis by reduction of the dislocation. On the contrary, with longstanding dislocations, neurological symptoms can last for months, even following volar surgical reduction of the dislocation with direct neurolysis of the median nerve. Tendon ruptures of the palmaris longus muscle or flexor pollicis longus (FPL) associated with a pseudoarthrosis of the carpal scaphoid with consequent hemorrhage and blood accumulation, might provoke median nerve compression. With recent fractures, early decompression and median nerve neurolysis is the only way to prevent latent forms of complex regional pain syndrome (CRPS type I).

Congenital Deformities and Anomalies

CTS is difficult to diagnose in children because its symptomatology is rare and vague. Sometimes, while the child is at school or is playing, a suspicion may arise due to a progressive loss of manual skills and grip, especially in absence of a specific traumatic event [16]. Those forms may be classified as idiopathic CTS, and are linked to a genetic origin and induced by edema or isolated swelling of the flexor tendon retinaculum in the absence of specific synovial inflammatory process-

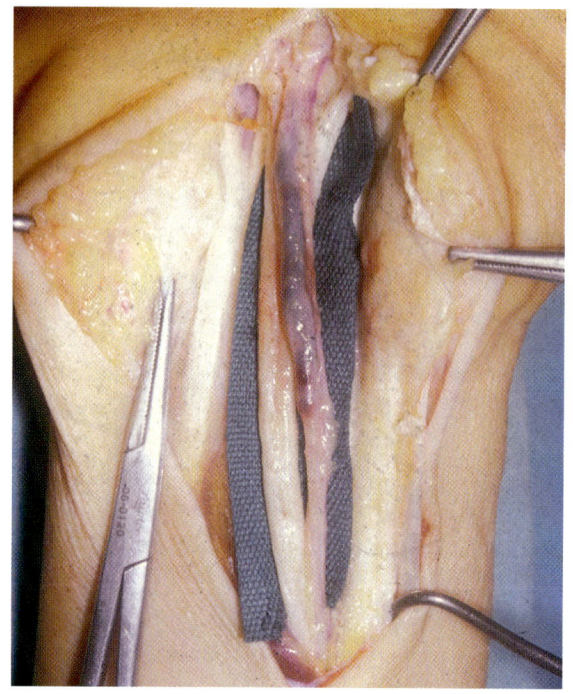

Fig. 13.1. Massive thrombosis of the median artery

es. Some forms are also associated with genetic and metabolic disorders. The excellent success rate of bone marrow transplants and recent achievements in cardiopulmonary support techniques have led to a remarkable increase of the life expectancy in children with mucopolysaccharidosis and mucolipidosis, who in the past where doomed to an average life span from one to a few decades. Therefore, more attention is addressed to secondary diseases such as CTS, which is determined by an accumulation of glycosaminoglycans in the flexor muscle retinaculum. Mental retardation, which is present in some forms of these diseases, in association with ocular and auricular disorders, are of primary clinical and prognostic interest even for the hand surgeon, since in these cases a diagnosis of median nerve compression and postoperative rehabilitation treatment are more demanding. Therefore, for diagnosis and surgical planning, any objective neurophysiologic anomaly and medical history and any clinical suspicions must be considered with great care. Macrodactyly [17], hamartoma, neurofibromatosis, and the Dejerine-Sottas syndrome are usually classified among the hereditary hypertrophic neuropathies [18] of the peripheral nerves and they are often associated with each other to the extent they are thought to be caused by an abnormal responsiveness of the organ to an unidentified trophic factor. In the Weill-Marchesani syndrome, local compression is caused by hypertrophy and thickening of the flexors retinaculum that is due to degeneration of the connective tissue [16]. Clinically, it is useful to evaluate the presence and severity of ocular disorders and of the epiphyseal dysplasia, which are responsible for reduced height and brachydactyly, with consequent joint stiffness, worsening a syndrome which is already quite complicated. The same reasoning applies to CTS in association with bone malformations such as Will-Leri pleonosteosis, where degeneration of fibrocartilage coexists with thickening of the retinaculum in addition to widening of the basis of the first metacarpus and flexion contraction of the thumb and of the long fingers. Melorheostosis is associated with index hypoplasia and Madelung's deformity with anterior carpal subluxation. Median nerve entrapment has also been described in association with constriction bands in the distal forearm. These entrapments demand an urgent fasciotomy in the case of a circumferential compression of the nerves as well as the vessels. The incidence of CTS in children is extremely low, and therefore it is very important to carefully study the underlying cause through an accurate clinical history and through an objective and scrupulous examination aimed at determining the presence of digital hypoplasia, deformities, pathognomonic type of facies, etc., in addition to the implementation of instrumental, radiological, and hematochemical investigations in tight collaboration with a geneticist.

Recurrent Focal Neuropathies

Recurrent focal neuropathies usually present as two main clinical pictures [18]. The first form is hereditary neuropathy of the brachial plexus, with episodes of hyposthenia anticipated by pain followed by spontaneous healing starting some months later, to be completed within 1 or 2 years. Normally, hypotelorism, syndactyly, and hyposomia are the dysmorphic signs of a genetic link.

The second form is a hereditary trend towards the onset of a compressive paralysis, appearing during sleep and following surgical procedures, with a paralysis which, instead of disappearing in a few minutes, lasts for several months. The sites are those typical of all compressive syndromes of the peripheral nerves: the radial nerve in the arm and the median nerve at the wrist. The hereditary signs can be represented by a cavus deformity at the foot and mallet toes. For such condition, a preventive policy based on patient discipline and self-management should be selected. The use of a tourniquet for potential focal neuropathy decompression or for treatment of noncorrelated pathologies must be avoided in order to prevent the onset of tourniquet paralysis described in such cases [19].

Connective Tissue Disorders

CTS has been frequently described in association with systemic diseases of connective tissue. In scleroderma [20, 21] and in systemic sclerosis [22–24] thickening of the connective tissue of the transverse ligament and nervous sheath, in association with vasculitic reactions and microangiopathies caused by perivasal, polymorphous, inflammatory infiltrates, account for the sudden neuropathy which accompanies and sometimes precedes systemic symptoms. In SLE (systemic lupus erythematosus) and in polyarteritis, the peripheral lesion is more frequently associated with retinopathy and vasculitis involving the central nervous system, which means that an early diagnosis and prophylaxis resorting to steroid therapy are required.

In rheumatoid arthritis [25–27] as well as in psoriatic arthritis and in mixed connective tissue disease [28], even severe carpal and radiocarpal synovitis, with frequent bilateral symptoms, contributes to increase the volume of the carpal tunnel. In mixed-connective diseases, sensory trigeminal neuropathy is the main symptom and requires an appropriate treatment with prednisone.

In rheumatoid arthritis, besides flexor tendon synovitis, also a proximal migration of the lumbrical muscle was described, due to the shortening of the metacarpal bones and subluxation of the metacarpo-phalangeal joints, leading to compression of the median nerve.

Endocrine Disorders

In patients with acromegaly [2, 29], CTS is not an infrequent event following both extrinsic processes such as excessive bone growth, thickening of the transverse ligament, soft tissue edema produced by an increase in the extracellular fluid, growth of perineural fibrous tissue, and intrinsic processes such as the endoneural fibrous proliferation (Fig. 13.2). In such cases, therapy aimed to reduce the growth hormone produced by the hypophysis can achieve a regression of the neurologic symptomatology of the median nerve, even if the neuropathy does not appear to be related to the blood level of the hormones. Surgical treatment must be planned early with the aim to decompress the carpal tunnel and to foster neurolysis, regardless of having been submitted to pituitary gland radiotherapy. Less frequently, compression of the median nerve is reported in association with hypothyroidism, as a consequence of fibrous degeneration of the carpal transverse ligament and of the peri- and endoneural [30–32] myxedematous infiltrate.

In such cases hormonal therapy helps relieve the symptoms, which disappear only when a prompt diagnosis and surgical decompression are established.

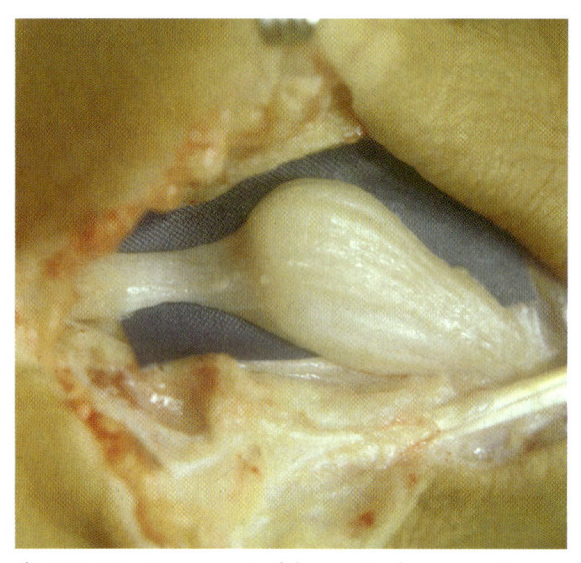

Fig. 13.2. Monstrous aspect of the proximal neuroma in a patient with acromegaly. Median nerve thickening and fibrosis with compression at the transverse ligament, which is also thickened

Infectious Diseases

The present century, characterized by a constant flow of racial migrations, has seen a recrudescence of tubercular infections and a reappearance of the obsolete granulomatous tenosynovitis of the flexor tendons as a potential rare cause for CTS. Indeed, the median nerve can be surrounded and compressed by granulomatous tubercular tissue. Besides a specific drug therapy, the opening of the tunnel in association with flexor tendon tenosynovectomy and removal of granulomatous tissue [33, 34] is required.

Likewise, histoplasmosis [35] can originally affect the carpal bones, and sarcoidosis [36] can exceptionally affect the tendinous sheaths of the flexor muscles, in the absence of generalized signs.

In the former, after a diagnosis confirmed by specific immunodiffusion tests of the *Histoplasma* antigens and wrist and chest x-rays, a surgical approach with removal of the tenosynovitic granulomatous tissue and curettage of the bone cystic areas must be implemented, supported by long-term drug therapy in order to reduce the risk of recurrence; in the latter, adjuvant steroid therapy is useful after tenolysis and neurolysis have been carried out.

On the other hand, patients with Hansen's disease [37] may present with intraneural abscesses. These abscesses represent a potential acute inflammatory reaction within a growing, cell-mediated immune process, which fosters an intrinsic compression of the nerve that requires epineurotomy to drain the abscess. Acute decompression is necessary when symptoms are very severe, and in these cases must routinely resort to therapy with thalidomide [31, 32].

Metabolic Diseases

Metabolic systemic disorders [31] leading to intracanalicular deposits represent another rare circumstance leading to CTS. In gout [38–41], calcinosis, and severe calcific [42] periarthritis, crystals of sodium urate, hydroxylapatite, and calcium pyrophosphate [43] are deposited on the volar surface of the carpal ligament, with consequent compression of the median nerve.

The same conditions are reproduced when intracellular deposits of glycosaminoglycans are concentrated in lysosomes in mucopolysaccharidosis and mucolipidosis [44]. In amyloidosis, deposits of beta-2-microglobulin are reported in hemolymph disorders and in patients undergoing hemodialysis [45, 46], homolateral to the shunt, with a consequent thickening of the flexor retinaculum and of the paratenon and epineurium. In such patients, median nerve neuropathy may be the first heralding symptom, because x-ray examination, which can detect radiopaque deposits is not customarily ordered for this entity. It is always advisable to combine release of the tunnel and tenosynovectomy with histopathologic exam of the material removed. Histologic characterization must be taken into account to modify the filters employed in case of hemodialysis, in order to reduce the blood level of amyloid and monocyte-macrophage cytokines.

Even in diabetes [31], besides the neuropathy related to the major pathology, flexor tenosynovitis along with microangiopathy is responsible for the onset of CTS.

All clinical suspicions must be confirmed through consultation with a neurologist and hematochemical and electromyographic exams. In such disorders, release of the carpal tunnel implies a careful epineurotomy of the median nerve, and in addition a flexor tenosynovectomy should be carried out as diabetic neuropathy belongs to the group of the edematous disorders.

Blood Coagulation Disorders

When severe venous thrombosis [47] is treated with heparin, whose action is enhanced by nonsteroidal anti-inflammatory drugs, neuropathies might occur along with this temporary iatrogenic blood disorder. The widespread use of anticoagulant drugs is aimed at preventing the onset of severe venous thrombosis, especially following hip prosthetic replacement. The onset of the neuropathy is abrupt. A burning pain affects fibers of different sizes, including the unmyelinated ones. One case of median nerve compression during the treatment of a postmyocardial infarction syndrome treated with warfarin has been reported. In such cases, anticoagulant therapy must be interrupted and, in the absence of an improvement of the symptoms, the spontaneous intraneural hematoma must be drained to relieve the pain. The same condition has been described in patients with classical hemophilia [48], in which epineurotomy and drainage of the hematoma is required. Functional recovery is related to the promptness of treatment.

Tumors

Intrinsic tumors of the nervous tissue constituents or extrinsic tumors within the carpal tunnel must be considered "space occupying" processes which compress and constrict the median nerve. Intrinsic tumors can be classified as follows: tumors with a proper nervous structure [32] and sheath tumor (neuroma, schwannoma, and neurilemmoma); tumors with a fibromatous structure (neurofibroma and outbreaks of macrodactyly or of Recklinghausen's disease); tumors derived from accessory and supply elements of the nerve (lipoma, hemangioma, etc.) and mixed tumors [49] (lipofibroma, ossifying fibrolipoma, lipofibromatous hamartoma, etc.). Among the extrinsic tumors, the osteoid osteoma [50, 51] of the capitate and lunate, causing edema of the perilesional soft tissues due to cortical and periosteal hypertrophy of the bone, synovial sheath osteochondroma and villonodular pigmented tenosynovitis,

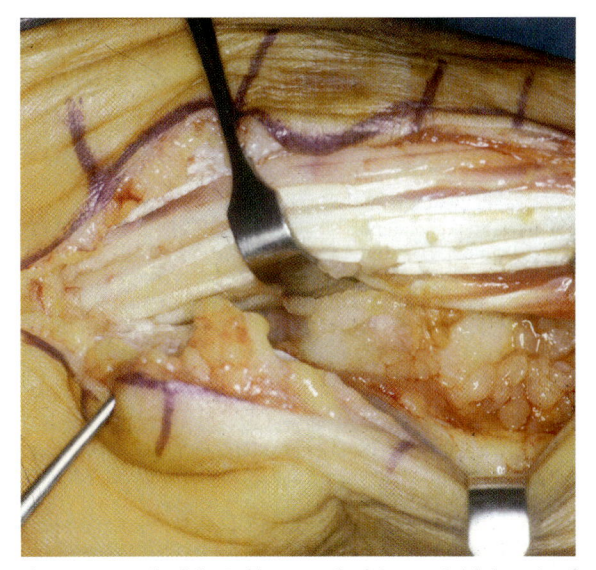

Fig. 13.3. Detail of the infiltrate and of the amyloid deposit of the carpal tunnel in a patient with lymphoma

as well as simple ganglions [52, 53] derived from the carpal joints can be encountered. Debulking of the tumor mass is the only therapeutic solution, even if in the intrinsic tumors not even an internal neurolysis with the aid of a microscope can guarantee a complete release of the nerve fascicles. Often we are forced to resort to a compromise surgery in order to avoid any further functional damage.

Needless to say, any tumor at this level must be treated with the general strategy procedures which apply to any tumor process.

Hemolymphopoietic tissue diseases are particularly interesting. In fact, B- and T-cell lymphomas can induce median nerve compressions in the wrist rather frequently for many different reasons: intracanalicular deposits of amyloid, mono- and polyclonal gamma globulins and infiltrates of neoplastic cells, especially of T cells [54]. Cases of neoplastic infiltrates of B cells, such as the case we described, in which removal of the infiltrate (Fig. 13.3) is invariably associated with a median nerve neurolysis are more rare.

In conclusion, rare causes of CTS may be of interest in every field of medicine, from internal medicine to the field of malformations and infections. The outcomes of a failed identification of such symptoms can be extremely serious in growing children, and the implemented treatment should always be related to the underlying pathology.

References

1. Phalen GS (1966) The carpal tunnel syndrome: Seventen years's experience in diagnosis and treatment of 654 hands. J Bone Joint Surg 48A: 211–228
2. Landi A, Schoenhuber R, Luchetti R (1995) Peripheral nerve injuries Microsurgery in orthopaedic practice. World Scient. Publishing
3. Luchetti R, Schoenhuber R, De Cicco G et al. (1989) Carpal-tunnel pressure. Acta Orthop. Scand 60: 397
4. Mantero R, Bertolotti P, Grandis C (1981) Trois cas rares de compression du nerf median dans le canal carpien. Ann. Chir 35: 9 bis: 804–806
5. Stevens J, Beard C, O'Fallon W et al. (1992) Conditions associated with carpal tunnel Syndrome. Mayo Clin. Proc 67; 6: 541–8
6. Schon R, Kraus E, Boller O et al. (1992) Anomalous muscle belly of the flexor digitorum superficialis associated with carpal tunnel syndrome: Case report Neurosurg. Vol 31,5: 969–871
7. Asai M, Wong ACW, Matsunaga T et al. (1986) Carpal tunnel syndrome caused by aberrant lumbrical muscles associated with cystic degeneration of the tenoynovium: A case report. J Hand Surg 11A: 218–221
8. Desajacques P, Egloff-Baer S, Roth G (1980) Lumbrical muscles and carpal tunnel syndrome. Electromyogr. Clin. Neurophysiol 20: 443–450
9. Jabaley ME (1978) Personal observations on the rule of the lumbrical muscles in carpal tunnel syndrome. J Hand Surg. Vol 3, 1: 82–84
10. Nather A, Pho RWH (1981) Carpal tunnel syndrome produced by an organising haematoma within the anomalous second lumbrical muscle. The Hand Vol 13, 1: 87–90
11. Catalano F, Fanfani F, Giani E (1986) L'arteria mediana e la sindrome del tunnel carpale. Riv. Chir. Mano 23: 429–433
12. Cristiani G, Marcuzzi A, Caroli A (1996) La nostra esperienza sulle fratture-lussazioni perilunari del polso. G.I.O.T 22, 513–524
13. Fikry T, Lamine A, Harfaoui A et al. (1993) Luxations perilunaires du carpe. Etude clinique (a propos de 39 cas).Acta Orthop. Belgica 59, 293–300
14. Lagur C, Peretti F, Barraud O et al. (1993) Luxations perilunaires du carpe. Interet du traitement chirurgical Rev. Chir. Orthop 79, 114–123
15. Vaccari A, Boselli F, Squarzina PB et al. (1989) Le lussazioni recenti, semplici e complesse, del carpo. G.I.O.T 61–72
16. Al-Quattan MM, Thomson HG, Clarke HM (1996) Carpal tunnel syndrome in children and adolescents with no history of trauma J Hand Surg 21B: 1: 108–111
17. Mirza MA, King ET, Reinhart MK (1998) Carpal tunnel syndrome associated with macrodactyly. J Hand Surg 23B: 5: 609–610
18. Windebank AJ (1977) Inherited recurrent focal neuropathies. In Dick T (ed): Peripheral neuropathy pp 1137–1148
19. Landi A, Saracino A, Pinelli M et al. (1995) Tourniquet paralysis in microsurgery. Annals Accademy of Med 24 (4): 89–93
20. Barr WG, Blair SJ (1988) Carpal tunnel syndrome as the initial manifestation of scleroderma. J Hand Surg 13 A: 3: 366–367
21. Thompson PD, Robertson GJ: Trigeminal neuropathy heralding scleroderma. J of Maine Medical Assoc 64; 123–124
22. Berth-Jones J, Coates PAA, Graaham-Brown RAC et al. (1990) Neurological complications of systemic sclerosis: A report of three cases and review of literature. Clin Exper Dermatol 15: 91–94
23. Kabadi UM, Sinkoff MW (1977) Trigeminal neuralgia in progressive systemic sclerosis. Postgraduate Medicine 61: 176–177
24. Machet L, Vaillant L, Machet MC et al. (1992) Carpal tunnel syndrome and systemic sclerosis. Dermatology 185: 101–103
25. Massarotti E (1996) Medical aspects of Rheumatoid Arthritis Hand Clinics Vol 12: 3: 463–475
26. Pierre-Jerome C, Bekkelund SI, Husby G et al. (1996) Bilateral fast MR imaging of the rheumatoid wrist. Clinical Rheumatol 15: 42–46
27. Sivri A, Guler-Uysal F (1998) The electroneurophysiological evaluation of Rheumatoid Arthritis patients. Clin. Rheumatol 17: 416–418
28. Vincent FM, Van Houtzen RN (1980) Trigeminal sensory neuropathy and bilateral carpal tunnel syndrome: the initial manifestation of mixed connective disease. J Neurol. Neuros. and Psychiatry 43: 458–460
29. Schiller F, Kolb FO (1954) Carpal Tunnel Syndrome in Acromegaly. Neurol 4: 271–282
30. Purnell DC, Daly DD, Lipscomb PR (1961) Carpal Tunnel Syndrome associated with mixedema. Arch. Int. Med 108: 751–756
31. Landi A, Luchetti R, Schoenhuber R (1989) Metabolic and neurophysiological correlations in carpal tunnel syndrome. J. West Pacif. Orthop. Assoc 26: 29
32. Landi A, De Luca S, Luchetti R et al. (1990) Particular aspects of lesions in continuity of peripheral nerves. J. West Pacif. Orthop. Assoc 27: 33
33. Lester B, Mayers MC (1964) Carpal Tunnel Syndrome secondary to Tubercolosis. Arch. Neurol. Vol 10 : 426–429
34. Mason ML (1934) Tuberculous Tenosynovitis of the Hand. Surg. Ginec. Obstet 59; 363
35. Care SB, Lacey SH (1998) Recurrent Hystoplasmosis of the wrist: A case report. J Hand Surg 23A: 1112–1114
36. Maj GE, Shambaugh W, Cirksena KL et al. (1964) Carpal Tunnel Syndrome as manifestation of Sarcoidosis. Arch. Int. Med. Vol 114; 830–833
37. Gaur SG, Kulshreshtha K, Swarup S (1994) Acute Carpal Tunnel Syndrome in Hansen's Disease. J Hand Surg 19 B; 286–287
38. Chuang HL, Wong CW (1994) Carpal tunnel syndrome induced by tophaceous deposits on the median nerve : Case report. Neurosurgery 34; 5: 919
39. Jacoulet P (1994) Double tunnel syndrome of the upper limb in tophaceous gout Annal. Chir. Main 13(1): 42–45
40. Kalia KK., Moossy J (1993) Carpal tunnel release complicated by acute gout Neuros 33(6): 1102–3
41. Pai C, Tseng C (1993) Acute carpal tunnel syndrome caused by tophaceous gout. J Hand Surg 18A; 4: 667–669
42. Knight DJ, Gibson PH (1993) Acute calcification and carpal tunnel syndrome" J Hand. Surg 18B; 3: 335–336
43. Verfaillie S, De Smet L, Leemans A et al. (1996) Acute carpal tunnel syndrome caused by hydroxyapatite crystals. J Hand Surg 21A: 3
44. Haddad FS, Jones DHA, Vellodi A et al. (1997) Carpal tunnel syndrome in the mucopolysaccharidoses and mucolipidoses. J Bone Joint Surg 4: 576–582
45. Musci S, Soglia S, Matarrese V et al. (1993) Responsabilità del fattore emodinamico nella genesi della sindrome del tunnel carpale nei pazienti emodializzati. Riv. Ital. Chir. Plast 25: 209–214
46. Vellani G, Dallari D, Fatone F et al. (1993) Carpal tunnel syndrome on Hemodialyzed patients. Chir. Org. Mov. LXXVIII, 15–18
47. Birch R, Bonney G, Wynnparry CB (1998) Iatropathic injury in surgical disorders of the peripheral nerves. In Birch R (ed), Churchill Livingstone pp 980–995
48. Parthenis DG, Karagkevrekis CB, Waldram M (1998) Von Willebrand's disease presenting as acute carpal tunnel syndrome. J Hand Surg 23B; 1: 114

49. Louis SD, Arbor A, Dick A (1973) Ossifyng lipofibroma of the median nerve J Bone Joint Surg. Vol. 55: 5: 1082–1084
50. Caserta S, Brambilla S, Lanzoni S et al. (1984) Rare localizzazioni dell'Osteoma Osteoide. Arch Ortop Reumatol 97 (I)
51. Herndon JH, Eaton RG, Littler JW (1974) Carpal Tunnel Syndrome. An Unusual presentation of Osteoid Osteoma of the capitate. J Bone Joint Surg 56 (A): 1715–1718
52. Brooks DM (1952) Nerve compression by single ganglia: A review of thirteen collected cases. J Bone Joint Surg 34 B: 391–400
53. Kerrigan JJ, Bertoni JM, Jagler SH (1988) Ganglion cystis and carpal tunnel syndrome. J Hand Surg 13A: 763–765
54. Chevalier X, Hermine O, Authier FJ et al. (1995) Carpal tunnel syndrome due "T" cell lymphoma: Arthritis Rheumatism 38: 11: 1707–1709

Part III

Treatment

Conservative Care for Carpal Tunnel Syndrome

J.S. Brault

Introduction

Carpal tunnel syndrome (CTS) is due to entrapment of the median nerve and is the most common form of compressive neuropathy affecting 1%–3% of the general population [1, 2]. Females in their fourth and fifth decades are four times more likely to suffer from CTS as opposed to men of the same age [3]. Symptoms often include paresthesias into the thumb, index, long and half of the ring finger, as well as pain in the hand, wrist, and occasionally the forearm [4]. These symptoms usually worsen at night and with repetitive, strenuous activities utilizing the hands. In severe cases, atrophy of the thenar musculature can be present [5]. The clinical diagnosis of CTS is generally straightforward; however, nerve conduction studies (NCS) and electromyogram (EMG) are often recommended to reliably confirm the diagnosis [6].

The natural history of this condition is not well understood, nor is there a universally accepted treatment of CTS. Individuals with severe CTS usually undergo surgical release of the transverse carpal ligament. Those with mild to moderate symptoms, or who are poor surgical candidates, are usually provided a course of conservative care. These conservative care measures range from activity modification, splinting, exercise, yoga, and oral medications to steroid injections. The effectiveness of these treatment measures for the management of CTS is uncertain.

The purpose of this chapter is to review conservative treatment measures and the evidence for their use.

Activity/Ergonomic Modification

The initial method of conservative treatment is to modify activities that may predispose an individual to CTS. Forceful, repetitive wrist motions have been associated with this condition. Several occupations, including food processing, manufacturing, logging, and construction work, have been associated with CTS [7, 8]. Although activity modification is typically the initial course of treatment, there is a paucity of research to support it.

The aim of activity modification is to maintain the wrist in a neutral position, to avoid strenuous repetitive activities, and to avoid vibration [9]. Ergonomic changes in the workplace to reduce repetitive motion have been employed. The literature available in this area is difficult to interpret. In two studies comparing ergonomic keyboards versus standard keyboards for the prevention of CTS, there have been mixed results. Rempel [10] demonstrated that there was a positive effect on hand function and pain with the use of ergonomic keyboards. Tittiranonda [11] demonstrated no significant benefit from the use of ergonomic keyboards on hand function or pain level.

Although activity modification has been used as a mainstay of carpal tunnel treatment, there has been very little research to support its use. It is still, however, considered a cornerstone of conservative treatment.

Splinting

Wrist splinting for individuals with CTS has been reported to decrease symptoms in 80% of patients within days [12]. Typically, splints are worn at night to prevent nocturnal symptoms, but can be utilized in the day and in the workplace to maintain the wrist in a neutral position.

There has been a multitude of splints used to reduce the symptoms of CTS.

These splints can be divided into two broad categories which include off-the-shelf and custom-made splints. Off-the-shelf splints are typically made of a neoprene derivative with Velcro closures. These splints often have a metal piece in the volar aspect to maintain the wrist in a static position. These maintain the wrist in a neutral to slightly extended position and restrict wrist flexion and extension (Fig. 14.1).

Custom-made splints are generally more comfortable for most patients due to decrease in bulk and a more precise fit. They are usually made out of a plastic polymer material that is held on to the wrist by Velcro straps. These volar wrist splints usually are extended into the palm to immobilize the wrist by preventing flexion and extension. They are typically more expen-

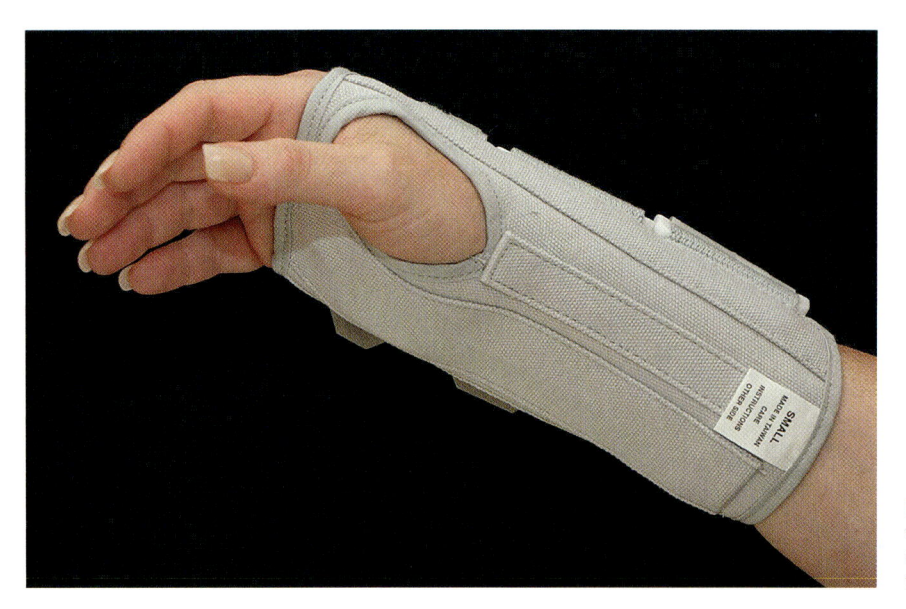

Fig. 14.1. Typical off-the-shelf wrist splint with a palmar metal stay to maintain the wrist in neutral

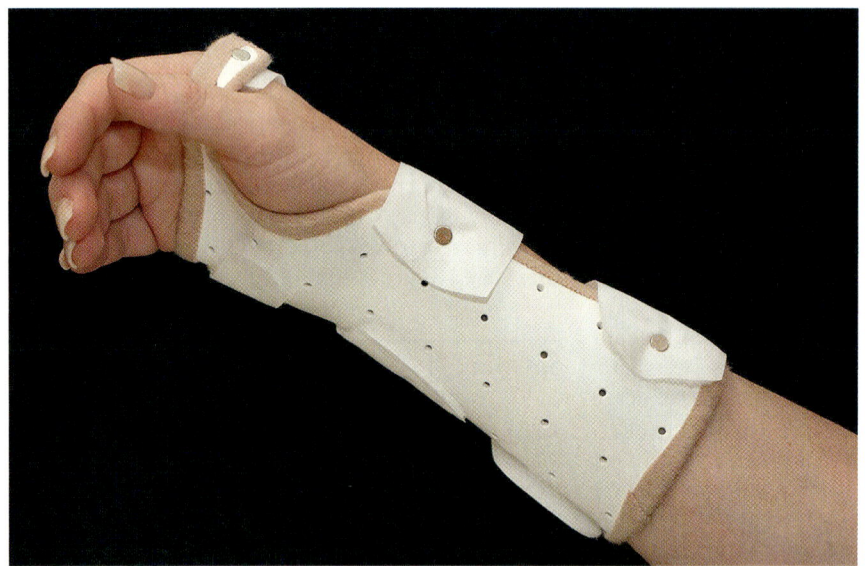

Fig. 14.2. Custom palmar wrist splint with the Metacarpal Phalanges (MCP) free

sive than off-the-shelf splints due to materials and time required to manufacture them (Fig. 14.2). Some custom wrist supports can be extended into the palm to maintain the metacarpophalangeal joint (MCP) in neutral. The splints are utilized for those individuals who have significant reproduction of their symptoms with a positive fist test. This test has been shown to bring the lumbricals into the distal carpal tunnel, resulting in symptoms [13]. By maintaining the MCPs in a neutral position, it is thought that the lumbricals are held outside of the carpal tunnel thus reducing symptoms and pressure within the tunnel (Fig. 14.3).

There has been a question as to the best position to splint the wrist. Burke [14] demonstrated that the neutral position was superior to 20° of extension in regard to nocturnal and overall symptomatology. This short 2-week trial demonstrated that the neutral position of the wrist was far superior to an extended position. Unfortunately, this was a short study and no long-term study has been subsequently attempted.

It has been shown that patients with shorter duration of CTS and less severe nocturnal symptoms do better with splinting [15]. Several randomized control trials have been performed on splinting of the wrists for CTS. Manente [16] evaluated the short-term effects of nocturnal splinting versus no treatment on nocturnal symptoms, hand function, and nerve conduction. In this short 4-week study, it was demonstrated that splinting was far superior to control at reducing predominantly nocturnal symptoms and improving hand function. Walker [17] evaluated full-time wrist splints versus nocturnal splinting only. In this 6-week study, it

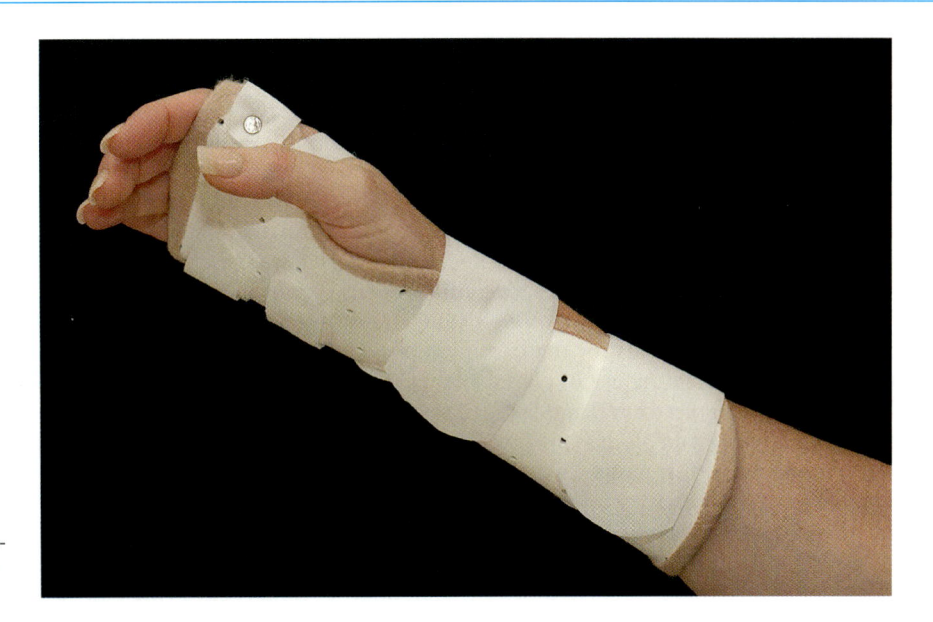

Fig. 14.3. Custom palmar wrist splint with the MCP immobilized to prevent lumbricals from traversing into the carpal tunnel

was demonstrated that there was no statistically significant difference between nocturnal and full-time splinting in regard to hand function and NCS.

Exercise/Modalities

There is also no universally accepted exercise program for the treatment of CTS. Several types of exercise, including nerve-gliding exercise and yoga, have been employed. Abalin [18] looked at nerve-gliding exercises where he had patients perform specific stretching maneuvers daily for 4 weeks. The control was a wrist splint only. They reviewed symptoms, hand function, grip strength, pin strength, and 2-point discrimination. No significant benefit was noted at the 4-week follow-up, with the exception of 2-point discrimination. Garfinkel [19] reviewed the efficacy of yoga versus wrist splint only. Patients performed yoga-type maneuvers with the upper extremity two times a week for 8 weeks. Although there was no significant benefit on nocturnal pain, Tinel's, grip strength, or nerve conduction studies, there was significant benefit at 4 weeks in regard to pain and Phalen's. This benefit was maintained at the 8-week follow-up.

Ultrasound therapy for the treatment of CTS has been utilized to reduce symptoms. Enbechler [20] performed a 8-week trial involving pulsed ultrasound versus placebo ultrasound. NCS, incidence of nocturnal wakening, sensation, and grip strength were followed. No significant benefit was noted in these parameters at 6 months. There was, however, a significant improvement in the general symptomatology of the patients at 6 months over the control group. Other studies involving ultrasound have also shown that there is short-term benefit with its use [21, 22].

Other modalities and alternative treatments that have been studied for the treatment of CTS include magnets, carpal bone mobilization, and laser. Carter [23] had patients wear magnetic devices for 45 min over the carpal tunnel and compared this to a placebo device. Follow-up at 2 weeks demonstrated no significant benefit in overall symptomatology. Tal-Akabi [24] evaluated the short-term effect of carpal bone mobilization versus no treatment. These carpal bone mobilizations were performed several times per week. There was no statistical improvement noted in pain, hand function, or active wrist motion. Aigner [25] studied the effect of treating laser acupuncture points in the upper extremity and compared this with placebo laser treatments. No significant difference in paresthesias or nocturnal pain at follow-up was identified.

Overall, there is limited evidence that ultrasound and yoga may improve short-term symptomatology. No study was carried out for greater than 6 months to evaluate the long-term benefit of these modalities.

Oral Medication

For years, the use of oral medications has been utilized to treat CTS. Medications, such as diuretics, nonsteroidal anti-inflammatories (NSAIDs), vitamin B6, oral steroids, and other medications have been studied for relief of symptomatology.

Chang et al. [26] evaluated the short-term effects of diuretics on CTS when compared to NSAIDs. This group was unable to identify any statistical significant difference in symptoms at 2–4 weeks of treatment. Pal [27] compared diuretics to placebo in a randomized, double-blind control trial that looked at symptom improvement and NCS changes at 4 weeks and 6 months of treatment. No statistically significant change was noted between placebo and diuretic therapy.

Stransky [28] compared 200 mg daily of vitamin B6 to placebo. At 10 weeks, a symptom questionnaire and NCS were performed. Again, no statistically significant changes were noted for vitamin B6 over placebo.

Oral steroids have long been used to treat CTS. Three randomized control studies, including Chang [26], Herowitz [29], and Hui [30] have demonstrated the benefit of oral steroids for the treatment of CTS. Chang [26] compared the use of prednisolone 20 mg/day for 2 weeks followed by 10 mg/day for 2 weeks with NSAIDS, diuretics, and placebo for 2 weeks. Outcomes were measured using a questionnaire rating pain, numbness, paresthesias, weakness, clumsiness, and nocturnal wakening on a 0–10 scale. There was a statistically significant improvement at 2- and 4-week follow-ups in the steroid group. Herowitz and Hui, utilizing prednisone for 2 weeks and 10 days respectively, demonstrated significant improvement in symptoms at 2 and 4 weeks of treatment.

Attempting to identify the optimal duration of treatment with oral steroids, Graham compared the use of prednisolone 20 mg/day for 2 weeks followed by 10 mg/day for 2 additional weeks with prednisolone 20 mg/day for 2 weeks followed by 2 weeks of placebo [31]. Symptoms were measured on a 10-point scale, and this group was unable to identify any benefit from the additional 2 weeks of oral steroids.

Double-blinded, randomized control trials do demonstrate that oral steroids seem to have a short-term benefit with CTS symptoms. Although the optimum oral steroid and dosage to be used remains controversial, the optimum duration appears to be 2 weeks of treatment. The other medications had no statistical effect on symptomatology at follow-up.

Corticosteroid Injections

Local corticosteroid injections for CTS have been utilized for years to alleviate symptoms. The effectiveness and duration of benefit from these injections have not been clearly outlined [32]. There is very little information as to the optimal corticosteroid to use, dosage, or location of the injection. It has been demonstrated that reoccurrence of symptoms after corticosteroid injection range from 8% to 100% [33]. Much of this depends on severity of symptoms, study design, and outcome measures. Patients with the most severe CTS generally derive the least benefit from steroid injections.

CTS injections can be performed in a variety of ways. One specific technique [34] can be performed to minimize potential injury to the median nerve. The palmar aspect of the wrist is cleansed and draped in a sterile fashion. A syringe containing a 2-ml solution of 1 ml of plain 1% lidocaine and 1 ml of a soluble corticosteroid, such as dexamethasone or triamcinolone, is utilized. The patient makes a loose fist. A 20-gauge, inch and a quarter needle is introduced ulnar to the palmaris longus and radial to the pisiform at the proximal wrist crease. Directing the needle at a 45° angle towards the MCP joint of the index finger, it is advanced 1 cm. The patient is asked to extend the fingers, and the movement of the tendons under the needle should be felt. After negative aspiration, the solution can be injected. If the patient experiences excessive pain or paresthesias, the needle should be withdrawn to the skin and redirected in an ulnar direction (see Fig. 14.4).

The effectiveness of corticosteroid injections versus other interventions for the treatment of CTS has been studied. Dammers [35] performed a randomized trial comparing 40 mg of methylprednisolone with 10 mg of lignocaine to 10 mg of lignocaine only injected 4 cm proximal to the wrist crease. At 1 month, individuals who had the corticosteroid injections had significant improvement in subjective reports of clinical severity. At 3 months, however, there was no statistical difference between the groups in clinical severity.

A double-blind, randomized comparison of local corticosteroid injection versus oral steroid injection was performed by Wong [36]. Corticosteroid injections included 15 mg of methylprednisolone and was compared to oral prednisolone 25 mg/day for 10 days. Primary outcome measures were pain, nocturnal paresthesias, weakness, clumsiness, and nocturnal wakening. At 2 weeks, there was no statistical difference between the two groups. At 8 and 12 weeks, however, the injections were statistically better than the oral prednisone. Unfortunately, this study was not carried out longer to determine if there was any ongoing benefit.

Celiker [37] performed an unblinded, randomized trial comparing injections to NSAIDs and splinting. This group injected 40 mg of prednisolone 4 cm proximal to the wrist crease. The primary outcome measure was the Symptom Severity Scale, NCS, VAS, Tinel's, and Phalen's tests. Outcomes were recorded at 2 weeks and 8 weeks. During the short follow-up periods, there was no statistical difference between corticosteroid injection alone versus NSAIDs and splinting.

The duration of benefit has not been systematically studied. Local corticosteroid injections appear to be superior to oral steroids for up to 3 months. No studies show, however, benefit from steroid injection greater than 3 months.

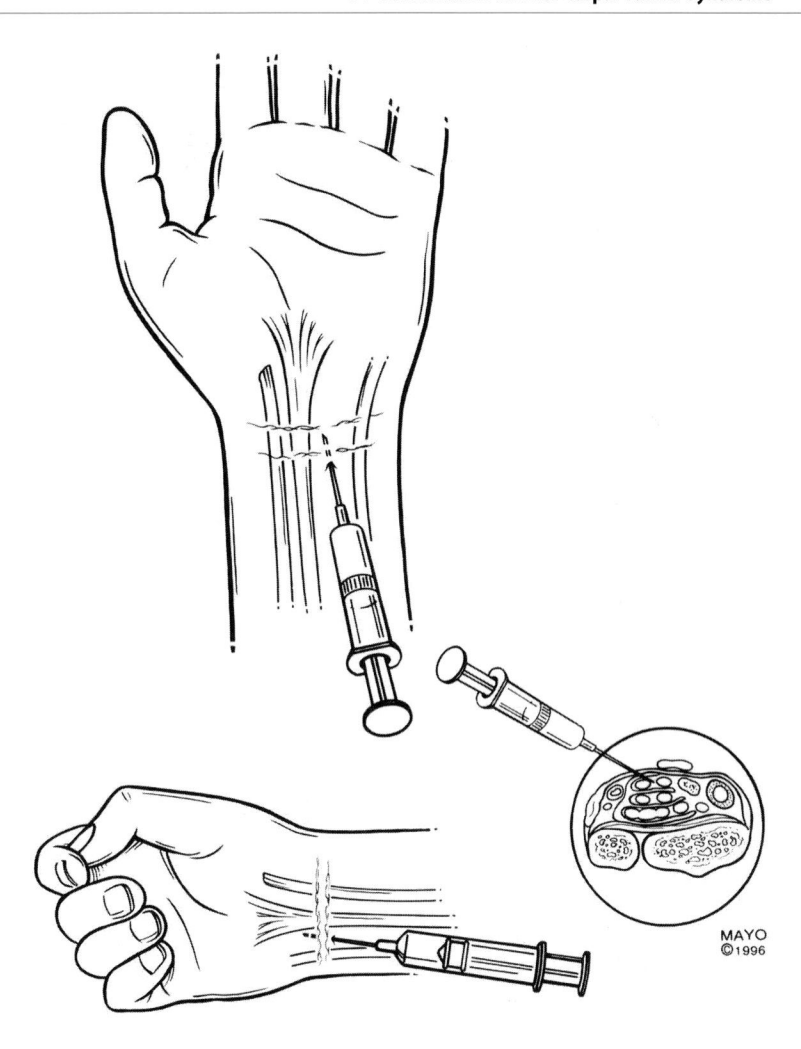

Fig. 14.4. Drawing of a carpal tunnel injection demonstrating the needle placement ulnar to the palmaris longus and passing obliquely towards the index finger MCP joint. The fingers are extended and the carpal tunnel is injected with solution

Conclusion

Conservative care measures are a viable consideration for individuals with mild to moderate CTS symptomatology or who are poor surgical candidates. There is strong evidence that corticosteroid injections and oral steroids do offer significant short-term benefits for CTS. Other treatments, such as splinting, ultrasound, yoga, and carpal bone mobilization offer benefits that are less consistent. A great deal of research needs to be performed to analyze other treatments that are employed for this condition.

References

1. Katz JNGR, Wright EA, Lew RA, Liang MH (1990) Reponsiveness of self-reported and objective measures of disease severity in carpal tunnel syndrome. Journal of Rheumatology 17: p. 1495–8
2. Levine DW, Koris MJ, Daltroy LH et al. (1993) A self-administered questionnaire for assessment of severity of symptoms and functional status in carpal tunnel syndrome. J Bone Joint Surg Am 75: p. 1858–92
3. Atroshi I et al. (1999) Prevalence of carpal tunnel syndrome in a general population. Jama 282(2): p. 153–8
4. Rempel D et al. (1998) Consensus criteria for the classification of carpal tunnel syndrome in epidemiologic studies. American Journal of Public Health 88(10): p. 1447–51
5. Szabo RM, Chidgey LK (1989) Stress carpal tunnel pressures in patients with carpal tunnel syndrome and normal patients. Journal of Hand Surgery – American Volume 14(4): p. 624–7
6. JC, S (1997) AAEM minimonograph 26: the electrodiagnosis of carpal tunnel syndrome. American Association of Electrodiagnostic Medicine. Muscle & Nerve 20(12): p. 1477–86
7. Bernard, BP (1997) Musculoskeletal disorders and workplace factors: a critical review of epidemiologic evidence for work-related musculoskeletal disorders of the neck, upper extremity and low back. Vol. 97–141. Cincinnati: National Institute for Occupational Safety and Health
8. Silverstein BA (1999) Work-related disorders of the back and upper extremity in Washington State 1990–1997, in SHARP technical report 40-2-1999. Sharp Program: Olympia, Wash.
9. Hagberg M, Kelsh M (1992) Impact of occupations and job tasks on the prevalence of carpal tunnel syndrome. Scand J Work Environ Health 18(6): p. 337–45
10. Rempel D et al. (1999) Effect of keyboard keyswitch design on hand pain. Journal of Occupational & Environmental Medicine. 41(2): p. 111–9

11. Tittiranonda P, Armstrong T, Burastero S (1999) Effect of four computer keyboards in computer users with upper extremity musculoskeletal disorders. Am J of Indust Med 35: p. 647–61
12. Burke DT, Stewart GW, Cambre A (1994) Splinting for carpal tunnel syndrome: in search of optimal angle. Archives of Physical Medicine & Rehabilitation. 75: p. 1241–4
13. Cobb TK, Cooney WP, Berger RA (1994) Lumbericle muscle incursion in the carpal tunnel during finger flexion. Journal of Hand Surgery – British Volume. 19(4): p. 434–8
14. Burke DT et al. (1994) Splinting for carpal tunnel syndrome: in search of the optimal angle. Archives of Physical Medicine & Rehabilitation. 75(11): p. 1241–4
15. Gerritsen AA, Scholten RJ, Bertelsmann FW et al. (2002) Splinting vs surgery in the treatment of carpal tunnel syndrome: a randomized control trial. JAMA 288(10): p. 1245–4251
16. Manente G, DiBlasio F, Staniscia T et al. (2001) An innovative hand brace for carpal tunnel syndrome: a randomized control trial. Muscle and Nerve, 2001. 24: p. 1020–5
17. Walker WC, Cifu DX, Swartz Z (2000) Neutral wrist splinting in carpal tunnel syndrome: a comparison of night-only vs full-time wear instructions. J of Phys Med and Rehab 81: p. 424–9
18. Akalin E et al. (2002) Treatment of carpal tunnel syndrome with nerve and tendon gliding exercises. American Journal of Physical Medicine & Rehabilitation. 81(2): p. 108–13
19. Garfinkel MS et al. (1998) Yoga-based intervention for carpal tunnel syndrome: a randomized trial. Jama. 280(18): p. 1601–3
20. Ebenbichler GR, Nicolakis P, Wiesinger GF et al. (1998) Ultrasound treatment for treating the carpal tunnel syndrome: randomised 'sham' control trial. British Medical Journal 316: p. 731–5
21. Koyuncu H, Sahin U, Togay P (1995) 3 MHz ultrasound applications in carpal tunnel syndrome. Fizik Tedavi ve Rehabilitasyon Dergisi 19: p. 141–5
22. Ozats O, Bora I, Kerim KM (1998) Ultrasound therapy effect in carpal tunnel syndrome. Archives of Physical Medicine & Rehabilitation. 79: p. 1540–4
23. Carter R, Aspy CB, Mold J (2002) The effectiveness of magnet therapy for the treatment of wrist pain attributed to carpal tunnel syndrome. Journal of Family Practic 51: p. 38–40
24. Tal-Akabi A (2000) An investigation to compare the effectiveness of carpal bone mobilisation and neurodynamic mobilisation as methods of treatment for carpal tunnel syndrome. Manual Therapy 5: p. 214–22
25. Aigner N, Petje G (1999) Results of laser-acupuncture in carpal tunnel syndrome: a prospective, randomised and blinded study. Deutsche Zeitschrift fur Akupunktur 40: p. 70–5
26. Chang MH, Lee SS, Ger LP, Lo YK (1998) Oral drug of choice in carpal tunnel syndrome. Neurology 51: p. 390–3
27. Pal B, Hossain MA, Wallace AS, Diffey BL (1988) Should diuretics be prescribed for idiopathic carpal tunnel syndrome? Results of a controlled trial. Clinical Rehabilitation 2: p. 299–301
28. Stransky M, Lava NS, Lasaro RP (1989) Treatment of carpal tunnel syndrome with vitamin B6: a double-blinded study. Southern Medical Journal 82: p. 841–2
29. Herskovitz S, Lipton RB (1995) Low-dose, short-term oral prednisone in the treatment of carpal tunnel syndrome. Neurology 45: p. 1923–5
30. Hui AC, Wong KS, Li E et al. (2001) Oral steroid in the treatment of carpal tunnel syndrome. Annals of Rheumatic Diseases 60(8): p. 813–4
31. BA G (2003) Two weeks of prednisolone was as effective as four weeks in improving carpal tunnel synmdrome symptoms. Journal of Bone & Joint Surgery – American 85(8): p. 1624–9
32. Marshall S, Ashworth N (2004) Local corticosteroid injection for carpal tunnel syndrome., in The Cochran Database of Systemic Reviews. The Cochran Library
33. Girlanda P, Venuto C, Mangiapane R, Nicolosi C (1993) Local steroid treatment in idiopathic carpal tunnel syndrome: short and long-term efficacy. Journal of Neurology 240: p. 187–190
34. RD B (1998) Carpal tunnel syndrome, in The Wrist: Diagnosis and Operative Treatment, LR Cooney WP, Dobyns JH, Editor. Mosby: St. Louis. p. 1197–1233
35. Dammers JW, Vermeulen M (1999) Injections with methylprednisolone proximal to the carpal tunnel: randomised double blind trial. British Medical Journal 319: p. 884–886.
36. Wong SM, Tang A, Ho PC (2001) Local vs systemic corticosteroids in the treatment of carpal tunnel syndrome. Neurology., 2001. 56: p. 1565–67
37. Celiker R (2002) Corticosteroid injection vs nonsteroidal antiinflammatory drug and splinting in carpal tunnel syndrome. Journal of Physical Medicine and Rehabilitation 81: p. 182–186

The Cutaneous Innervation of the Palm and Its Implications During Carpal Tunnel Release Surgery

M.M. Tomaino

Introduction

The evolution of the technique of carpal tunnel release reflects growing awareness of the cutaneous innervation of the palm and its implication on postoperative scar tenderness. The palmar cutaneous branch of the median nerve (PCBMN) has received the most attention in past reports addressing local complications during carpal tunnel release [1–3]. Several anatomical dissections have demonstrated the course of this nerve and underscored its vulnerability during surgical approaches to the carpal tunnel near the thenar crease [4–6].

Nevertheless, scar sensitivity and "pillar pain" in the thenar and hypothenar eminences continue to compromise postoperative patient satisfaction following otherwise successful carpal tunnel release [2, 3, 7]. Indeed, at late postoperative follow up, Cseuz et al. noted that 36% of their patients had unpleasant scar sensitivity despite an appropriately placed incision [8], and Katz et al. reported a 26% incidence of palmar scar discomfort and a 16% incidence of pillar pain in a group of 19 patients at an average of 2.7 years following carpal tunnel release [9].

Although the cause of these symptoms has remained somewhat elusive, explanations have included neuroma formation secondary to division of cutaneous nerves, postoperative edema, and a change in the structural anatomy secondary to division of the transverse carpal ligament itself. Regardless, a number of limited open incisional [10–12] and endoscopic techniques [13–15] have been developed to limit violation of the interthenar palmar skin. Until recently, the innervation of the palmar skin has been relatively under investigated compared to the PCBMN and the palmar cutaneous branch of the ulnar nerve (PCBUN) [16], but data currently exists which supports the concept that injury to small nerves in the interthenar area may occur during carpal tunnel release [17, 18]. This data and its implications on the selection of incisions for carpal tunnel surgery are discussed in the remainder of this chapter.

Incision Selection: Historical Review

Underscoring the ramifications of injuring the PCBMN, in 1973 Taleisnik recommended an incision in line with the ulnar aspect of the ring finger [4]. He was the first to demonstrate that the PCBMN divided into one or more somewhat smaller ulnar branches as well as radial branches directed toward the thenar area, and that the former actually perforated the transverse carpal ligament to lie amongst the layer of longitudinal and oblique fibers where the end of the palmaris longus tendon fused with the palmar fascia. The incision he recommended, therefore, was designed to avoid sectioning interthenar skin and transverse carpal ligament for that reason. Notwithstanding the relative rarity of a true PCBUN [16–19], Taleisnik's incision increased the risk of injuring these branches. In that light, Engber and Gmeiner recommended an incision in line with the ring finger ray axis in an attempt to avoid injury to both ulnar and median palmar cutaneous nerves [16].

In fact, there may be no true "internervous plane" in the palm. In 1996, Martin et al. reported their findings following dissection of 25 cadaveric hands [20]. In 16 (64%), an incision in the axis of the ring finger would likely have encountered at least one branch of the ulnar-based cutaneous innervation to the palm. These authors hypothesized that the decreased levels of discomfort in patients undergoing endoscopic carpal tunnel release may be in part due to the preservation of the crossing cutaneous nerves.

Current Anatomical Studies and Implications on Incision Selection

Although Biyani et al. expressed skepticism regarding the association of a proximal interthenar carpal tunnel skin incision and postoperative scar tenderness, having immunohistochemically demonstrated comparable numbers of free nerve endings in both the proximal and distal palm [21], they may have underestimated the differences in exposure between these two areas of the palm during functional activity. For example, during gripping and other functional activities, the heel of the palm is far more vulnerable to pressure than the more distal portion. In 1996, DaSilva et al. clearly demonstrated that open release of the carpal tunnel jeopardizes very small terminal branches of the PCBMN and postulated that this may be responsible for postoperative soft tissue pain [18]. These investigators performed a detailed anatomic, histologic, and immunohistochemical study of the PCBMN and its distal arborization in 12 fresh human cadaveric hands. They showed that small unmyelinated fibers terminated in the superficial loose connective tissue of the transverse carpal ligament, and that there were no nerve fibers detected in the deep, dense collagen aspect of the ligament. Based on their findings, they recommended that the skin incision during open carpal tunnel release be placed along the axis of the ring finger to avoid these superficial branches [18].

Watchmaker et al. confirmed Taleisnik's original admonition that an incision made in the thenar crease would frequently lead to PCBMN injury [22]. Their investigation was the first to demonstrate that the projection of the ring finger axis changes depending on whether the finger is in flexion or extension. They reported that the PCBMN extends ulnar to the axis of the ring finger when determined with the finger flexed into the palm. By contrast, when the axis of the ring finger is drawn with the ring finger extended, it projects in a more ulnar direction. In this case the PCBMN was found an average of 9 mm radial to this axis (range 1 to 16 mm). In light of the variability of superficial landmarks and the influence of flexion and extension on ring finger axis, they recommended that the interthenar depression be used as a constant landmark in planning carpal tunnel incisions. They showed that the PCBMN was found an average of 4–5.5 mm radial to the interthenar depression (range 0–12 mm) and in no case did it travel ulnar to it. They recommended that incisions be placed approximately 5 mm ulnar to the interthenar depression extending distally in the direction of the third web space.

The most comprehensive anatomic study of the cutaneous innervation of the palm was performed by Martin et al. in 1996 [20]. Twenty-five fresh-frozen cadaveric hands were dissected and the cutaneous branches of the median and ulnar nerves were described relative to an incision for carpal tunnel release in the axis of the ring finger – although it was not mentioned whether the finger was flexed or extended [20]. In a single specimen, the PCBMN was isolated as it crossed the incision, and in another two specimens the terminal branches of the nerve were identified at the margin of the incision. In four hands, a classic palmar cutaneous branch of the ulnar nerve was found an average of 4.9 cm proximal to the pisiform and in ten, a nerve of Henle rose an average of 14.0 cm proximal to the pisiform and traveled with the ulnar neurovascular bundle to the wrist flexion crease. In 24 specimens, at least one transverse palmar cutaneous branch was identified originating at an average of 3 mm distal to the pisiform within Guyon's canal. In 16 specimens, an incision in the axis of the ring finger would have encountered at least one branch of the ulnar-based cutaneous innervation to the palm.

In a similar light, Matloub et al. detailed anatomy of the palmar cutaneous nerves and discussed its clinical implications in 1998 [19]. These authors concluded that incisions along the axis of the ring finger are safer than more radial incisions, but acknowledged that among the 40 fresh-frozen cadaver hands that they dissected, injury would have occurred in one quarter of the specimens. Because of their concern that all "standard" incisions for carpal tunnel release endanger the cutaneous innervation, they recommended two minimal incisions or a single short incision parallel and 10–15 mm ulnar to the thenar crease [19].

Ruch et al. have provided the most recent analysis of the innervation of the palm [23]. Cutaneous nerves were localized and quantitated not only by longitudinal axis, but also by proximity to the distal palmar crease and tissue layer in an attempt to identify an incision that would avoid injury to the palmar branches. Ten cadaveric palms were harvested en bloc, fixed at physiologic tension, and prepared for histologic examination. The nerves were counted and classified by their size and location within each tissue layer and longitudinal axis as well as by proximal, middle, and distal locations within each axis [23]. As with Biyani et al. [21], the mean number of large nerves identified within regions of the palm did not differ based on longitudinal location within each axis. The longitudinal axes used for identification of tissue samples included the index/long finger web space, the long finger axis, the long/ring finger axis, and the ring finger axis. Tissue layers included skin, fat, palmaris brevis muscle, and transverse carpal ligament.

With regard to tissue layer, these authors identified on average 9.8 large nerves within the subcutaneous fat compared with a mean of 3.2 nerves located in the palmaris brevis, and only 0.6 nerves within the transverse carpal ligament. With respect to axis, the total number of large nerves across tissue layers was significantly greater in line with the index/long finger web space than in the long/ring finger web space. Furthermore, the long/ring finger web space had a significantly decreased number of larger nerves across tissue layers compared to the index/long finger web space and the axis of the ring finger. These authors concluded that the long/ring finger web space had the lowest innervation density and suggested that the ideal location for an incision at the base of the palm would be in the long/ring finger web space longitudinal axis.

Summary

Historical and contemporary anatomical studies have detailed the palmar cutaneous anatomy and allowed recommendations regarding the ideal incision for open carpal tunnel surgery. There appears to be no "internervous plane." Nevertheless, studies by Ruch et al. [23] and Watchmaker et al. [22] suggest that an incision slightly ulnar to the interthenar depression minimizes the risk of injury to small cutaneous nerves.

In 1998, Tomaino and Plakseychuk [24] evaluated the feasibility of identifying and preserving cutaneous palmar nerve branches during open carpal tunnel release using an incision in the long/ring finger axis, as recommended by Ruch [23]. A single palmar cutaneous nerve was identified crossing the incision in 16 of 34 hands (47%) (Fig. 15.1). More importantly, these authors demonstrated that it was possible to perform carpal tunnel release while preserving such crossing nerves, and that no patient experienced either pillar pain or scar tenderness postoperatively [24]. Similarly, Watchmaker et al. evaluated 23 patients following carpal tunnel surgery using an incision 5 mm ulnar to the interthenar depression and reported that 15 of 16 non-workers-compensation patients stated that their incision was completely pain free within 3 weeks of surgery [22].

It appears, therefore, that carpal tunnel release through an open incision need not necessarily be complicated by postoperative scar discomfort and pillar pain. An understanding of the cutaneous innervation of the palm may improve patient satisfaction following open surgery. An incision made in the third/fourth web axis, preferably in line with the radial aspect of the extended ring finger, is recommended. Such an incision will resemble Watchmaker et al.'s recommendation that the incision be placed 5 mm ulnar to the interthenar depression [22]. In light of the presence of nerve fibers in the palmaris brevis muscle, it is probably advantageous to avoid cutting this structure if not necessary.

References

1. Brown RA, Gelberman RH, Seiler JG et al. (1993) Carpal tunnel release. J Bone Joint Surg. 75A:1265–1275
2. Mac Donald RI, Lichtman DM, Hanlong JJ et al. (1978) Complications of surgical release for carpal tunnel syndrome. J Hans Surg. 3:70–76
3. Louis DS, Greene TL, Noellert RC (1985) Complications of carpal tunnel surgery. J Neurosurg. 62:352–356
4. Taleisnik J (1973) The palmar cutaneous branch of the median nerve and the approach to the carpal tunnel. J Bone Joint Surg. 55A:1212–1217
5. Naff N, Dellon AL, MacKinnon SE (1993) The anatomical course of the palmar cutaneous branch of the median nerve, including a description of its own unique tunnel. J Hand Surg. 18B:316–317
6. Hobbs RA, Magnussen PA, Tonkin MA (1990) Palmar cutaneous branch of the median nerve. J Hand Surg. 15A:38–43
7. Al-Qattan MM, Bowen V, Manktelow RT (1994) Factors associated with poor outcome following primary carpal tunnel release in non-diabetic patients. J Hand Surg. 19B:622–625
8. Cseuz KA, Thomas JE, Lambert EH et al. (1966) Long-term results of operation for carpal tunnel syndrome. May Clin Proc 41:232–241
9. Katz JN, Fossell KK, Simmons BP et al. (1995) Symptoms, functional status and neuromuscular impairment following carpal tunnel release. J Hand Surg. 20A:549–555

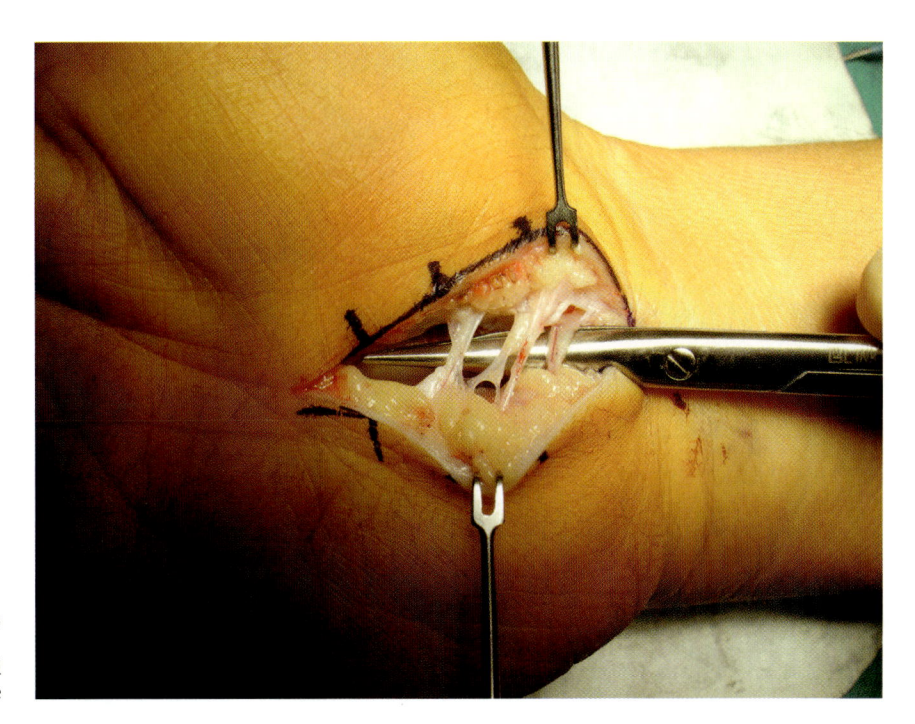

Fig. 15.1. Crossing cutaneous branch of the median nerve in the proximal incision used for open carpal tunnel release

10. Bromley GS (1994) Minimal-incision open carpal tunnel decompression. J Hand Surg. 19A:119–120
11. Citron ND, Bendall SP (1997) Local symptoms after open carpal tunnel release. A randomized prospective trial of two incision. J Hand Surg. 22B:317–321
12. Biyani A, Downes EM (1993) An open twin incision technique of carpal tunnel decompression with reduced incidence of scar tenderness. J Hand Surg. 18B:331–334
13. Chow JCY (1989) Endoscopic release of the carpal ligament: A new technique for carpal tunnel syndrome. Arthroscopy 5:19–24
14. Agee JM, McCarroll HR, Tortosa RD et al. (1992) Endoscopic release of the carpal tunnel: A randomized prospective multicenter study. J Hand Surg. 17A:987–995
15. Brown MG, Keyser B, Rothenberg ES (1992) Endoscopic carpal tunnel release. J Hand Surg. 17A:1009–1011
16. Engber WD, Gmeiner JG (1980) Palmar cutaneous branch of the ulnar nerve. J Hand Surg. 5:26–29
17. Wheatley MG, Hall JW, Faringer PN (1996) Are the palmar cutaneous nerves safe during standard carpal tunnel release? Ann of Plast Surg. 37:251–253
18. DaSilva MF, Moore DC, Weiss APC et al. (1996) Anatomy of the palmar cutaneous branch of the median nerve and clinical significance. J Hand Surg. 21A:639–643
19. Matloub HS, Yan J-G, Mink Van Der Molen AB et al. (1998) The detailed anatomy of the palmar cutaneous nerves and its clinical implications. J Hand Surg. 23B:373–379
20. Martin CH, Seiler JG, Lesesne JS (1996) The cutaneous innervation of the palm: An anatomic study of the ulnar and median nerves. J Hand Surg. 21A:634–638
21. Biyani A, Wolfe, K, Simison AJM et al. (1996) Distribution of nerve fibers in the standard incision for carpal tunnel incision for carpal tunnel decompression. J Hand Surg. 21A: 855–857
22. Watchmaker GP, Weber D, Mackinnon SE (1996) Avoidance of transsection of the palmar cutaneous branch of the median nerve in carpal tunnel release. J Hand Surg. 21A: 644–652
23. Ruch DS, Marr A, Holden M et al. (1999) Innervation density of the base of the palm. J Hand Surg. 24A:392–397
24. Tomaino MM (1998) Plakseychuk A. Identification and preservation of palmar cutaneous nerves during open carpal tunnel release. J Hand Surg. 23B:607–608

Traditional Technique: Wrist-Palm Incision

G. Cristiani, M. Marcialis

Introduction

The history of carpal tunnel syndrome (CTS) and its treatment begins in 1913, when Marie and Fox [1], after an autopsy of a patient having bilateral atrophy of the thenar muscles, recommended, in such cases, a surgical treatment of nerve decompression dissecting the transverse ligament. In 1930, Learmonth [2] described the first case of surgical release of TCS.

In 1966, Phalen [4] reported the first important series of surgical procedures for TCS: 654 operations undergone in 439 patients.

Various surgical incisions have been described by many authors: S-shaped, palmar extended toward the wrist in various manners: zigzag, transverse, longitudinal, etc. Milford 1963 [5], Phalen 1966 [4], Inglis 1972 [5], Taleisnik 1973 [6], Bonola 1981 [5], Razemon 1982 [5], and Eversman 1982 [5] (Fig. 16.1).

For many years most surgeons used a long skin incision and a radical decompression: not just a simple ligament dissection but also the intra- and extrafascicular neurolysis, together with complete tenosynovectomy of the flexor tendons.

Various problems with this technique were described by many authors [7–8]: skin adhesions; neuro-dermo-desis phenomenon; small, painful neuromas; algo-paresthesias; and a long recovery time.

All these problems produced another evolution of the surgical technique and the internal neurolysis was definitively abandoned.

The surgical technique that we've been using for the last 20 years in hundreds of cases, being traditional and following the historical principles of TCS treatment [2, 9], is a new modification of the above-described technique.

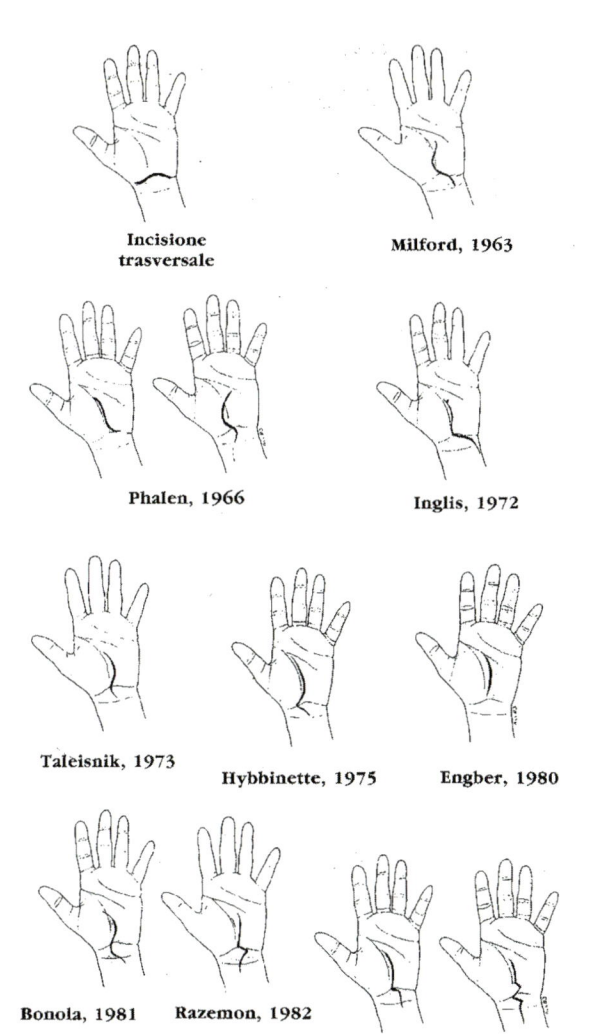

Surgical Technique

This technique requires brachial plexus anesthesia and a tourniquet at the base of the arm.

We perform a distal-proximal skin incision from the radial margin of the hypothenar eminence 3–4 cm toward the base of the thenar eminence, deviating ulnarly again at the wrist (Fig. 16.2).

We make a complete longitudinal dissection of the transverse ligament (Fig. 16.3). Then, we approach the median nerve and we check it proximally and distally to the skin incision; using smooth scissors, we carefully dissect part of the palmar aponeurosis distally and the residual of carpal transverse ligament and antebrachial

Fig. 16.1. Skin incisions

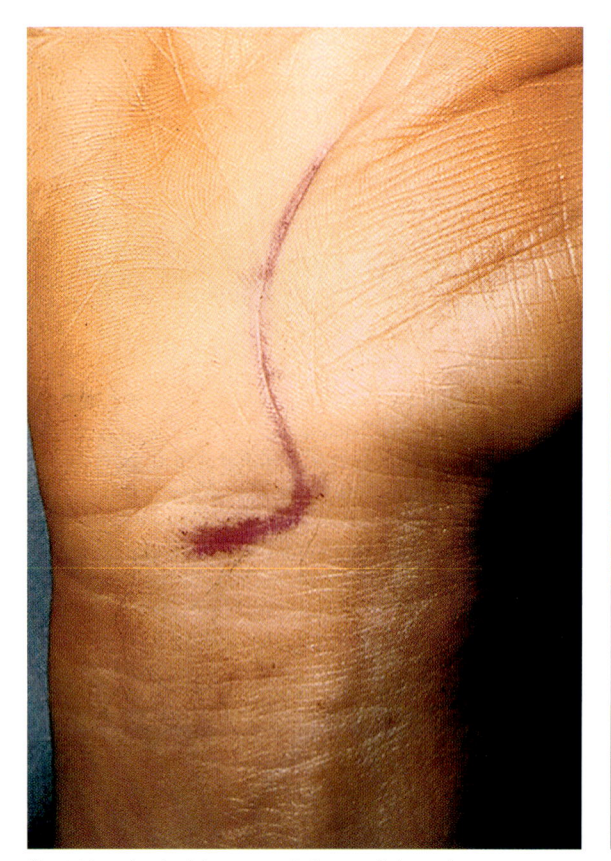

Fig. 16.2. Palm incision extended toward the wrist

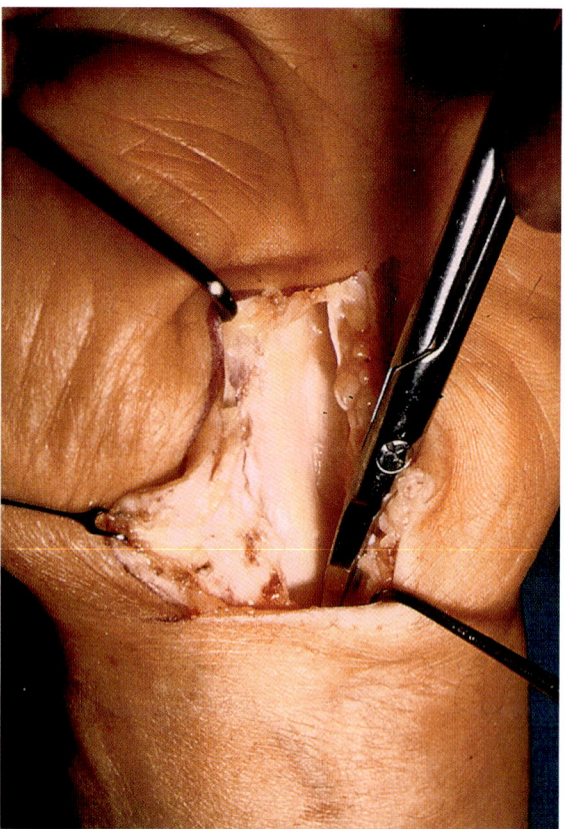

Fig. 16.3. Complete longitudinal dissection of the carpal transverse ligament

fascia proximally. Next, we examine the nerve, evaluating how much it is compressed and if there are anatomical or pathological anomalies. After that, we gently push the nerve radially and we explore the floor of the tunnel: if an hypertrophic tenosynovial tissue is present, we perform a limited tenosynovectomy just to reduce the volume of the tunnel contents. Only in a limited number of advanced cases is external neurolysis requested.

We usually check the conditions of the motor branch and the cutaneous branches (when present).

After taking off the tourniquet, a careful and complete hemostasis is performed.

Finally, we suture the skin using resorbable 4/0 suture (Vicryl rapid).

A passing drain strip and elastic bandage are applied.

After 24 h, we take off the drain strip and change the dressing.

One week later we change the dressing. Two weeks later we take off the bandage and residual suture.

Indications

1. All those cases in which, for age, general conditions, or activity, cosmetic appearance or fast recovery are not considered the most important goal.
2. In those cases in which the preoperative clinical examinations (EMG, x-rays, Echo, MRI, etc.) make us suspect the presence of anatomical or pathological anomalies [10–11] of the median nerve or of the internal or external tunnel structures (tumors or pseudo-tumors, muscle or nerve anomalies, double nerve, etc.) (Figs. 16.4–12).
3. In those cases in which, together with CTS, there is a systemic disease such as rheumatoid arthritis, diabetes, amyloidosis (in dialyzed patients), multiple neurofibromatosis, etc.
4. When the blood coagulation is abnormal and a specially accurate hemostasis is required.
5. In case of recidivism or when, in advanced cases, due to thenar atrophy and motor paralysis, a tendon opposition transfer could be indicated in the same operation.

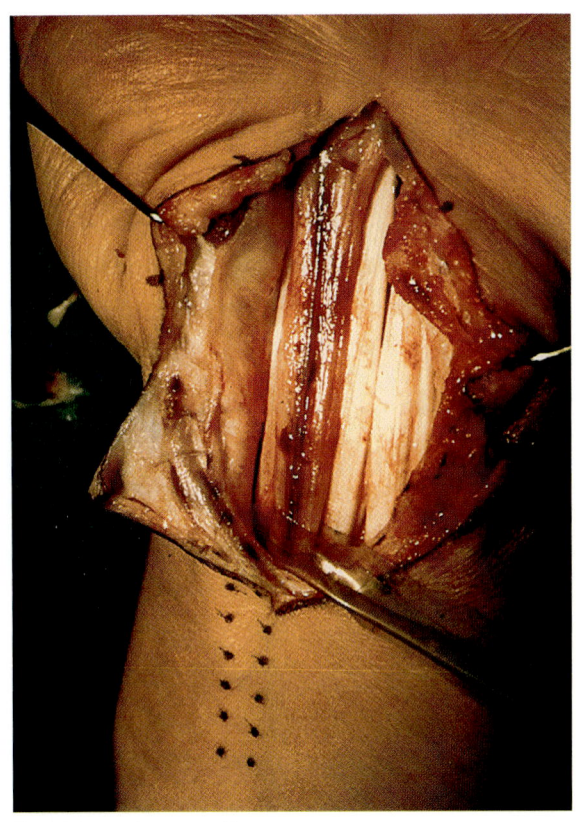

16 Traditional Technique: Wrist-Palm Incision 117

Fig. 16.4. Persistent median artery

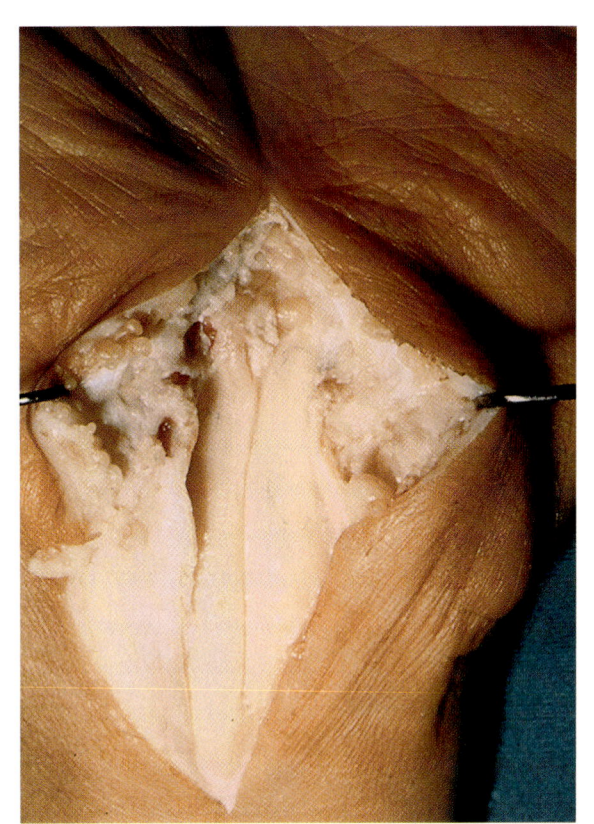

Fig. 16.5. Doubled median nerve with same caliber

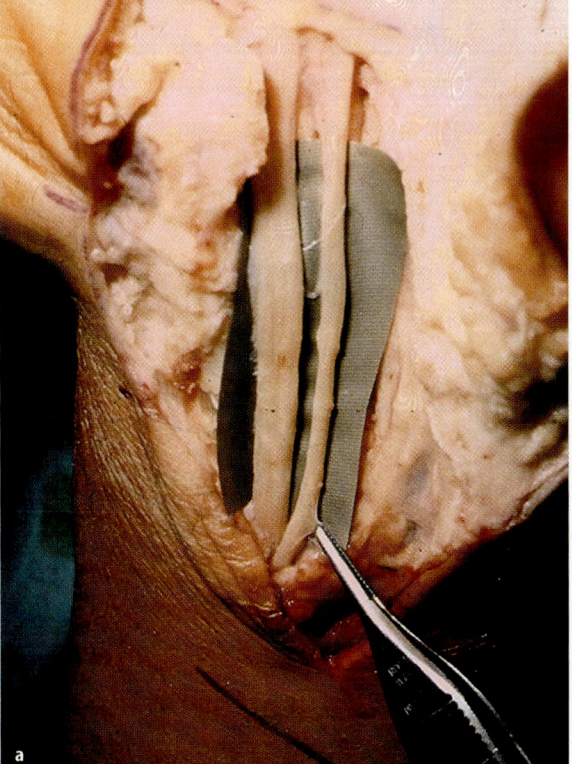

Fig. 16.6. Doubled median nerve with different caliber

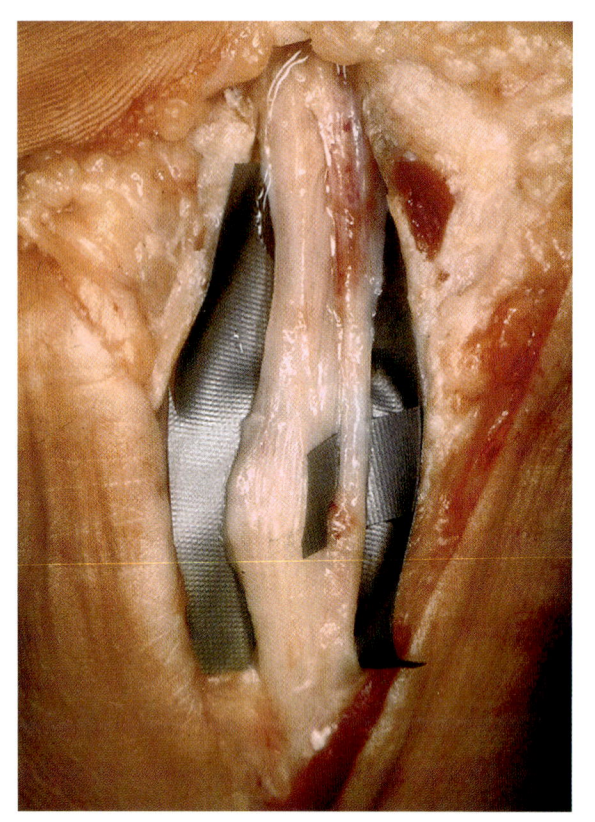

Fig. 16.7. Fork anomaly of the nerve

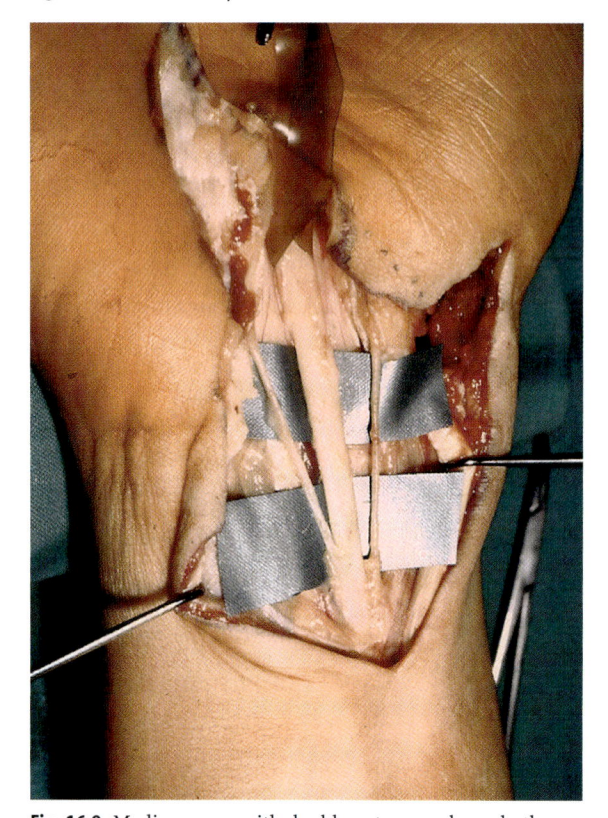

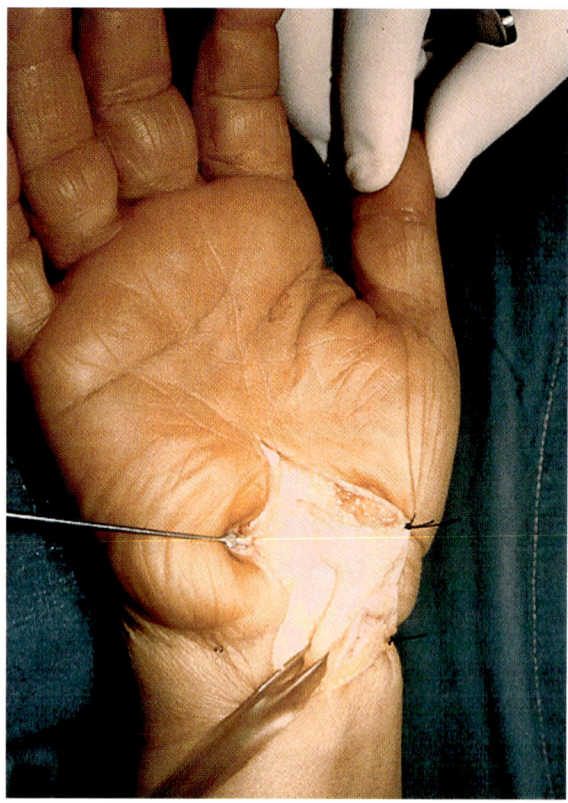

Fig. 16.8. Origin and direction anomaly of the motor branch

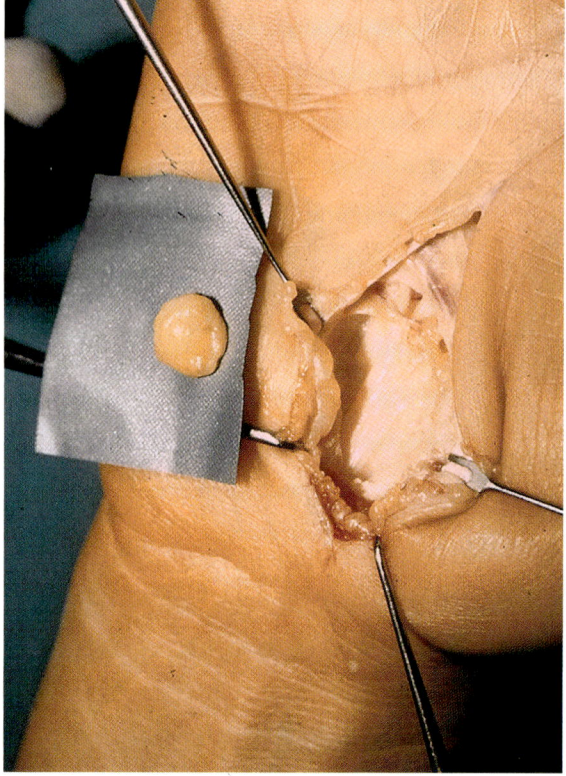

Fig. 16.9. Median nerve with double cutaneous branch: thenar and hypothenar

Fig. 16.10. Lipoma inside the carpal tunnel, close to the median nerve

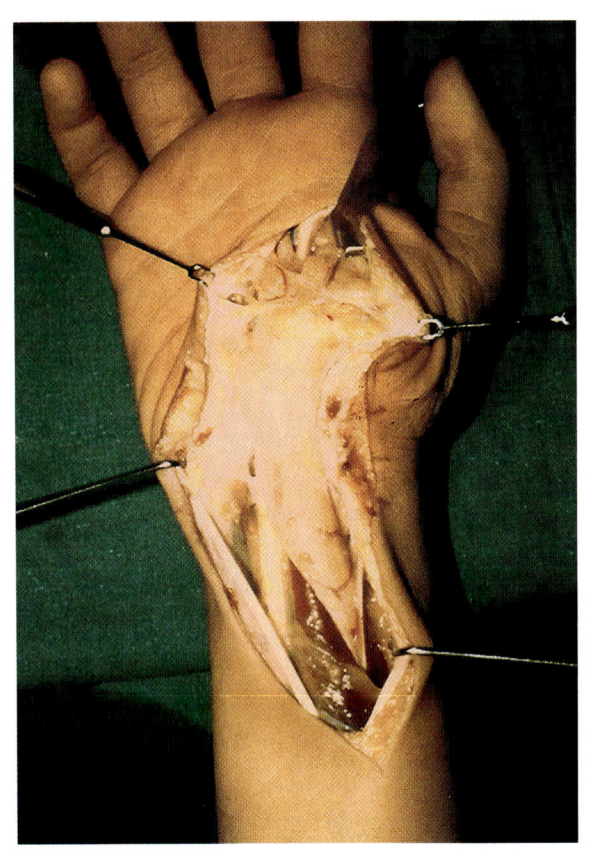

Fig. 16.11. Lipofibroma of the median nerve

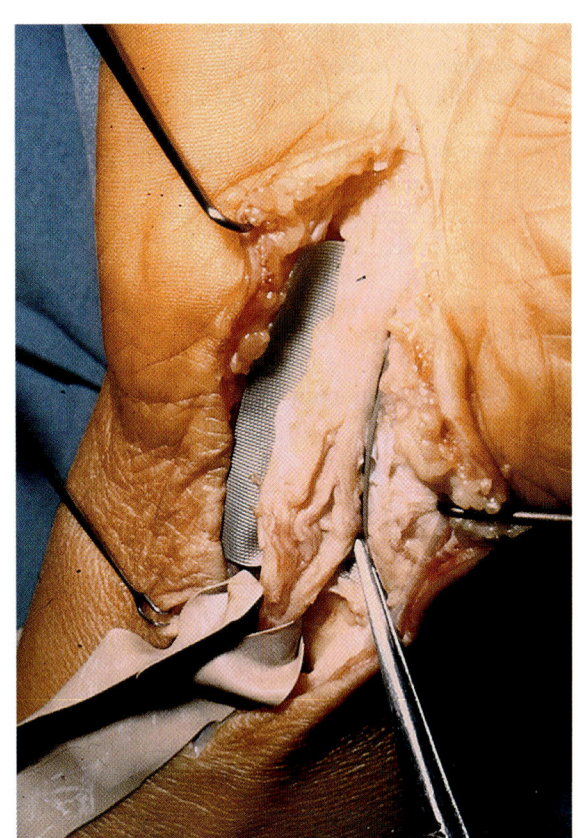

Fig. 16.12. Neurofibroma of the median nerve

Contraindications

Generally, there are no absolute contraindications, because this procedure usually produces good results and patient satisfaction. However, when a patient needs (for age, position, or activity) a very fast recovery and a better cosmetic result, we consider the use of more recently developed endoscopic or mini-invasive techniques particularly useful.

Complications

If the technique is carefully performed, generally, there are no complications; however, in a limited number of cases, we have observed hypertrophic scarring together with some hyperesthesia.

In almost all cases, physiotherapeutic treatment of the scar produces better results.

For these reasons, the social cost of the procedure, due to late recovery and return to work, is rather high.

Author's Suggestions

In general, I suggest that this operation never be undervalued because, although it is very common and could therefore seem to be simple and banal, it is often the case that unusual anatomical or pathological situations exist. Great care must be used to avoid iatrogenic damages, unexpected by the patients, which can result in serious legal consequences.

In particular, I suggest that during the operation the following steps be taken:

- Dissect the transverse ligament longitudinally, along its ulnar margin; cut off a small longitudinal strip of it, avoiding the closure of the tunnel during the scar period and the subsequent risk of recurrences.
- Always explore the nerve proximally and distally and check, with your finger, the complete dissection of all the subcutaneous structures, which are possible causes of residual nerve compression.
- Do not move up completely the nerve – it may damage the cutaneous branches. Instead, move it toward the radial side together with flexor tendons, thereby preserving the motor branch.

- The operation should be performed with axillary block anesthesia, thereby avoiding surrounding the tissue with anesthetic liquid and the possible nerve damage caused by the needle.
- Always use a tourniquet at the base of the arm.
- Take great care with the hemostasis, waiting a few minutes after tourniquet removal, because of reactive hyperemia.

Postoperative Care

Always use a passing drain strip to be removed after 24 h.

Rehabilitation Protocol

Three to four weeks after surgery, the patients start automassages on the scar twice a day with cortisone cream. Later on, ultrasound and physical therapy can be suggested until complete recovery.

References

1. Marie P, Foix C (1913) Atrophie isolee de l'eminence thenar d'origine nevritique, role du legamente anulaire anterieur du carpe dans la pathogenie de la lesion Revue. Neurol 21:647
2. Learmoth JR: The principle of decompression in the treatment of certain deseases of peripheral nerves. Surg. Clin. North Am. 13: 905, 933
4. Phalen GS (1966) The Carpal Tunnel Syndrome. Seventeen years experience in diagnosis and treatment of six hundred fifty-four hands J Bone Joint Surg 48A:211
5. Bertolotti P (1993) Sindromi da intrappolamento dell'arto superiore. Fondazione Savonese per gli studi sulla mano, 81 – 121
6. Taleisnik J (1973) The palmar cutaneous branch of the median nerve and the approach to the carpal tunnel. J Bone Joint Surg. 55A:121
7. Cacialli S, Grazzini S (1983) Analisi dei risultati sfavorevoli nel trattamento chirurgico della Sindrome del Tunnel Carpale. Riv. Chir della Mano Vol 20, 421 – 425
8. Crandal RE, Weeks PM (1988) Multiple nerve disfunction after carpal tunnel release. J Hand Surg.13A, 584 – 589
9. Amadio PC (1992) The Mayo Clinic and Carpal Tunnel syndrome. Mayo Clin. Proc.67:42
10. Delcroix G (1965) Su alcuni casi di variazione del nervo mediano alla regione del polso. Riv.Chir.Mano, 3, 228 – 230
11. Lanz U (1977) Anathomical variations of the median nerve in the carpal tunnel, J Hand Surg 2;53

Chapter 17

Palmar Incision

R. Luchetti

Introduction

A vast amount of medical literature has been written concerning surgical approaches for transverse carpal ligament (TCL) sectioning [1–19].

Surgical incisions that are localized to the wrist-palm area have replaced the single palmar incision. The choice of a surgical approach that is shorter and where the incision site will be located depends on various factors: (1) explicit knowledge of the physiopathology in relation to median nerve compression at the carpal canal (anatomical correspondence between nerve compression site and palm-wrist cutaneous projection; Figs. 17.1–17.3); (2) an increase in the frequency of both early onset and moderate level carpal tunnel syndrome (CTS) surgeries; (3) an increased request by the patient for aesthetic-functional aspects of the scar.

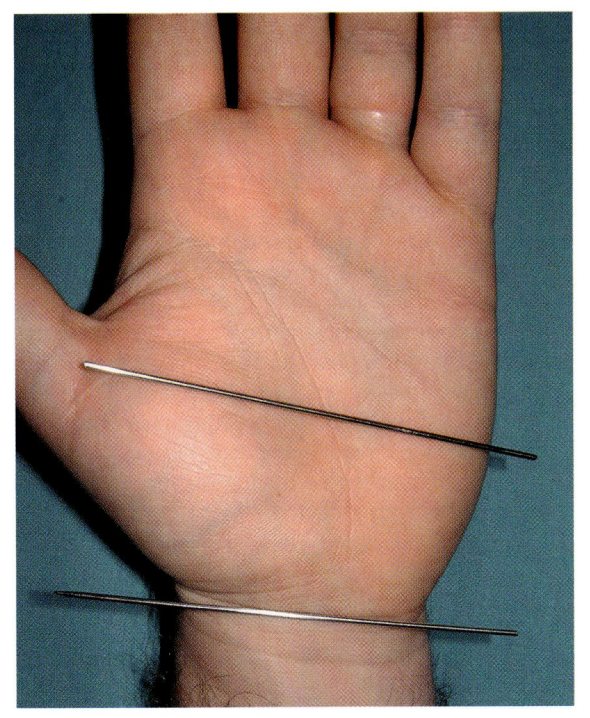

Fig. 17.1. Skeletal demarcation x-ray taken in anterior-posterior, proximal-distal projections of the carpal canal

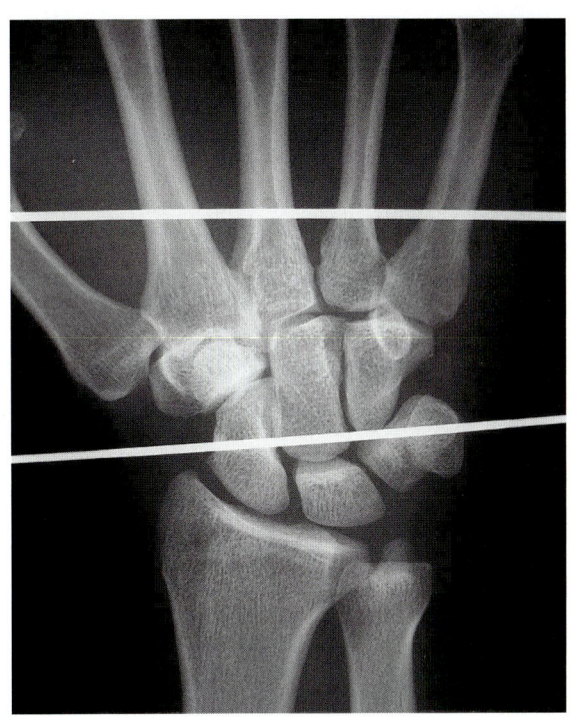

Fig. 17.2. Skeletal demarcation x-ray taken in lateral, proximal, and distal projections of the carpal canal

In relation to the palmar approach, Ariyan [1] and Nigst [20] recommend curvilinear and longitudinal incision on or parallel to the thenar crease that passes over the palm ulnarly along the fourth ray axis (Fig. 17.4). The incision extends over the base of the hand and curves ulnarly before reaching the wrist. Its extension is optional for 1–2 cm at the wrist. The TCL and antebrachial fascia is sectioned for 3 cm up until the distal flexor wrist crease. The bottom of the canal should be inspected thoroughly for possible abnormalities or masses. Excision of the tendon sheath is not performed except when hypertrophy is present due to rheumatoid arthritis.

Taleisnik [19] begins the incision at the interthenar fold, in the middle of the palm, and continues proximally up until where the ulnar margin of the fourth ray intersects the distal wrist crease (see Chap. 16). The

122 III Treatment

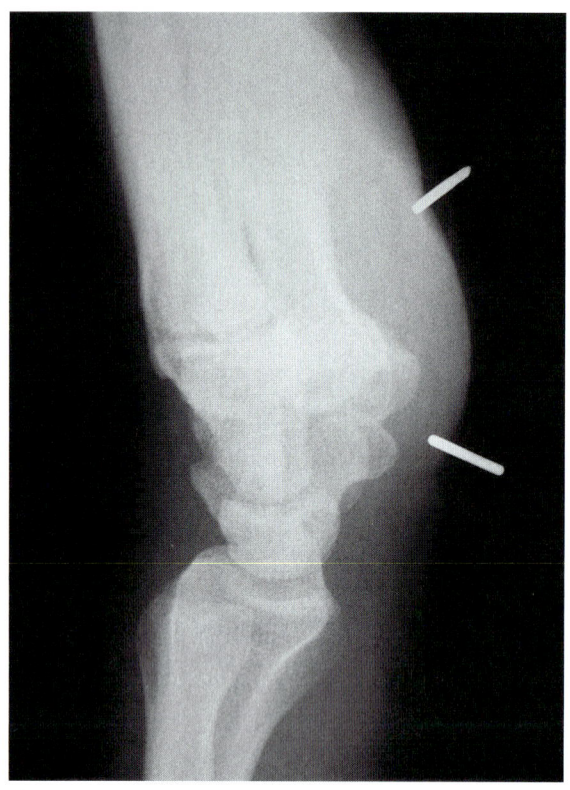

Fig. 17.3. Cutaneous palmar-wrist limits of the carpal canal

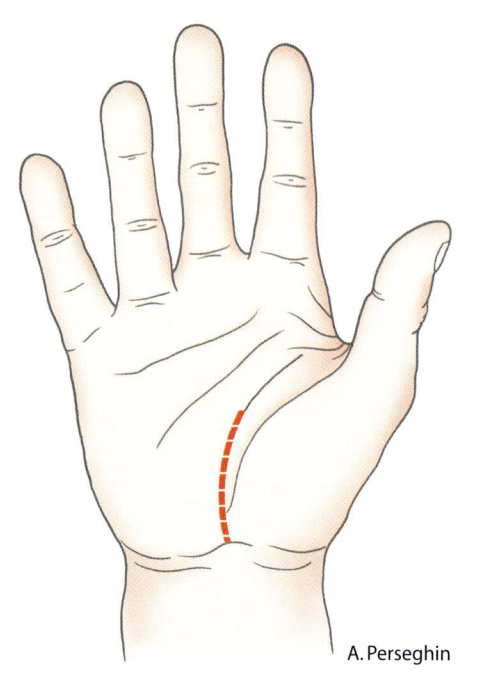

Fig. 17.4. Cutaneous incision according to Ariyan and Nigst [1, 20]

TCL is isolated and divided longitudinally near the point where the adipose tissue is encountered and wraps itself around the superficial vascular palmer arch. A more proximal exposure can be made, if necessary, at the wrist, by extending the incision proximally in an ulnar direction.

Gelberman [21] advises that a purely palmar approach should be performed (similar to that which has been described by Connolly [22]. The proximal reference point can be found by flexing the fourth finger towards the distal wrist crease. Once identifying this point, one traces a cutaneous incision line, in a curved projection, along the fourth ray. It is advisable to move lateral to this line for both the cutaneous incision and its underlying exposure. The cutaneous incision line is ulnarly located with respect to the thenar crease and is located 2 mm ulnarly to the fourth ray. An optical magnification of 3.5 is used during the dissection. As soon as the skin is incised, the surgeon should be extremely careful to look for eventual sensitive branch anomalies that cross over the same incision line (see Chap. 15). As soon as the proximal margin of the TCL is isolated, sectioning is begun along the fourth ray. The distal half of the TCL is sectioned in layers. One should also be extremely careful when sectioning the midpalmar adipose tissue that surrounds the superficial vascular arch. Therefore, the antebrachial fascia should be sectioned for 2–3 cm. The external margins of the TCL are raised towards the thenar muscles and the median nerve is detached from the TCL; thorough checking of the compression site and the epineurium's thickness should always be done. The tissue should be infiltrated with 1% lidocaine without epinephrine before removing the tourniquet and suturing the skin. A volar splint is then applied positioning the wrist at 30° of extension.

Author's Preferred Technique

The anesthetic technique used in this surgery is chosen at the discretion of the surgeon, anesthesiologist and patient. The surgery is begun only once ischemia has been achieved in the upper extremity by using a proximally placed upper arm tourniquet. A single surgeon, with the help of a surgical nurse, can perform the surgery. The surgical instruments that are needed (Fig. 17.5) for this type of surgery are: a scalpel (blade no. 15), two hooks, two tweezers (one anatomical and one surgical) a pair of blunt scissors, a small elevator, and a surgical marker for tracing the incision line. A "lead hand" blocking device is useful for positioning the hand and fingers and a bipolar coagulator is necessary for obtaining hemostasis.

The incision begins in the midpalm and is directed towards the fourth ray, immediately under the palmar flexor crease, and proceeds proximally to the distal flexor wrist crease. The incision is made in a straight line, sometimes curvilinear at the lunar concavity (Fig. 17.6).

17 Palmar Incision 123

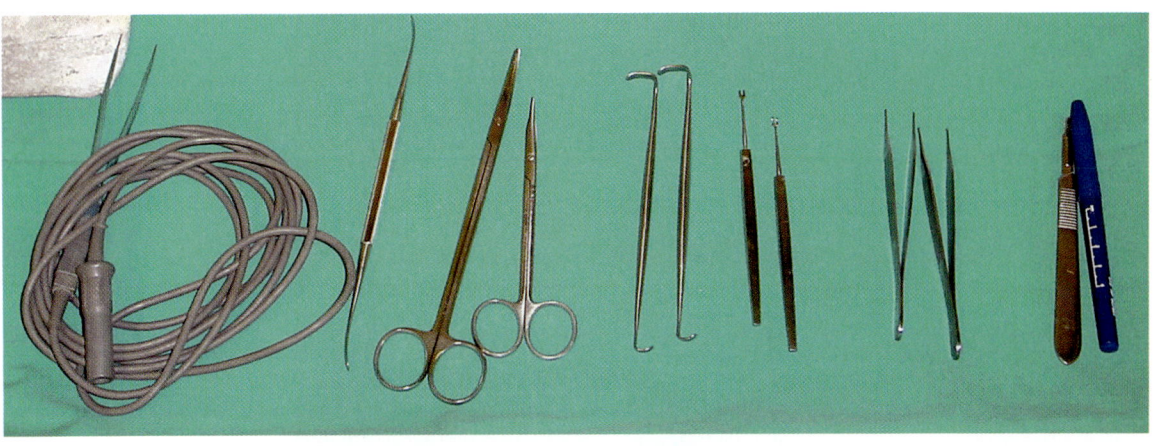

Fig. 17.5. Instruments that are used in the surgical treatment of carpal tunnel syndrome

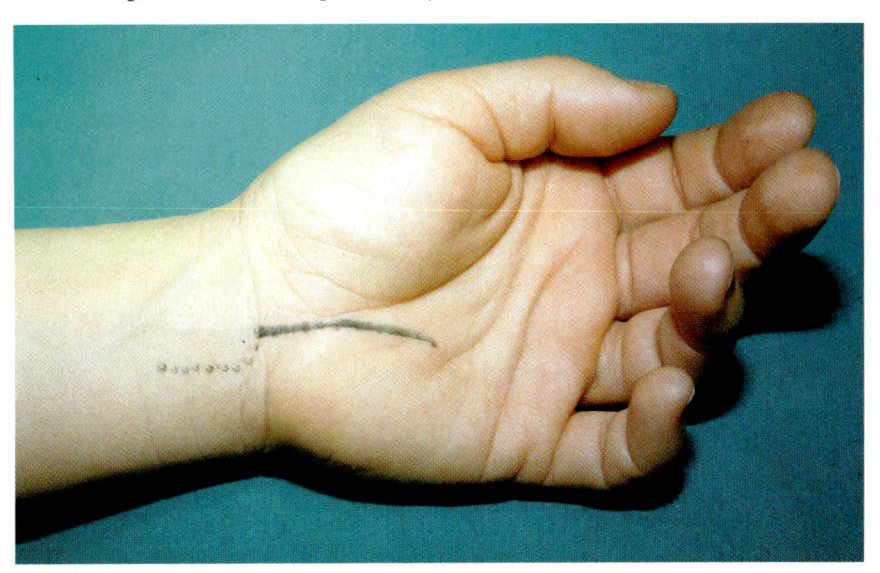

Fig. 17.6. Cutaneous incision

In order to better expose the underlying structures, the two hooks are applied to the skin. An ocular magnifying instrument is used in order to more easily see the terminal sensitive branches of the palmar cutaneous and median nerve [23, 24] or branches of the ulnar nerve [25] and therefore they can be protected from unnecessary injury (Figs. 17.7, 17.8). In the central tract, central-proximal to the site of the incision, preligamentous adipose tissue is found and should be sectioned, protecting the eventual neurosensitive underlying structures. Hemostasis is accurately performed for each layer, above all, in the adipose tissue area. At this point, the ulnar hook is exchanged with a spatula in order to open the surgical field guaranteeing a broader visual field and therefore greater protection to the surrounding structures. Proceeding in a distal-proximal direction, the palmer fascia that covers the branch of the palmer arch, which comes off the ulnar artery, is sectioned. Even this fascia is incised and the ulnar artery is exposed before the superficial arch. The vascular structures are placed aside ulnarly and protected. At this point, at the TCL level, an incision is made that has a slightly conical shape at the surgical distal aperture. The ligament incision is done on the ulnar side, towards the hook of the hamate. The first structures that border and come out of this area are the fifth finger flexor tendons (Figs. 17.9–17.13). It is important to be careful during the sectioning of this part of the TCL in this area, because frequently one can encounter the terminal branches of the median nerve and eventual anastomoses of the ulnar nerve (Fig. 17.14). The incision proceeds in a proximal direction and one can appreciate the change in consistency of the ligament. It is usually thicker in this area. The procedure is considered finished when one reaches the proximal end of the TCL which is in correspondence to the distal wrist crease. At this point, one should continue subcutaneously and start to section the antebrachial fascia for some centimeters. Two hooks are applied to the proximal margins of the incision moving the skin so that the surgeon can

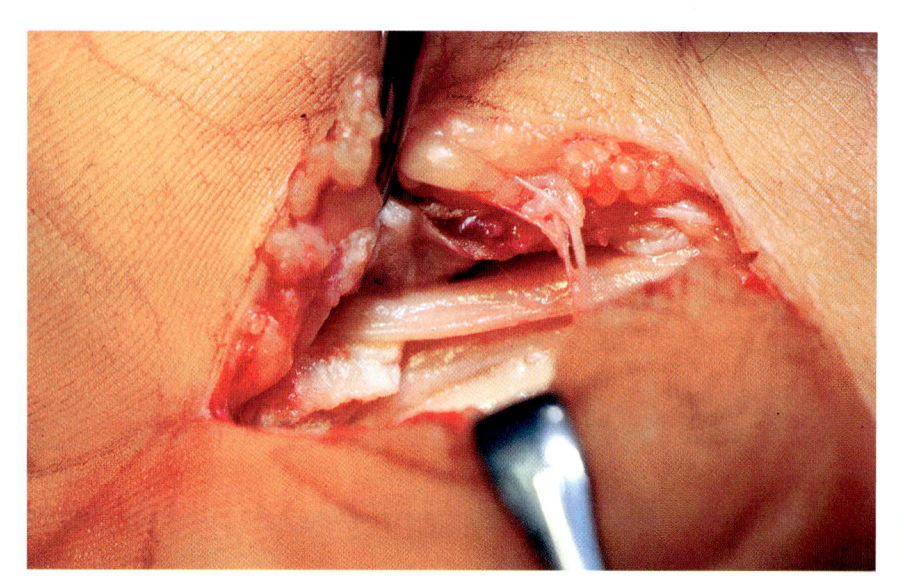

Fig. 17.7. Surgical findings regarding the sensitive branch through a cutaneous incision

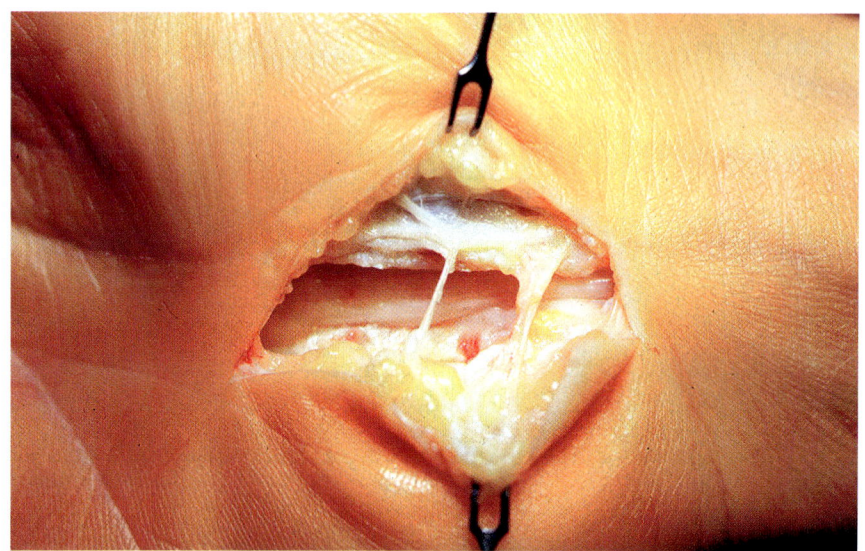

Fig. 17.8. Surgical findings regarding two sensitive branches through a cutaneous incision

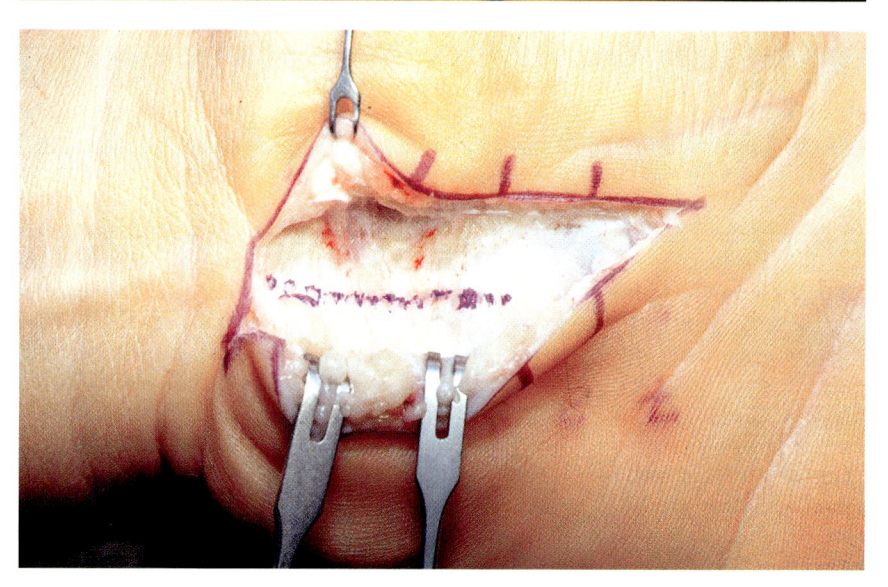

Fig. 17.9. The incision site for the transverse carpal ligament

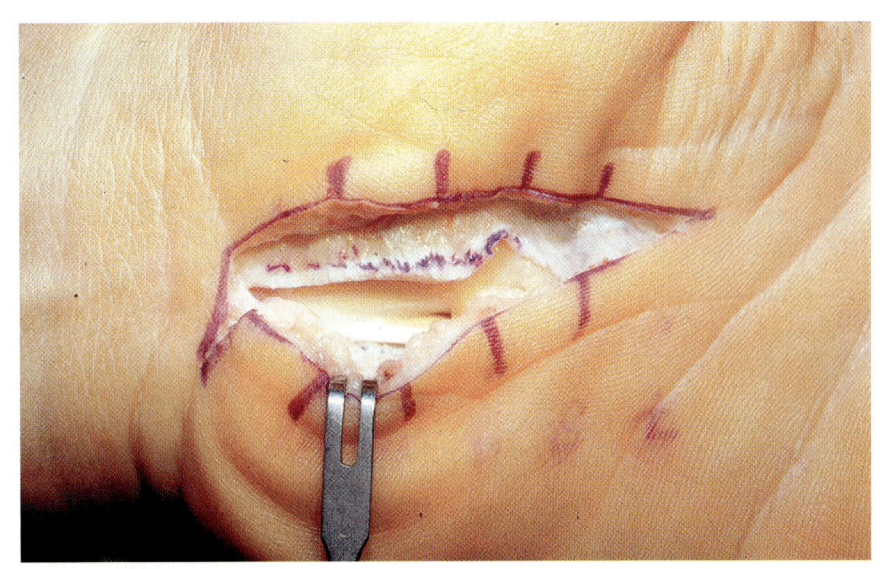

Fig. 17.10. Ligament sectioning

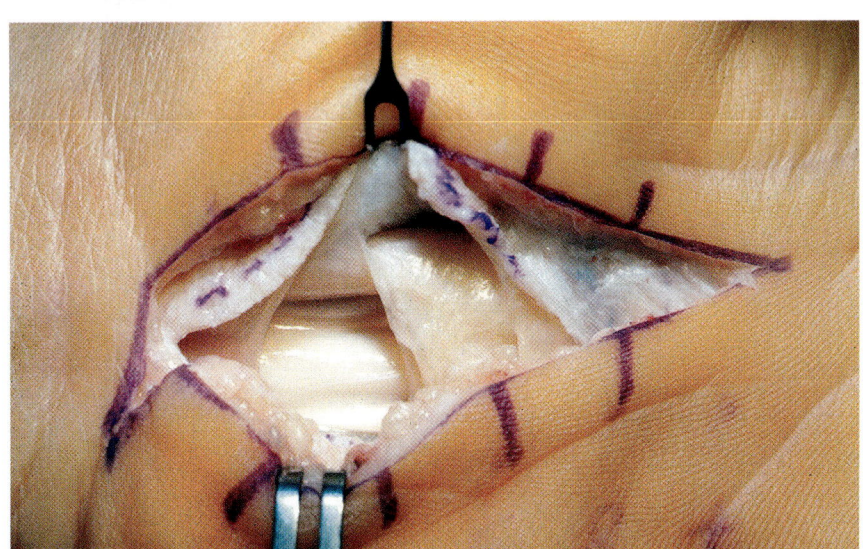

Fig. 17.11. Median nerve adhesion to the deep layers of the transverse ligament

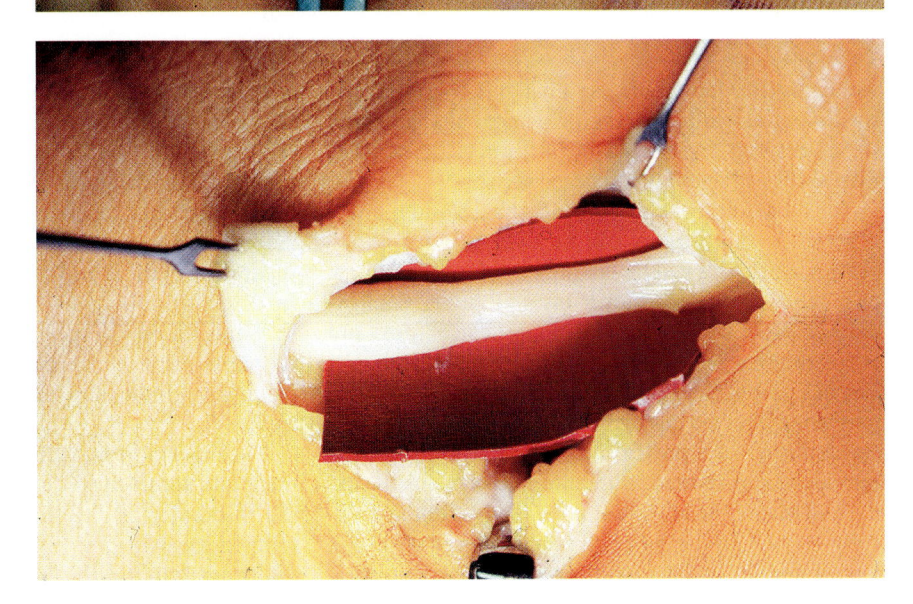

Fig. 17.12. Exposure of the median nerve with highlighter; note the double compression site

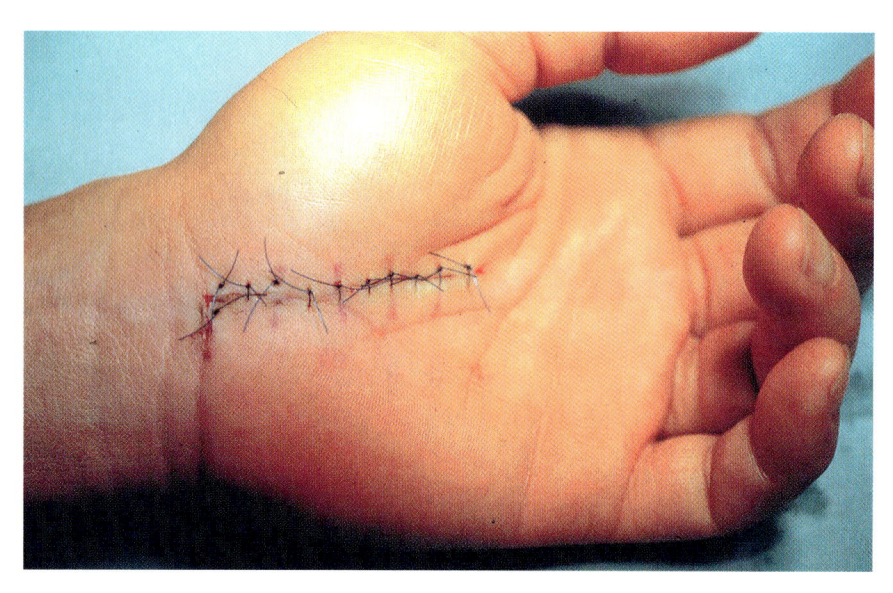

Fig. 17.13. Cutaneous suture

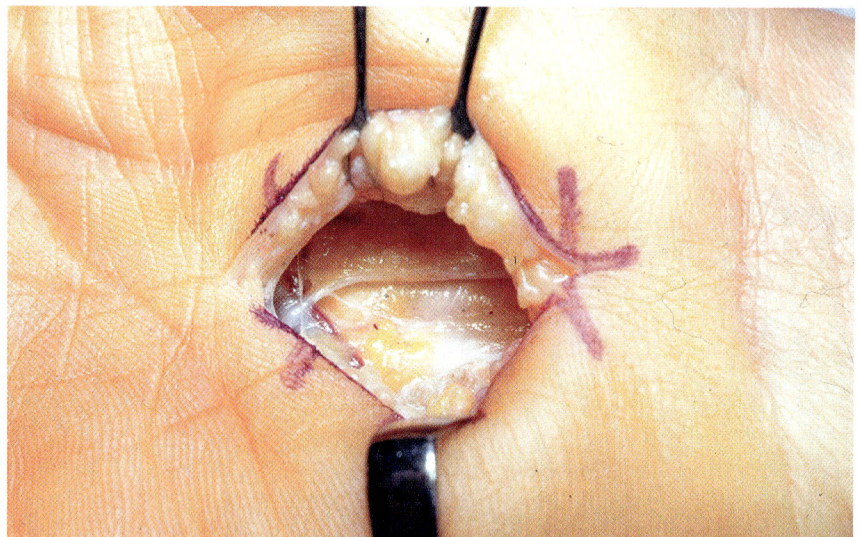

Fig. 17.14. Distal anastomosis between the median and ulnar nerve

see the fascia. One should use small, blunt-ended scissors when carefully moving or detaching anatomical structures that are located in this area. The fascia is then sectioned with blunt, curved scissors.

For those surgeons who already have good manual experience, this surgery can be done using a no. 15 blade scalpel. The two hooks raise up the skin and expose the fascia: a separator is inserted under the ligament in order to separate the adherent structures and to create a space in order to introduce the scalpel blade. The flat part of the blade is introduced with the sharp part being directed towards the ulnar side and one delicately pushes in a proximal direction. The superficial traction that is created by the two hooks opens the canal and favors the entrance of the blade without difficulty. As soon as the entire blade has entered the canal, it is rotated 90° so that its cutting edge is positioned vo-larly and pressure is placed in a superior direction. In this way the blade cuts in an upward direction, thus sectioning the tissue without ripping it. At the end of the procedure the complete release of both the retinaculum and antebrachial fascia is determined. By using a palpator introduced in a palm-wrist direction, the surgical separation of these two structures is tested with a back (proximal-distal) maneuver. Resistance must not be encountered during the back maneuver. If resistance is encountered, it is mandatory to reperform or to complete the retinaculum and/or antebrachial fascia release.

The median nerve is frequently adherent to the ligament and sometimes it is so tenaciously adherent that the thickening of the surrounding structures, which wrap themselves around it, are similar to the actual median nerve canal itself. The nerve is delicately detached from the ligament by using blunt-ended scissors, taking the utmost care not to injure surrounding nerve structures that come off of the median nerve itself. These nerve structures can correspond to an anomaly of the palmer cutaneous nerve's sensitive branch, which comes off any part of the median nerve, even the ulnar side, its most distal portion, or off a motor accessory anomaly or a communicating ulnar nerve. These above-mentioned anomalies could perforate the ligament and represent an adherent point on the median nerve, which leads to a compressive pathology. Another important nerve structure that must be checked is the anatomical branch of the median nerve that can come off the ulnar nerve [26] just as it exits from the canal.

The median nerve is carefully checked at the same time that the surgeon performs this maneuver or immediately thereafter. If the fascicular nerve structure is not recognizable and a thickening of its most external sheath has occurred, an epineurotomy is indicated. This delicate technical procedure on the median nerve must be performed on its ulnar side in order to make sure that it is free and that eventual adhesions along the scar tract do not form. If the two scar incisions (ligament and epineurium) correspond, it is highly possible that scar adhesions can form and restrict the nerve gliding. If the nerve's fascicular structures are recognizable, then this technical procedure is not necessary.

We do not perform epineurectomy or internal neurolysis without very specific motives. These procedures can provoke phenomenon of nerve devascularization and iatrogenic injury. If these procedures must be done, then optical magnification of the surgical field is imperative.

The anomalous nerve branches are carefully sectioned and then freed from their passage along the ligament. This is done in order to avoid median nerve adhesions from forming, and causing eventual residual CTS. The motor branch is systematically located in order to verify its position. If the passage is extraligamentous it is sufficient enough to check its integrity, but if it is intraligamentous then it is better to perform a decompression by sectioning the ligament, as has been previously described for the anomalous branches. If a prestenotic thickening has occurred, then an epineurectomy is indicated.

The nerve is checked in order to see how it glides in a longitudinal direction [27–29]. The nerve can be exposed by using tweezers and hooking the skin so that the TCL's radial flap can be raised, the perineural tissue can be tractioned, and the part of the median nerve that is located in the proximal area is exposed. If necessary, an epineurotomy is performed in this area. If there are doubts as to the nerve's integrity, due to the presence of a lateral neuroma and a constrictive stenosis, we advise that the skin incision is widened in order to directly expose the nerve and efficiently treat the immediate condition.

At the end of the procedure, the tourniquet is removed and an accurate hemostasis is performed. The skin is sutured with Nylon or Dermalon 4/0 or 5/0. A small, plastic drain is inserted and is usually removed during the first postoperative medication, which is done 1 or 2 days after. A light, nonconstrictive elastic bandage is applied and the fingers are left free to move. Generally, we do not use wrist immobilization splints, but the patient is instructed not to flex the wrist and to immediately begin mobilizing the fingers in all directions.

Additional Technical Procedure

Guyon Tunnel Decompression

In 1973, Sedal [30] reported on the presence of superficial palmar arch anomalies of the ulnar nerve in 40% of CTS patients. On the basis of these findings, many hand surgeons uphold the usefulness of performing a decompression of the ulnar nerve in Guyon tunnel at the same time that the median nerve is being decompressed in the carpal tunnel.

In 1985, Silver and colleagues [31] evaluated the effects of carpal tunnel decompression on patients with documented neuro-electrical abnormalities of the median and ulnar nerve. A significant percent of these cases had clinical signs of ulnar nerve compression at the wrist. After the decompression was performed, only in the carpal tunnel and not in the Guyon tunnel, 89% of the cases demonstrated an improvement in their symptoms in the ulnar nerve distribution territory. Based on these findings, one can conclude that decompression of the Guyon tunnel is not always necessary during a CTS median nerve decompression. A recent morphological study has demonstrated that the dimension and the shape of the Guyon canal undergoes modifications after a decompression of the carpal canal is performed. MRI exams have demonstrated that the ulnar canal increases in diameter from a triangular to an oval shape.

These results sustain observations that have been made by Silver. The TCL fibers extend ulnarly towards the hook of the hamate and form the ceiling of the Guyon tunnel. The sectioning of the TCL fibers from the ulnar side reduces the tension of the Guyon tunnel fibers.

This additional procedure is suggested only in conditions where there are accurate clinical signs of ulnar nerve compression within the Guyon tunnel.

Synovectomy

Flexor tendon synovectomy is not indicated if cell proliferation is not present, as is usually associated with and found in cases with rheumatoid arthritis.

No complications have been yet reported due to the lack of flexor tendon vaginal removal during the treatment of idiopathic CTS [21].

Postoperative Care Suggested by the Author

The hand should be placed in a position which aids in venous return (above the level of the heart), whether the patient is standing or lying down. The patient is educated, immediately postoperatively to begin moving the fingers, elbow, and shoulder throughout the day. The wrist and fingers can be moved contemporaneously, but the hand and wrist should not undergo resistive strains.

The drain is removed during the first medication. The patient should change medications and perform tepid water baths with a gentle disinfectant (1 spoon of Amuchina for 1 l of water). The bath should last 20 min and the patient should move the wrist and fingers back and forth, as well as open and close the fist in the water. The only movement to be avoided is wrist flexion. Once the hand is removed from the water, it should be thoroughly dried with a sterile gauze and wrapped in a light elastic bandage. Other medicinal ointments do not need to be applied. The postoperative medical treatment is characterized by the administration of a large spectrum antibiotic for 3 days and an anti-inflammatory. The sutures are removed on the 8th to 9th postoperative day. The baths should continue for another additional week. Progressively, the patient is educated to use the hand in their activities of daily living, but without excessively overloading it. Three weeks after operation the patient can begin progressive resistive activities, and return to work is usually by the 6th week, when they can fully load the wrist and hand.

In cases where there is excessive edema or the initial signs of reflex sympathetic dystrophy, the patient is sent to a specialized hand therapist and compressive bandages are applied to aid in stimulating venous return, and a specific hand therapy program is initiated to prevent the onset of finger and wrist rigidity (see Chap. 36 entitled "Postoperative Treatment of Carpal Tunnel Syndrome After Median Nerve Decompression (Open Field or Endoscopic Technique)").

Summary and Suggestions

The surgery is almost always performed by brachial plexus anesthesia or local anesthesia. In the latter, the presence of a liquid anesthetic in the treatment site can slow down the surgical maneuver.

The tourniquet that is used to provoke ischemia of the upper extremity is well tolerated for 15 min; this is a sufficient amount of time for the entire surgery to be performed.

The surgical incision is based on the presence of two nerve structures: the palmar cutaneous and the motor branch of the median nerve [32]. The sensitive branch, anomalies, and the ulnar nerve [25] can cross the incision site, as well as the palmar cutaneous nerve [23], and they can cause pain in the scar site. For this reason, it is of utmost importance that once the skin incision has been made, the surgeon carefully distinguishes these structures and protects them from injury. Sectioning of the TCL can be initiated proximally or distally because it will be sectioned completely. The sectioning of the antebrachial fascia for 2–3 cm is facultative, but advised. The sectioning of the ligament must be as ulnarly located as possible. It maintains a protective function for the pulley system even after it has been sectioned, even if the canal changes its dimensions. Postoperative reduced grasp strength can be totally recuperated within 6 months from the time of surgery.

Carpal tunnel decompression is sufficient in the treatment of a median nerve compression within the carpal canal. Gelberman [34] has demonstrated that a simple decompression has healing effects on the CTS-afflicted patient without necessitating direct surgical maneuvers to the nerve itself (such as a neurolysis). These same results have been reconfirmed by the studies that have been conducted by Mackinnon [35] and Dellon [36]. However, it is important to remember that a thickened epineurium should be reconstructed and it is useful to perform an epineurotomy in order to decompress the fascicles. Myers [37] has demonstrated that endoneural pressure can be elevated if there is an external compression and it will remain high even after a reduction of the external pressure, like that which happens after a decompression [38, 39]. The site of the epineurotomy must be performed ulnar to the nerve [40].

Excision of the tendon sheath is reserved for only hypertrophic-hyperplastic cases, such as those found in rheumatoid arthritis.

The median nerve should be completely checked once the incision is made by applying a longitudinal traction to it while flexing the wrist and fingers, thus exposing it both proximally and distally at the canal. This maneuver should be performed with extreme care and delicacy. The surgeon can also perform an ulterior epineurotomy both proximal and/or distal to the exposed nerve when performing this maneuver

The motor branch is always checked in case it has been compressed in association with or isolated from the median nerve compression [21]. If neglected at this level, the median nerve decompression will not be sufficient to restore a thenar muscle defect.

References

1. Ariyan S, Watson HK (1977) The palmar approach for the visualization and release of the carpal tunnel. An analysis of 429 cases. Plast Reconstr Surg 60, 539–547
2. Crow RS (1960) Treatment of the carpal tunnel syndrome. Br Med J 1, 1611–1615
3. Cseuz KA, Thomas JE, Lambert EH et al. (1941) Long-term results of operation for carpal tunnel syndrome. Mayo Clin Proc 41, 232–241
4. Dahlin LB, Danielson N, Ehira T et al. (1986) Mechanical effects of compression on peripheral nerves. J Biochem Eng 108, 120
5. Denman EE (1981) The anatomy of the incision for carpal tunnel decompression. Hand 13, 17–28
6. Eboh N, Wilson DH (1978) Surgery of the carpal tunnel. Technical note. J Neurosurg 49, 316–318
7. Freshwater MF, Arons MS (1978) The effect of various adjuncts on the surgical treatment of carpal tunnel syndrome secondary to chronic tenosynovitis. Plast Reconstr Surg 61, 93–96
8. Harris CM, Tanner E, Goldstein MN, Pettee DS (1979) The surgical treatment of the carpal tunnel syndrome correlated with preoperative nerve conduction studies. J Bone Joint Surg 61A, 93
9. Hoppenfeld S, deBoer S (1984) Surgical Exposures in orthopaedics: the anatomic approach. Philadelphia: JB Lippincott, 154–157
10. Hunt WE, Luckey WT (1964) The carpal tunnel syndrome. Diagnosis and treatment. J Neurosurg 21, 178–181
11. Loong SC, Seah SC (1971) Comparison of median and ulnar sensory nerve action potentials in the diagnosis of the carpal tunnel syndrome. J Neurol Neurosurg Psychiatry 34, 750
12. MacDonald RI, Lichtman DM, Hanlon JJ, Wilson JN (1978) Complications of surgical release for carpal tunnel syndrome. J Hand Surg 3, 70–76
13. Milford L (1987) Carpal tunnel and ulnar tunnel syndromes and stenosing tenosynovitis. In: Edmondson AS, Crenshaw AH, eds. Campbell's operative orthopaedics. ed 7. St Louis: CV Mosby, 459–461
14. Mitz V, LeViet D, Vilain R (1982) Syndrome du canal carpien. Incision esthetique. Nouv Presse Med 11, 2353–2354
15. Phalen GS (1966) The carpal tunnel syndrome. Seventeen years experience in diagnosis and treatment of 654 hands, J Bone Joint Surg 48A, 211
16. Phalen GS, Gardner WJ, LaLonde AA (1950) Neuropathy of the median nerve due to compression beneath the transverse carpal ligament. J Bone Joint Surg 32, 109–112
17. Rowland SA (1974) A palmar incision for release of the carpal tunnel. Clin Orthop 103, 89–90
18. Szabo R (1989) Nerve compression syndromes: diagnosis and treatment. Thorofare, Nj: Slack
19. Taleisnik J (1988) Fracture of the carpal bones. In: Chapman MW, ed. Operative orthopaedics. Philadelphia: JB Lippincott 1346–1348
20. Nigst H (1992) The carpal tunnel syndrome. Operative technique for surgical decompression. Orthop and Traumat 1, 122–129
21. Gelberman RH, North ER (1991) Carpal tunnel release. Open release of transverse carpal ligament. In: Operative nerve repair and reconstruction. Gelberman RH (ed). Philadelphia: JB Lippincott, 899–912
22. Connolly WB (1984) Treatment for carpal tunnel syndrome. London: Wolfe
23. Taleisnik J (1973) The palmar cutaneous branch of the median nerve and the approach to the carpal tunnel. An anatomical study. J Bone Joint Surg 55A, 1212–1217
24. Tomaino MM, Plakseychuk A (1998) Identification and preservation of palmar cutaneous nerves during open carpal tunnel release. J Hand Surg. 23B:607–608
25. Enberg WD, Gmeiner JG (1980) Palmar cutaneous branch of the ulnar nerve. J Hand Surg 5, 26–29
26. Ferrari GP, Gilbert A (1991) The superfcial anastomosis on the palm of the hand between the ulnar and median nerves. J Hand Surg 16B, 511–514
27. McLellan DL, Swash M (1976) Longitudinal sliding of the median nerve during movements of the upper limb. J Neurol Neurosurg Psychiatry 39, 566–570
28. Wilgis M (1986) The significance of longitudinal excursions in peripheral nerves. Hand Clin 2, 761–768
29. Millesi H, Zock G, Rath Th (1990) The gliding apparatus of peripheral nerve and its clinical significance. Ann Hand Surg 9, 87–97
30. Sedal L, McLeod JG, Walsh JC (1973) Ulnar nerve lesions associated with the carpal tunnel syndrome. J Neurol Neursurg Psychiatry 36, 118–123
31. Silver MA, Gelberman RH, Gellman H et al. (1985) Carpal tunnel syndrome: associated abnormalities in ulnar nerve function and the effect of carpal tunnel release on these abnormalities. J Hand Surg 10A, 710
32. Kuhlmann NR, Tubiana R, Lisfranc R (1978) Apport de l'anatomie dans la comprehension des syndromes du canal carpien et des sequelles des interventions decompressives. Rev Chir Orthop 64, 59
33. Gellman H, Kan D, Gee V et al. (1989) Analysis of pinch and grip strength after carpal tunnel release. J Hand Surg 14A, 863–864
34. Gelberman RH, Pfeffer GB, Galbraith RT et al. (1987) Results of treatment of severe carpal-tunnel syndrome without internal neurolysis of the median nerve. J Bone Joint Surg 69A, 896–903
35. Mackinnon SE, O'Brien JP, Dellon AL et al. (1988) An assessment of the effects of internal neurolysis on a chronically compressed rat sciatic nerve. Plast Reconstr Surg 81, 251–258
36. Dellon AL, Mackinnon SE (1988) Surgery of peripheral nerves. New York, Thieme
37. Myers RR, Heckman HM, Powell HC (1983) Endoneurial fluid is hypertonic. result of microanalysis and its significance in neuropathy. J Neuropathol and Exper Neurol 42, 217–224
38. Lundborg G, Myers P, Powell H (1983) Nerve compression injury and increased endoneurial fluid pressure: a "miniature compartment syndrome". J Neurol Neurosurg Psych 46, 1119–1124
39. Lundborg G (1988) Nerve injury and repair. New York Churchill Livingstone
40. Carroll RE, Green DP (1972) The significance of the palmar cutaneous nerve at the wrist. Clin Orthop 83, 24–27

18 Open Carpal Tunnel Release with a Short Palmar Incision and No Specialized Instruments Combined with a Rehabilitation Program for Early Return to Activity

P.A. NATHAN

Outcomes from surgical procedures are assessed by the extent to which symptoms are relieved and patients can resume the normal activities of daily living, including gainful employment. Optimally, surgery satisfies the criteria of the Three Es: it has a limited impact on health care resources and causes little disruption to human anatomic structures (*economy*); it consists of methods that can be performed competently, with few difficult surgical skills (*efficiency*); and it accomplishes its intended purpose, which is relief of symptoms and restoration of function (*effectiveness*). A simplified approach to open release of the carpal tunnel (OCTR), with a short palmar incision, satisfies these criteria. This approach is consistent with today's trend for minimally invasive surgical procedures.

Technical aspects of OCTR with short palmar incision, along with a program for postoperative rehabilitation, are discussed in this chapter. We have found that a combined surgery-postoperative rehabilitation program achieves favorable outcomes with only minimal disruption to patients' normal daily routines [14]. A review of private and workers' compensation patient records from our clinic indicates that patients who undergo OCTR with short palmar incision followed by postoperative rehabilitation can, on average, return to modified or regular work by the end of the first week or during the second week after surgery.

Implementation of OCTR with Short Palmar Incision

As endoscopic carpal tunnel release (ECTR) techniques became available they were reported to provide rapid recovery and decreased postoperative pain and functional limitations [4]. This was during a period when it was common to use longer incisions, which at times extended into the distal forearm, for OCTR. The less rapid recovery time from OCTR was thought to be secondary to the longer lengthof the incision. This was felt to result in more incisional soft tissue discomfort and pillar pain than ECTR, and in turn delayed resumption of normal hand activities. The abbreviated recovery times reported in response to ECTR prompted us to ask if decreasing the length of the open surgical incision could improve recovery time from OCTR. The key to achieving a more rapid recovery appeared to be in reduction of intraoperative trauma to skin and subcutaneous tissues.

The proximal margin of the transverse carpal ligament is at the distal wrist crease, and the ligament extends 2–3 cm into the palm. We felt initially that a shorter incision could theoretically compromise vision intraoperatively and thus increase the risk for nerve injury or incomplete release of the transverse carpal ligament. In practice we have not encountered these complications.

Indications/Contraindications and Complications

We have used a procedure involving a short (2 cm) palmar incision for OCTR for 14 years. This surgical approach has been effective, even in the presence of severe conduction abnormalities of the median nerve that include involvement of the motor fibers. A slightly longer incision may be indicated for surgical re-release of the carpal tunnel, as the anatomical structures in the area of the carpal tunnel may be poorly defined, or when a need for synovectomy is anticipated, as in comorbid conditions such as rheumatoid arthritis. Though we have not encountered intraoperative complications when using OCTR with short palmar incision, the incision can be lengthened during OCTR if the surgeon desires a full view of the nerve.

Complications associated with CTR are well known and can include, in the worst case, injury or transection of the median nerve. Injury to the median nerve has not occurred in our patients as a result of OCTR with short palmar incision even though direct vision of the median nerve is more restricted than in OCTR with a longer incision. Others who perform OCTR with a short or mini incision have reported a similar level of satisfaction with the procedure. In a study of 104 patients (149 hands) Klein et al. demonstrated that good functional outcomes can be achieved safely even when the OCTR incision is decreased to 1.0 cm [11].

Electrodiagnostic tests that include use of the serial incremental technique of Kimura, which assesses 1-cm segments of the median nerve [9], can identify the precise location(s) of median nerve conduction abnormalities during clinical diagnostic work-up for carpal tunnel syndrome (CTS). Through analysis of results from use of this technique, we found that the segment of the median nerve at or just distal to the distal end of the carpal tunnel was affected by slowing most frequently. We found the segment of the nerve within the carpal tunnel was affected less often, and the segment of nerve proximal to the tunnel was affected least [15]. The finding that the median nerve was not compromised proximal to the tunnel suggested that it is not necessary to extend the surgical incision into the distal forearm and cut the antebrachial fascia.

Surgical Anesthesia

OCTR with short palmar incision is performed in an outpatient setting with local block and tourniquet control. The procedure begins with injection of 5–7 cc of 1.0% Xylocaine, without epinephrine, at the level of the distal wrist crease. The needle is positioned subcutaneously between the thenar and hypothenar masses just proximal to the distal wrist crease and directed in a distal course subcutaneously across the wrist crease and through the area where the incision will be made. As the injection progresses the skin becomes distended and assumes a slightly blanched appearance. The injection anesthetizes all soft tissues, including the ligament, in the surgical area. A tourniquet on the upper arm is inflated to 250 mm Hg once injection of the anesthesia agent and prepping are complete. The tourniquet is not released until the surgical incision is closed and dressings are applied. Average tourniquet time is less than 10 min.

The anesthetic effect achieved by the injection is sufficient to prevent discomfort, even if the surgeon accidentally touches the median nerve when the ligament is being released.

Instrumentation and Surgical Technique

OCTR with short palmar incision is performed with loupe magnification (×2.5) and with basic surgical instruments. The instruments include an Adson forceps; no. 3 scalpel (blade handle); no.15 blade; a Weitlaner self-retaining skin retractor; tenotomy scissors with a long shaft and blunt, curved tip; and a Ragnell right-angle retractor.

Specific techniques are used to minimize the possibility of injury to the median nerve and excessive trauma to adjacent structures [13]. An incision is initiated through the skin and the most superficial subcutaneous tissues. A self-retaining retractor is placed within the incision, under sufficient tension to offer good exposure and to separate the tissues. Next, using a reverse blade technique in which the blade (no.15) is turned upward, the tissues are pressed downward with the back of the blade while elevating the tip and gently pushing forward with the sharp upraised tip to dissect the tissues (Fig. 18.1).

This technique avoids unwanted cuts of superficial veins and cutaneous nerves. Once the transverse/volar carpal ligament is cleared of the overlying, more super-

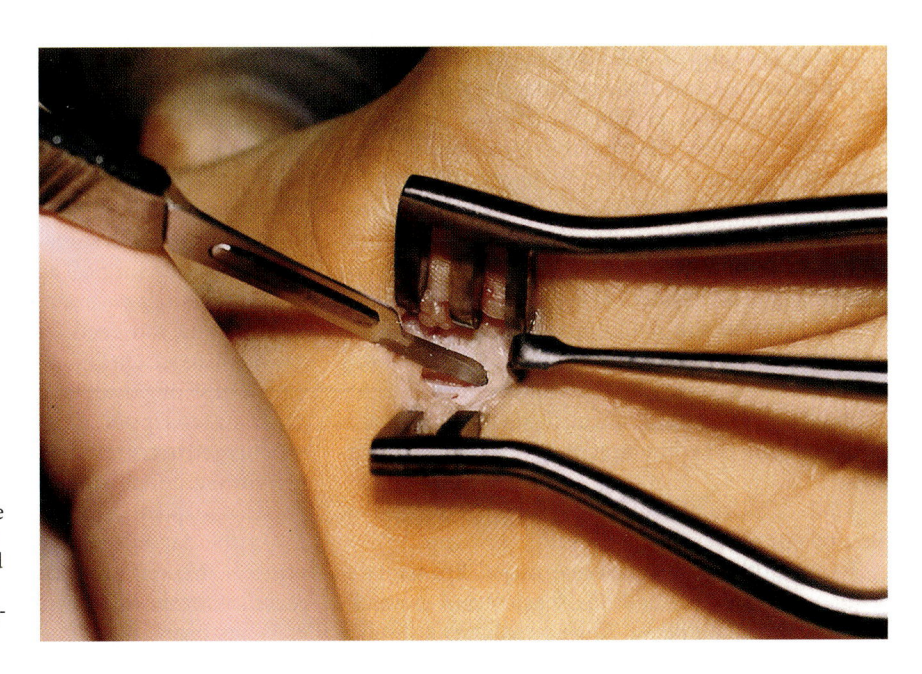

Fig. 18.1. The back of the scalpel blade is pressed down against the ligament. The handle of the scalpel is grasped in the dominant hand and stabilized with the fingers of the nondominant hand while pushing forward and upward with the sharp tip of the blade to cut the ligament

ficial soft tissues, the ligament is incised with the same technique: back of blade down, pressed into the ligament, and pushing forward and upward with the sharp tip to cut the ligament (Fig. 18.1). The scalpel handle is gripped with the dominant hand. A finger of the surgeon's nondominant hand is positioned under the blade handle to achieve more precise control as the ligament is cut. This prevents accidental cuts of the nerve during ligamental dissection if a patient under local block moves the hand.

After the ligament has been penetrated, cutting through the ligament continues distally to the point where it blends into the palmar fascia. At this point there is no longer any fascial structure, and a small amount of fat tissue is present. Vision in this area is facilitated by use of a Ragnell right-angle retractor to lift and extend the skin at the distal end of the incision. The point at which distal dissection stops is well proximal to the superficial palmar arterial arch. Infrequently the motor branch of the median nerve is found to protrude through the ligament in the line of dissection or to cross the volar surface of the sensory bundles of the nerve. The reverse blade technique is useful for preventing injury to the motor branch of the nerve in either circumstance.

Upon completion of the distal dissection attention is given to the proximal aspect of the incision. Visualization is improved with a Ragnell retractor placed at the proximal margin of the incision to lift the subdermal tissue. The exposed proximal portion of the ligament is cut under direct vision, also with reverse blade technique. The palmaris brevis muscle seen proximally can often be retracted and need not be divided. The remaining portion of the proximal dissection requires use of the long, blunt tenotomy scissors due to limitations in space and vision. Visualization of the proximal dissection is improved if the surgeon's chair is repositioned toward the end of the operating table so that vision can be directed proximally, into the area under dissection. Complete release of the entire proximal portion of the ligament is confirmed when the tip of the tenotomy scissors can be passed subcutaneously from the distal forearm across the wrist to the point of the incision. An outline of the curved tip of the scissors can be seen on the skin surface of the forearm and also felt by palpating the skin 1–3 cm proximal to the distal wrist crease. The scissors are pulled back slowly through the tunnel area and out into the open incision. During this process any uncut ligamental structures can be felt and cut with the scissors, without direct vision.

A 2.0 cm incision is sufficiently long to permit complete release of the median nerve.

Transection of the transverse carpal ligament relieves compression of both the sensory and motor fibers of the median nerve. It is unnecessary to isolate the motor branch of the median nerve even if median motor conduction abnormalities have been identified on electrodiagnostic tests. In our experience the presence of conduction defects of the motor fibers of the median nerve indicates a more chronic or severe neuropathic process that involves the main bundle of mixed sensory and motor fibers; it does not indicate a particular compression of the motor branch of the median nerve at a site separate from the median nerve in the tunnel.

Histological examinations [6, 8] have demonstrated that there is rarely hypertrophy of synovial tissue. We do not recommend synovectomy except possibly in patients who present with tissue hypertrophy from rheumatoid arthritis. In our experience epineurotomy is also not indicated as there is no evidence that constriction of the epineurium is a primary problem. Epineurotomy may actually be detrimental as opening of the epineurium removes the physiological barrier of the median nerve. Borisch and Haussman found no advantage in clinical or neurophysiological outcome from CTR combined with epineurotomy when compared to CTR (without epineurotomy) in a group of 273 patients [1]. In a meta-analysis that compared global outcomes of patients receiving CTR with global outcomes of patients who received CTR and epineurotomy or neurolysis, patients who received only CTR tended to have better global outcomes than those who had concomitant epineurotomy or neurolysis. The authors concluded that these additional procedures are potentially harmful for most patients with CTS [3].

Immediate Postoperative Rehabilitation

The surgical site is injected with 2.0 cc of 0.5% Marcaine immediately after closing the skin, for pain reduction, and the surgical wound is dressed with a sterile pad and a soft gauze wrap, with some compression. The tourniquet is released only after the dressings are applied. Splints are not used as we have found them to cause secondary soft-tissue tightness that can restrict wrist motion and in some cases adherence of the median nerve in the surgical area.

The dressings are examined before patients leave the hospital and loosened or redressed, as necessary, to avoid constriction, which we have found to be a common cause of postoperative discomfort. Patients are given a prescription for pain medication but they are encouraged to try to achieve a satisfactory level of comfort from a nonprescription pain reliever such as ibuprofen or aspirin.

On the day after surgery patients are started in a physical therapy program of gentle range-of-motion exercises for the hand, wrist, and elbow and specific exercises to promote gliding of the median nerve through the surgical area. Patients are also instructed in a self-administered home program of edema control, wound care, nerve gliding exercises, and range-of-motion exercises for the wrist and hand.

Following the first visit to physical therapy, patients are seen every 2–4 days to monitor progress and to advance postoperative rehabilitation. When discomfort from a surgical incision inhibits active use of the hand, a program of sterile whirlpool and assisted stretching exercises is used to improve range of motion and to facilitate wound healing. Gradually-progressive strengthening exercises are instituted approximately 3–5 days after surgery, along with incorporating these exercises into the self-administered home care routine.

Surgical sutures are removed approximately 10 days after surgery. Ultrasound and soft tissue mobilization techniques are administered to the proximal palm if pillar pain is present. Patients are monitored closely to assess progress in range of motion, strength, and level of comfort. Occupational requirements are evaluated frequently. Patients are released to gainful employment when it is felt that strength, range of motion, and hand comfort have increased to a level where modified or regular work can be performed comfortably and safely.

Return-to-Work Intervals

We have found resumption of normal activities of daily living and gainful employment to be affected by insurance type (workers' compensation versus private/Medicare/welfare). In our experience, patients who receive workers' compensation benefits generally have a longer recovery period, regardless of occupation. In a 1993 retrospective study of CTR patients who underwent OCTR with short palmar incision followed by early postoperative rehabilitation, we reported a 10-day average return-to-work interval for private patients and 21 days on average for workers' compensation patients [14]. We have since further decreased the period of postoperative recovery for both groups. Others have also found workers' compensation patients to take longer to return to work following carpal tunnel release surgery [2, 7].

In our clinical experience patients who undergo bilateral OCTR with short palmar incision, at the same surgical setting, recover in the same time period, on average, as patients who undergo unilateral surgery. Reduction in postoperative recovery intervals appears to involve multiple factors associated with the surgical program. Prior to scheduling OCTR we prepare patients for the surgical process and the postoperative rehabilitation phase. We explain that surgery is not debilitating and that the surgical event will not appreciably disrupt the activities of daily living and the normal enjoyment of life.

Patients are released from the hospital within an hour after surgery. Before patients leave the hospital they are given a printed hand diagram that illustrates how to loosen or cut the dressings if they become too tight. We contact the patients at home, by telephone, later in the same day to address any concerns that have arisen, such as excessive pain or swelling, which is often secondary to tight surgical dressings.

The first postoperative office visit occurs on the day after surgery, associated with a physical therapy session, as described in this chapter. Close patient monitoring through physical therapy, office visits, and frequent telephone contact continues throughout the postoperative recovery period. We encourage employers to develop modified work programs or to restrict work hours, if needed, to assist patients in early return to work.

Summary

Review of current literature demonstrates that proponents of ECTR continue to favor this approach for early recovery [12, 19] and for cost effectiveness in an employed population (but not in general population as a whole) [16]. Findings such as these must be weighed against increasing numbers of reports that cite advantages of OCTR compared to ECTR. Kiymaz et al. have reported that OCTR appears to be safer, as ECTR leads to more frequent neurovascular injuries [10]. In a comparison of ECTR and OCTR patient groups, Uchiyama et al. found less risk of nerve damage in OCTR and that OCTR patients improved slightly faster than those who had ECTR [20]. Reviewers of 16 ECTR and OCTR studies concluded that none of the existing alternatives to OCTR seemed to offer better clinical outcomes in the short or long term [17]. Ferdinand and MacLean found that ECTR did not afford any significant advantage in return of hand strength and function, and operation time was slightly slower than OCTR [5]. Further, Serra-Renom et al. support a "short-incision" approach for OCTR, reserving the classic longer incision for reoperations [18].

OCTR with short palmar incision is an uncomplicated, reliable, and safe technique that can be performed unilaterally or bilaterally in the same surgical setting, with minimal instrumentation. Trauma to the skin and subcutaneous tissues is limited, postoperative rehabilitation is generally uncomplicated, and resumption of the normal activities of daily living and gainful employment can occur soon after surgery. An early, active postoperative rehabilitation program further increases the likelihood for an optimal outcome.

Based on our experience, recovery time from OCTR with short (2-cm) palmar incision can be as efficient as that from ECTR, with less risk for injury than ECTR.

We recommend OCTR with short palmar incision for surgeons interested in a procedure that can be performed economically and efficiently and that provides patients with an effective result.

References

1. Borisch N, Haussmann P (2003) Neurophysiological recovery after open carpal tunnel decompression: comparison of simple decompression and decompression with epineurotomy. J Hand Surg 28(5)B:450–4
2. Carmona L, Faucett J, Blanc PD, Yelin E (1998) Predictors of rate of return to work after surgery for carpal tunnel syndrome. Arthritis Care Res 11(4):298–305
3. Chapell R, Coates V, Turkelson C (2003) Poor outcome for neural surgery (epineurotomy or neurolysis) for carpal tunnel syndrome compared with carpal tunnel release alone: a meta-analysis of global outcomes. Plast Reconstr Surg 112(4):983–990
4. Chow JC (1989) Endoscopic release of the carpal ligament: a new technique for carpal tunnel syndrome (1989) Arthroscopy 5(1):19–24
5. Ferdinand RD, MacLean JG (2002) Endoscopic versus open carpal tunnel release in bilateral carpal tunnel syndrome. A prospective, randomized, blinded assessment. J Bone Jt Surg 84B(3):375–9
6. Fuchs P, Nathan P, Myers L (1991) Synovial histology in carpal tunnel syndrome. J Hand Surg 16A:753–758
7. Hallock GG, Lutz DA (1995) Prospective comparison of minimal incision "open" and two-portal endoscopic carpal tunnel release. Plast Reconstr Surg 96(4):941–7
8. Kerr C, Sybert D, Albarracin N (1992) An analysis of the flexor synovium in idiopathic carpal tunnel syndrome: Report of 625 cases. J Hand Surg 17 A: 1028–30
9. Kimura J (1979) Carpal tunnel syndrome: localization of conduction abnormalities within distal segment of median nerve. Brain 102:619–635
10. Kiymaz N, Cirak B, Tuncay I, Demir O (2002) Comparing open surgery with endoscopic releasing in the treatment of carpal tunnel syndrome. Min Invasive Neurosurg 45(4): 228–30
11. Klein RD, Kotsis SV, Chung KC (2003) Open carpal tunnel release using a 1-centimeter incision: technique and outcomes for 104 patients. Plast Reconstr Surg 111(5): 1616–1622
12. Mackenzie DJ, Hainer R, Wheatley MJ (2000) Early recovery after endoscopic vs. short-incision open carpal tunnel release. Annals of Plast Surg 44(6):601–4
13. Nathan P: Instruments in hand surgery (1984) In: Birch R, Brooks D (eds) Operative Surgery: The Hand, 4th edn, Butterworths, London pp 1–11
14. Nathan P, Meadows K, Keniston R (1993) Rehabilitation of carpal tunnel surgery patients using a short surgical incision and an early program of physical therapy. J Hand Surg 18A:1044–1050
15. Nathan P, Srinivasan H, Doyle L, Meadows K (1990) Location of impaired sensory conduction of the median nerve in carpal tunnel syndrome. J Hand Surg 15B : 89–92
16. Saw NL, Jones S, Shepstone L et al. (2003) Early outcome and cost-effectiveness of endoscopic versus open carpal tunnel release: a randomized prospective trial. J Hand Surg 28B(5):444–9
17. Scholten RJ, Gerritsen AA, Uitdehaag BM et al. (2002) Surgical treatment options for carpal tunnel syndrome. Cochrane Database of Systematic Reviews (4):CD003905
18. Serra-Renom, Jose M, Benito J, Rubio J (2002) Carpal tunnel release through a short incision: an update. Plast Reconstr Surg 110(3):859
19. Trumble TE, Diao E, Abrams RA, Gilbert-Anderson MM (2002) Single-portal endoscopic carpal tunnel release compared with open release: a prospective, randomized trial. J Bone Jt Surg 84-A(7):1107–15
20. Uchiyama S, Toriumi H, Nakagawa H et al. (2002) Postoperative nerve conduction changes after open and endoscopic carpal tunnel release. Clin Neurophys 113(1):64–70

Chapter 19

The Mini-Invasive Technique for Carpal Tunnel Release: Open Approach with Converse Fiberoptic Light Retractor

P. Di Giuseppe

Introduction

Carpal tunnel syndrome (CTS) requires a different surgical treatment depending on the clinical stage. In the first stage, which is defined as irritative or initial, a simple release by division of the transverse carpal ligament (TCL) is indicated; in the second stage, sensory or intermediate, some cases require a flexor synovectomy in association with external neurolysis; in the third stage, paralytic or terminal, a synovectomy, an opposition transfer, and even an internal neurolysis may be necessary [1]. In the last 30 years surgical treatment of CTS has changed because of acquired experience and availability of new technical devices. In the 1970s, when microsurgery became common in surgical practice, many surgeons suggested epineurectomy associated with internal neurolysis. This indication was then limited to fibrotic epineurium. In the 1980s, short incisions, with a simple division of the TCL became popular, with the purpose of reducing complications, followed by endoscopic division of the TCL in the 1990s. Early diagnosis was at the basis of this evolution. The endoscopic technique (ET), has the main advantages of shortening the skin incision and obtaining an early return to work; on

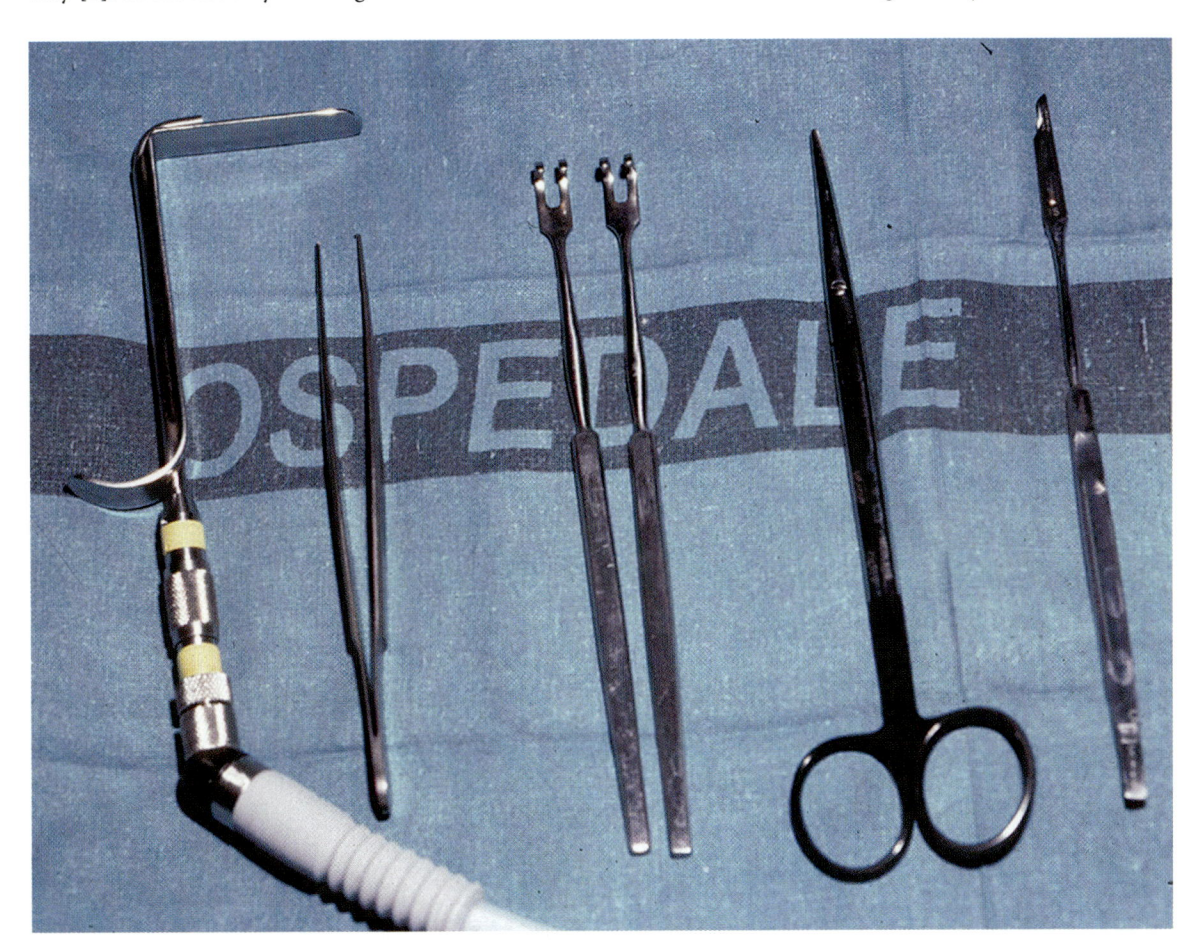

Fig. 19.1. The Converse Fiberlight retractor

the other hand, it is more expensive and implies the risk of major complications [3–5]. After the development of the endoscopic technique, a different solution has been researched [2–4].

Mini-Invasive Technique

In the 1990s a controversy developed between supporters of the open methods and supporters of the endoscopic methods [5–12]. Several nonendoscopic mini-invasive methods proposed are demonstrating the need for reducing the scar-related problems of the open methods and obtaining an early functional recovery, such as after endoscopic surgery, while still maintaining the simplicity and safety of the open methods [13]. By considering the pros and cons of these techniques, in 1993 I looked for an alternative mini-invasive method, through a short incision, like that used in ET, but with the possibility of a traditional division of the TCL with an ordinary scalpel, with the benefit of direct viewing of the median nerve (MN).

This was possible thanks to a particular retractor with fiberoptic light, designed by Converse for maxillofacial surgery (Fig. 19.1). The technique and first clinical series observations were presented at the 6th Congress of the IFSSH in Helsinki (July 1995) [1] and first results during the 3rd FESSH Congress in Paris (April 1996).

Operative Technique

The following points are marked on the skin to define the carpal tunnel (Fig. 19.2):

(a) The two proximal bone pillars: the scaphoid tubercle and the pisiform.
(b) The bisection of the opposition skin crease and the edge of the thenar eminence, marking the origin of the MN motor branch and the distal radial side of the tunnel.
(c) The ulnar side of the fourth finger, as ulnar limit of the tunnel.
(d) The ulnar edge of the palmaris longus tendon for the subcutaneous tunnel to protect the palmar branch of the MN.
(e) The incision, 2 cm long, is placed centrally to the tunnel, parallel to the opposition crease, starting from the distal limit of the tunnel.

Under tourniquet control the skin is incised, and the distal part of the TCL is approached and transected (Fig. 19.3), while directly viewing the underlying MN. The division of the exposed part of the TCL has to be completed under direct viewing. Then a subcutaneous tunnel on the ulnar side of palmaris gracilis tendon has to be made using Metzenbaum scissors (Fig. 19.4), 5 cm long and large enough to insert the retractor. After placing the retractor with fiberoptic light (Fig. 19.5), the proximal part of the TCL and antebrachial fascia is divided in continuity in a distal-to-proximal direction, as in the open technique, using a no. 15 blade. We can see the TCL and the MN almost as in the open tech-

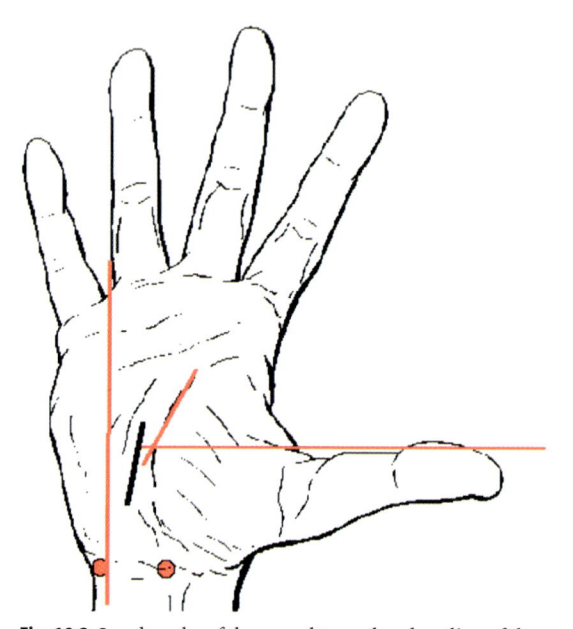

Fig. 19.2. Landmarks of the carpal tunnel and outline of the cutaneous incision

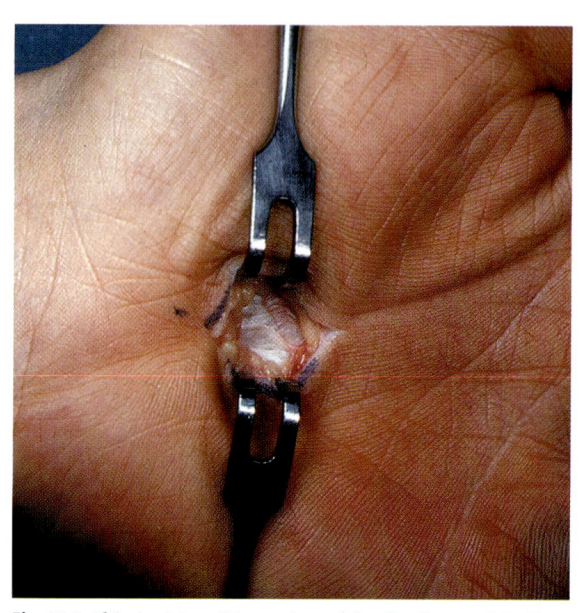

Fig. 19.3. Skin incision. Direct view of the distal part of the ligament

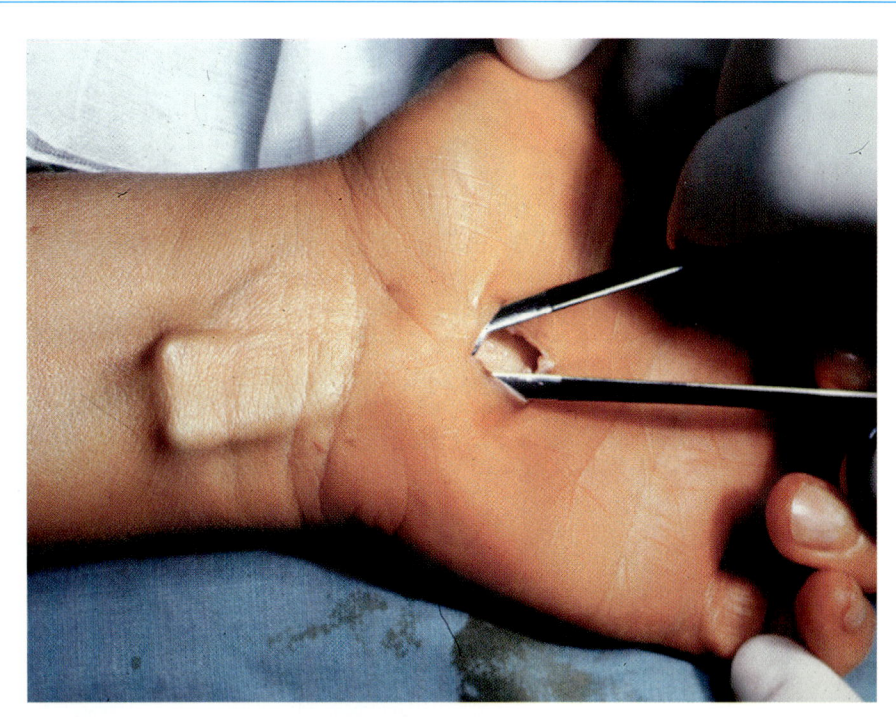

Fig. 19.4. Subcutaneous tunnel, made by blunt dissection with scissors

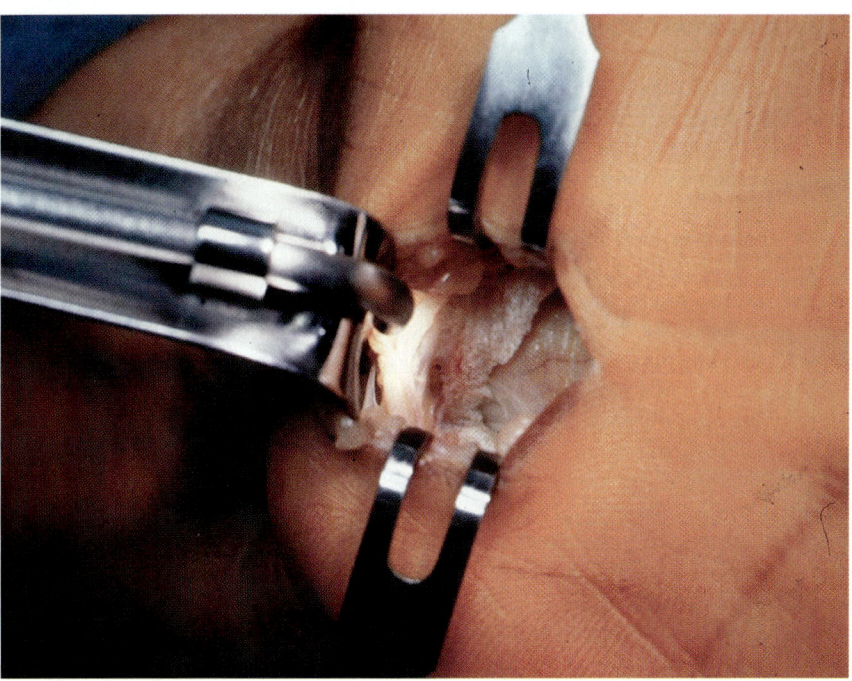

Fig. 19.5. The retractor with fiberoptic light is inserted in the subcutaneous tunnel to obtain the best view

nique (Fig. 19.6). We complete the division of the distal part of the antebrachial fascia with scissors, paying attention to separate, by blunt dissection, the underlying nerve. We carry out an external neurolysis of the MN with the same scissors and we verify the complete MN release. After removing the tourniquet, we check hemostasis and insert a drain. It consists of a sheaf of four threads draining by capillarity. For bandages we use dry soft gauzes and a cotton-padded gauze to absorb any possible hematic drainage and protect the hand from traumas. The bandages have to be comfortable with the wrist kept in light extension to prevent carpal tunnel inner structure from subluxation between the edges of the divided TCL. The bandages have to be slightly elastic to help hemostasis. The splint placed on the dorsal face of the wrist allows free finger movement just after the operation. The surgical procedure takes 10–15 min.

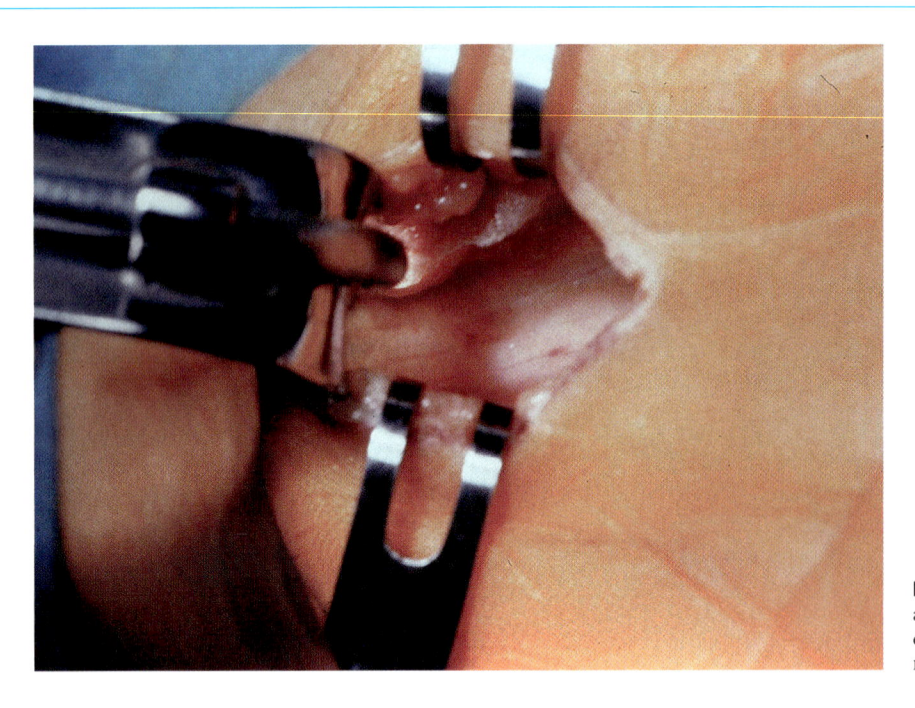

Fig. 19.6. Checking the nerve after the ligament has been completely divided. External neurolysis is possible

Comments and Conclusions

When a mini-invasive technique is proposed to a patient, the possibility of changing to open method has to be considered, informing the patient, if intraoperative findings requires it. From this point of view this technique is more elastic than endoscopic ones.

The incision is made in the central part of the palm, corresponding to the distal, narrowest portion of the carpel tunnel, where the motor branch of the MN emerges towards the thenar muscles. Particular care is taken in dividing the distal part of the TCL due to possible anomalies of MN motor branch. We must find and identify the motor branch before carrying on surgery.

The subcutaneous tunnel allows insertion of the retractor valve with free movement of the patient's hand to obtain the best view (Fig. 19.5). The most important point is that the TCL subcutaneous division is carried out with a scalpel as in the open technique. We verify the complete division of the TCL and the condition of the MN. If we find an important thickening of flexor synovial sheaths, we will lengthen the incision and practice the traditional open technique, because our mini-invasive technique allows only a partial synovectomy.

The mini-invasive open technique with fiberoptic light allows a short palmar incision (2–2.5 cm long, depending on skin elasticity); it is safe, allowing the TCL section and MN motor branch control under direct vision with just a subcutaneous dissection to insert the retractor, so that the carpal tunnel itself is not instrumented. Moreover, being similar to the open technique, it doesnot require particular training, and allows MN external neurolysis, inspection of flexor synovial sheaths, and the option of using the open technique where necessary. It takes about 5 min of ischemia.

It is important to pose the right indication, that is, a CTS in the irritative or early sensitive stage, on the basis of a clinical and electromyographic diagnosis. In some cases, I believe a larger open approach is indicated, for example: with very young patients, when anatomical anomalies are suspected, when expanding masses are present, in case of late paralytic stage or recurrence, in patients affected by rheumatoid arthritis or in dialysis treatment, and finally in posttraumatic cases.

References

1. Codega G (1987) La Patologia Moderna del Polso. Sindromi canalari e loro trattamento chirurgico. Piccin Ed., Padova
2. Di Giuseppe P, Ajmar R (1995) Surgical treatment for carpal tunnel syndrome by mini-invasive method. A personal technique. Proc. 6TH Congress I.F.S.S.H. – Helsinky, July 3–7, 519–522
3. Lee H, Jackson TA (1996) Carpal tunnel release through a limited skin incision under direct visualization using a new instrument, the carposcope. Plast Reconstr Surg 98 :313
4. Serra JMR, Benito JR, Monner J (1997) Carpal tunnel release with short incision. Plast Reconstr Surg 99 :129
5. Ablove RH, Peimer CA, Diao E et al. (1994) Morphologic changes following endoscopic and two-portal subcutaneous carpal tunnel release. J Hand Surg 19A : 821–826
6. Erdmann MWH (1994) Endoscopic carpal tunnel decompression. J Hand Surg 19B :5–13
7. Agee JM, Peimer CA, Pyrek JD, et al. (1995) Endoscopic carpal tunnel release : a prospective study of complications and surgical experience. J Hand Surg 20A :165–171
8. Bande S, DE Smet L, Fabry G. (1994) The results of carpal tunnel release : open versus endoscopic technique. J Hand Surg 19B :14–17

9. Lee H, Masear VR, Meyer RD et al. (1992) Endoscopic carpal tunnel release: a cadaveric study J Hand Surg 17A:1003–1008
10. Kelly CP, Pulisetti D, Jamieson AM (1994) Early experience with endoscopic carpal tunnel release. J Hand Surg 19B:18–21
11. Friol JP, Chaise F, Gaisne E (1994) Decompression endoscopique du nerf median au canal carpien. Ann Chir Main (Ann Hand Surg) 13 (3): 162–171
12. Brown RA, Gelberman RH, Seiler JG, et al. (1993) Carpal tunnel release. J Bone and Joint Surg 75A:1265–1275
13. Richter VM, Bruser P (1996) Surgical treatment of carpal tunnel syndrome: a comparison between long and short incision and endoscopic release. Handchir Mikrochir Plast Chir 28(3):160–166
14. Ajmar R, Fassi P, Alemanni A, et al. (1995) Controllo del trattamento della sindrome del tunnel carpale differenziato per stadi. Revisione di 657 casi. Riv Chir Riab Mano Arto Sup., 32(1): 45–51

20 The Indiana Tome for Carpal Tunnel Release

B.J. Wilhelmi, W.P. Andrew Lee

History

Consequent to persistent debate over endoscopic versus open carpal tunnel release, a minimally invasive technique was developed which combines the reduced tissue trauma and postoperative morbidity of endoscopic release with the simplicity and safety of the traditional open technique. After Chow described an endoscopic technique of carpal tunnel release in 1989, several modifications of his approach were developed including the use of video equipment for visualization of the transverse carpal ligament and specially designed instruments [1–8]. The clinical efficacy of the endoscopic release was found to be equivalent to that of open carpal tunnel release [4, 9, 10]. Proponents of endoscopic release claim a reduction in postoperative morbidity as less tissue is surgically violated [11, 12]. A multicenter randomized prospective study comparing open and endoscopic carpal tunnel releases showed greater grip and pinch strength and less scar and pillar tenderness at various early postoperative period in patients who underwent endoscopic release [4]. In addition, endoscopic patients were found to have earlier return to activities of daily living (median 5 days versus 13 days) and to work (16.5 days versus 45.5 days) [4]. Another multicenter randomized prospective study corroborated the findings of less scar tenderness and reduced time out of work (median time of 14 days versus 28 days) in patients following the endoscopic procedure [9]. Additionally, the advantages of both one- and two-portal endoscopic releases compared with open release in postoperative parameters of tenderness, grip and pinch strength, as well as return to normal activities were demonstrated in another study [10].

Despite these reported advantages with endoscopic release, its role in the operative treatment of carpal tunnel has not been uniformly accepted. Critics of the endoscopic approach claim that the required elaborate and expensive equipment required renders this simple procedure cumbersome and costly. As with any endoscopic procedure, there is a steep learning curve for development of required technical skills and ability to efficiently use the video equipment [13–15]. Many reports recommend practice of this technique on cadavers before clinical use [13–15]. Most importantly, there have been many reported complications of this procedure, including neuropraxia [4, 6, 9, 14], transection of median nerve or its branches [9, 17, 18], ulnar nerve [19], and superficial palmar arch [9, 18, 20]. Incomplete division of the transverse carpal ligament has also been noted in cadaveric studies and clinical series [13, 15, 19–23]. Thus, the reported advantages of endoscopic carpal tunnel release must be weighed against potential injury to adjacent neurovascular structures [24–25].

Accordingly, we describe a technique of carpal tunnel release through a small palmar incision utilizing a carpal tunnel tome or Indiana tome designed by James W. Strickland (Indianapolis, IN) for this purpose to combine the advantages of the endoscopic and open approaches to carpal tunnel release [26] (Fig. 20.1).

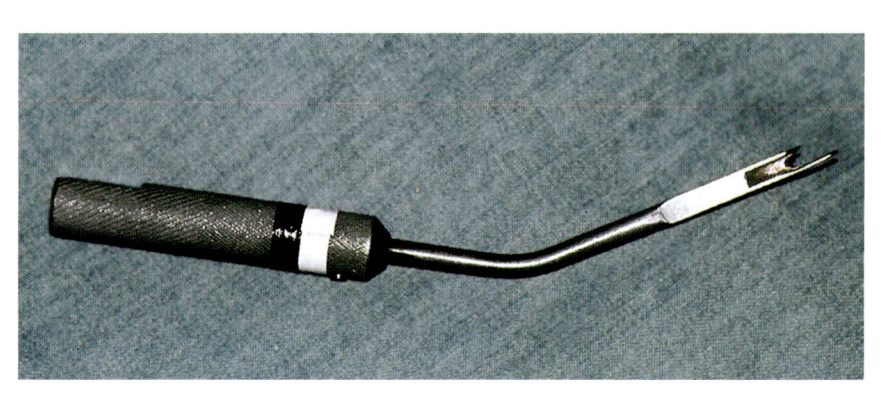

Fig. 20.1. The original carpal tunnel tome

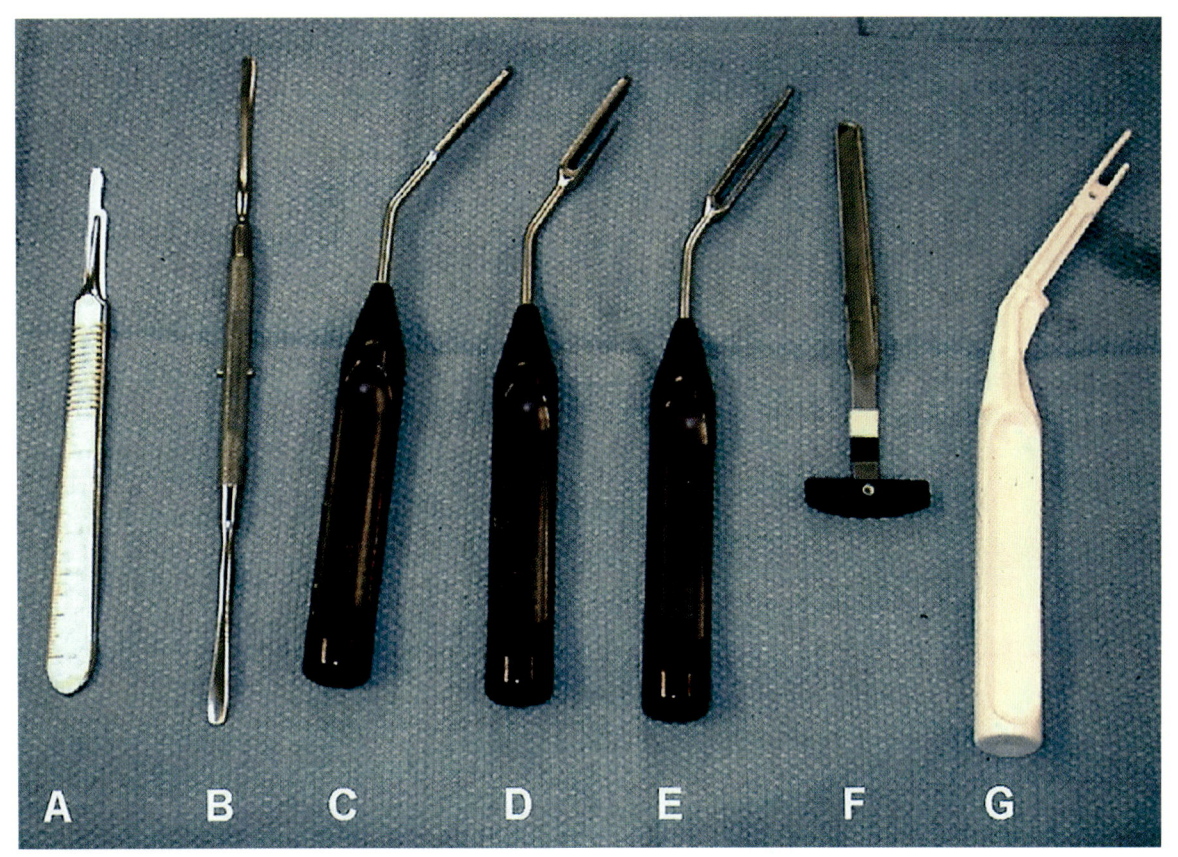

Fig. 20.2.A–G The instruments used for limited incision carpal tunnel release, in order of use from left to right: **A** No. 15 blade; **B** Freer elevator; **C** transverse carpal ligament elevator; **D** small volar/dorsal transverse carpal ligament elevator; **E** large volar/dorsal transverse carpal ligament elevator; **F** nerve protector; **G** disposable carpal tunnel tome

This technique was first evaluated in a cadaver model, which demonstrated preservation of the aponeurotic layer at the convergence of thenar and hypothenar muscular fascia and the palmar aponeurosis as with the endoscopic technique [26]. Additionally, this anatomic study confirmed adjacent neurovascular structures to be at a safe distance from ligament release using the appropriate landmarks and this technique [26]. Clinically, 694 carpal tunnel releases with the tome were reported with only two complications and 92.2% complete resolution of symptoms [26]. Furthermore, since the original description of this minimally invasive technique, it has evolved to include several modifications, including the development of specialized instruments such as a transverse carpal elevator, small and large volar/dorsal transverse carpal elevator, nerve protector, and a disposable Indiana tome (Fig. 20.2).

Indications

This limited incision technique can be used for all patients with carpal tunnel syndrome. Exceptions are those with recurrent or refractory symptoms following previous release, and those with concomitant tenosynovitis (such as in rheumatoid arthritis) requiring tenosynovectomy.

Technique

The procedure is usually performed under local anesthesia with 8 cc of 1% lidocaine and 0.25% bupivacaine in equal mixture, injected into the volar wrist as a median nerve block and along the longitudinal axis of the predicted location for the palmar incision. Then a tourniquet is placed on the upper arm. The hand and forearm are exsanguinated with Esmarck bandage and the tourniquet is inflated. A 1.0- to 1.5-cm longitudinal incision is made along the third web space, starting distally at the level of Kaplan's cardinal line (Fig. 20.3). The incision is deepened until the palmar aponeurosis is identified. A Miltex self-retaining retractor is inserted to optimize exposure. At this point only the exposed palmar aponeurosis is incised. This allows for deeper placement of the self-retaining retractor thus providing for exposure and identification of neurovascular anomalies. The distal edge of the transverse carpal ligament

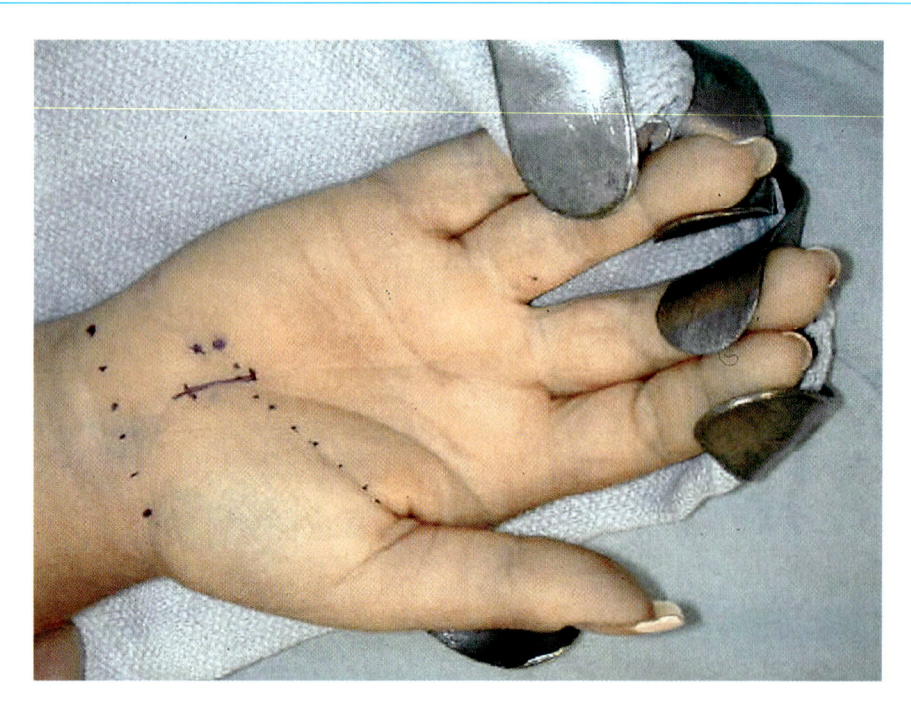

Fig. 20.3. The volar surface of the hand demonstrating use of landmarks for performance of incision. This (1.0–1.5 cm) longitudinal incision is based along the third web space with the distalmost edge at the Kaplan's cardinal line

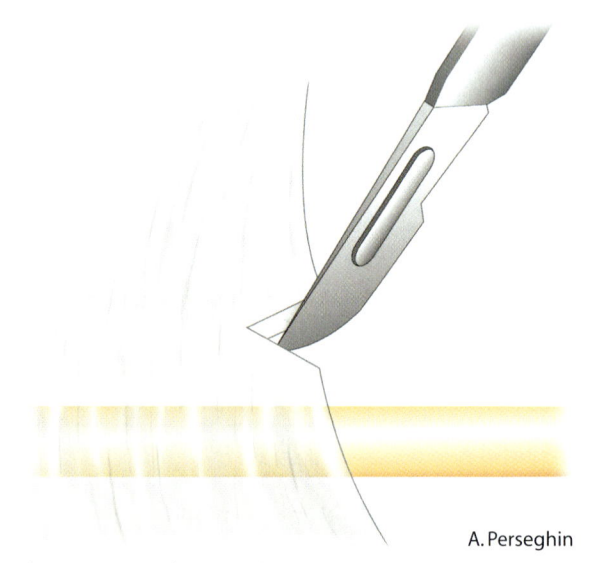

Fig. 20.4. 5-mm division of the distal-most edge of the transverse carpal ligament with the no. 15 blade. The underlying median nerve in the carpal tunnel is identified

is then located. About 5 mm of the distal edge of the transverse carpal ligament is divided with a no. 15 blade under direct vision (Fig. 20.4). This allows access to the carpal canal and exposure of the median nerve. Then a blunt Freer elevator is placed dorsal to or under the ligament and carefully advanced proximally along the longitudinal axis of the third web space with the wrist in mild extension (Fig. 20.5). Then a transverse carpal elevator (Instrument C in Fig. 20.2) is passed in the distal-to-proximal direction in the same plane as the Freer elevator (Fig. 20.6). Next, the small and large dorsal/volar transverse carpal elevators (Instruments D and E in Fig. 20.2) are used to free tissues volar and dorsal to the transverse carpal ligament, advancing in the distal-to-proximal direction until resistance is met (Fig. 20.7). The use of gradually larger blunt instruments provides for safe dissection and dilation of the planes volar and dorsal to the transverse carpal ligament, while preserving the aponeurotic layer at the convergence of thenar and hypothenar muscular fascia and the palmar aponeurosis. At this point, with the wrist in mild extension, the nerve protector (Instrument F in Fig. 20.2) is carefully advanced proximally into the plane developed dorsal to or under the transverse carpal ligament (Fig. 20.8). This nerve protector is advanced proximal to the distal wrist crease, which can be confirmed by palpation of the tip. Then, the disposable Indiana Tome is engaged into the volar groove of the nerve protector against the distal undivided edge of the transverse carpal ligament (Fig. 20.9). The Indiana Tome is then firmly advanced proximally to divide the transverse carpal ligament and distal antebrachial fascia (Fig. 20.10). The Indiana Tome should not be passed again, as with releasing the carpal ligament the carpal canal enlarges and other structures could theoretically migrate over the nerve protector into the path of the Indiana Tome. Wide separation of the radial and ulnar edges of the divided transverse carpal ligament can be seen and the carpal tunnel content is inspected. The skin is closed with 4-0 nylon sutures in a horizontal mattress fashion (Fig. 20.11). A soft dressing is applied to the proximal palm and wrist and reinforced with an Ace wrap. The patient is discharged home following the procedure, and is instructed to avoid strenuous activities only.

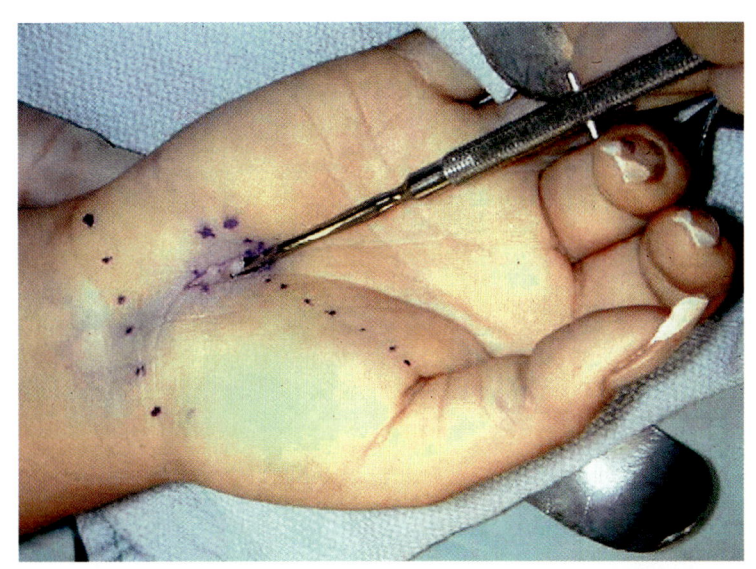

20 The Indiana Tome for Carpal Tunnel Release 143

Fig. 20.5. Freer elevator being passed in the proximal direction developing the plane under or dorsal to the transverse carpal ligament

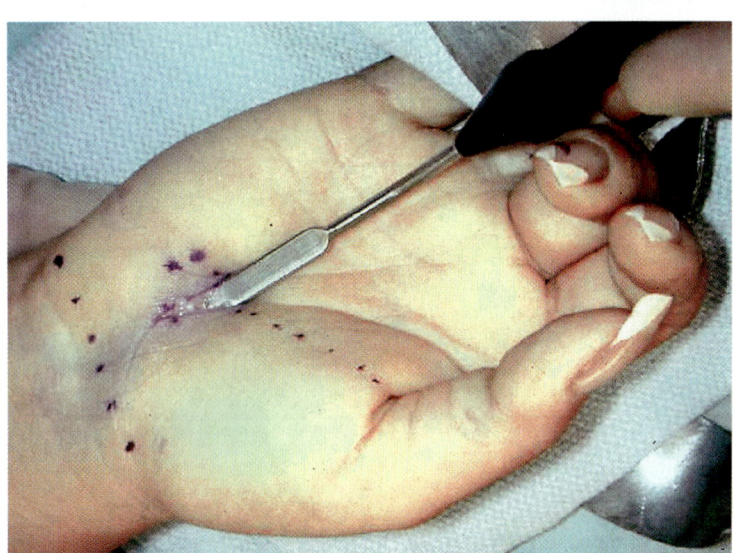

Fig. 20.6. Transverse carpal elevator passed under transverse carpal ligament in same plane as Freer

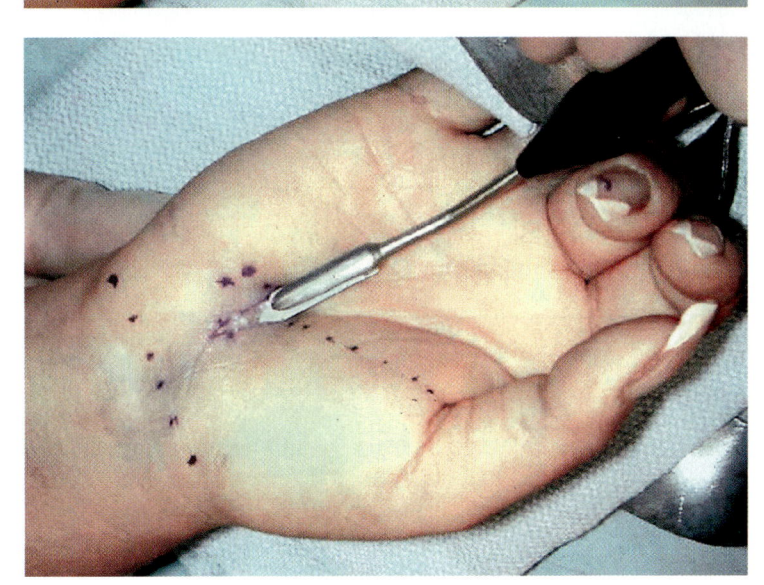

Fig. 20.7. The volar/dorsal transverse carpal elevator dilating planes volar and dorsal to the transverse carpal ligament

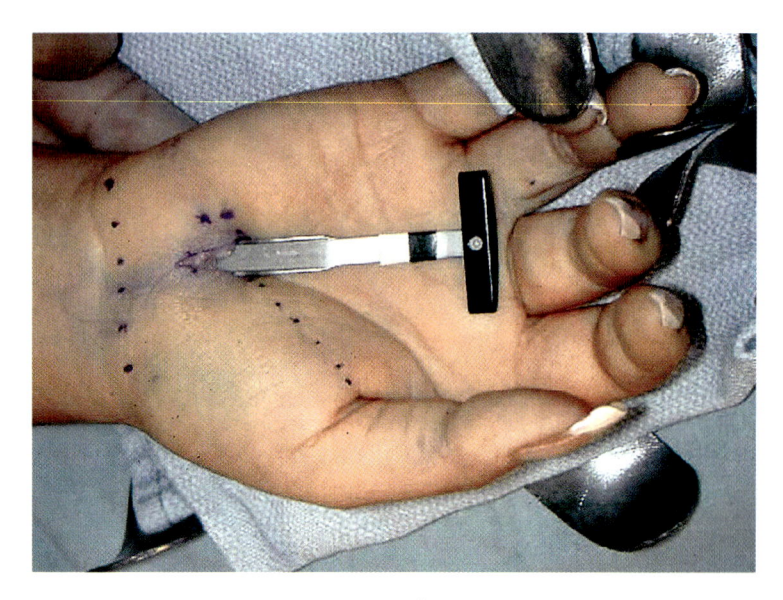

Fig. 20.8. The nerve protector being placed dorsal or under the transverse carpal ligament, advanced proximally until tip palpated at wrist crease

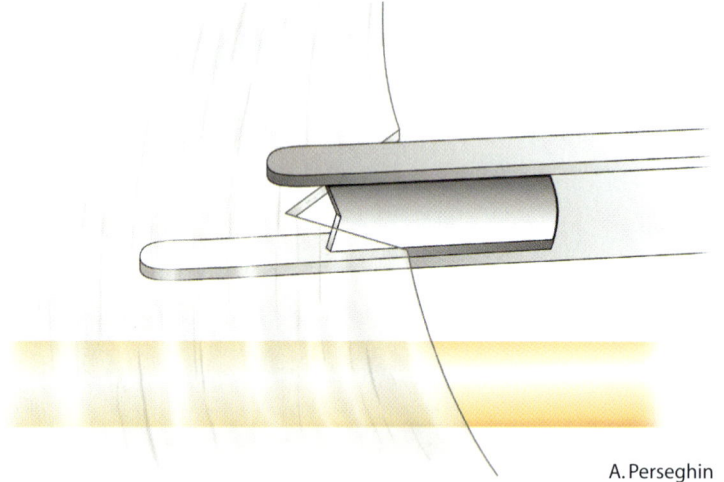

Fig. 20.9. The tome is firmly engaged against the distal undivided edge through the volar groove of the nerve protector

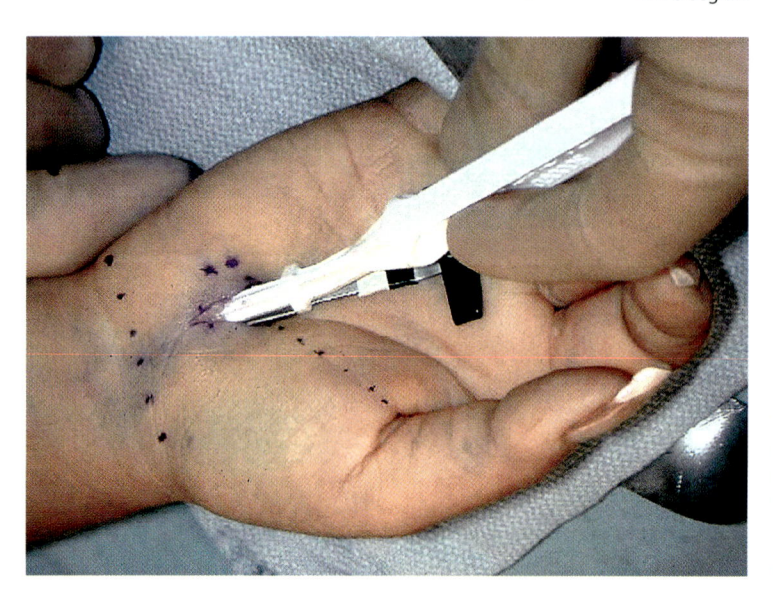

A. Perseghin

Fig. 20.10. The disposable Indiana Tome is placed into the volar groove of the nerve protector and engaged to the distal edge of undivided transverse carpal ligament. Then the tome is firmly advanced proximally to divide the ligament and distal antebrachial fascia

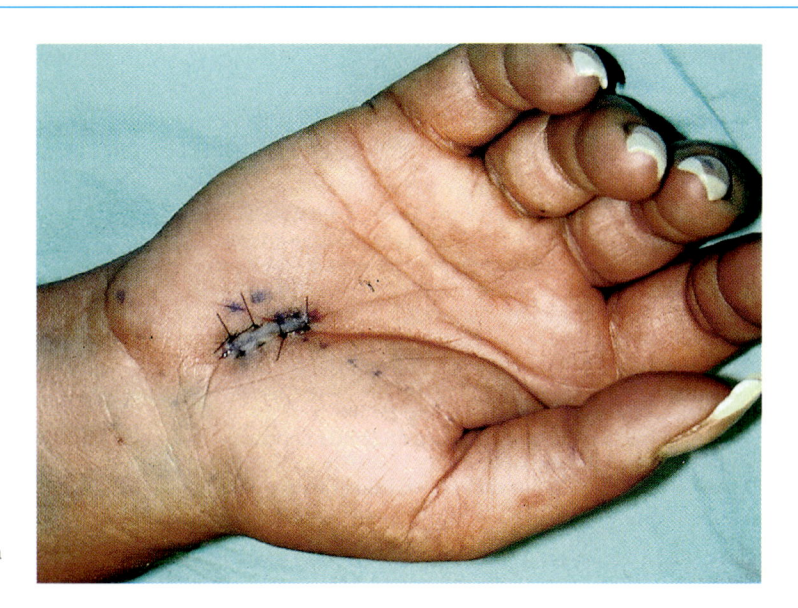

Fig. 20.11. The skin is closed with 4-0 nylon in a horizontal fashion

Advice

Technical tips that can help avoid problems with the use of this technique include precise placement of the incision along the third web space to avoid thenar branch of median nerve. Using a distally placed limited incision instead of a proximal incision at the wrist level allows for direct inspection of the liable neurovascular structures which are located in the distal-versus-proximal limited incision approach. Only longitudinal structures consistent with fibers of the palmar aponeurosis should be divided in deepening the incision to avoid injuring anomalous neurovascular structures at the distal edge of carpal ligament along confluence of the third web and Kaplan's line. The gradual dilation of the carpal canal with blunt instrumentation should be carefully passed through the same path/plane. This allows for preservation of the thenar and hypothenar fascial convergence and the palmar aponeurosis, which may be responsible for the quicker postoperative recovery seen with the endoscopic technique. Most importantly, a second pass with the tome should not be attempted, as with releasing the carpal ligament the carpal canal enlarges and other structures could theoretically migrate over the nerve protector into the path of the Indiana Tome. In fact, no complications occurred after recognizing this risk and avoiding the second pass. This tome with a blunt bottom edge designed to lie beneath the transverse carpal ligament is essential for this limited incision technique. Other instruments such as scissors could potentially catch the epineurium and lead to median nerve injuries.

Complications

Two complications were encountered in using this technique for 694 carpal tunnel releases, including partial median nerve laceration (20%) and a complete nerve transection. The latter occurred in an elderly woman with a previous Colles' fracture and altered carpal anatomy. Both complications took place during the early portion of the patient series and were the result of an attempted second pass of the tome. Since the maneuver was abandoned and avoided, no complications have occurred.

Rehabilitation

The patient is instructed to maintain the postoperative dressing and to begin immediate active finger motion with the dressing in place. The patient returns to office at 10–14 days for suture removal.

Conclusion

Carpal tunnel release with the Indiana Tome via limited palmer incision is a technically simple procedure that causes tissue trauma equal to or less than that produced by any endoscopic method while preserving all structures attributed to quicker postoperative recovery. A midpalm versus wrist incision allows direct visualization of neurovascular structures at risk.

References

1. Chow JCY (1989) Endoscopic released of the carpal ligament: a new technique for carpal tunnel syndrome. Arthroscopy 5:19
2. Okutsu I, Nonomiya S, Takatori Y et al. (1989) Endoscopic management of carpal tunnel syndrome. Arthrocopy5: 11
3. Resnick CT, Miller BW (1991) Endoscopic carpal tunnel release using the subligamentous two-portal technique. Contemp. Orthop. 22: 269
4. Agee JM, McCarroll HR, Tortosa RD et al. (1992) Endoscopic release of the carpal tunnel: a randomized prospective multicenter study. J. Hand Surg. 17A: 987
5. Menon J (1993) Endoscopic carpal tunnel release: a single portal technique. Contemp. Orthop. 26: 109
6. Brown MG, Keyser B, Rothenberg ES (1992) Endoscopic carpal tunnel release. J. Hand Surg.17A: 1009
7. Mirza MA, King ET, Tanveer S (1995) Palmar uniportal extrabursal endoscopic carpal tunnel release. Arthrocscopy 11: 82
8. Preibler, P (1995) Endoscopic release of the transverse carpal ligament in palmar-dorsal direction. Med. Orth. Tech. 115: 68
9. Brown RA, Gelberman RH, Seiler JG III et al. (1993) Carpal tunnel release: a prospective, randomized assessment of open and endoscopic methods. J. Bone Joint Surg. 75A: 1265
10. Palmer DH, Paulson JC, Lane-Larsen CL et al. (1993) Endoscopic carpal tunnel release: a comparison of two techniques with open release. Arthroscopy. 9: 498
11. Chow JCY (1990) Endoscopic release of the carpal ligament for carpal tunnel syndrome: 22 month clinical result. Arthroscopy 6: 288
12. Chow JCY (1992) Pro: endoscopic carpal tunnel release. American Academy of Orthopedic Surgeons Bulletin 12
13. Lee DH, Maeser VR, Meyer RD et al. (1992) Endoscopic carpal tunnel release: a caveric study. J. Hand Surg. 17A: 1003
14. Newmeyer WL (1992) Thoughts on the technique of carpal tunnel release (Editorial). J. Hand Surg. 17A: 985
15. Rowland EB, Kleinert JM (1994) Endoscopic carpal tunnel release in cadavers: an investigation of the results of twelve surgeons with this training model. J. Bone Joint Surg. 76A: 266
16. Agee JM, Peimer CA, Pyrek J, Walsh WE (1995) Endoscopic carpal tunnel release: a prospective study of complications and surgical experience. J. Hand Surg. 20A: 165
17. Feinstein PA (1993) Endoscopic carpal tunnel release in a community-based series. J. Hand Surg. 18A: 451
18. Murphy RX Jr, Jennings JF, Wukich DK (1994) Major neurovascular complications o endoscopic carpal tunnel release. J. Hand Surg. 19A: 114
19. Nath RK, Mackinnon SE, Weeks PM (1993) Ulnar nerve transection as a complication of two-portal enodscopic carpal tunnel release: a case report. J. Hand Surg. 18A: 896
20. Seiler JG III, Barnes K Gelberman RH, Chalidapong P (1992) Endoscopic carpal tunnel release: an anatomic study of the two-incision method in human cadavers. J. Hand Surg. 17A: 996
21. Levy HJ, Soifer TB, Kleinbart FA et al. (1993) Endoscopic carpal tunnel release: anatomic study. Arthroscopy 9: 1
22. Schwartz JT, Waters PM, Simmons BP (1993) Endoscopic carpal tunnel release: a cadaveric study. Arthroscopy 9: 209
23. Kelly CP, Pulsietti D Jamieson AM (1994) Early experience with endoscopic carpal tunnel release. J. Hand Surg. 19B: 18
24. Jabaley ME (1993) Single portal endoscopic carpal tunnel release Commentary). Contemp. Orthop. 26: 115
25. Fischer TJ, Hastings HII (1996) Endoscopic carpal tunnel release: Chow technique. Hand Clin. 12: 285
26. Lee WPA, Strickland JW (1998) Safe carpal tunnel release via a limited palmar incision. Plast. Reconstr. Surg. 101: 418

Alternative Techniques and Variants: Double Approach – Proximal and Distal Mini-Incisions

M. Corradi

Introduction

The surgical technique of double access with proximal and distal mini-incision does not have a clear paternity, and therefore cannot be attributed to one single author [1–4]. This appears in literature in the period that follows the introduction of the endoscopic technique [5] and takes advantage of certain specific characteristics of said technique and, at the same time, of the open technique. This methodology uses two incisions similar to those used in the endoscopic technique [6], thus avoiding problems due to pain during the healing process of the skin. At the same time, by means of the distal incision, a view is obtained of the components of the carpal tunnel (median nerve and flexor tendons), which would not be possible with the endoscopic technique, but only with the open technique.

Technique

The operation is carried out under local anesthetic with the injection of about 8–10 cc of lidocaine at 2% [7] in the region of the palm along the axis of the fourth finger, starting from the fold of the wrist.

The operating field is rendered bloodless by means of the application of a tourniquet to the forearm with pressure not exceeding 70 mmHg over the patient's maximum pressure [8]. The application of the tourniquet to the forearm permits an endurance which is 45% longer than when positioned on the arm and is less painful both during use and immediately after removal [9].

The distal incision is made between the hamate and the proximal palmar crease and has a longitudinal course of about 1.5–2 cm in the direction of the axis of the fourth finger (Fig. 21.1).

The Kaplan line helps to identify the area of the distal incision, which begins exactly at the confluence of the same line with the hook of the hamate and the axis of the fourth finger. By means of distal incision and dissection by scissors of the aponeurotic tissue, the distal part of the transverse carpal ligament can be reached.

At this point, the presence of any synovitis of the flexors should be verified; a situation which contraindicates the use of the mini-incision technique. In this

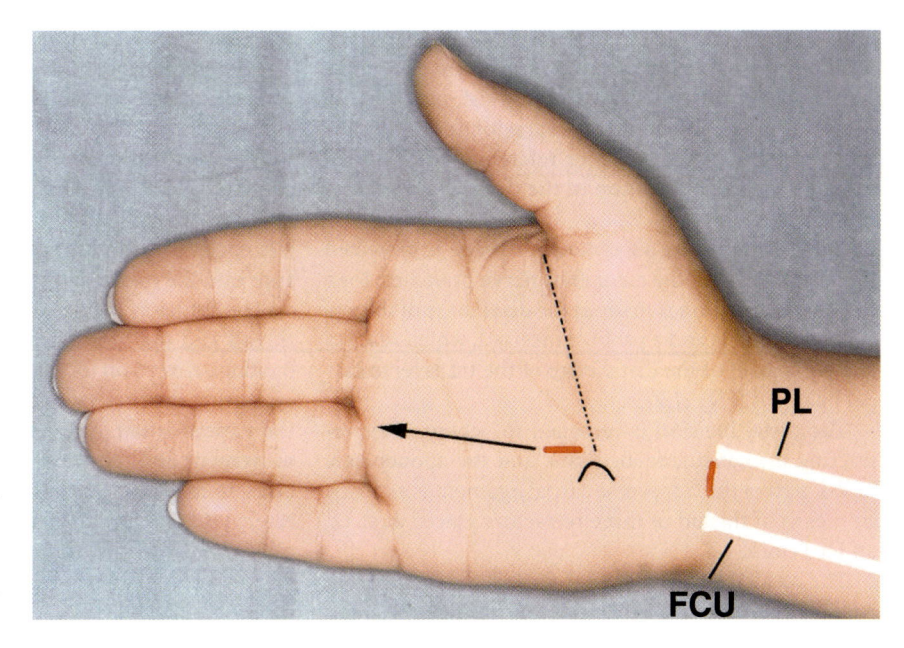

Fig. 21.1. Distal and proximal mini-incision (*red lines*) Kaplan line (*dotted line*), axis of fourth finger (*arrow*). FCU, flexor carpi ulnaris; PL, palmaris longus

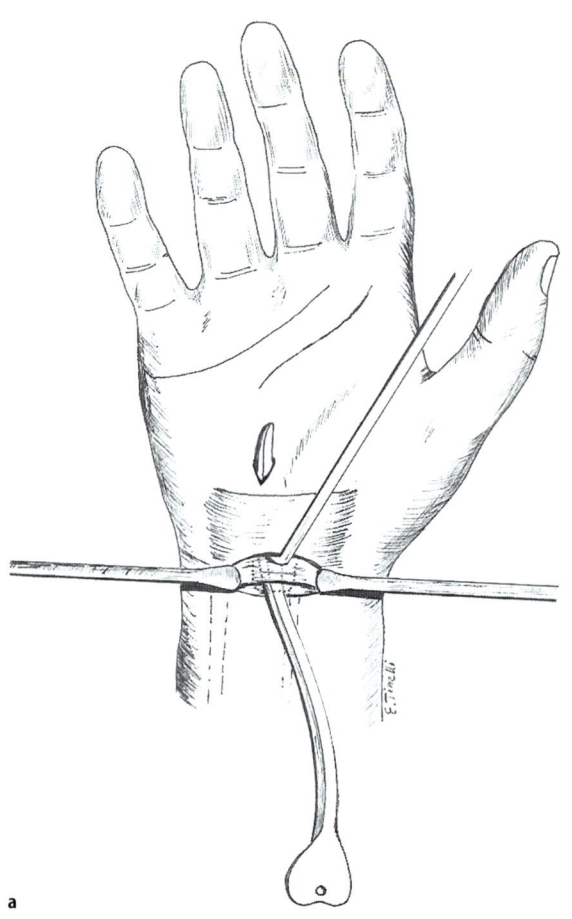

Fig. 21.2. Graphic representation (**a**) and operating field (**b**) of probe which goes through the two accesses

case, starting from the distal incision, it is possible to widen the operating field, extending it in the proximal direction towards the fold of the wrist.

The proximal transverse incision is about 1 cm in length, just above the crease of the wrist, between the flexor carpi ulnaris and the palmaris longus; in the absence of the latter as point of reference, the incision should be in radial position to the flexor carpi ulnaris (Fig. 21.1).

Using scissors, the subcutaneous tissue is dissected to avoid damaging the cutaneous nerve branches; then a U-shaped incision is made at the distal base of the anti-brachial fascia and a probe is inserted, which reaches and comes out of the distal edge of the transverse carpal ligament (Fig. 21.2).

The distal incision is returned to, where, after retracting the subcutaneous tissue and the aponeurotic fascia, part of the transverse carpal ligament is exposed by means of the aid of three retractors placed at 9, 12, and 3 o'clock.

The retractor placed at 12 o'clock is the longest and permits the skin and subcutaneous tissue to be lifted and protected; thus the transverse ligament can be safely separated by means of straight scissors, in distal-proximal direction (Fig. 21.3).

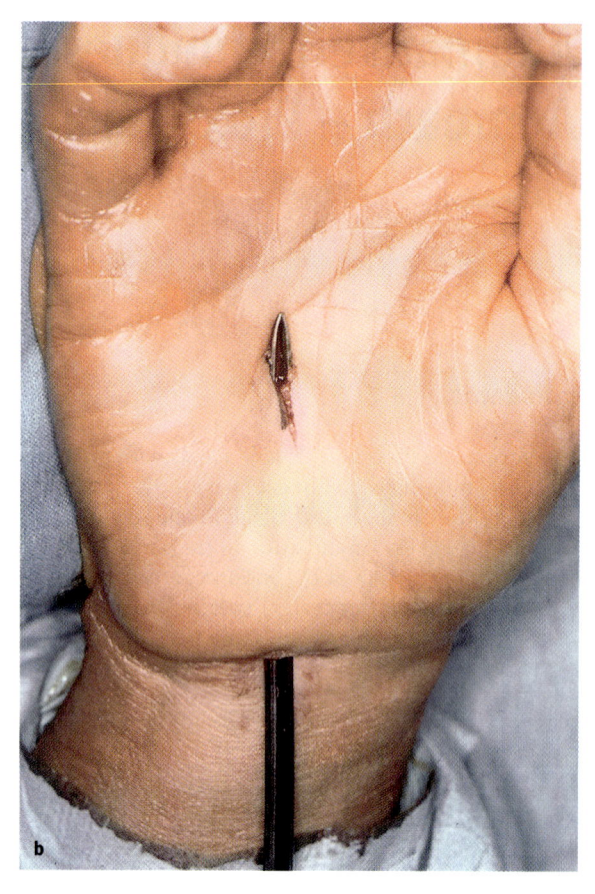

The most proximal part of the ligament is not easily reached by distal incision, and it is therefore often necessary to complete the dissection of the ligament in the proximal-distal direction from the proximal incision.

The median nerve can be protected not only by a probe, but also, alternatively, by a Freer-type dissector [2].

Once the section of the transverse ligament has been completed, the effective opening of the carpal canal must be ascertained by a direct view and the *geyser-effect* obtained from the saline solution injected at pressure into the incisions [4].

The suture of the skin is carried out with a 5-0 nylon thread and the dressing with gauze and a soft, elastic bandage is kept on for 10–12 days.

During the first 3 weeks of the postoperative period, the patient is taught to check the edema, to maintain movement and, above all, by means of specific exercises, to move the tendons and the median nerve separately [10]. Patients are finally allowed to use their grip after about 8 weeks from the operation.

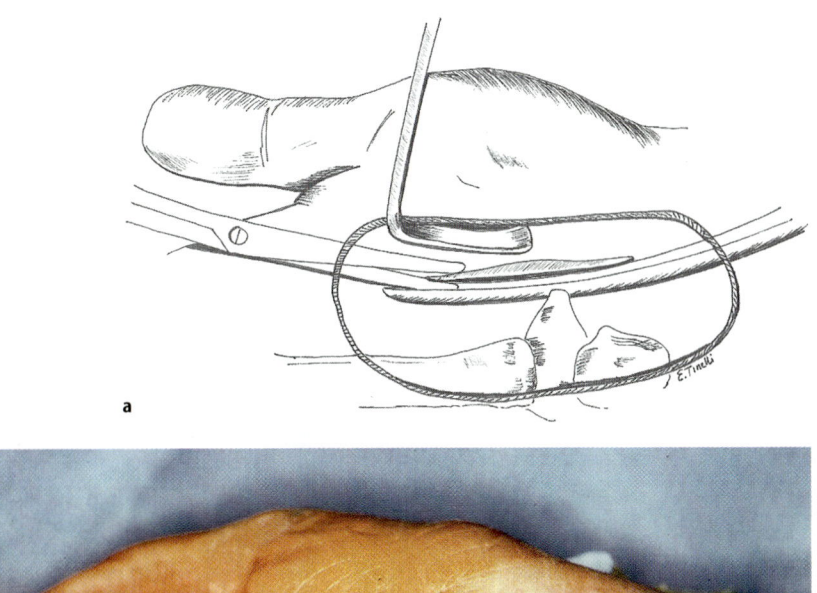

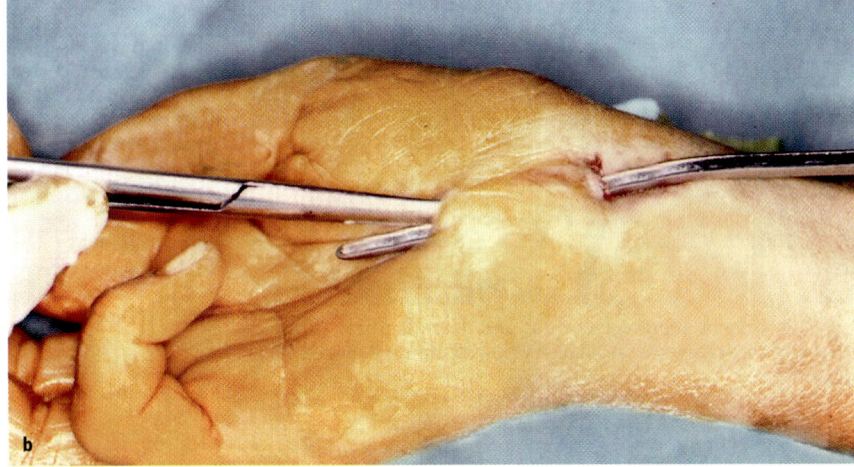

Fig. 21.3. Graphic representation (**a**) and operating field (**b**) section of the transverse carpal ligament with scissors

Discussion

The decompression technique of the carpal tunnel, still the most used today, is the open technique, by means of a single longitudinal incision on the course of the transverse ligament, with the direction along the axis of the fourth finger [11].

The results are optimal as regards the disappearance of the symptoms, and complications are not frequent, but a considerable scar may remain and pillar pain on the thenar and hypothenar area can last for several months. This problem seems to have been resolved with the introduction of the endoscopic technique; however, the benefits of lesser surgical trauma and quicker resumption of work are in contrast with the high cost of the material and the difficulty of the method. Furthermore, neuro-vascular complications and the incomplete section of the ligament are not infrequent, especially during the learning period [12].

The double proximal and distal mini-incision technique represents a valid alternative in view of the effectiveness of the results on pain, the low cost, and the lack of complications. The reduction in pain is partly due to the position of the incisions, which allows a part of the skin to be left intact, the part considered an area of contact of the wrist in many manual activities, thus permitting a quicker resumption of work. Furthermore, the possibility of a direct view of the transverse carpal ligament and of the anatomical structures contained in the carpal canal reduces the risk of complications to the minimum.

Once the distal incision has been carried out and part of the transverse ligament has been opened, the contents of the carpal canal can be inspected, to see if there is tenosynovitis of the flexors or any other pathology; in which event, the access can be lengthened proximally, before the proximal incision is carried out.

Severe forms with atrophy of the thenar muscles represent other contraindications to the double mini-incision technique, by acute carpal tunnel syndrome and by relapses.

Some alterations, recently made to the original technique, make the operation of the double access with mini-incision even more comfortable for the patient, and simpler and safer for the surgeon. Above all, use of the tourniquet can be avoided, which is often a cause of pain and is tolerated only for a brief period of time.

The use, as anesthetic, of mepivacaine hydrochloride (Carbocaine®) at 1% or 2% with adrenalin con-

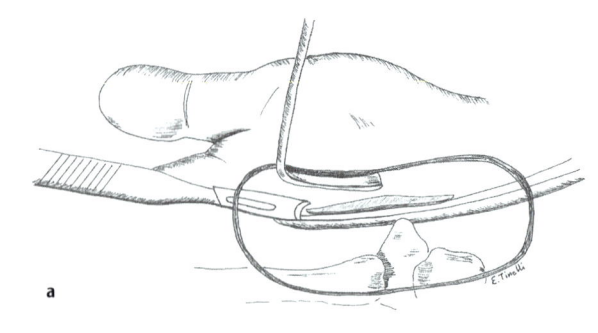

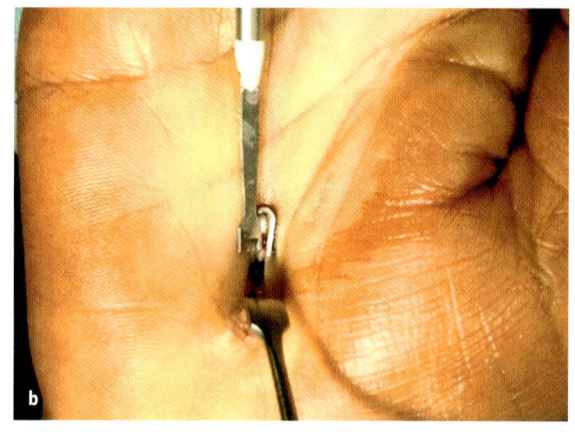

Fig. 21.4. Graphic representation (**a**) and operating field (**b**) section of the transverse carpal ligament with crescent-shaped blade

cenration at 1:200,000 (or 1:100,000), permits a good anesthetic and an operating field which is sufficiently bloodless, thanks to the adrenalin vasoconstrictor [13, 14].

At the level of the distal incision, the space may be found to be very limited, and therefore it can be difficult to succeed in dissecting the carpal ligament with scissors: a lancet with a crescent-shaped blade represents a very effective solution and furthermore permits an easier cut (Fig. 21.4).

In conclusion, compared to the other techniques of decompression of the carpal canal, the double access with proximal and distal mini-incision is easy to carry out, uses equipment of limited cost and which is easy to obtain, and, finally, permits a rapid recovery in function and of work activity.

Acknowledgements. I would like to thank Dr. Ettore Tinelli for the illustrations.

References

1. Szabo R (1998) Entrapment and compression neuropathies: Bower's limited incision technique. In Green D (ed): Operative Hand Surgery. 4th ed. New York. Churchill Livingstone vol 2, p 1413
2. Beckenbaugh R (1998) Carpal tunnel syndrome: release through two nonpalmar incisions. In Cooney W (ed): The Wrist. St.Louis, Mosby vol 2, p 1218
3. Biyani A, Downes E (1993) An open twin incision technique of carpal tunnel decompression with reduced incidence of scar tenderness. J Hand Surg 18B:331–334
4. Wilson K (1994) Double incision open technique for carpal tunnel release:an alternative to endoscopic release. J Hand Surg 19A:907–912
5. Chow JCY (1989) Endoscopic release of carpal ligament:a new technique for carpal tunnel syndrome. Arthroscopy 5: 19–24
6. Chow JCY (1994) Endoscopic carpal tunnel release:two portal technique.Hand Clin 10:637–646
7. Altissimi M, Mancini GB (1988) Surgical release of the median nerve under local anesthetic for carpal tunnel syndrome. J Hand Surg 13B;395–396
8. Khuri S, Uhl R, Martino J, Whipple R (1994) Clinical application of the forearm tourniquet. J Hand Surg 19A: 861–863
9. Hutchison DT, McClinton MA (1993) Upper extremity tourniquet tolerance. J Hand Surg 18A :206–210
10. Baxter-Petralia P (1990) Therapist's management of carpal tunnel syndrome. In Hunter-Schnider-Mackin-Callahan (eds): Rehabilitation of the hand:surgery and therapy.3rd ed. St.Louis, Mosby pp 640–646
11. Taleisnik J (1973) The palmar cutaneous branch of the median nerve and the approach to the carpal tunnel:an anatomical study. J Bone Joint Surg 55A:1212–1217
12. Deune G, Mackinnon E (1996) Endoscopic carpal tunnel release. The voice of polite dissent. Clin Plast Surg 23:487–505
13. Gibson M (1990) Outpatient carpal tunnel decompression without tourniquet: a simple local anaesthetic technique. Ann R Coll Surg Engl 72:408–409
14. Tzarnas CD (1993) Carpal tunnel release without a tourniquet. J Hand Surg 18A:1041–1043

Anatomic Landmarks for Endoscopic Carpal Tunnel Release

T.K. Cobb, W.P. Cooney

Introduction

The use of topographic landmarks and other anatomic considerations have been shown to reduce the incidence of complications, as well as the learning curve, associated with endoscopic carpal tunnel release [1]. This technique was based on findings of several anatomic studies [2–6]. The purpose of this chapter is to outline the anatomic approach to endoscopic carpal tunnel release and discuss the pertinent anatomy.

Anatomy

The carpal canal is a fibro-osseous canal which has traditionally been defined by the following borders: hamate hook, tubercle of trapezium, scaphoid tubercle, and pisiform. We now know that the hamate hook is not the distal extent of the canal. The flexor retinaculum extends approximately 1 cm distal to the hamate hook [5]. The canal is hour-glass shaped with the most constrictive portion lying at the level of the hamate hook [6]. This anatomic relationship is consistent with the experimental findings of Luchetti et al., who found the central region at the level of the hamate hook t generate the highest pressures within the canal [7].

The flexor retinaculum consists of three parts [6] (Fig. 22.1). The central part is defined by its attachment to the pisiform, hamate hook, scaphoid tuberosity, and ridge of trapezium. Most of the radial fibers originate from the trapezium deep to the thenar musculature. A narrow strip of fibers (approximately 20%) arises from the scaphoid tubercle. On the ulnar aspect, the fibers arise from the pisiform to form a distinct head. An interval exists between these fibers and those that arise from the hypothenar muscles. The hamate hook lies at the apex of this interval. This portion of the flexor retinaculum is 1.24 ± 1.3 cm in length [5].

The proximal segment of the flexor retinaculum has inconsistent boundaries. The thickness of this segment varies considerably among different specimens [5]. This segment is fused to and inseparable from the antebrachial fascia [5, 6].

The distal segment of the flexor retinaculum con-

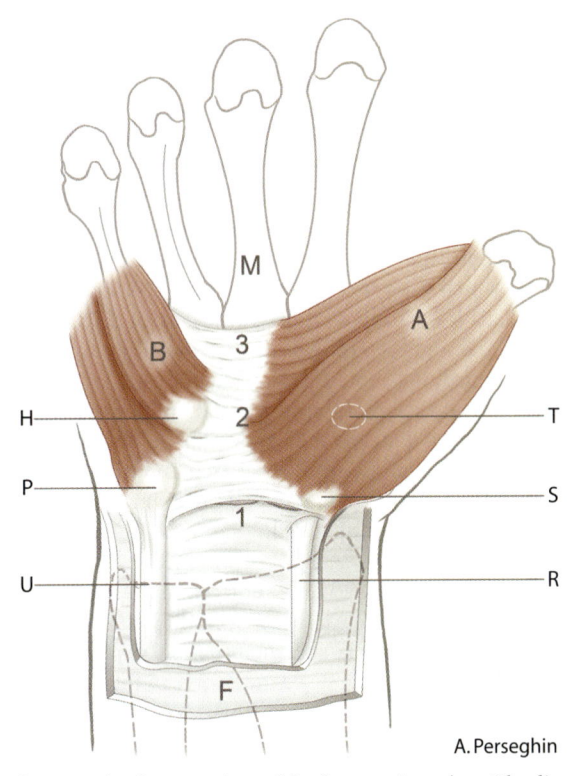

Fig. 22.1. The three portions of the flexor retinaculum. The distal segment of the flexor retinaculum (3) consists of a thick aponeurosis between the thenar (A) and hypothenar (B) muscles. The middle segment of the flexor retinaculum is the true transverse carpal ligament defined by its attachments to the pisiform (P), hamate hook (H), tubercle of the trapezium (T), and tubercle of the scaphoid (S). The proximal segment of the flexor retinaculum (1) courses deep to the flexor carpi ulnaris (U) and flexor carpi radialis (R). This segment is much thinner than the middle and distal segments of the flexor retinaculum. Antebrachial fascia (F) and third metacarpal (M) are shown. (From [6])

sists of an aponeurosis between the thenar and hypothenar muscles [6]. The hypothenar muscles (opponens digiti minimi and flexor digiti minimi brevis) originate from the ulnar aspect of the aponeurosis, whereas the thenar muscles (flexor pollicis brevis muscle and to a lesser degree abductor pollicis brevis and opponens pollicis) originate from the radial side of this aponeurosis. This portion of the flexor retinaculum has a mean length of 0.99 ± 0.13 cm [5].

Technique

The modified technique begins by first localizing the hamate hook by drawing a line from the central aspect of the base of the ring finger to the distal flexor crease of the wrist at the junction of the ulnar and middle third (Fig. 22.2). A second line is drawn from the proximal flexor crease of the palm in line with the central aspect of the index finger to the pisiform bone. The hook of the hamate is marked at the junction of these two lines [1].

The estimated position of the hook of the hamate is useful during the surgical procedure with respect to three important anatomical observations (Fig. 22.3): the distal aspect of the flexor retinaculum lies 1 cm distal to the hamate hook; the flexor retinaculum should be released just radial to this point; the median nerve and its recurrent branch occupy the central and/or radial aspect of the canal and are to be avoided; a trocar passed into the carpal canal will palpate the hamate hook, which is a very rigid structure and easily identified. This is in sharp contrast to the lack of distinct ulnar border and the probe passing to the ulnar aspect of the hamate hook should one accidentally enter Guyon's canal. The position of the superficial arch lies approximately 2.5 cm distal to the hamate hook. The approximate positions of the superficial arch and distal extent of the retinaculum are marked on the palm of the hand prior to proceeding with surgical intervention (Fig. 22.4).

The carpal canal should be entered in the central aspect in the distal forearm because in the distal forearm the antebrachial fascia and the proximal aspect of the flexor retinaculum are fused anteriorly in the region of the palmaris longus tendon [6] (Fig. 22.5). On the ulnar aspect, these fascial planes separate. The ulnar artery and nerve and the tendon of the flexor carpi ulnaris lie between these two fascial planes. A probe placed between these two fascial planes (near the tendon of the flexor carpi ulnaris) will be advanced into Guyon's space, whereas a probe placed into the proximal aspect of the carpal tunnel (near the palmaris longus tendon) will be advanced into the carpal tunnel. Proper identification and incision through the antebrachial fascia are important in preventing accidental entry into Guyon's space. The ulnar border and roof of Guyon's space will be soft and have the consistency of a prune in comparison to the palpably dense hamate hook on the ulnar border of the carpal canal and the rigid washboard effect of the undersurface of the retinaculum within the carpal tunnel.

The ulnar artery may overlie the ulnar border of the flexor retinaculum and may be at risk during endoscopic carpal tunnel release [2] (Fig. 22.6). The position of the ulnar neurovascular bundle within the carpal ulnar neurovascular space (Guyon's canal) should be understood during endoscopic carpal tunnel release to avoid potential injury to the ulnar neurovascular bundle. The nerve is generally anterior or ulnar to the hamate hook but the artery is often immediately superficial to the flexor retinaculum lying within a fat-filled space. Because of this position, we have recommended not applying pressure to the palm of the hand when the release is performed. Pressure applied to the palm of the hand could inadvertently press the ulnar artery against the flexor retinaculum and increase the potential of injury.

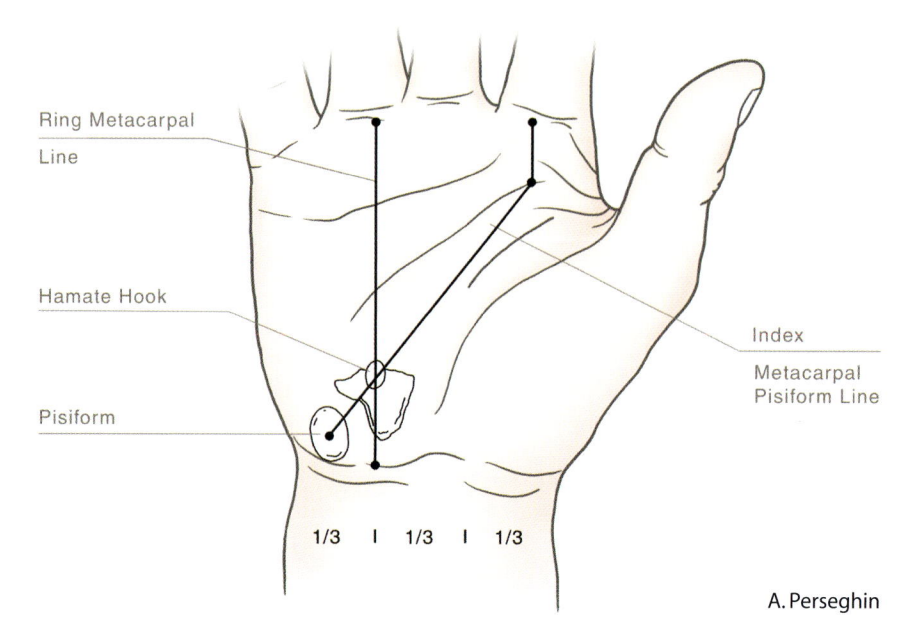

Fig. 22.2. Technique for estimating position of hook of hamate. *One line* is drawn from base of ring finger to junction of ulnar and middle thirds of distal flexor crease of wrist. A *second line* is drawn from proximal flexor crease of palm in line with central aspect of index finger (or index metacarpal bone) to pisiform bone. Estimated position of hook of hamate is at the junction of these two lines. (By permission of Mayo Foundation for Medical Education and Research. All rights reserved [4])

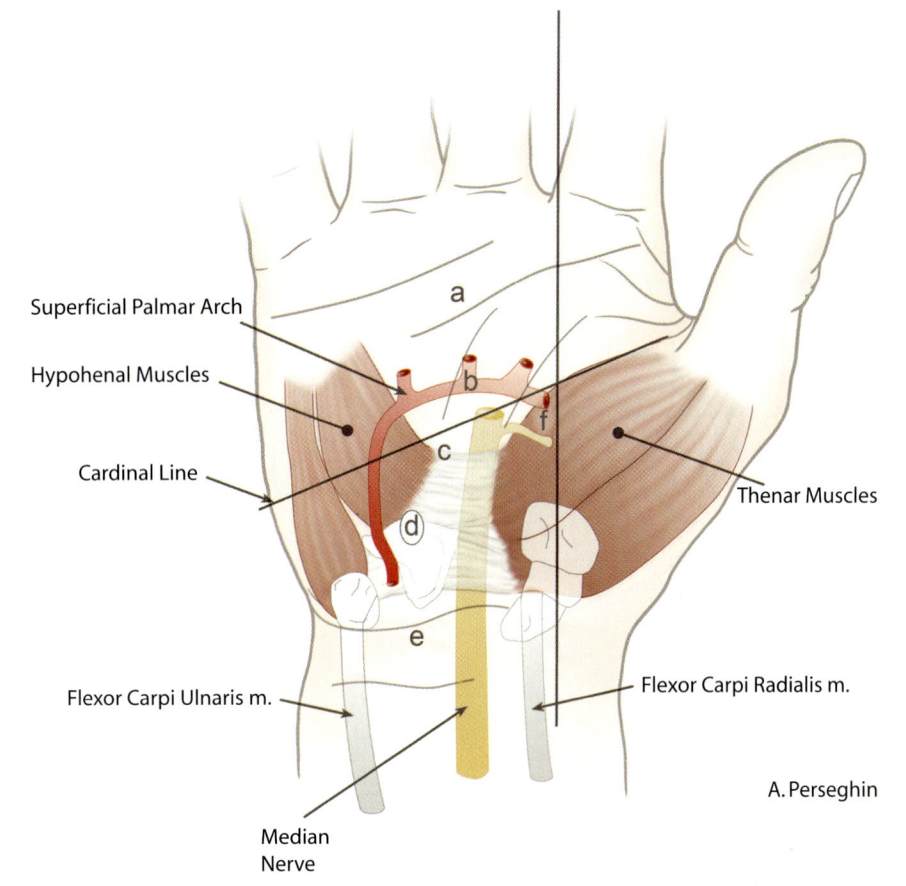

Fig. 22.3. Relative position of the flexor retinaculum and superficial palmar arch in relation to topographic markings. (*a*) Proximal palmar crease of hand; (*b*) superficial arch; (*c*) distal extent of flexor retinaculum; (*d*) hook of hamate; (*e*) distal flexor crease of wrist; (*f*) site of entry of recurrent branch of median nerve into thenar muscles. (By permission of Mayo Foundation for Medical Education and Research. All rights reserved [5])

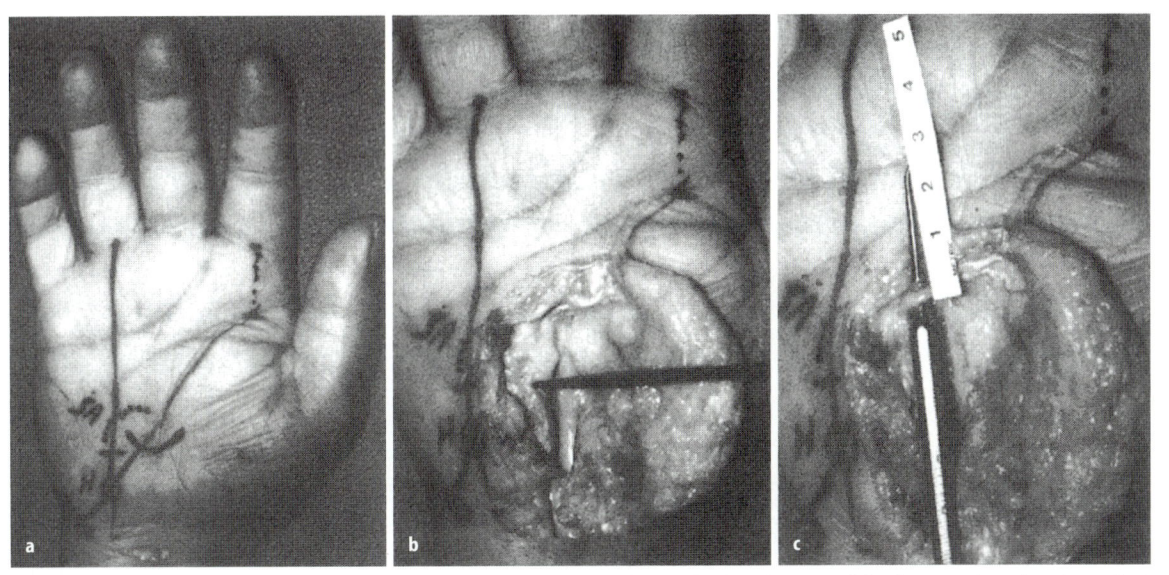

Fig. 22.4. a Cadaver hand marked before endoscopic carpal tunnel release. The distal aspect of the flexor retinaculum is marked 1 cm distal to the hook of the hamate (*H*). The *dotted line* (*SA*) is the estimated position of the superficial palmar arch, 2.7 cm distal to *H* and 4.7 cm distal to the distal flexor crease of the wrist. **b** Same hand after endoscopic carpal tunnel release. The skin and superficial tissue have been removed to expose the flexor retinaculum. A probe marks the distal aspect of the flexor retinaculum. The transverse mark on the ring finger metacarpal line (1 cm distal to *H*) accurately localizes the position of the distal extent of the flexor retinaculum. **c** Same hand with probe placed under superficial palmar arch. Note that the level of this structure was accurately estimated (*SA* in **a**). *P*, pisiform

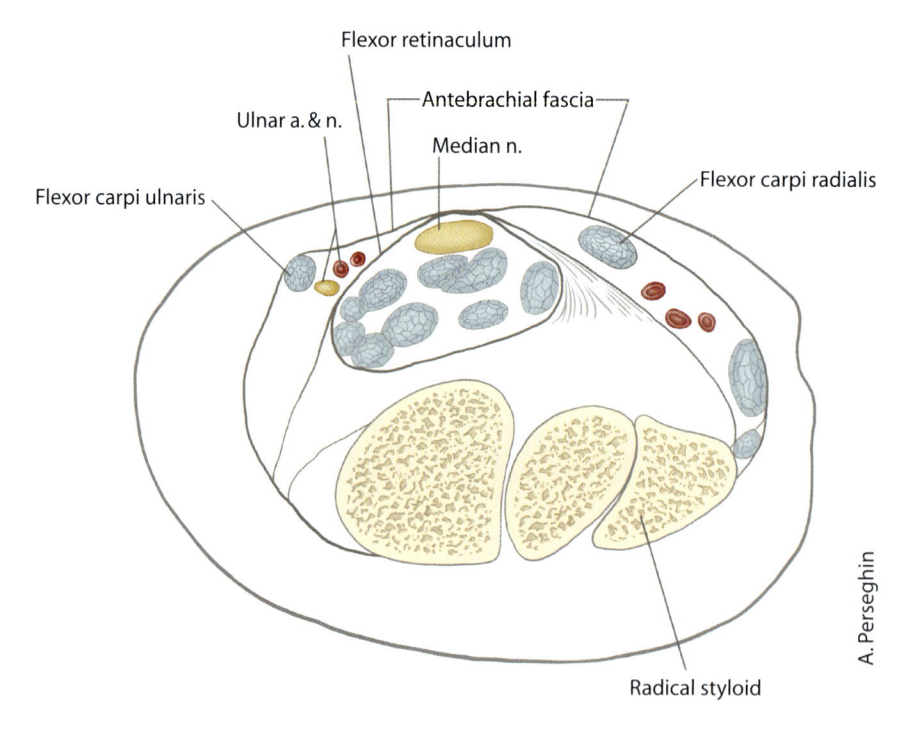

Fig. 22.5. Transverse section of wrist at distal radial styloid. Nine flexor tendons and median nerve are enclosed in proximal aspect of carpal tunnel. Proximal portion of flexor retinaculum is fixed to antebrachial fascia anteriorly and split medially and laterally. Note how anterior approach through antebrachial fascia in central aspect of wrist in region of palmaris longus tendon results in simultaneous section of proximal portion of carpal canal. A more medial approach near the tendon of flexor carpi ulnaris results in entry into proximal aspect of Guyon's canal. (By permission of Mayo Foundation for Medical Education and Research. All rights reserved [2])

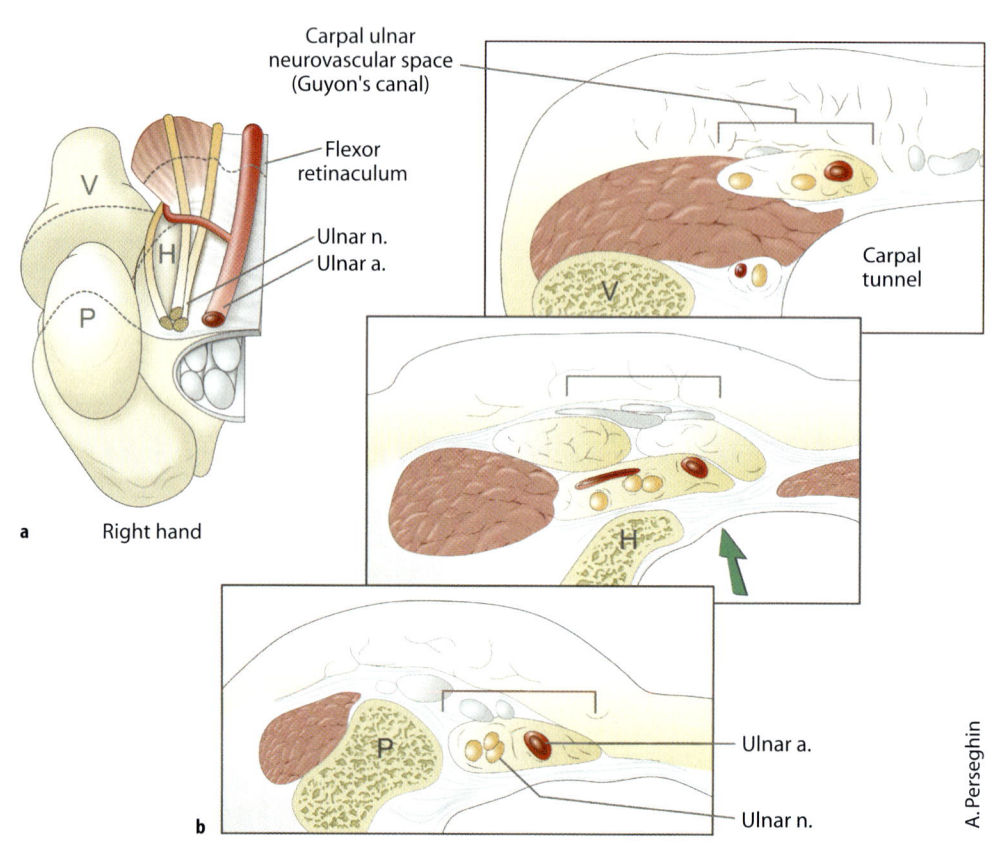

Fig. 22.6. Carpal ulnar neurovascular space. (**a**) Space viewed from proximal to distal. (**b**) Transverse sections at level of pisiform (*P*), hook of hamate (*H*), and fifth metacarpal (*V*). *Arrow* shows approximate location of endoscopic release of the flexor retinaculum (transverse carpal ligament). Note potential vulnerability of ulnar artery. This specimen does not have a segmental carpal ulnar neurovascular space roof. *A*, artery; *n*, nerve. (By permission of Mayo Foundation for Medical Education and Research. All rights reserved [3])

Please note that the estimated positions of the distal aspect of the retinaculum as well as the superficial arch are the only estimates and that variations will exist. They do, however, provide some guidelines with respect to the anticipated position of these structures and give some guidance during endoscopic carpal tunnel release.

References

1. Cobb TK, Knudson GA, Cooney WP (1995) The use of topographical landmarks to improve the outcome of Agee endoscopic carpal tunnel release. Arthroscopy: The Journal of Arthroscopic and Related Surgery 11(2):165–172
2. Cobb TK, Carmichael SW, Cooney WP (1996) Guyon's canal revisited: An anatomic study of the carpal ulnar neurovascular space. J Hand Surg 21A:861–869
3. Cobb TK, Carmichael SW, Cooney WP (1994) The ulnar neurovascular bundle at the wrist: A technical note on endoscopic carpal tunnel release. J Hand Surg 19B:24–26
4. Cobb TK, Cooney WP, An KN (1994) Clinical location of hook of hamate: A technical note for endoscopic carpal tunnel release. J Hand Surg 19A(3):516–518
5. Cobb TK, Cooney WP, An KN (1993) Relationship of deep structures of the hand and wrist to topographical landmarks. J Clin Anat 6:300–307
6. Cobb TK, Dalley BK, Posteraro RH, Lewis RC (1993) Anatomy of the flexor retinaculum. J Hand Surg 18A:91–99
7. Luchetti R, Schoenhuber R, De Cicco G et al. (1989) Carpal tunnel pressure. Acta Orthop Scand 60:397–399

23 Endoscopic Carpal Tunnel Release

J.C.Y. Chow, A.A. Papachristos

History of the Endoscopic Release of Carpal Ligament

When I began working on my technique in 1985, I was unaware that Dr. Ichiro Okutsu in Japan and Dr. John Agee in California were both working on similar goals at approximately the same time. Through trial and error of different approaches, a major breakthrough for the development of a slotted cannula came sometime in late 1986. After 4–5 months of persistent practice on cadavers, the procedure was completed in May 1987 and it was first applied to a patient later in September of the same year. Afterwards, there were continuous efforts for the improvement of this procedure. During the 1988 AANA Annual Spring Meeting, President Dr. George Schonholtz made a Presidential address regarding the past, present, and future for arthroscopy. He also presented one of Dr. Okutsu's slides that he had brought back from Japan, depicting a view of the carpal ligament through a plastic tube. I believe that nobody else in that meeting, except Dr. Schonholtz and I, had previously seen the palmar aspect of the transverse carpal ligament. Also this was the first presentation at an official meeting revealing an endoscopic view of the carpal ligament. At the same time, it was Dr. Schonholtz who predicted that endoscopic release of the carpal ligament would be developed in the near future. The first two reports in the literature regarding the Endoscopic Carpal Tunnel Release, written by Dr. Okutsu and myself separately, were published in the March issue of Arthroscopy Journal in 1989. Also, my conference paper on Endoscopic Carpal Tunnel Release was first presented at the 1990 Arthroscopy Association of North America's Annual meeting in Orlando, Florida. This paper was based on clinical results of first 149 cases since I had begun performing this specific type of endoscopic surgery on a regular basis. In the fall of the same year, Dr. John Agee presented a conference paper on the clinical results of his multicenter study at the 1990 American Society for Surgery of the Hand Annual Meeting in Toronto, Canada. Therefore, three different surgical techniques of endoscopic carpal ligament release were developed in distinct locations worldwide aiming at the same idea of minimal incision in the palm region for the surgical treatment of carpal tunnel syndrome. There has been increasing interest, and a log to debate among surgeons, since the publishing of the three original endoscopic carpal ligament release techniques. Several modifications and variations to the three original ideas have been made since their initial demonstration

Chow Technique

Set Up

The patient is placed in a supine position and a hand table is used. Two video monitors are preferred, although some surgeons perform the procedure with only one. One monitor should face the surgeon and the other should face the assistant. The surgeon sits on the ulnar side of the patient and the assistant faces the surgeon. Standard preparations and draping are performed as usual (Fig. 23.1).

Anesthesia

Local anesthesia and intravenous medication are recommended for the procedure. The use of local anesthesia allows the patient and surgeon to communicate. An alert patient is able to give the surgeon the appropriate information in case of any anatomical variance of nerve structure during the procedure [5–9]. Usually, when the patient first comes into the room, 1–2 mg of Versed (midazolam hydrochloride; Roche, Nutley, NJ) is given intravenously to help the patient relax and be more comfortable during the preparations and draping. 200–500 µg of Alfenta (alfentanil hydrochloride; Janssen Pharmaceutica, Piscataway, NJ) is given intravenously when the surgeon begins to mark the hand. This is a short-acting analgesia with a peak action of 5–10 min. Normally, the surgical time of the procedure is less than 10 min. An injection of 1% Xylocaine (lidocaine; Astra, Westboro, MA) without epinephrine is used at the entry and exit portals, but only in the skin to avoid affecting the nerve by penetrating deeply.

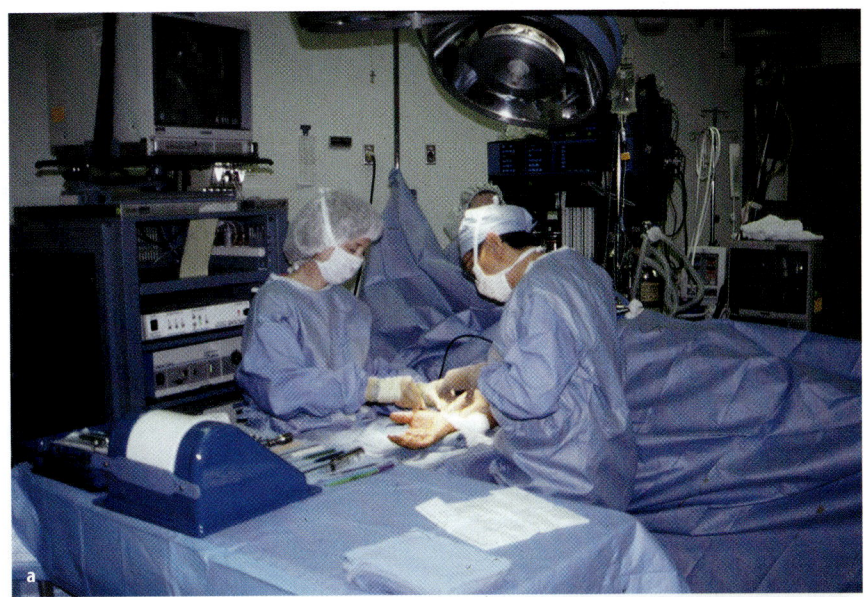

Fig. 23.1. a The patient is placed in a supine position. The surgeon sits on the ulnar side and the assistant faces the surgeon. Two video monitors are used, one each facing the surgeon and assistant. **b** The instrumentation for endoscopic carpal ligament release

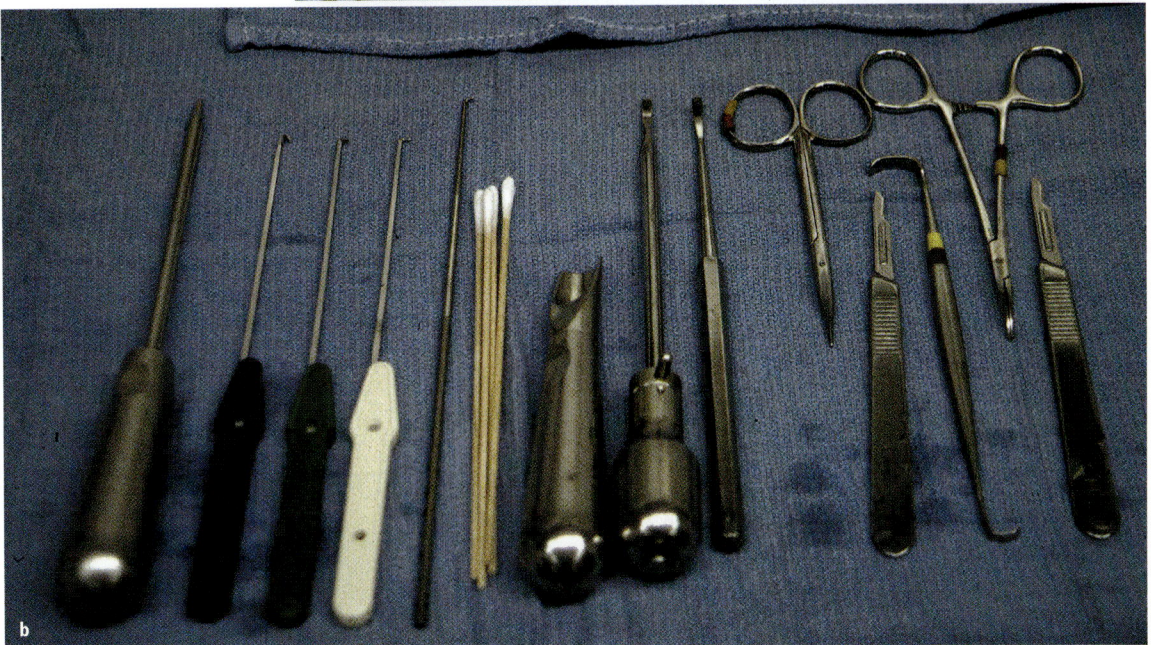

Entry Portal

The proximal end of the pisiform is palpated and marked with a small circle. A 1.5–2 cm line is drawn radially from the proximal pole of the pisiform, depending on the size of the hand. A second line is drawn approximately 0.5 cm proximally to the end of the first line, keeping to a 1:3 ratio with the first line. A small, dotted line, approximately 1 cm (7–10 mm) in length, is drawn from the end of the second line to create the entry portal (Fig. 23.2a, c). If the palmaris longus is present, the center of the entry portal should be located at the ulnar border of the palmaris longus.

Exit Portal

With the thumb in full abduction, a line is drawn from the distal border, perpendicular to the long axis of the forearm. The second line is drawn from the third web space, parallel to the long axis of the forearm. These two lines should be at a right angle. A line bisecting the right angle between these two lines is drawn extending 1 cm proximally from its vertex to locate the distal portal (Fig. 23.2b, c). The surgeon should be able to palpate the hook of hamate. The exit portal should fall into the soft spot in the center of the palm and line up with the ring finger. The conjunction of the entry and exit por-

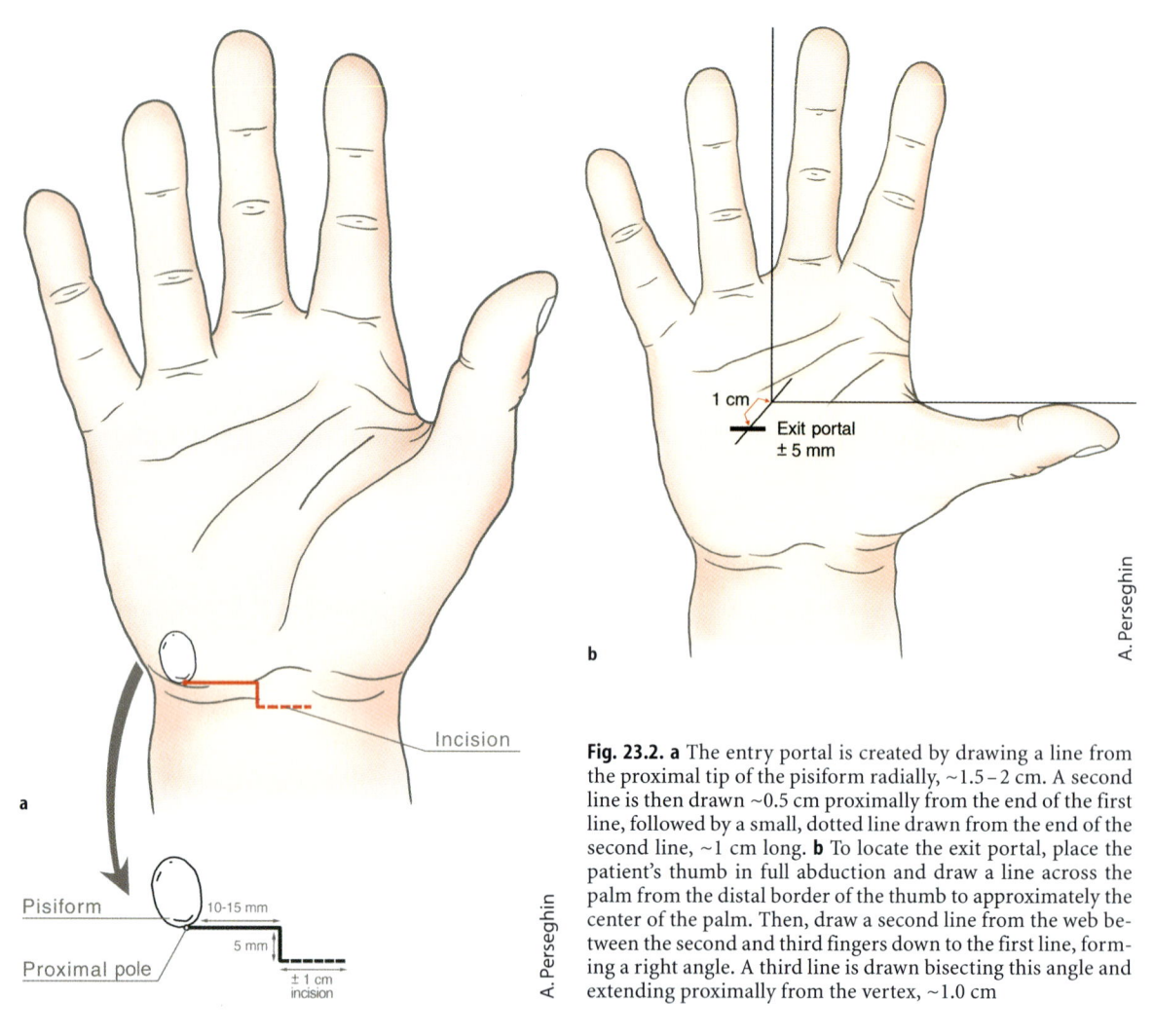

Fig. 23.2. a The entry portal is created by drawing a line from the proximal tip of the pisiform radially, ~1.5–2 cm. A second line is then drawn ~0.5 cm proximally from the end of the first line, followed by a small, dotted line drawn from the end of the second line, ~1 cm long. **b** To locate the exit portal, place the patient's thumb in full abduction and draw a line across the palm from the distal border of the thumb to approximately the center of the palm. Then, draw a second line from the web between the second and third fingers down to the first line, forming a right angle. A third line is drawn bisecting this angle and extending proximally from the vertex, ~1.0 cm

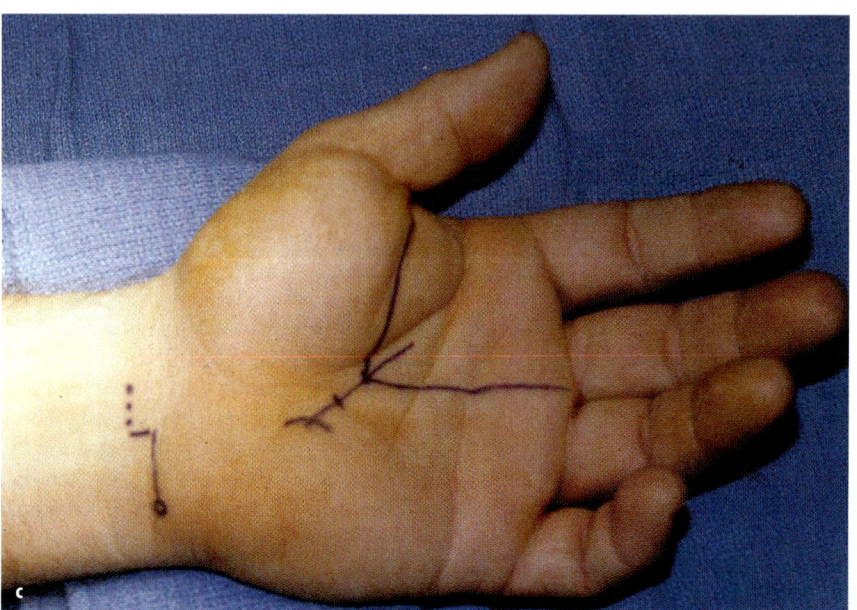

c The entry and exit portals

tals should follow the long axis of the forearm and be just radial to the hook of hamate (Fig. 23.3).

Procedure

The 1% Xylocaine is injected at both the entry and exit portals, approximately 1–2 cc to proximal portal and 3–4 cc to the distal one due to the higher degree of sensitivity on the palmar region. A small, transverse 1 cm (7–10 mm) incision is made at the entry portal mark. A hemostat is used for blunt dissection. Small digital nerves and vessels are retracted away [10–16]. A tourniquet is normally not required if this dissection is handled properly. The fascia, with it's distinguished fibers, should be visible. A knife is used to make a small, longitudinal opening. This cut is extended with small, Stephen's curved tenotomy scissors. If the palmaris longus is present, the longitudinal cut should be along the ulnar border of the palmaris longus. Care should be taken as, sometimes, there are two layers of fascia. Both layers must be cut and the ulnar bursa should be seen from underneath. With the small retractors, the distal border of the skin is lifted to create a vacuum that will separate the carpal ligament and the ulnar bursa. A curved dissector is used to gently push through a thin membrane and enter the carpal canal. When the dissector is maneuvered back and forth, the rough undersurface of the carpal ligament which is de-

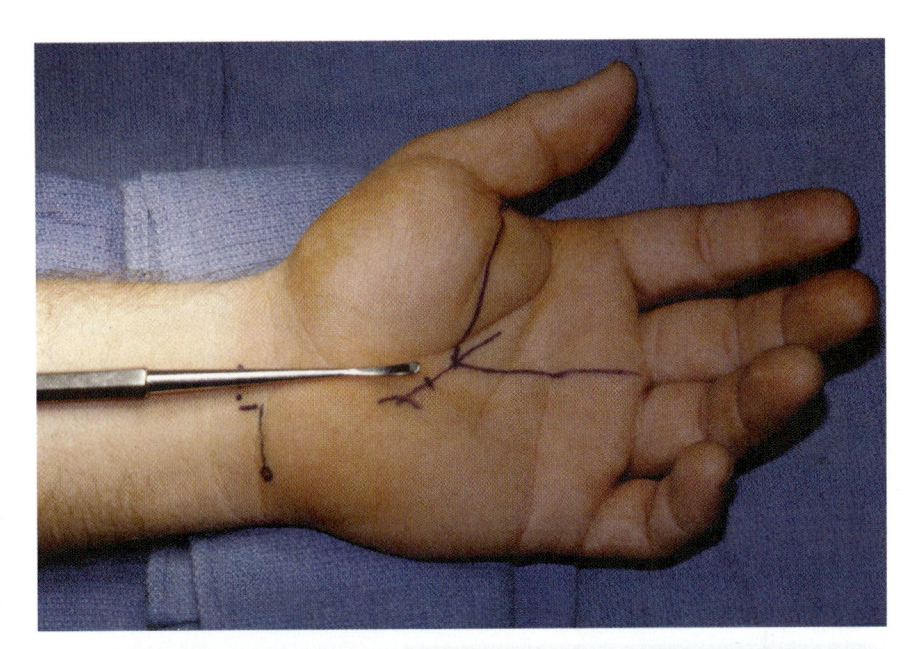

Fig. 23.3. The conjunction of the entry and exit portals should follow the long axis of the forearm and be radial to the hook of hamate

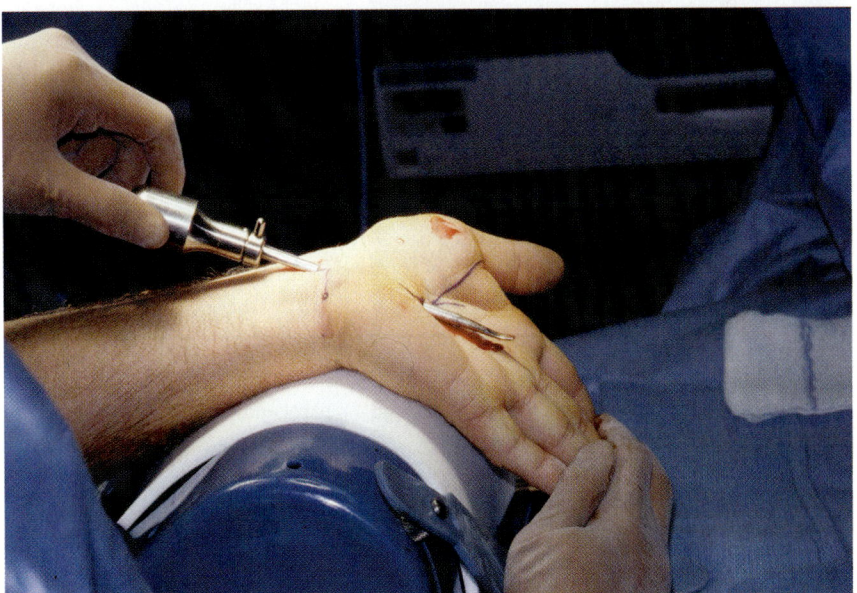

Fig. 23.4. The slotted cannula assembly is advanced through the distal portal and patient's hand is stabilized in the hand holder

scribed as "washboard" or "railroad track" affect, can be felt. Then a curved dissector/slotted cannula assembly unit is slipped under the carpal ligament. With the tip of this unit touching the hook of hamate, the surgeon picks up the patient's fingers and hand and, while maintaining this position, gently hyperextends the fingers and wrist. The assistant brings the hand rest down so that the patient's hand rests comfortably on the frame. The slotted cannula assembly is gently advanced distally, pointing toward the exit portal. A small, transverse or oblique, incision is made cutting only the skin. Arch suppressors are used to press down the structures and the assembled unit exits through the distal portal (Fig. 23.4). The trocar is then removed so that the slotted cannula remains in position under the carpal ligament. The hand is then stabilized on the hand holder.

Ligament Cutting Technique

With the scope in the proximal opening of the slotted cannula and the instrumentation in the distal opening, the distal border of the carpal ligament is identified with the use of a probe (Fig. 23.5). The probe can also be used to palpate any non-ligamentous structure to ensure that it is not the median nerve. Any abnormal sensation in the patient's hand should alert the surgeon and in the presence of any doubts the cannula should be removed and reinserted. The probe knife is used to make the first cut, cutting distally to proximally (Fig. 23.6a, b). Any anatomical structure beyond the distal border of the carpal ligament should not be excised. The scope is withdrawn proximally about 1 cm (10 mm) and the triangle knife is used to make a small

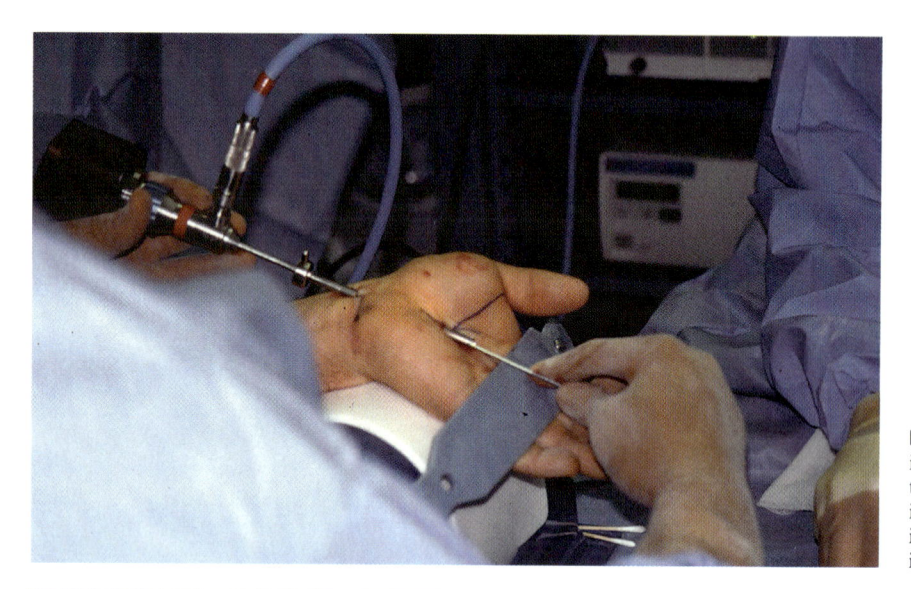

Fig. 23.5. The scope is placed in the proximal opening of the slotted cannula and the instrumentation is brought in through the distal opening

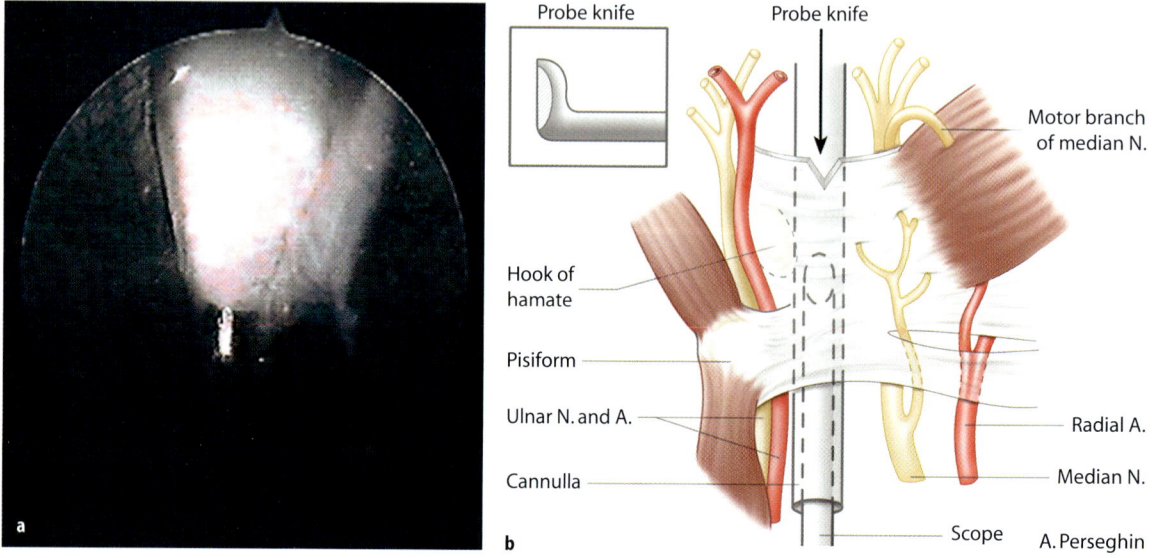

Fig. 23.6. a, b The distal border of the carpal ligament is identified and the probe knife is used to make the first cut distally to proximally

23 Endoscopic Carpal Tunnel Release   161

opening in the midsection of the carpal ligament (Fig. 23.7a, b). The retrograde knife is brought in and placed in the second cut. Once the retrograde knife is well seated, it is pulled distally to join the first two cuts (Fig. 23.8a, b). At this point, the distal portion of the carpal ligament is completely released.

The scope is removed from the proximal opening of the slotted cannula and inserted in the distal one (Fig. 23.9). The view on the screen now forms a mirror effect. The surgeon should realize that the previous ulnar side has become the radial side. By moving the scope proximally and distally, the previous distal cut is identified. The probe knife is inserted and any soft tissue present, usually a thin synovial membrane, is retracted to identify the proximal border of the carpal ligament. A small cut is then made with the probe knife pulled proximally to distally (Fig. 23.10a, b). The probe knife is withdrawn and the retrograde knife is inserted and seated in the proximal edge of the distal cut. It is then pulled proximally to join the proximal cut to completely excise the proximal carpal ligament (Fig. 23.11a, b). The surgeon can use the triangle knife,

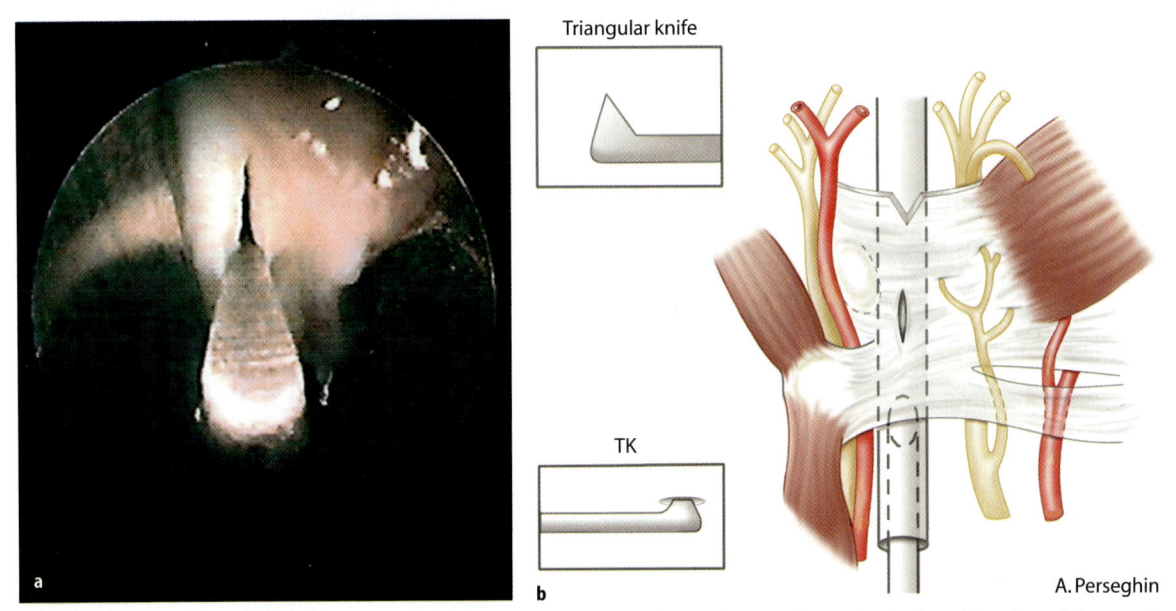

Fig. 23.7. a, b The scope is withdrawn ~1 cm and the triangle knife is used to make a small opening in the midsection of the carpal ligament

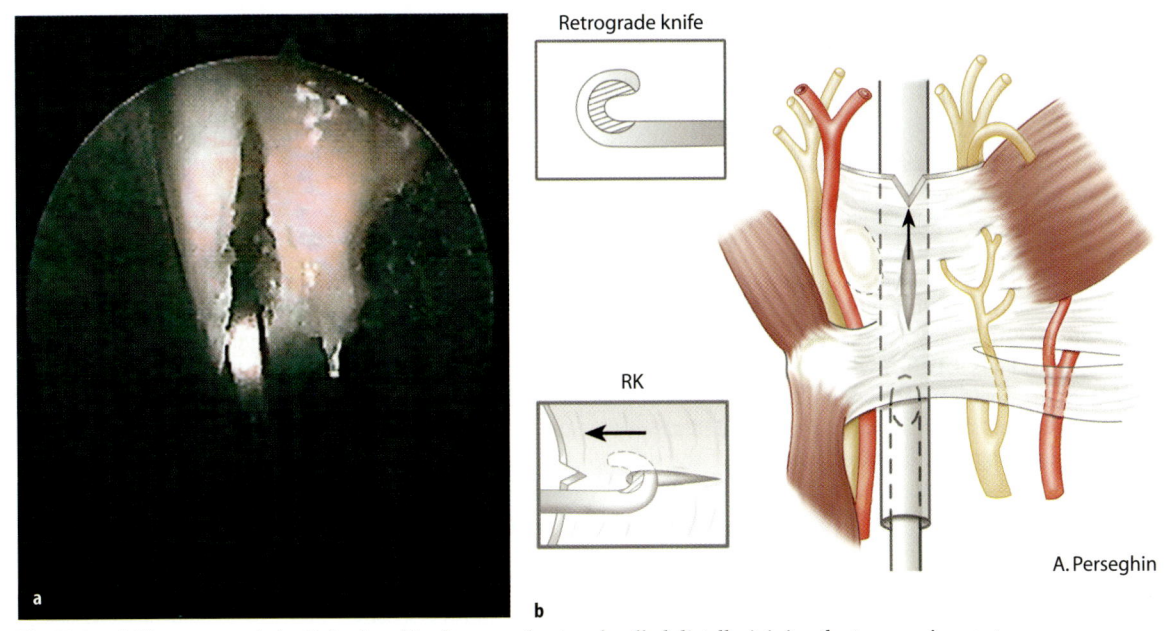

Fig. 23.8. a, b The retrograde knife is placed in the second cut and pulled distally, joining the two previous cuts

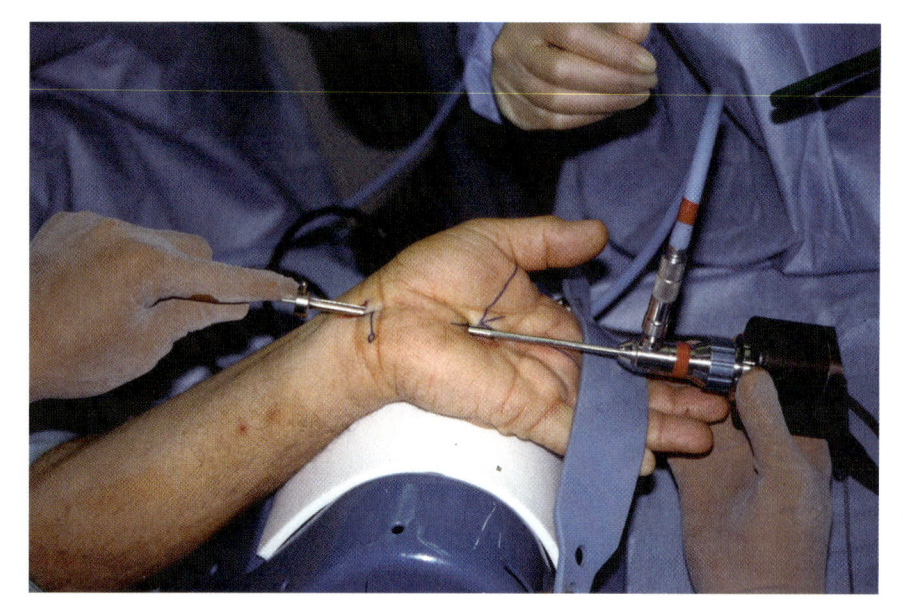

Fig. 23.9. The scope is switched from the proximal to the distal opening of the slotted cannula

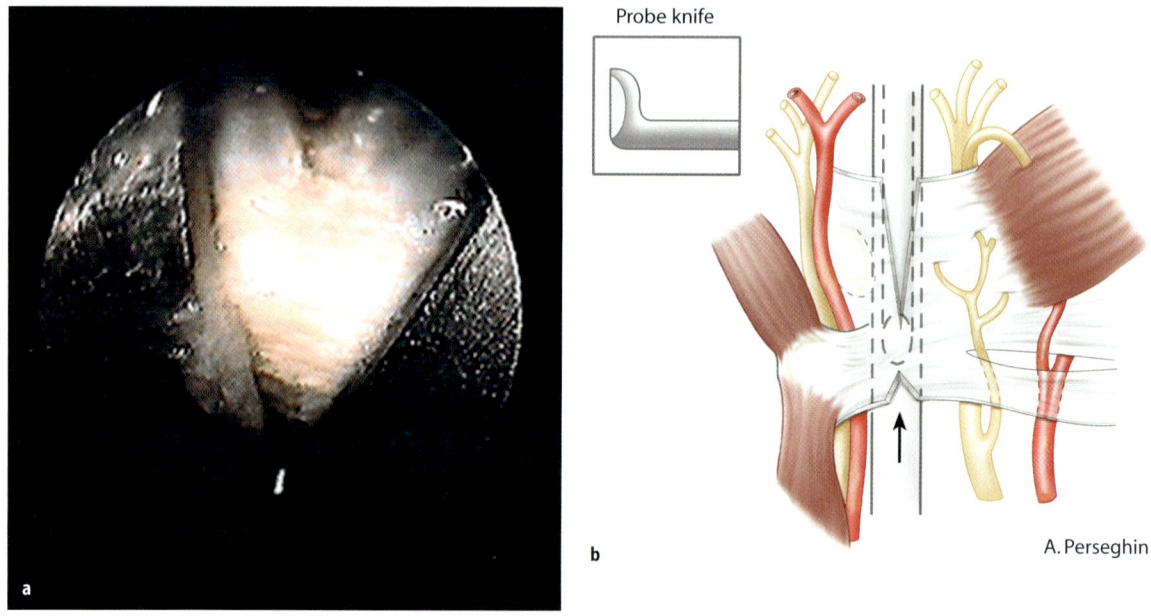

Fig. 23.10. a, b The previous performed distal transection can be viewed through the arthroscope. The proximal edge of the carpal ligament is identified and the probe knife is used to make a small cut, proximally to distally

or any other of the instrumentation knives that feels appropriate, to release any fibers that may have remained in place until he is satisfied with a complete release.

Due to the position of the hand, the cut edges of the carpal ligament should spring apart and disappear from the opening of the slotted cannula. If the edges can still be seen through the opening, the release is incomplete. While the assistant fully abducts the patient's thumb, the uncut portion of the ligament can be identified and the surgeon can complete the transection. By rotating the slotted cannula, the completely cut ligament can be seen endoscopically. After the transection of the carpal ligament, a soft tissue layer could always be found volarly to the carpal ligament that bridges the thenar and hypothenar musculature. This structure should be preserved as well as the opponens digiti minimi and the palmaris brevis muscle, if present. This thin, soft tissue layer from the thenar to the hypothenar muscles will prevent bowstringing of the flexor tendon and preserve the muscle strength. There is seldom any bleeding and only one suture is required for closing each portal (Fig. 23.12). Immediately after the surgical procedure, the surgeon can examine the patient while the sterilized environment has been kept. If any intra-

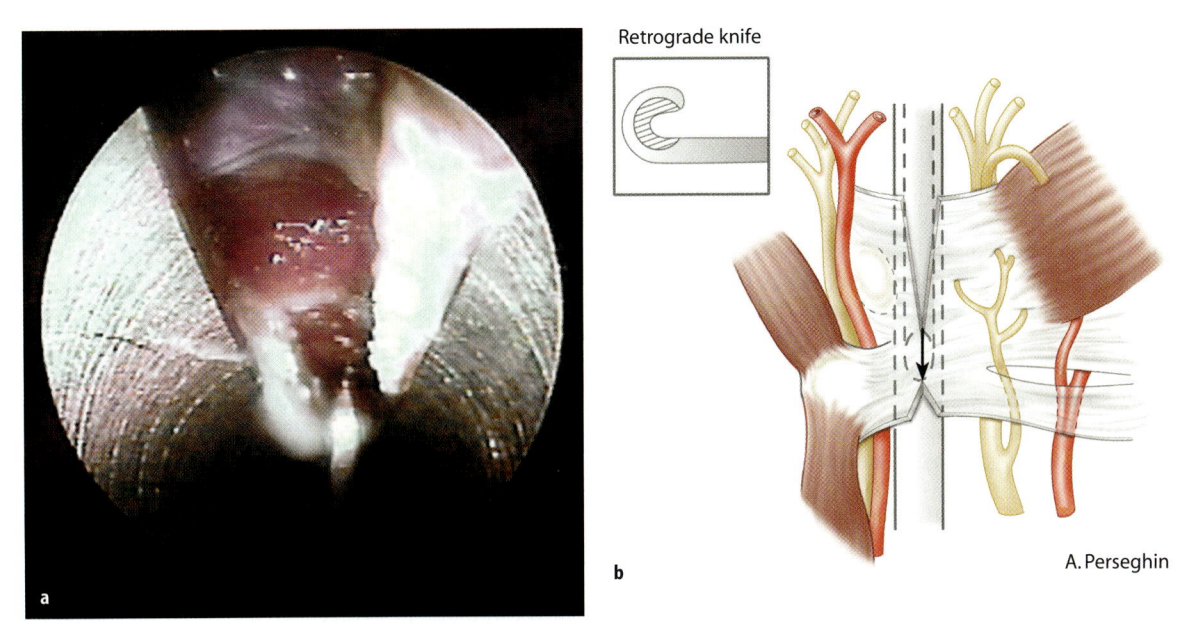

Fig. 23.11. a, b The retrograde knife is inserted and seated in the proximal edge of the distal cut, then pulled proximally to complete the transection of the remaining proximal portion of the carpal ligament

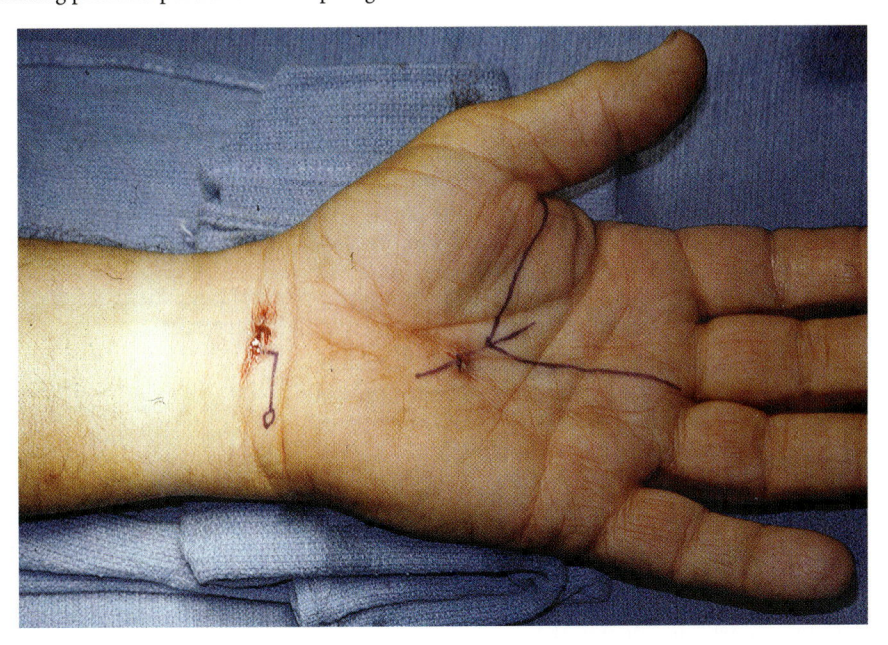

Fig. 23.12. Only one suture is required to close the surgical wound at each portal

operative complications have occurred, which may necessitate exposure of the hand, it can be performed at the same time.

Postoperatively, active exercise begins immediately. The patient is advised to avoid heavy lifting or pushing down on the palm region until the discomfort disappears, usually in 2–3 weeks. Active motion of the fingers decreases the formation of scar tissue in the wrist region; therefore, adhesions on the tendons or nerves at the surgical site are avoided. Sutures are usually removed in 1 week. If patients engage in heavy lifting activities soon after surgery, they may experience some swelling and prolonged pain in the palm region. If these occur, fluidotherapy treatment for 20 min per day can help to decrease the discomfort within 2 weeks.

Normally, the carpal ligament does not have a rich blood supply or nerve fiber distribution; therefore, cutting only the carpal ligament definitely decreases postoperative pain, bleeding, and scarring. The palmaris longus tendon extension and muscle fibers are preserved by the endoscopic technique, which prevents bowstringing of the flexor tendon and the median nerve, as well as preserving the pinch and grip strength [17–21].

Alternative Chow Technique

A Special Design for Hand Surgeons

Many hand surgeons are very uncomfortable with the blind insertion of the trocar exiting distally without seeing the distal superficial palmar arch and distal digital nerve; therefore, they may want to make the distal portal larger in order to identify these structures prior to introducing the slotted cannula. This alternative technique is designed for those surgeons who are willing to take the time to explore the distal portal, especially for a hand surgeon who uses loupe magnification. So that the important distal structures can be seen, the slotted cannula would be placed in the same way but inserted in a manner distally to proximally.

Procedure: The setup and marking of the portal setups would be the same as described previously. It depends upon the surgeon's preference whether a regional block or local anesthesia is used; however, we strongly recommend the use of local anesthesia for the same reason mentioned above. The entry portal for this alternative technique is made with a small oblique incision (1 – 1.5 cm) over the distal palm region at the mark for the exit portal in the above method. Magnified loupes are used while carefully dissecting down to identify the superficial palmar arch curving ulnarly to radially. Further careful dissection allows the identification of the median or digital nerve in the area.

The distal carpal ligament is identified and the slotted cannula, curved side pointing upwards, is inserted under the carpal ligament. The assembly should be touching the hook of hamate, gliding proximally. The "washboard" texture of the carpal ligament should be palpable with the curved dissector as the cannula is aimed towards the center of the wrist and the exit portal. The exit portal should be on the ulnar border of the palmaris longus, if it exists; otherwise, it should be aimed towards the center of the wrist marked as previously described, approximately 0.5 – 1.0 cm proximal to the flexor wrist crease. The fingers and the rest of the hand is then hyperextended and the hand is placed in the hand holder. The surgeon should be able to palpate the curved dissector tip. A small transverse incision is then made and the slotted cannula assembly is brought outside proximally. The rest of the procedure and cutting techniques can be carried out as previously described.

17 Years' Experience and Clinical Results

From September 1987 through April 2005, in Mt. Vernon, Illinois, 3,536 wrists of 2,479 patients underwent endoscopic release of the transverse carpal ligament for the treatment of carpal tunnel syndrome using the dual portal Chow technique. A total of 330 wrists – or 232 patients – were lost to final follow-up evaluation either because they were deceased or had moved without a forwarding address and thus, 3,206 wrists of 2,247 patients comprise our actual study population. Of these, 1,434 were females and 813 were males. Their ages ranged from 14 to 96 years, with a mean of 52 years. All of the patients in this series were carefully examined for other associated problems, including cervical radiculopathy, thoracic outlet syndrome, double crush syndrome, and other systemic diseases such as rheumatoid arthritis, hypothyroidism, lupus, and diabetes. All of the patients exhibited classical carpal tunnel syndrome symptoms including diminished sensation accompanied eventually by numbness and tingling to the median nerve distribution at wrist and hand, nocturnal pain and paresthesias, decreased pinch and grip strength, weakness of the thenar musculature, and persistent waking up during the night. The duration of the symptoms ranged from 1 month to 45 years, with the majority (95%) having a positive Nerve Conduction Velocity test. The follow-up range was 4 months to 17 years. The majority (93%) of the patients were completely asymptomatic or had minor symptoms after the endoscopic release of carpal ligament. There were 18 cases of recurrence, for a rate of 0.6%. There were also 24 cases with residual symptoms following the endoscopic release of the carpal ligament, for a failure rate of 0.7%.

References

1. Chow JCY (1989) Endoscopic Release of the Carpal Ligament: A New Technique for Carpal Tunnel Syndrome; Arthroscopy 5:19-24
2. Okutsu I, Nonomiya S, Takatori Y, Ugawa Y (1989) Endoscopic Management of Carpal Tunnel Syndrome; Arthroscopy 5;11
3. Chow JCY (1990) Endoscopic Carpal Tunnel Release – Clinical Results of 149 Cases; Presented at the 9th Annual AANA Meeting, Orlando, FL, April 26 – 29
4. Agee JM, Tortsua RD, Palmer CA, Berry C (1990) Endoscopic Release of the Carpal Tunnel: A Prospective Randomized Multicenter Study; Presented at the 45th Annual Meeting of the American Society of the Hand, Toronto Canada, September 24-27
5. Caffee HH (1979) Anomalous Thenar Muscle and Median Nerve: A Case Report; J Hand Surg; 4:446
6. Ogden J (1972) An Unusual Branch of the Median Nerve; JBJS;54-A(8)
7. Papathanassiou BT (1968) A Variant of the Motor Branch of the Median Nerve in the Hand JBJS [Br];50:156
8. Lanz U (1977) Anatomical Variations of the Median Nerve in the Carpal Tunnel; J Hand Surg [AM];2:44
9. Eiken O, Carsta N, Eddeland A (1971) Anomalous Distal Branching of the Median Nerve; Scand J Plast Reconstr Surg Hand Surg 5:149
10. Carroll RE, Green DP (1972) The Significance of the Palmar Cutaneous Nerve at the Wrist; Clin Orthop 83:24

11. Taleisnik J (1973) The Palmar Cutaneous Branch of the Median Nerve and the Approach to the Carpal Tunnel; JBJS[Am]; 55: 1212–7
12. Kessler I (1969) Unusual Distribution of the Median Nerve at the Wrist; Clin Orth & Rel Res 67:124–126
13. Kleinert, J (1990) The Nerve of Henle; J Hand Surg (Am) 15:784
14. Shimizu K, Iwasaki R, Hoshikawa H, Yamamuro T (1988) Entrapment Neuropathy of the Palmer Cutaneous Branch of the Median Nerve by the Fascia of Flexor Digitorum Superficialis; J Hand Surg 13A:581-3
15. Enger WD, Gmeiner JG (1980) Palmar Cutaneous Branch of the Ulnar Nerve; J Hand Surg 5:26
16. Ritter MA (1973) The Anatomy and Function of the Palmar Fascia; Hand 5:263–7
17. Shrewsbury MM, Johnson RK, Ousterhout DK (1972) The Palmaris Brevis-A Reconsideration of Its Anatomy and Possible Function; JBJS[Am];54:344–8
18. Viegas S, Pollard A, Kaminksi K (1992) Carpal Arch Alteration and Related Clinical Status After Endoscopic Carpal Tunnel Release; J Hand Surg; 17A:1012-6
19. Garcia-Elias M, Sanches-Freijo J, Salo J, Lluch A (1992) Dynamic Changes of the Transverse Carpal Arch During Flexion-Extension of the Wrist: Effects of Sectioning the Transverse Carpal Ligament; J Hand Surg 17A:1017-9
20. Richman JA, Gelberman RH, Rydevik BL et al. (1989) Carpal Tunnel Syndrome: Morphologic Changes After Release of Transverse Carpal Ligament; J Hand Surg [Am];14:852-857
21. Seradge H, Seradge E (1989) Piso-Triquetral Pain Syndrome After Carpal Tunnel Release; Journal of Hand Surgery 14A: 858–862

24 Endoscopic Technique: The Gilbert Technique (or Technique by Two Different Portals)

F. Brunelli, C. Spalvieri, A. Gilbert, M. Merle

History

Until 1950 the treatment of carpal tunnel syndrome (CTS) was not treated seriously, but then Phalen suggested as a treatment the dissection of the annular anterior carpal ligament [1].

Even if we can say that in most cases there is an improvement, quite often the patient feels pain for some weeks or months, particularly pain in the area of the lower part of the hand, which is frequently followed by a significant loss of power. Furthermore, this operation is followed by inflammation caused by the cicatrix, which can be very painful because of iatrogenic damage of the ramus cutaneus palmaris of the median nerve. To prevent this kind of inconvenience Chow [2], Okutsu [3], and Agee [4] suggested endoscopic treatment of the CTS. The results of the first cases were very interesting in relation to improvement after the operation and recovery, but on the other hand, there was an unacceptable percentage of complications such as nerve, artery, and tendon damage. The technique we are presenting makes an easy and secure endoscopic dissection of the annular anterior carpal ligament possible using specific instruments.

Technique

The operation takes place with axillary or block anesthesia of the median nerve at the distal third of the forearm. After having pumped out the blood of the arm so it gets swollen and before skin incision, a styptic loop is put at the beginning of the arm (close to the shoulder).

This incision is performed on the anterior aspect of the wrist and it is 1.5 cm proximal to the wrist joint. It starts on the level of the internal side of the palm tendon and goes towards the ulnar and it is about 2 cm long (Fig. 24.1). Before the dissection of the superficial aponeurosis, a longitudinal vein should be isolated and if possible kept safe. This vein is in the middle of the cut. Once the aponeurosis is opened you can identify the tendon flexor and the median nerve. There are four different spatulas to choose from according to the dimension of the tunnel. When the spatula is introduced

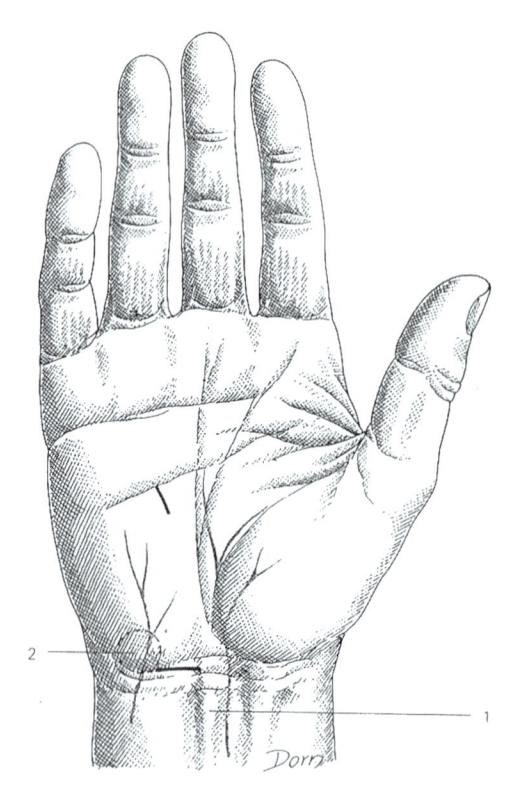

Fig. 24.1. The two incisions to enter for the endoscopic treatment of carpal tunnel syndrome. (*1*) tendon of the palmar gracile; (*2*) Pisiform. (From [18])

in the canal it creates a free operation space. The spatula is introduced horizontally and then turned out 90° to move the tendon flexor and the median nerve. The second cannula is then introduced with a distance of 2 cm between the inner side of the guiding spatula and the hook of hamate. The extended hand is lying on a movable metallic support and as the hand gets stretched more and more, the mandrel gets closer to the annular anterior carpal ligament and it takes out the synovial tissue, if there is a lot of it. The carpal tunnel is formed in such a way that the entrance of the mandrel is in the axis of the fourth ray but the hook of hamate changes its direction and it goes obliquely in a radial direction. Therefore, the exit of the probe out of the tunnel is in

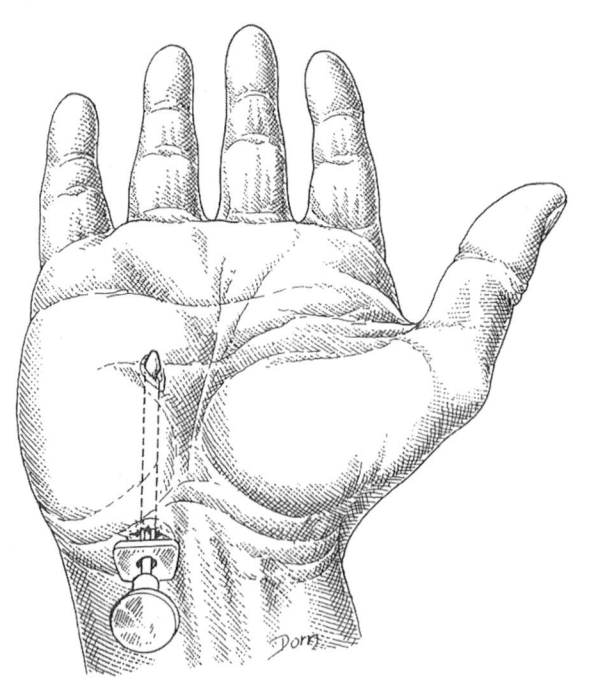

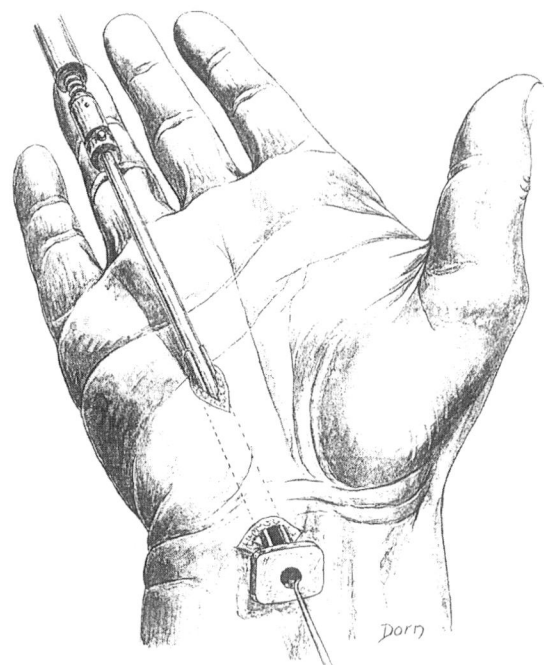

Fig. 24.2. The cannula probe with its mandrel is entered in proximal-distal way. (From [18])

Fig. 24.3. The endoscope is entered in proximal-distal direction in the probe. (From [18])

the axis of the third ray; if it gets too close to the ulnar, there is a risk of penetrating the canal of Guyon. The head of the mandrel can be palpated at the level of the palm. At the distal end of the tunnel the pressure of the thumb by the surgeon helps to make it immediately superficial and to move the superficial arch and the dividing branches of the median nerve. The second little incision is made vertically on the tip of the trocar on palm level. Now the aponeurosis gets moved in such a way so that the exit of the trocar can be performed without inclusion of the digital nerve of the third finger, which is extremely vulnerable in that area. An endoscope connected to a video camera replaces the mandrel and is inserted in the probe in a distal-proximal direction (Fig. 24.2, 24.3). The transversal direction of the annular anterior carpal ligament fiber and the correct position of the endoscope can be followed now on the monitor. At this point it is important to make sure that there is no interposition of tendon flexor or synovial fringe which could passively move the fingers. Abduction of the thumb makes it possible to keep the median nerve on the radial side of the carpal tunnel. If there is no clear view of the transversal ligament fiber because of synovial accretion, it would be better to reinsert the trocar and use its top to stimulate the ligament. This way the endoscope and the video camera are reintroduced in the probe. Sectioning of the ligament is performed in a distal-proximal direction using a knife with a curved blade under the control of the endoscope. It is introduced as close as possible with the point of the knife pointed down. Slowly it slides to the point where it can be seen through the camera and is turned 180° to connect it to the distal margin of the ligament. The permanent visual control allows the surgeon to see the section of the ligament and the interposition of subcutaneous adipose cell tissue. If the diastase is performed well, it is sufficient to pass once, then the endoscope is taken off and the mandrel is reinserted in the probe. At this point it is possible to see, through transillumination, if the ligament has been sectioned correctly. A last verification can be obtained by pointing the point of the mandrel up and letting it slide in distal-proximal direction. This makes it possible to see and feel the blunt point of the mandrel sliding directly under the skin and to make sure that no ligament tissue is left which could put pressure on the nerve. In case of an excessive synovitis it is possible to perform a partial synovectomy of the flexors. This is done through a 5-cm incision on the anterior aspect of the wrist pulling the different tendons or tendon groups with a blunt hook knife to free them from the hypertrophic synovium. The cutaneous incision is sewn with two or three stitches using a rapidly resorbent thread. To protect the wrist from the first dressing, which is placedon the third day after the operation, it is enough to use a simple pressure bandage without any orthesis. Later on a simple plaster is put on the wound and the patient is asked to be careful with movements. The only limitation of movement is the postoperative pain.

Indications and Contraindications

The endoscopic treatment of CTS is indicated for most of the patients, no matter what stage of the syndrome. Ideally, this technique should be performed at an early stage, but it can be performed at a later stage using amyotrophia if intraneural neurolysis does not demonstrate any effect on the external neurolysis (obviously this can be done only with an open surface). Therefore, this technique can be performed on every patient with an idiopathic CTS if the aspecific synovitis has reactive, hormonal, or professional origins, but also if the syndrome is accompanied by systematic illnesses like diabetes or amyloid disease.

Contraindications are rare and concern the following cases:

- Syndromes which need a complete synovectomy such as in the case of rheumatic arthritis.
- Compression because of pyogenic synovitis.
- Syndromes with any kind of etiology which requires an exact exploration of the content and the contenting area.
- In cases of palindromia where postoperative accretion can be a risk for endoscopic surgery.
- In cases of younger and older children where an abnormal compression must evoke suspicion.
- Finally, in the case of all patients where the intraoperative endoscopic treatment does not identify correctly the ligament in its whole length and where structure finds itself between the probe and the ligament fiber, even though everything has been performed as described above. In these cases you should not hesitate to change and work according the traditional technique.

Results and Complications

Endoscopic surgery of the carpal tunnel makes it possible for the hand to recover very fast. Generally speaking, pain in the elbow and the shoulder, and waking up at night disappear immediately. In some cases paresthesias might persist for a changeable period, depending on the time and the stage of the compression of the nerve before the operation (an approximate prognosis might be given based on the electromyographic exam before the operation). In most cases the patient is able to flex and extend the fingers already the first day after the operation and after the first dressing 3 days after the operation, the daily routine can be carried out almost normally. Strength is gained quicker than after the traditional treatment with an open surface: after 15 days, the hand gains 60% of the strength it had before the operation (with the open technique this is hardly possible after the same time because of pain). After 21 days 78% of strength is gained; with the traditional technique only 28% is gained. After 45 days, strength gained for both techniques is comparable.

Possible complications have been well described in international specific literature. It is important to know this literature and to understand that endoscopic surgery of the carpal tunnel is not a "simple" operation. A lack of experience of the surgeon can create serious complications concerning the nerve, tendon, and arterial sectioning [5–10], but we would like to focus on two minor complications which appear relatively often and about which the patient has to be informed preoperatively. Too often patients think that the operation is easy, fast, and that they will not suffer for a long time.

Thirty percent of the cases feel pain on the palm of the hand (pillar pain), followed by swelling because of inflammation for some weeks or even months. This pain does not allow the patient to force the hand, especially if they have to move the wrist or push with the lower part of the hand. The reason for this pain is still not clear. Certainly the sectioning of the ligament provokes a transformation from a concave to a convex structure and the two margins of the sectioned ligament are positioned directly under the skin. This can provoke a painful inflammation. For the time being it is difficult to foresee and prevent this kind of pain. Maybe the conservation of the superficial aponeurosis fiber could reduce the amplitude, but at the same time it would reduce clearance and support recurrence.

In a relatively high percentage of patients (about 5%) it is possible to notice local paresthesia on the ulnar inclination of the third finger and on the radial of the fourth finger. Generally, it disappears a couple of days after the operation, but in some cases (0.5%) it can be very painful for weeks or months [11–13]. In few cases the pain remains permanently [14, 15]. The paresthesia is probably caused by a direct traction of the probe on the common digital nerve of the third interdigital space or by a indirect traction on a anastomotic branch placed at the exit of the tunnel between the median and the ulnar nerve [16]. This complication represents a real problem for endoscopic surgery compared to the traditional technique and to avoid it is rather difficult because of anatomic variations which are difficult to judge using the endoscope. In any case, this problem appears also after having performed the "open" technique [17], even if in fewer cases.

Advice and Tricks

Even though the mentioned technique is effective and reliable, some advice and tricks should be given based on the experience of surgeons who have performed many decompressions of the median nerve using the endoscopic technique.

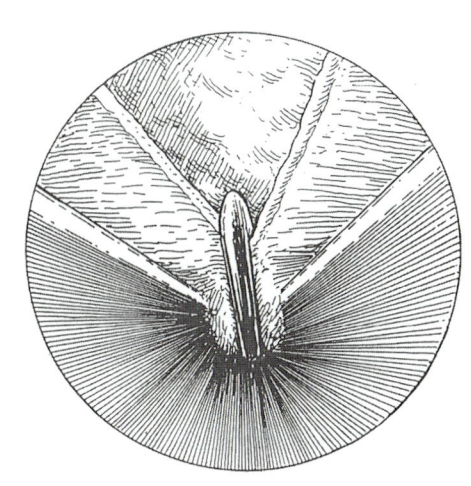

Fig. 24.4. Once the annular ligament is identified due to its transversal fiber the special bistoury is introduced and the sectioning of the ligament is performed under constant control through the endoscope. (From [18])

Whoever decides to follow this procedure from the very beginning is going to ask the following questions:

Did I introduce the probe and its mandrel in the right place?

Actually there are two possible mistakes that can occur: The probe might have been introduced in the canal of Guyon (this presents the danger of damaging the nerve or the ulnar artery) or into the subcutaneous tissue. For an expert surgeon it is clear when the probe with its mandrel has "entered" into the tunnel but for someone using this technique for the first time it might not be as clear. When introducing the probe correctly in the canal resistance can be felt, but then it slides down easily. If the probe is positioned incorrectly resistance can be felt all the way. If it is positioned superficially it can be palpated under the skin all the way and not only at the exit of the tunnel. After having cut the skin at the wrist transversally it is suggested to cut the brachial aponeurosis and the annular ligament 2 cm longitudinally with scissors. Check the content of the tunnel, and before entering with the trocar use big, blunt scissors to enter. Stay close to the edge of the ligament until you clearly feel the exit at the distal margin of the tunnel.

Is it only the ligament that is being sectioned?

If you have a clear endoscopic view of the annular anterior carpal ligament transversal fiber through the probe, then that is an ideal intraoperative situation (Fig. 24.4). In that case, there are no doubts because everything that is transversely oriented and presents a fibrous structure can be sectioned without hurting important parts. It can happen that the view is not as clear because of synovial proliferation on top of the canal or because of interposition of different structures like ten-

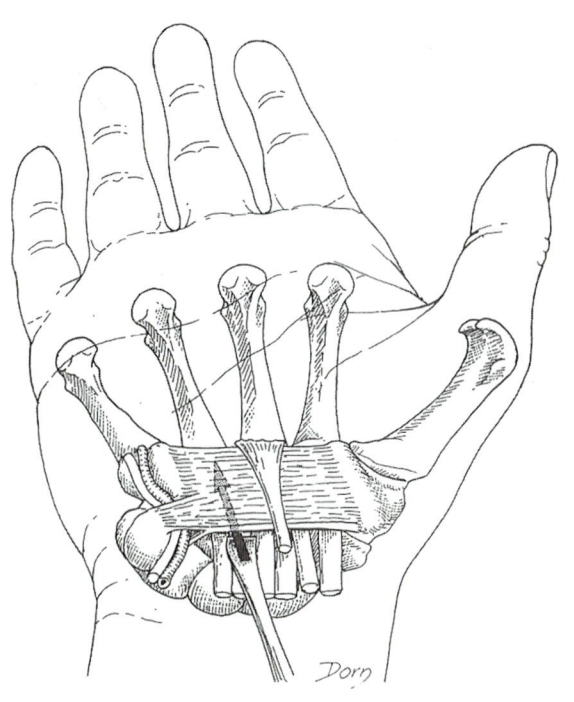

Fig. 24.5. If there is no clear view of the ligament, the deep part of it is scraped and cleaned from synovial accretion using a spatula. (From [18])

dons or the medial nerve. In that case, it is better to take the probe out and continue carefully with a spatula to scratch the deep aspect of the ligament (Fig. 24.5). If after having done so there still is no clear view, it is better to continue according to the traditional technique.

Is the ligament completely sectioned?

This is the most common question using a technique with only one entrance. Actually, the advantage of using the described technique is the ability to identify and isolate the complete ligament from two incisions, i.e., to section it in a complete way. Generally speaking, we can say that the tunnel has been opened correctly if the patient does not complain anymore about pain and awakenings during the night as he/she used to have before the operation at the first clinical control 3 days after the operation (even if paresthesias remain).

Conclusion

The decompression technique of the CTS with a double entrance is reliable by now because of:

- An empty operation space due to a prepared path
- An articulated support of the forearm which allows the extension of the wrist
- Atraumatic and optic instruments which assure a perfect view of the annular carpal ligament

The endoscope with an oblique view makes it possible to adjust to most of the endoscopic cameras. Its special design makes it stable inside the cannula probe.

Respecting the operation protocol makes this surgery reassuring, comfortable, and fast.

References

1. Phalen GS (1966) The carpal tunnel syndrome: seventeen years experience in diagnosis and treatment of six hundred and fifty-four hands. J Bone Joint Surgery 48A: 211–28
2. Chow JCY (1989) Endoscopic release of carpal tunnel ligament: a new technique for carpal tunnel syndrome. J. Arthroscop Rel Surg 5: 19–24
3. Okutsu I, Niomiya S, Takatori Y (1989) Endoscopic management of carpal tunnel syndrome. Arthroscopy 11–18
4. Agee JM, McCarrol HR, Tortosa RD et al. (1992) Endoscopic release of carpal tunnel: a randomised prospective multicenter study. J Hand Surg 17A: 987–95
5. Feinstein AP (1993) Endoscopic carpal tunnel release in a community-based series. J Hand Surg 18A: 451–4
6. Kelly CP, Pulisetti D, Jamieson AM (1994) Early experience with endoscopic carpal tunnel release. J Hand Surg 19B: 18–21
7. Lee DH, Masear VR, Meyer RD et al. (1992) Endoscopic carpal tunnel release: a cadaveric study. J Hand Surg 17A: 1003–8
8. Luallin SR, Toby EB (1993) Incidental Guyon's canal release during attempted endoscopic carpal tunnel release: an anatomical study and report of two cases. J Arthroscopy Rel Surg 9: 382–6
9. Murphy RX, Jennings JF, Wukich DK (1994) Major neurovascular complications of endoscopic carpal tunnel release. J Hand Surg 19A:114–8
10. Shinya K, Lanzetta M, Conolly WB (1995) Risk and complications in endoscopic carpal tunnel release. J Hand Surg 20B: 2: 222–7
11. Foucher G, Allieu Y, Balmann B (1993) Endoscopic release of the carpal tunnel median nerve using Ageès technique 80 cases. Chirurgie Endoscopique 2: 9–13
12. Tennent TD, Goddard NJ (1997) Carpal tunnel decompression: open vs endoscopic. Br J of Hospital Medicine 58: 11: 551–4
13. Jacobsen MB, Rahme H (1996) A prospective, randomised study with an independent observer comparing open carpal tunnel release with endoscopic carpal tunnel release . J Hand Surg 21B: 2: 202–4
14. Le Nen D, Rizzo Ch, Brunet PH (1998) Neurolyse du nerf median au poignet selon la technique endoscopique à deux voies. Ann Chir Main 17: 3: 221–31
15. Friol JP, Chaise F, Gaisne E, Bellemere PH (1994) Decompession endoscopique du nerf median au canal carpien, a pros de 1400 cas. Ann Chir Main 13: 3: 162–71
16. Ferrari GP, Gilbert A (1991) The superficial anastomosis on the palm of the hand between the ulnar and the median nerves. J Hand Surg 16B: 511–4
17. May JW, Rosen H (1981) Division of the sensory ramus communicans between the ulnar and median nerve: a complication following carpal tunnel release. J Bone Joint Surgery 63A:5: 836–8
18. Tubiana G-M, Martin D (Eds.) (1999) An Atlas of Surgical Techniques for the Hand and Wrist. Lippencott, Williams and Wilkins

Endoscopic Carpal Tunnel Release

C.A. Peimer, R.K. Brown

It was probably inevitable that the trend toward endoscopically guided and similar methods utilizing smaller skin incisions, and offering the opportunity for faster healing times, would include decompression of the median nerve for carpal tunnel syndrome (CTS) that is unresponsive to conservative care. The interest in endoscopic methods for carpal tunnel release (CTR) has been motivated by the desire to minimize or eliminate the need for potentially tender and troublesome incisions in the palmar skin. In 1989 Okutsu and colleagues reported a technique they originated for performing carpal tunnel releases utilizing the "universal subcutaneous endoscope" [1]. Fifty-four hands in 45 patients with CTS had decompression by their method under local anesthetic, with reported excellent clinical and postoperative electrodiagnostic results. These authors concluded that endoscopic carpal tunnel release by their technique was both effective and safe. An editor's note accompanying Okutsu's article expressed "doubts as to the wisdom of using arthroscopic [sic] carpal tunnel release." Sixteen years later, endoscopic techniques for carpal tunnel release are used widely, but in some quarters similar doubts and hesitancy remain; and the scientific basis for such fears continues to be debated.

In the USA, several commercially available systems for performing endoscopic carpal tunnel release are available; there are two truly original designs: one using a single-portal technique (Carpal Tunnel Release System, MicroAire Surgical Instruments, Charlottesville, VA, USA) and the other using two incisions (ECTRA II, Smith & Nephew, Andover, MA, USA). Both techniques employ fiberoptic lights and video-endoscopes to send real-time images from inside the carpal canal to a television monitor. Guided by these images, (as with any arthroscopic surgical method) the surgeon isolates and then divides the transverse carpal ligament in order to enlarge the canal and thereby decompress the median nerve [2–10].

Indications and Contraindications

The indications for endoscopic carpal tunnel release (eCTR) are, in fact, no different than those for performing an historically-traditional open method carpal tunnel release (oCTR) [2–7, 9, 10]. None of the endoscopic systems are appropriate for visual "exploration" of the carpal tunnel; rather, the endoscope is used to allow a limited external (volar region) dissection while fully visualizing the transverse carpal ligament (TCL) prior to and during its division. The contraindications for endoscopic method release include circumstances in which the canal contents or the median nerve must be dissected and/or explored (e.g., for a space-occupying lesion that is compressing the nerve, when a prolific inflammatory tenosynovitis is present, or when fluid [pus or hematoma] must be evacuated. Acute carpal tunnel syndrome, in the setting of a distal radius fracture, or associated with a compartment syndrome of the hand or forearm, may be a relative contraindication to eCTR for these reasons. Recurrent carpal tunnel syndrome in a patient who has had previous release (by any method), and may have fibrosis that limits full and "safe" visualization of the TCL with protection of the median nerve can also be considered another relative contraindication as well [8, 11, 12].

Anatomy

In the forearm, the median nerve courses distally between the flexors digitorum superficialis and profundus. As it nears the wrist, the nerve moves volarly (i.e., it becomes more superficial), to lie just beneath the antebrachial fascia, between the tendons of flexor digitorum superficialis and the flexor carpi radialis, and deep to the palmaris longus tendon, when that latter structure is present. The median nerve enters the carpal tunnel in its most palmar and radial quadrant, and shares this space with nine digital flexor tendons to the fingers and thumb. The three walls of the carpal tunnel are formed by the volar arch of the carpal bones. The roof of the carpal tunnel (on its palmar aspect) is the transverse carpal ligament, which is also known as the flexor retinaculum. On its radial margin, the TCL attaches to the scaphoid tuberosity and the beak of the trapezium. On the ulnar side, the TCL attaches to the pisiform and the hook of the hamate (hamulus). The proximal edge of the TCL is continuous with and blends into the antebrachial fascia (both arising embryologically from mesoderm), is deep to the palmar fascial (arising from ectoderm), which is itself continuous proximally with the palmaris longus tendon.

Rotman and Manske studied the anatomic structures in close proximity to an endoscopic carpal tunnel release device [13]. They concluded that insertion of the endoscope into the carpal tunnel in line with the ring finger (fourth ray) axis maximizes the distance between the endoscope and the median nerve, and from the superficial palmar (arterial) arch, thereby lessening the risk of injury to these two structures. They noted a separate fascial layer immediately palmar to the TCL, derived continuously from the thenar and hypothenar muscle fascia, as well as from the dorsal fascia of the palmaris brevis overlying Guyon's canal, and contiguous with the palmaris longus tendon. These fibers did not appear to be part of either the palmar fascia or the palmaris brevis, but rather corresponded to the intact (transverse) collagen fibers clearly seen intraoperatively after endoscopic TCL release.

Single-Portal Technique (Modified from Agee)

This method of TCL division was designed with the intention of avoiding a palmar skin incision in the palm and its associated morbidity [2–4]. The endoscopic instrument has a disposable, retractable blade assembly which is operated with a triggered pistol-grip handle. The handle and cutting blade may be easily rotated to permit surgery on either the right or the left hand. The original device was redesigned shortly after its introduction to permit clear visualization of the cutting blade as it is deployed to divide the TCL.

The operating room is organized to allow the surgeon a comfortable, unimpeded, direct view of the television monitor while operating, as is typical for any endoscopic surgical method. The surgery may be performed – at the preference of the patient and surgeon – under general, regional, or local anesthetics, with tourniquet control. The upper extremity is prepped and draped free; the arm is exsanguinated and a pneumatic tourniquet inflated *before* infiltrating with anesthetic to avoid blood-staining at the injection site. Using a large volume of local anesthetic may impair the view through the endoscope by unnecessarily increasing fluid within the canal (we typically use a total of <6 ml). A 1.5–2.0 cm transverse incision is made in the nonglabrous skin of the most distal volar forearm, proximal to the palm, in or just proximal to the distal flexion crease of the wrist. The glabrous palmar skin is far less mobile and more difficult to dissect than at the preferred site, where longitudinal exposure in the deep tissues is easily achieved through a limited skin incision. The incision is begun at the radial margin of the palmaris longus tendon, if present, and is continued ulnarly. Blunt, spreading longitudinal dissection is done in the subcutaneous layer, deep and *ulnar* to palmaris longus (thereby staying out of the territory of the palmar cutaneous branch of the median nerve which is located between palmaris and flexor carpi radialis), to expose and visualize the antebrachial fascia. A distally-based flap of antebrachial fascia is begun with a longitudinal incision beneath the palmaris, then elevated from tenosynovium and the median nerve beneath, and then incised sharply on its other two sides. A small, blunt spatula elevator is used to dissect adherent flexor tenosynovium, also known as the ulnar bursa, off the deep (dorsal) surface of the antebrachial fascia and contiguous TCL, staying in line with the fourth ray. The leading distal edge of the proximal antebrachial fascia is divided subcutaneously in the volar midline with blunt dissecting scissors, up to a point about 3–5 cm proximal to the area of carpal tunnel dissection in order to gain more space. A series of progressively larger blunt probes ("dilators") is available for insertion into the carpal tunnel for the purpose of facilitating insertion of the endoscopic device, and importantly – further verifying entry in line with the fourth ray axis. The endoscope is then inserted into the carpal tunnel in line with the fourth ray, in the most palmar and ulnar quadrant, as experimental evidence earlier cited indicates that this is the safest orientation and position for the endoscope [13]. It is also important to verify that insertion of the endoscope is radial to the hook of the hamate, to avoid entering Guyon's canal. The dorsal surface of the TCL should be clearly visualized endoscopically (Fig. 25.1), with the dense, transverse fibers having a washboard-like appearance. If this is not what is seen, the endoscope should be removed (Fig. 25.2) and properly reinserted. When the tenosynovium in the carpal canal has not been well cleared, or there is residual fluid within the canal, additional blunt dissection of flexor tenosynovium off the dorsal surface of the TCL is done. If the "transverse" fibers seem sparse, widely spaced and interspersed with fat, it is likely that the scope lies ulnar to the hamulus and fourth ray, palmar to the carpal canal, and is actually within Guyon's canal.

When a clear view of the TCL is achieved, the distal edge of the TCL is identified easily. A fingertip lightly tapping or pressed gently onto the palmar skin at the estimated location of the distal edge of the TCL can be helpful for this endoscopic visualization. Indentation and motion of the softer, yellowish subcutaneous tissues will be seen through the endoscope just distal to the rigid distal edge of the TCL. The cutting blade of the

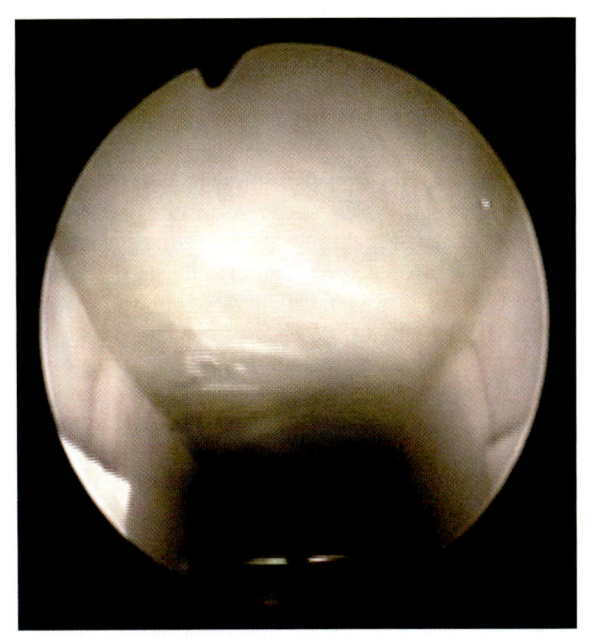

Fig. 25.1. TCL endoscopic view at the beginning of its release

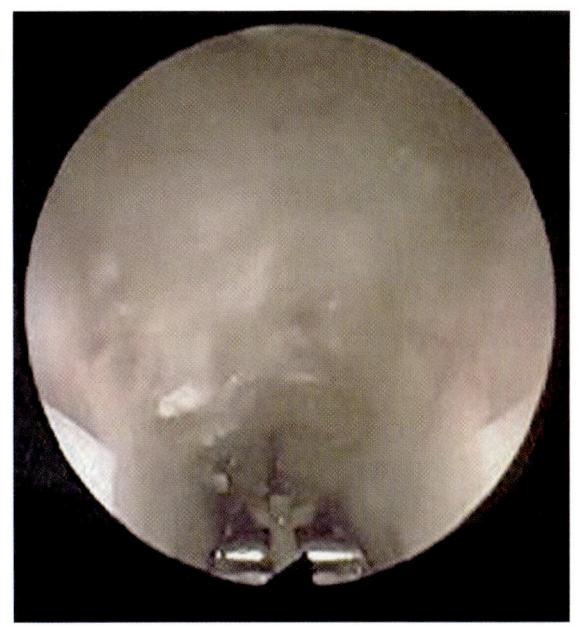

Fig. 25.2. TCL endoscopic view in which the dorsal surface is not clearly visualized

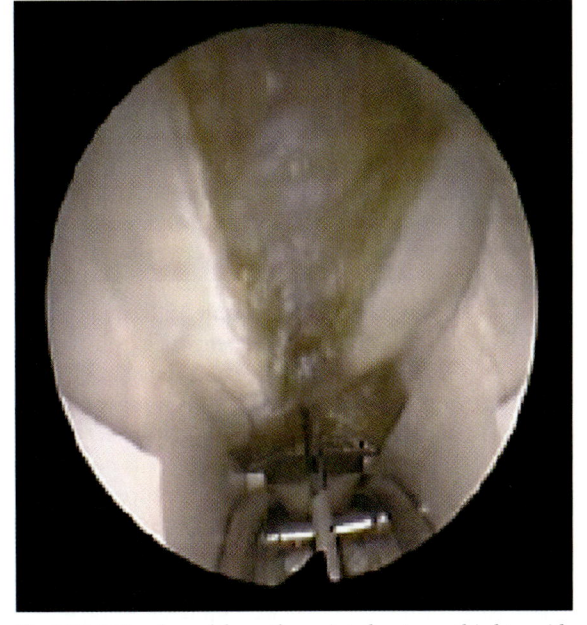

Fig. 25.3. TCL released from the point about one third to midway between the proximal and distal edges of it

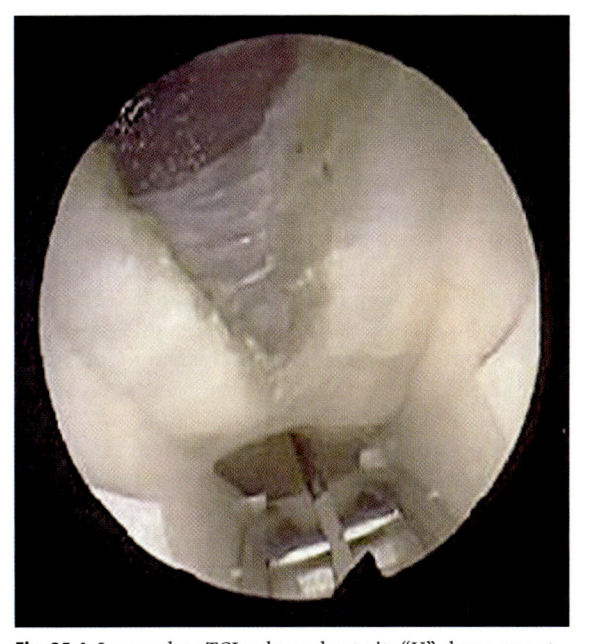

Fig. 25.4. Incomplete TCL release due to its "V" shape aspect

device is deployed at the distal edge by depressing the trigger fully, and the device is then slowly withdrawn proximally to a point about one third to midway between the proximal and distal edges of the TCL (Fig. 25.3). With the trigger released and the cutting blade retracted, the endoscope is advanced again distally and the incised portion of the TCL is inspected for any remaining intact (generally, superficial) TCL fibers. Undivided fibers of the TCL (Fig. 25.4) can be incised with one or more additional distal-to-proximal passes with the endoscope in the distal half of the canal [4]. Incising *only* the distal half of the TCL at first helps avoid the visibility problem of fatty midpalm tissues hanging down between the cut edges of the TCL in the middle of the canal, and obscuring the view of the cut, or uncut, ligament through the endoscope. When division of the distal half of the TCL is complete, the endoscope is positioned barely distal to the most proximal portion of

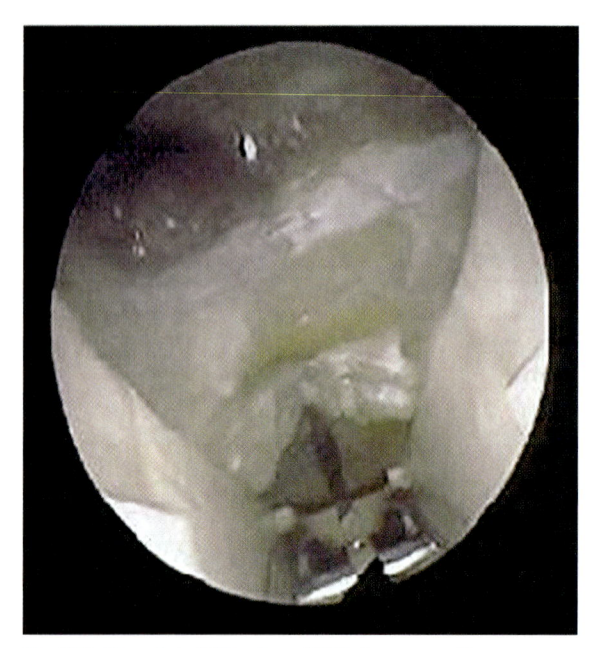

Fig. 25.5. Complete TCL release ("U" shape aspect)

the cut ligament, the blade is deployed, and the scope is withdrawn proximally to the proximal edge of TCL. With the blade retracted, the scope assembly is reinserted, the entire incised TCL is inspected, and any remaining intact fibers are divided.

With complete division of the TCL, the cut edges separate widely enough that both leaves can no longer be seen at the same time through the endoscope (Fig. 25.5). Importantly, the most distal edge of each cut leaf of TCL will hang freely and separately. The canal will now be – and feel – much larger, and light transmission through palmar skin is increased. A small right-angled blunt retractor can be used after endoscope removal to inspect the proximal 50%–75% of the carpal tunnel under direct vision, in order to further confirm satisfactory wide separation of the cut edges of the TCL [10, 11], verify the absence of masses or other pathology, and assure that the condition of the nerve and tendons in the tunnel and entire zone of surgical dissection remain virginal (prior to closure).

The distally-based ("handle") flap of antebrachial fascia is now excised. After irrigation, the tourniquet is deflated and hemostasis is obtained. We close the skin with buried absorbable monofilament sutures, or just use interrupted, 4-0 plain gut as a skin suture. A sterile dressing is applied. We provide the patient with a canvas cock-up splint purely for comfort, for use as desired. The wrist may be splinted initially, according to the preference of the surgeon, but wrist extension is not required due to the advantageous postrelease tendon biomechanics with endoscopic CTR, which leaves intact extra-ligamentous palmar tissues that significantly diminish flexor bowstringing [14].

We generally schedule patients for a postoperative visit in hand therapy 5–8 days after surgery to make sure that all dressings are removed, a band-aid applied to the incision, and motion started in the hand. Some patients, especially the more elderly and disabled, will benefit from supervised therapy visits over the next few weeks, but most patients merely need reassurance and encouragement; splint use is entirely optional and only for comfort; activities are resumed as soon as the patient wishes once the wound is healed. Patients are seen by the physician at about 2 and 8 weeks post surgery; and then followed as needed depending on the specifics of the case.

Efficacy

The reported peer-reviewed long-term clinical results, for symptom-relief after endoscopic carpal tunnel release, performed by experienced surgeons trained in one or more of these techniques, are little different from those after open carpal tunnel release [1–10, 15]. The principal benefit of endoscopic technique release seems to be the reduction in the morbidity associated with a sizable incision in the palm, and a faster, more comfortable postoperative recovery, as is typical for smaller incisions and scope-based surgical methods in all anatomic locations and with surgical specialties. Reported time off work is generally much less in non-worker's compensation cases, slightly less in the litigating and workers' compensation patients; but, in certain reports the times have not differed when endoscopic and open releases were compared [16, 17].

Postoperative tenderness in the proximal palm, also known as "pillar pain," is a recognized, frequent, and annoying but self-limited consequence of carpal tunnel release surgery, but one that can cause considerable delay in the postoperative recovery, return to work, and other normal activities of daily living. The exact origin of pillar pain is not understood, and there is no widely accepted system for its grading or measurement [18, 19]. Published studies, and our own 17 years of experience support that there is a marked and more rapid reduction in pillar pain and palm soreness after endoscopic carpal tunnel release as compared to open release [2, 6, 9, 10, 15, 17], but agreement on this issue is not universal [20, 21]. Further to the point, the value in patients with systemic diseases and those requiring rapid recovery of hand use for weight-bearing has also been documented [18, 19].

Complications

The reported complications of both open and endoscopic release range from failure to fully decompress the median nerve, to partial and complete transections of the median, ulnar, radial, palmar cutaneous, and any/all palmar digital and motor nerves and their various branches in the forearm and hand [4, 21–24]. It is always advisable for the surgeon to tell patients that they reserve the option of converting the endoscopic release to an open release if all of the conditions for a safe and effective, complete endoscopic-method release are not fulfilled intraoperatively. We never cut when we can not see everything that must be seen, at all times. The surgeon must be able to see what s/he is doing (and not doing, or shouldn't be) – whether using an endoscope, a microscope, loupes, or just his/her eyes.

Authors' Recommendations

On balance, we find that, for the vast majority of our patients, endoscopic method carpal tunnel release affords a significantly more comfortable and shorter short-term course and an equally effective long-term recovery and improvement when CTR surgery is required. The single-portal endoscopic methodology in this location is not overly challenging compared to arthroscopic surgeries in the upper and lower limbs, and we find that – for ourselves as well as residents and fellows whom we train – the intellectual and technical skills for safe eCTR are not difficult to acquire. Speaking personally, we believe that the "learning curve" is best surmounted by starting with training, practice on cadaver surgeries if possible, and/or direct operative experience with someone seasoned in the particular, specific methodology and equipment to be employed; but this kind of an approach to a new operative technique or method is neither unique nor even new advice. As with all technologically-dependent surgeries (i.e., endoscope, microscope, laser, etc.), attention to equipment details and their function is of import almost equal to meticulous anatomic technique. In any event, the caveats against attempting surgical release in a fluid-filled, fogged, or otherwise obscured field are, in truth, no different than for any or all such procedures. After all, did we not all swear, *primum non nocere*?

We continue to use, teach, and advocate single-portal endoscopic method carpal tunnel release because, while it is equally effective in decreasing pressure within and increasing volume of the canal as compared to open and other limited incision methods, it is just more comfortable for our patients, affording the same symptom relief and a return to required and daily activities in a much shorter timeframe without adding complications or dangers. In addition, the experimentally-proven endoscopic method's biomechanical advantage of significantly lessening palmar migration of the median nerve and flexor tendons [11] is useful to remember for those who work with their hands (especially for tasks in palmar flexion, where a tendon pulley mechanism is important to retain). At the end of the day, no amount of fancy technology and surgical enhancements will ever eliminate the need for care, skill, and prudent judgment.

References

1. Okutsu I, Ninomiya S, Takatori et al. (1989) Endoscopic management of carpal tunnel syndrome. Arthroscopy 5: 11–18
2. Agee JM, McCarroll HR, Tortosa RD et al. (1992) Endoscopic release of the carpal tunnel: a randomized prospective multicenter study. J Hand Surg 17A: 987–995
3. Agee JM, McCarroll HR, North ER (1994) Endoscopic carpal tunnel release using the single proximal incision technique. Hand Clinics 10:647–659
4. Agee JM, Peimer CA, Pyrek JD, Walsh WE (1995) Endoscopic carpal tunnel release: a prospective study of complications and surgical experience. J Hand Surg 20A:165–171
5. Chow JCY (1989) Endoscopic release of the carpal ligament: a new technique for carpal tunnel syndrome. Arthroscopy 5:19–24
6. Chow JCY (1990) Endoscopic release of the carpal ligament for carpal tunnel syndrome: 22 month clinical result. Arthroscopy 6:288–296
7. Chow JCY (1994) Endoscopic carpal tunnel release. Hand Clinics 10:637–646
8. Berger RA (1994) Endoscopic carpal tunnel release. A curent perspective. Hand Clinics 10:625–636
9. Hasegawa K, Hashizume H, Seneda M et al. (1999) Evaluation of release surgery for idiopathic carpal tunnel syndrome: Endoscopic versus open method. Acta Med Okayama 53(J):179–83
10. Trumble TE, Diao ED, Abrams RA, Gilbert-Anderson MM (2002) Single-portal endoscopic carpal tunnel release compared with open release: a prospective, randomized trial. J Bone Joint Surg 84A: 1107–15
11. Varitimidis SE, Herndon JH, Sotereanos DG (1999) Failed endoscopic carpal tunnel release. Operative findings and results of open revision surgery. J Hand Surg 24(BE): 465–67
12. Peimer CA, Farber JM. Recurrent carpal tunnel syndrome: who needs repeat surgery? J Hand Surg (submitted)
13. Rotman MB, Manske PR (1993) Anatomic relationships of an endoscopic carpal tunnel device to surrounding structures. J Hand Surg 18A:442–450
14. Brown RK, Peimer CA (2000) Digital flexor tendon mechanics after endoscopic and open carpal tunnel releases. J Hand Surgery 25A:112–119
15. Povlsen B, Tegnell I, Revell M et al. (1997) Touch allodynia following endoscopic (single portal) or open decompression for carpal tunnel syndrome. J Hand Surg 22(BE): 325–327
16. Jacobsen MB, Rahme H (1996) A prospective, randomized study with an independent observer comparing open carpal tunnel release with endoscopic carpal tunnel release. J Hand Surg 21(BE):202–204
17. Ferdinand RD, MacLean JG (2002) Endoscopic versus open carpal tunnel release in bilateral carpal tunnel syndrome. A prospective, randomized, blinded assessment. J Bone Joint Surg 84(B): 375–79
18. Belcher HJ, Varma S, Schonauer F (2000) Endoscopic carpal tunnel release in selected rheumatoid patients. J Hand Surg 25(BE):451–52
19. Ludlow KS, Merla JL, Cox JA et al. (1997) Pillar pain as a

complication of carpal tunnel release: a review of the literature. J Hand Ther 10:277–282
20. Szabo RM (1999) Nerve Compression Syndromes, in Light TR (ed): Hand Surgery Update 2. Rosemont, IL, American Academy of Orthopaedic Surgeons p.189
21. Lee DH, Masear VR, Meyer RD et al. (1992) Endoscopic carpal tunnel release: a cadaveric study. J Hand Surg 17A:1003–1008
22. Hulsizer DL, Staebler MPS, Weisss APC, Akelman E (1998) The results of revision carpal tunnel release following previous open versus endoscopic surgery. J Hand Surg 23A: 865–869
23. Palmar AK, Toivonen DA (1999) Complications of endoscopic and open carpal tunnel release. J Hand Surg 24(A): 561–65
24. Boeckstyns ME, Sorensen AI (1999) Does endoscopic carpal tunnel release have a higher rate of complications than open carpal tunnel release? An analysis of published series. J Hand Surg 24(BE):9–15

Endoscopic Carpal Tunnel Release: Menon's Technique

P.G. Castelli, A. Dell'Uomo, C. Ferrari

Endoscopic carpal tunnel release described by Jay Menon [14, 15, 22] (Loma Linda University, California USA) is an original one-portal release technique of the carpal tunnel ligament (CTL) developed after the first one-portal release techniques introduced by Okutsu and Agee [2–4, 8].

The technique is characterized by:

1. Oblique incision line
2. Progressive carpal tunnel dilatation
3. Use of an original cannula
4. Continuous visualization of distal edge of LTC during the time of release
5. Proximo-distal section of LTC

The technique is indicated in most cases of CTS. Severe CTS isn't a contraindication, and internal neurolysis does not seem to be more effective than endoscopic release in cases of thenar hypotrophy or severe weakness [19].

Indications are idiopathic and overstress syndromes, CTS in diabetes and other peripheral neuropathies, and in hemodialyzed patients (without severe flexors tenosynovitis).

ContraindicationContraindications are:

1. Recurrence of CTS and CTS after surgical treatment of the volar side of the wrist, for risk of iatrogenic injuries for synechias of previous scar
2. When CTS treatment requires an associated flexors synovectomy (rheumatoid arthritis, gout, amyloidosis)
3. CTS after wrist fractures
4. Isolated compression of motor branch of median nerve
5. Thenar hypotrophy when Camitz or Thompson's procedures are indicated
6. Acute or tubercular tenosynovitis
7. Acute compression of median nerve
8. Insufficient intraoperative visualization of ligament or intraoperative finding of anatomical anomalies that need to be converted at an open treatment [11, 20]

Relative contraindications are children with possible congenital anomalies [7]

Preoperative electromyography and standard and axial x-rays are performed in all cases. Sometimes an ultrasound scanning of the median nerve under the ligament [6, 9, 16, 17] (high frequency from 7.5 to 12 MHz – longitudinal and transverse dynamic scanning) and only occasionally a wrist MRI are performed.

Instrumentation

The surgical disposable kit (Concept Carpal Tunnel Relief Kit, Linvatec) consist of five instruments:

1. Two blunt rods (5.5–7 mm diameter) to enlarge the CT
2. A closed and blunt-end, grooved cannula with D-shaped cross section (7 mm diameter), with trocar (4 mm diameter)
3. Scalpel Smillie-like with curved blade and blunt corners (Figs. 26.1, 26.2)

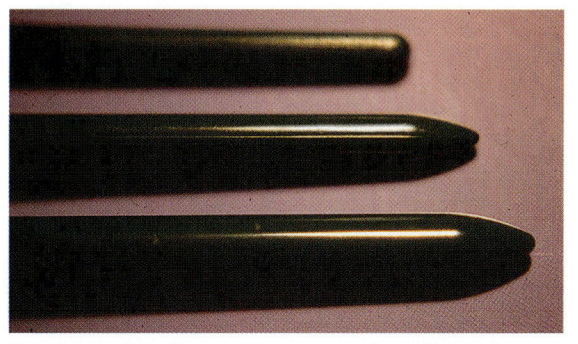

Fig. 26.1. Rods and trocar (4–5, 5–7 mm) to enlarge CT

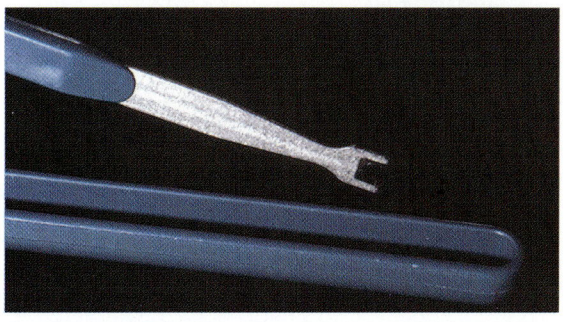

Fig. 26.2. Original D-shaped grooved cannula (cross section 7 mm) and scalpel

Common arthroscopic instrumentation is required:

1. A 4-mm rod-lens telescope (30° oblique lens)
2. Video-camera, couplers, and monitor
3. A little probe

Surgical Anatomy

Treatment is usually performed under local anesthesia (3 cc of 1% Xylocaine without Epinephrine is used at entry portal and 3–4 cm distally along the volar side of carpal tunnel), sometimes under brachial plexus block or retrograde venous anesthesia. Tourniquet is employed for 4–6 min.

In all cases the surgeon should first draw all anatomical landmarks on the volar skin to identify the distal margin of CLT and the operative area of cutting cannula:

1. The pisiform (P).
2. Kaplan's line (from first interdigital space in abduction of the thumb to ulnar side of the hand, side by side with proximal palmar plica). The line runs 5–8 mm distally to the pisiform [24].
3. A second line is drawn proximally from the ulnar side of the ring finger to the wrist: the intersection with the Kaplan's line (U) identifies the apophysis of hamatus, ulnar distal insertion of CLT (Fig. 26.3).
4. Intersection between thenar plica and Kaplan's line mark the area where the motor branch of median nerve bends proximally as recurrent branch (m).
5. A last line runs proximally from the radial side of the ring finger to the palmaris longus.

The two lines that run side by side all along the proximal projection of the ring finger mark a real binary as a safety operative area to avoid iatrogenic injuries (Fig. 26.4).

Wrist is extended 30°–40° to retract flexor tendons dorsally within the carpal canal.

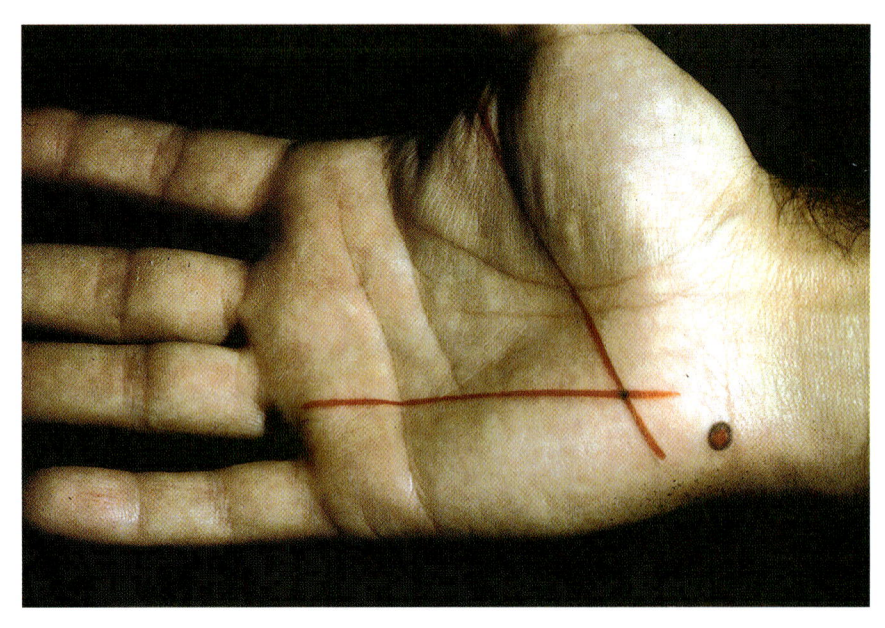

Fig. 26.3. Landmarks of the distal edge of the CTL (pisiform, Kaplan's line, line drawn proximally from the ulnar side of the ring finger to the wrist)

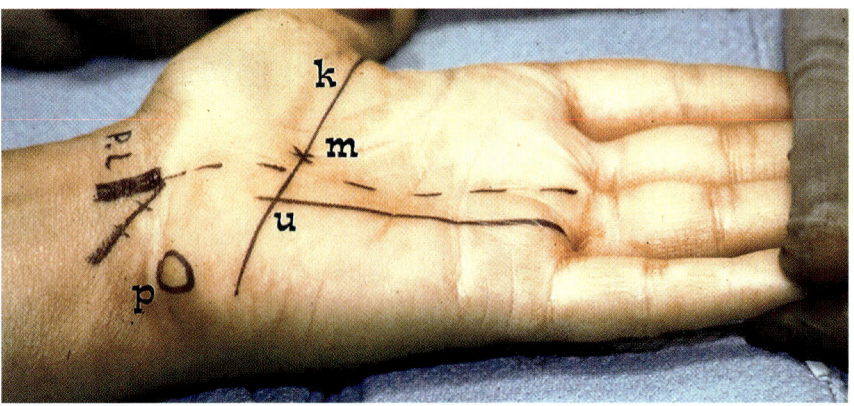

Fig. 26.4. Landmarks request for release (line drawn proximally from the radial side of the ring finger to the wrist and safety area)

Surgical Technique

A 1-cm oblique incision is performed at the ulnar side of the palmaris longus, proximally to the distal wrist plica, or, in the absence of the palmaris longus, at the ulnar side of the line that runs along the radial side of the ring finger. The oblique incision is easily extended distally on the volar side to convert at an open release if per operative visualization of LCT is insufficient.

Transverse fibers of antebrachial fascia, distally jointed to the CTL, are sectioned along their direction. A constant, little venous branch is cauterized.

Fascial fibers are raised and a 4 mm trocar and 5.5 and 7 mm rods are gently introduced to progressively enlarge the carpal tunnel.

Rods are gently rotated during insertion to detach the synovia from the dorsal surface of the CTL, then the grooved cannula with trocar is inserted into the tunnel, the groove at the volar side.

The anatomic area distally to the edge of the CTL presents narrow margins [10, 12] (sensitive branch of ulnar nerve and its anastomotic branch with median nerve, which runs side to side with superficial palmar arch, and third interdigital nerve) (Fig. 26.5).

The shape of the carpal tunnel shifts radially the tip of the cannula, during introduction (Fig. 26.6). Then

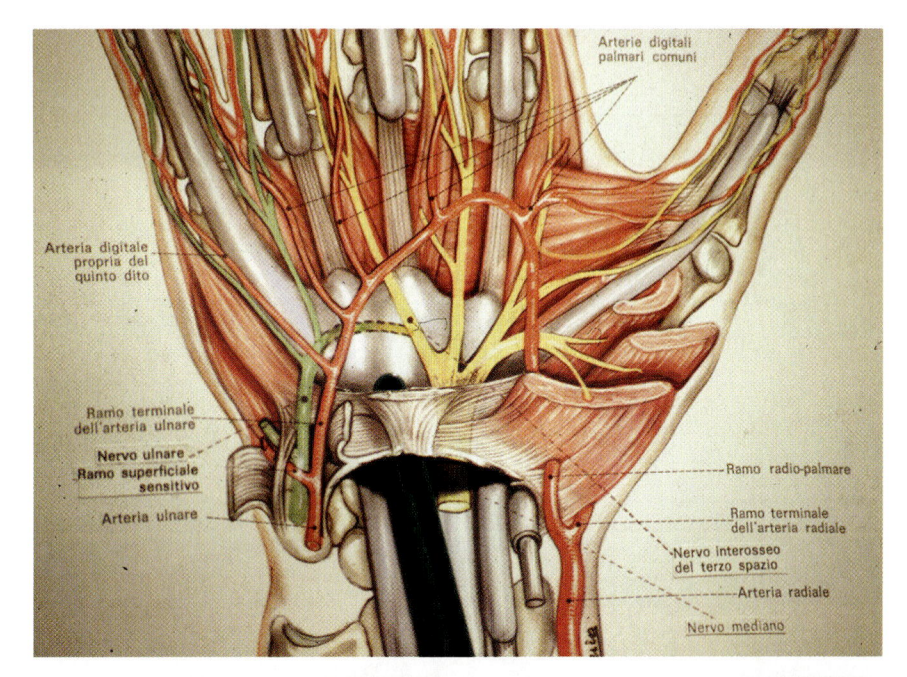

Fig. 26.5. Anatomic area where the tip of the cannula protrudes

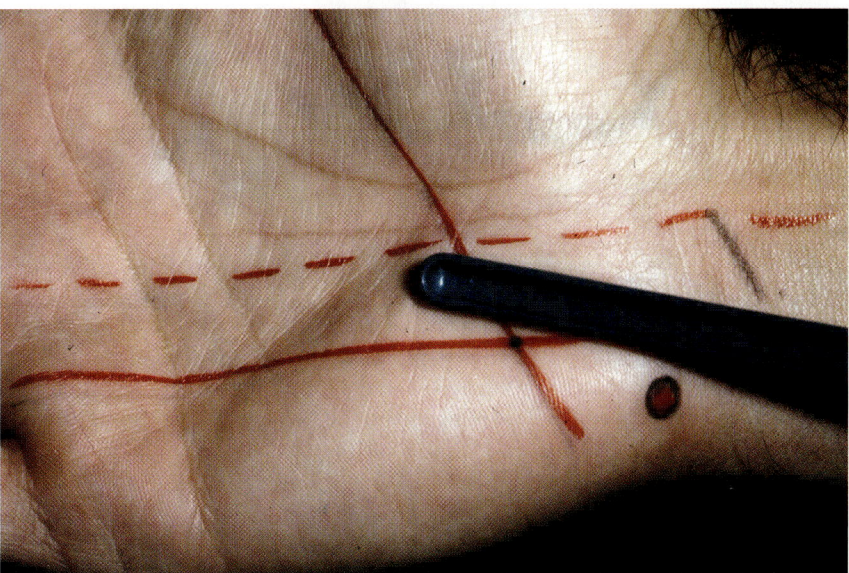

Fig. 26.6. Natural position of the cannula into the CT

180 III Treatment

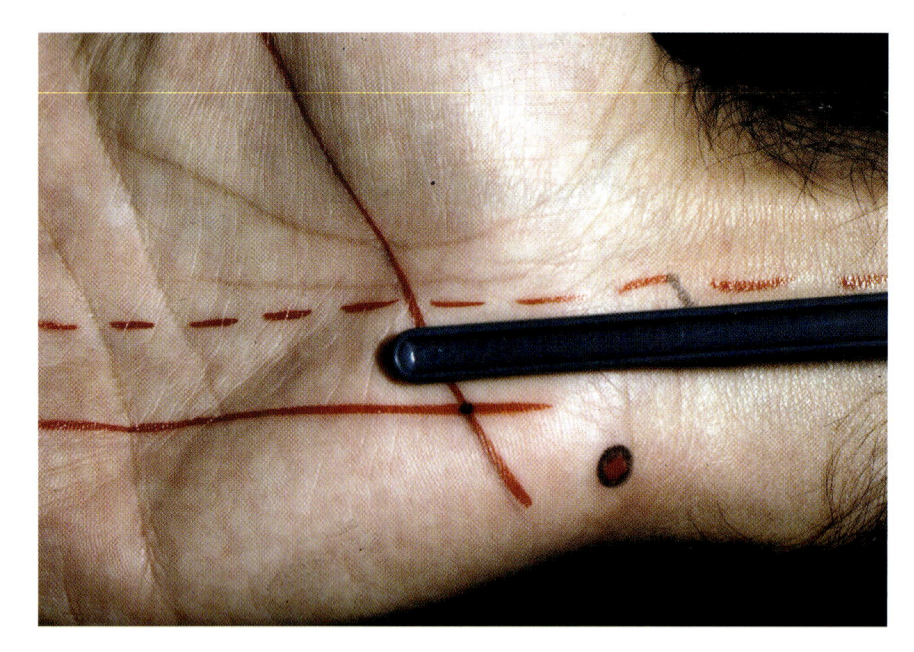

Fig. 26.7. After insertion into the CT, the cannula is positioned in the safety area and protrudes beyond the distal edge of the CTL only 3–4 mm

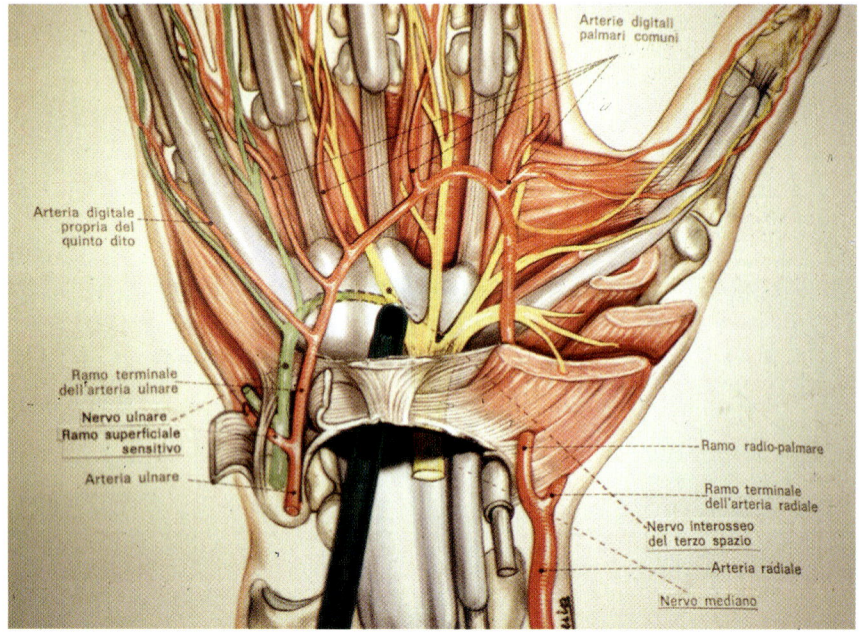

Fig. 26.8. Release performed with the cannula out of the safety area or with its tip beyond the distal edge of the CTL is dangerous

the cannula is inserted and the surgeon pushes radially the proximal end of the cannula, so the distal tip shifts at the ulnar side, in the safety binary on the fourth ray, in contact with the apophysis of the hamatus (Fig. 26.7). An insufficient ulnar shift of the cannula may cause injuries to the third interdigital nerve (Fig. 26.8).

It's very important to avoid pushing hard on the rods or cannula distally across the edge of ligament: the tip of the cannula is easily palpated under the ligament and it passes only 4–5 mm from the Kaplan's line along the safety binary (Fig. 26.5).

The D-shaped cross section and the volar groove stabilize the cannula into the tunnel, adherent to the ligament, thereby avoiding preoperative rotations and penetration of synovia in the cannula's groove.

Then, the trocar is removed and a 4-mm rod-lens telescope at a 30° angle is introduced in the cannula with the 30° lens obliquely turned in the volar side to visualize the transverse fibers of the CTL. The distal edge of the ligament is easily examined for the presence of palmar fatty tissue, a good landmark of the end of the CTL (Fig. 26.9).

A percutaneous 25-G needle is inserted under endoscopic control on the distal edge of the ligament (Fig. 26.10): it's the real landmark during the release.

Sometimes fatty tissue fills the distal part of the CT

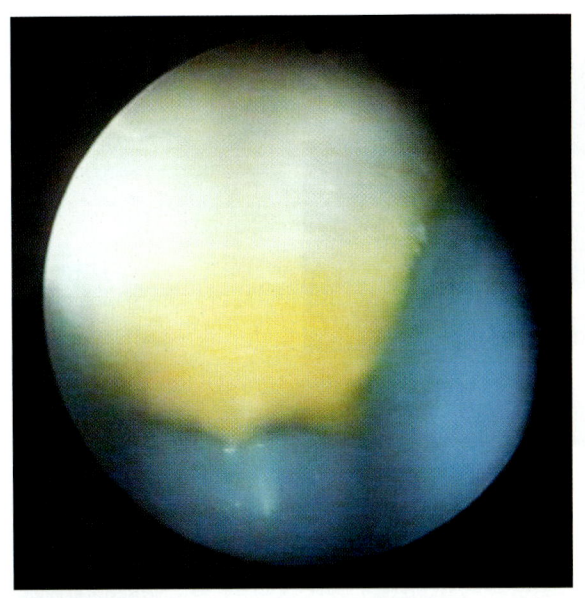

Fig. 26.9. Fatty tissue at the distal edge of the CTL

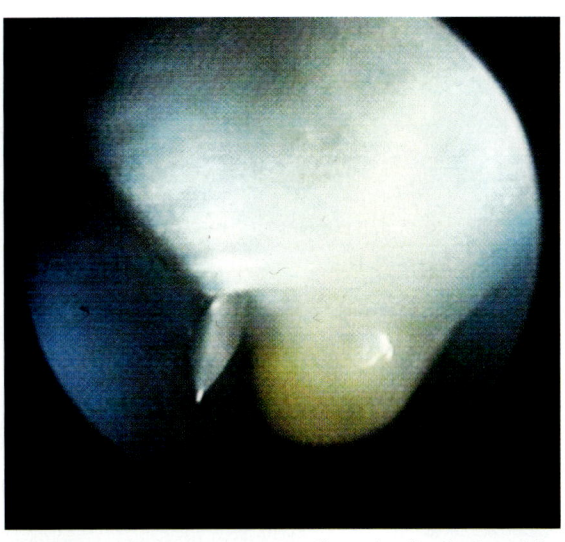

Fig. 26.10. Percutaneous 25-G needle at the distal edge of the CTL

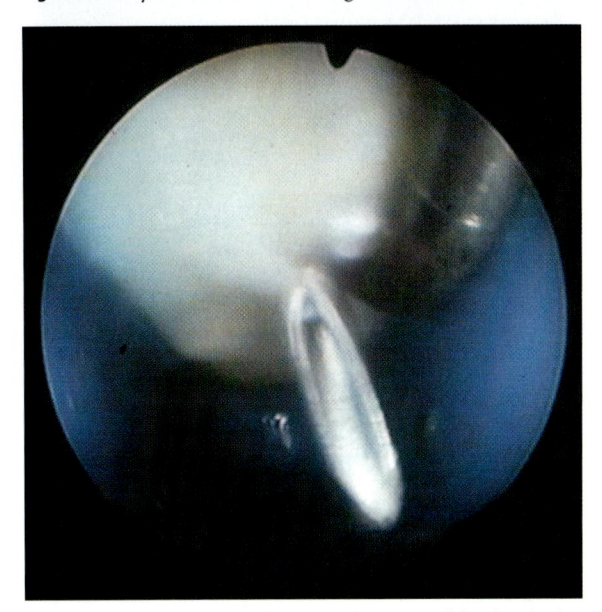

Fig. 26.11. A probe check of the exact location of the distal edge of the CTL

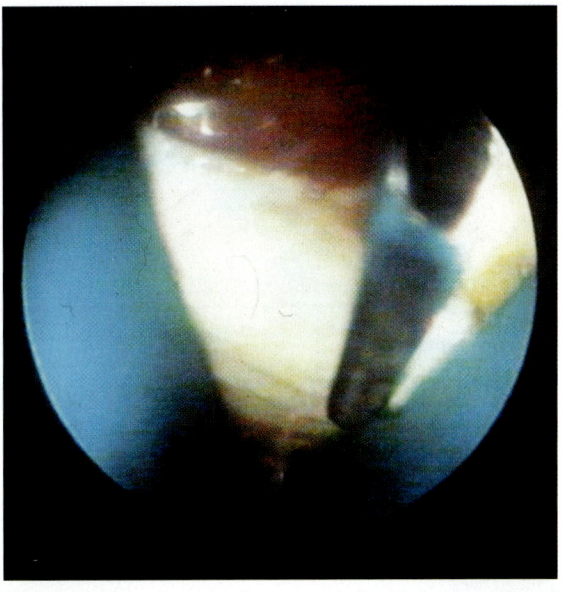

Fig. 26.12. Then the scope is retracted, the blade is positioned on the proximal edge of the CTL for proximo-distal release

causing insufficient visualization of the ligament: a little probe can gently push away the tissue to visualize with certainty the distal edge of the CTL (Fig. 26.11). The arthroscope's light across the skin is unreliable to identify the distal end of release.

The arthroscope is then retracted to visualize the proximal edge of the ligament: the curved blade of the scalpel is positioned on the proximal fibers (Figs. 26.12, 26.13) and gently pushed distally to section the ligament under endoscopic control (Fig. 26.14) until the fibers of the distal edge are cut, at the level of the percutaneous needle.

The closed blunt tip of the cannula stops the blade (Fig. 26.15), with a really certain and complete release (Fig. 26.16).

Only transverse fibers are sectioned. All the fibers of palmaris fascia and palmaris brevis are preserved (Fig. 26.17) to avoid insertion of thenar and hypothenar muscles (easy recovery) and scar formation in subcutaneous (cause of pillar pain).

When the visualization of the CTL is incomplete or insufficient, the treatment is converted in an open release.

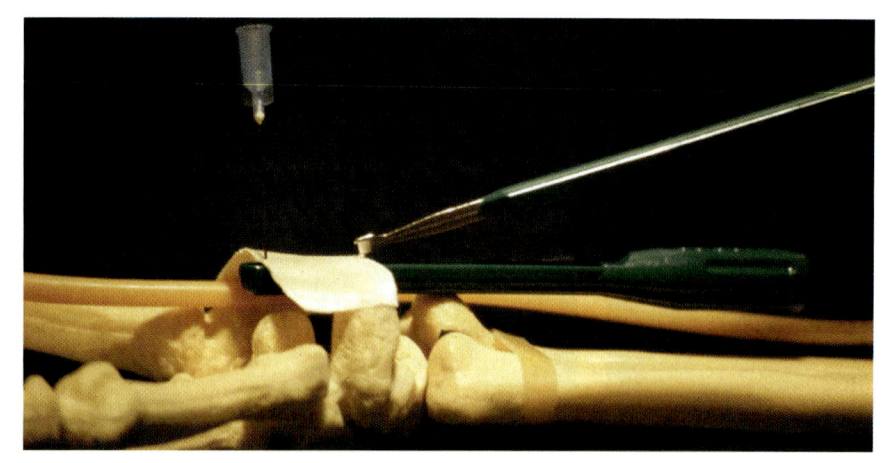

Fig. 26.13. Surgical instrumentations kit

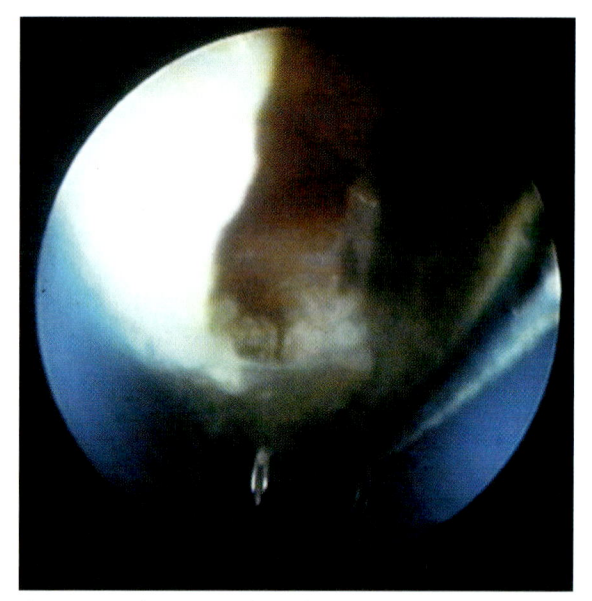

Fig. 26.14. Release is performed: percutaneous needle at the distal edge of the CTL during the treatment

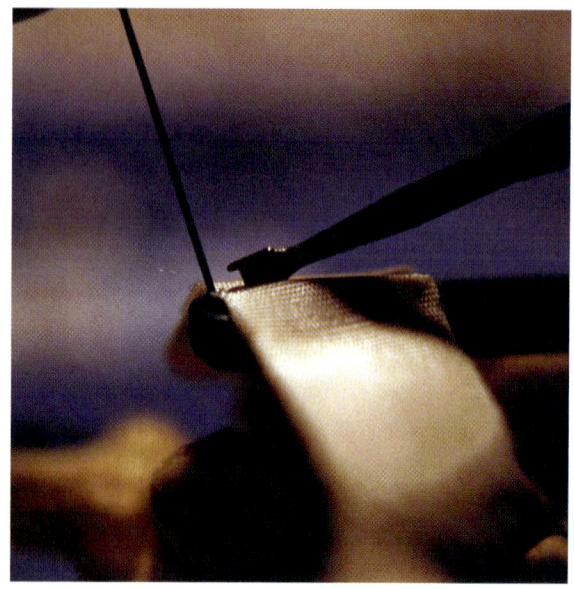

Fig. 26.15. Position of instruments at the distal edge of the CTL

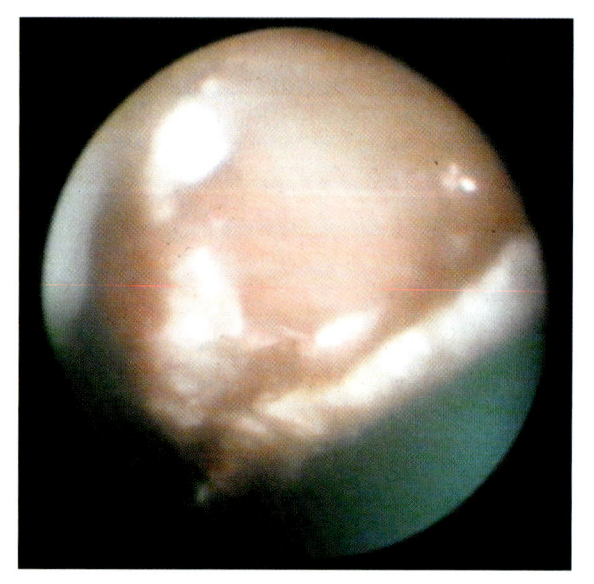

A little probe checks the quality of release and the needle is removed. The cannula is gently rotated to visualize the sectioned edges of the ligament (Fig. 26.18). Then the cannula and the tourniquet are removed and a compressive hemostasis is performed for 1–2 min.

The incision is closed (Nylon 5.0) and a compressive bandage is applied.

◁
Fig. 26.16. Complete release

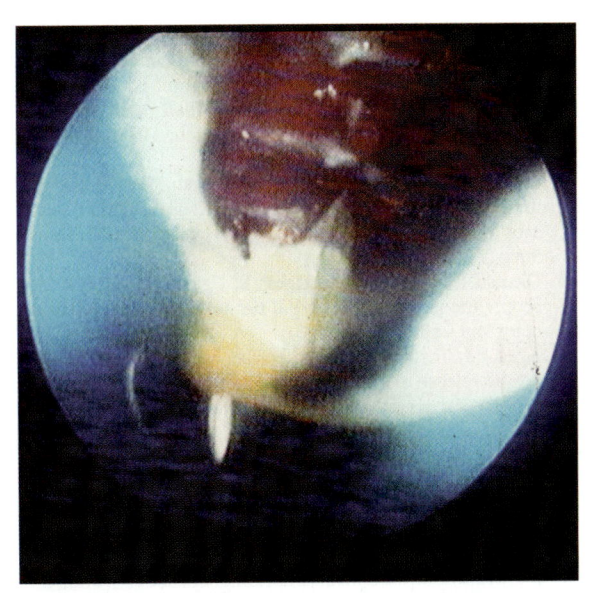

Fig. 26.17. During release fibers of palmaris brevis are preserved

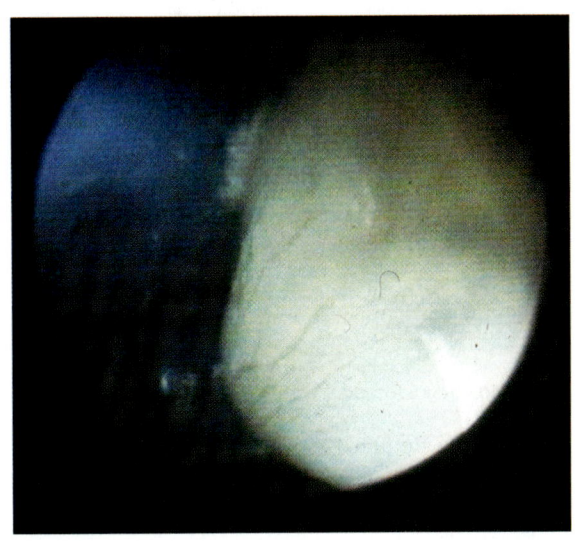

Fig. 26.18. Needle is removed. The cannula is gently rotated to check the edges of the section. The median nerve is visible

Postoperative Treatment

The compressive bandage is removed after 4–5 days. Chow [24] recommends, after an endoscopic release, a dorsal splint with gently dorsal flexion of the wrist for 1 week.

Flexion and extension of the fingers are recommended immediately.

Resumption of work is possible after 2–3 weeks.

Results

Five hundred fifty-one cases of CTS in 398 patients were treated by Menon's endoscopic release from 1992 to 1998. In 538 cases in 385 patients aged 23–84 (median age 48 years old) release was performed. One hundred forty-three patients were heavy workers; preoperative pain and/or paresthesias were present in all cases from 6 to 48 months.

Twelve cases were excluded from valuation because the endoscopic release was converted in open release during the treatment: in 9 cases for insufficient visualization of the CTL, and in 3 cases for anatomic anomalies (presence of flexor muscle in the CT). One patient with an uncertain nervous injury was excluded for low compliance and psychic disorder.

Postoperative pain was not important in all cases.

Patients were valuated at 1, 2, 3, 6, 9, 12 and 24 weeks from the treatment.

Pain and/or paresthesias decreased or disappeared after 3 weeks in 80% of cases. Restoration of strength was complete after 3 weeks in 70% of cases and after 6 weeks in 90% of cases.

Resumption of regular activity was possible after 4 weeks in 80% of patients, resumption of heavy work in 80% of patients from 4 to 6 weeks.

The results of the treatment were excellent (complete recovery) or good (absence of pain and/or paresthesias, very small weakness and/or alteration of two-point Dellon's test) at follow-up in 90% of cases. Ninety percent of patients were satisfied with treatment.

Complications

In 24 cases paresthesias were increased postoperatively in middle and ringer fingers: in 20 cases symptoms disappeared after 10–15 days, in 4 patients after 2–4 months. Probably a third interdigital nerve apraxia was caused by a compressive effect of the cannula All these cases were treated in the first 2 years [21, 23]. No severe nervous branch injuries occurred in any patients.

A hematoma occurred only in 1 case, 2 days after release.

In 6 cases (4 diabetics) the results of release were considered insufficient due to persistence of symptoms and an open release was performed 4–7 months after the endoscopic treatment: in 3 cases the endoscopic section of the ligament was complete and in 3 cases incomplete. After open treatment the 3 cases of insufficient release and 1 case of complete release had a complete recovery.

To consider a release effective only because the there is a complete section of the ligament is questionable: in a cadaver study Lee [10] demonstrated after endoscopic release in 60% of cases a section of only two thirds of the TL.

In 5 cases a postoperative severe hypothenar pillar pain occurred and disappeared only after 2–3 months.

No infections or bow-stringing flexors effect were present in the study.

Discussion

Among the endoscopic release techniques, the Menon's one-portal technique is preferable because:

1. The oblique incision is easily extendable in the palmar side if an open release is required.
2. Progressive dilatation and cleaning of the CT with atraumatic introduction of the cannula is possible.
3. The proximo-distal sectioning by a curved blade avoids possible traction injuries caused by a hook blade in case of an insufficient visualization of the distal edge of the TL during a retrograde release.
4. Correct positioning of the cannula and percutaneous needle avoids injuries to the anastomotic ulnar branch (present in 80% of cases) [1, 18], which is a risk in two-portal techniques [13, 19].
5. The distal edge of the TL is visualized during the entire release by the percutaneous needle.
6. The D-shaped cross section cannula is in tight contact with the ligament, without penetration of synovia in the cannula's groove.
7. After release, the section of the CT is greatly increased. In 18 cases, an MR study was performed preoperatively and 8 weeks and 8–10 months after treatment [25]: in all cases no significant variations of carpal bony arch were detected, but the antero-posterior cross section increased, changing from an oval to a round section, for volar translation of a flexors neo-retinaculum. In these cases, an early postoperative MR showed, after endoscopic release, a lesser volar shift of the median nerve than after open release.
8. Postoperative lack of pain is related to preservation of rich skin innervation and poor innervation of the CTL [5].

Problems with techniques are related to incorrect positioning of the cannula in the safety area due to:

1. Incorrect positioning of landmarks
2. Protrusion of the distal tip of the cannula beyond the distal edge of the CTL
3. Radial bending of the distal tip of the cannula
4. Deep sectioning of fascial or subcutaneous tissue

In our experience more frequent complications seem related to an incorrect positioning of the cannula into the carpal tunnel (distal protrusion or lateral bending). The risk of iatrogenic injuries decrease with surgical experience [13].

References

1. Meals RA, Shaner M (1983) Variations in the digital sensory patterns. A study of the ulnar nerve-median nerve, palmar, communicating branch. J Hand Surg 8: 411–414
2. Okutsu I, Ninomya S, Hanamaka T et al. (1989) Measurement of pressure in the carpal canal before and after endoscopic menagement of carpal tunnel syndrome. J Bone J Surg (A) 71:679–683
3. Okutsu I, Ninomya S, Takatori L, Ugawa Y (1989) Endoscopic menagement of carpal tunnel syndrome. Arthroscopy 5:11–18, 1989
4. Agee JM, Tortosa RD, Palmer CA, Berry C (1990) Endoscopic release of carpal tunnel: a prospective randomized multicenter study. 45th Annual Meeting of ASSH, Toronto, Canada
5. Chow J (1990) Endoscopic release of carpal ligament for carpal tunnel syndrome: 22-month clinical result. Arthroscopy 6: 288–296
6. Milbrandt H, Calleja E, Quayuli SA (1990) Sonography of the wrist and hand. Radiology 30: 360–365
7. North ER: Endoscopic carpal tunnel release (1991) in Gilbermann RH (ed): Operative nerve repair and reconstruction. J.B. Lippincott – Raven, 913–920, Philadelphia
8. Agee JM, Mc Carrol HR, Berry C et al. (1992) Endoscopic release of carpal tunnel: a randomized prospective multicenter study. J Hand Surg 17A 987–995
9. Buchberger W, Judmaier W, Birbamber E (1992) Carpal tunnel syndrome: diagnosis with high-resolution sonography. Am J Roentegenlogy 159: 793–798
10. Lee DH, Masear VR, Meyer RD et al. (1992) Endoscopic carpal tunnel release: a cadaveric study. J Hand Surg 17A,1003–1008
11. Scoggin JF, Whipple TL (1992) A potential complication of endoscopic carpal tunnel release. Arthroscopy 8: 363–365
12. Levy HJ, Seifer TB, Kleibart FA (1993) Endoscopic carpal tunnel release: an anatomic study. Arthroscopy 9: 1–4
13. Luchetti R, Pederzini L, Soragni O et al. (1993) La sindrome del tunnel carpale. Decompressione endoscopica secondo Chow e secondo Agee. Riv Chir Riab Mano Arto Sup 30 (2): 163–175
14. Menon J (1993) Endoscopic carpal tunnel release. A single portal thecnique. Contemp Orthop 2:109–116
15. Menon J (1993) Endoscopic carpal tunnel release. Current status. J Hand Therapy 6: 139–144
16. Nakamichi K, Tachibana S (1993) Ultrasonography in the diagnosis carpal tunnel syndrome caused by an occult ganglion. J Hand Surg 18: 174–175
17. Nakamichi K, Tachibana S (1993) The use of ultrasonography in detection of synovitis in carpal tunnel syndrome. J Hand Surg 18: 176–179
18. Schwartz JT, Waters PM, Simmons BP (1993) Endoscopic carpal tunnel release: a cadaveric study. Arthroscopy 9: 209–213
19. Thomas C, Merle M, Gilbert A (1993) Endoscopic surgical treatment of carpal tunnel syndrome in Tubiana R (ed) The Hand, vol. 4, WB Saunders Co., Philadelphia
20. Wolf AW, Packard S, Chow J (1993) Transligamentous motor branch of the median nerve discovered during endoscopically assisted carpal tunnel release. Arthroscopy 9:222–223
21. Castelli PG, Ferrari C (1994) Sindrome del tunnel carpale. Confronto tra trattamento a cielo aperto e decompressione endoscopica Riv Chir Riab Mano Arto Sup 31 (2), 157–161
22. Menon J (1994) Endoscopic carpal tunnel release: preliminary report. Arthroscopy 10:31–38

23. Castelli PG, Ferrari C (1997) Evaluation of one portal endoscopic release in treatment of CTS. 3rd Congress of E.F.O.R.T. Barcelona
24. Chow J: Carpal tunnel release (1997) in J. McGinty (ed): Operative Arthroscopy. (2nd Edition), JB Lippincott – Raven
25- Dell'Uomo A, Mastantuono M (1997) Endoscopic carpal tunnel release by Menon single portal technique: clinical and MRI evaluation after 120 cases. J Hand Surg (B) vol 22B:42

27 The Distal Single Incision Scope-Assisted Carpal Tunnel Release – Thirteen-Year Follow-Up Results

M. A. Mirza, M.K. Reinhart

Introduction

Carpal tunnel syndrome (CTS) was first recognized by Sir James Paget in 1854 and continues to attract considerable attention in contemporary orthopedics [18]. Learmonth first described surgical decompression of peripheral nerves in the 1930s while Phalen's contributions to the clinical evaluation of CTS began in the 1950s [9, 20, 21]. Known both as the most researched and most common peripheral nerve entrapment neuropathy, the incidence of CTS continues to increase [6]. According to data reported by the National Institute for Occupational Safety and Health (NIOSH), roughly 60% of all work-related illnesses are "disorders associated with repeated trauma" [16]. In addition, with about 50% of all CTS cases being work related, return to work can reflect significant costs to industries [22]. Postoperative scar/pillar tenderness and/or weakness of pinch and grip strength are often variables that delay the return to work [1].

When conservative management including the use of nonsteroidal anti-inflammatory drugs (NSAIDS), splinting, and/or cortisone injection fail to alleviate CTS, surgical decompression of the median nerve may be indicated. The most widely accepted surgical approach is to make a curved incision in the palm, which is extended into the distal forearm. Such an open technique has resulted in a median return to work of 46.5 days [1]. Endoscopic techniques for carpal tunnel release (CTR) include two-portal procedures, proximal uniportal incision techniques, and the single distal incision technique [1, 2, 4, 12, 14, 15, 17, 19, 23,]. Overall, these techniques have resulted in a faster return to work, less scar tenderness, and an earlier return of grip strength.

The distal, single incision, scope-assisted carpal tunnel release was first described in 1993 [13]. Its technique, evolution, and early postoperative results have been previously reported [13–15].

Study Protocol

Subjective symptoms of pain, tingling, numbness, burning, and swelling were recorded for each patient by using preoperative and postoperative questionnaires. Patients rated their symptoms as: none; mild, not interfering with normal activities or job function; moderate, occasionally curtailing normal activity or job function; or severe, significantly interfering with normal activity or job function. Two-point discrimination and single-trial grip, lateral, and precision pinch strengths were recorded by using the Jamar hand dynamometer and Jamar hydraulic pinch gauge.

Postoperative measurements are scheduled at 10-day, 4-week, 8-week, 6-month, and 1-year intervals. Four-year follow-up data were available in some patients who were also analyzed. The subjective symptoms, grip, and lateral and precision pinch strengths were recorded at the times noted above. Palpated scar, radial pillar, and ulnar pillar tenderness levels were recorded as none, slight, moderate, or severe. The return-to-work date was documented. The insurance type was classified as "Workman's Compensation" or "Other," and the employment type was classified into "white collar" or "other." Housewives were classified as "other" and retired patients were classified as "white collar" with respect to their employment status.

Operative Technique

Surgery is performed on an outpatient basis by using intravenous regional anesthesia (Bier block) and a forearm tourniquet. The hand is first placed on the AM Surgical arm support table. Two lines are then drawn in the palm (Fig. 27.1), one in a transverse orientation along the distal border of the abducted thumb and one in a longitudinal orientation from the third web space; both lines should intersect as illustrated. Two additional longitudinal lines, each about 2.5 cm in length, are then drawn on the distal forearm, one along the flexor carpi ulnaris tendon and the other along the palmaris longus tendon. If the palmaris longus tendon is absent, the midline of the wrist is used. An "X" is drawn mid-

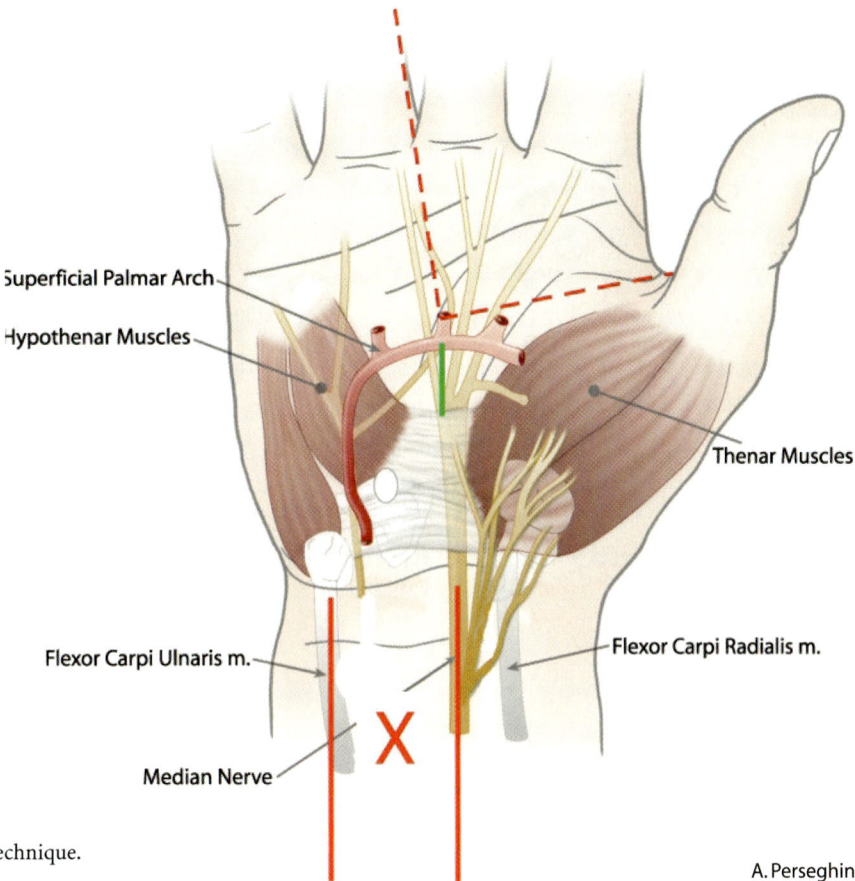

Fig. 27.1. Distal single incision technique. (Courtesy of AM Surgical)

A. Perseghin

way between those two lines. At 0.5 cm proximal to the intersecting palm lines, a 1.5-cm longitudinal incision is made, usually in or along the thenar crease (Fig. 27.1). The incision is subsequently deepened to expose the palmar fascia, which is then divided longitudinally. Once the incision is complete, the very distal edge of the transverse carpal ligament (TCL) as well as the fat pad that is present at the distal edge of the TCL is exposed. The palmar arch should now be identified. At this point in the procedure it is imperative to identify the median nerve branch to the third web space, otherwise, look for the median nerve itself if the nerve has not divided. At this time, a special effort should be made to identify the communicating branch of the ulnar nerve, and any aberrant motor branch variants, if present. Blunt dissection with a curved clamp is then undertaken to create a pathway underneath the TCL, staying ulnar to the median nerve.

By using a specially designed hand table,[1] the hand is then elevated and the wrist is extended to facilitate the dissection of the extrabursal subligamentous path (Fig. 27.2). This is accomplished by introducing a curved dissector into the carpal canal, palmar to the ulnar bursa, while hugging the under surface of the TCL. The dissector is then advanced to the "X" mark at the wrist – one should not feel undue obstruction. The dissector is then removed. The obturator-cannula-dissector assembly is now introduced into the pathway created by the dissector. The assembly is then guided midway between the two longitudinal lines on the forearm so as not to damage the median or ulnar neurovascular structures. At this point, the obturator is removed from the slotted cannula and a 4-mm, 30° standard scope is introduced. This standard arthroscope is now used as an endoscope for this technique. Once in place, the endoscope permits thorough visualization of the transverse fibers of the flexor retinaculum. It is of paramount importance to identify these transversely oriented fibers. If fluid or fat globules obstruct the visualization, withdraw the endoscope and introduce a sterile cotton-tipped applicator to clear the obstruction(s) and enhance visualization. If there is any synovial membrane obstructing the visualization of the transverse fibers, repeat the process by reintroducing the clamp and spreading to allow for the reintroduction of the dissector. Reintroduce the obturator-cannula-dis-

---
[1] Hand Table 9500, A.M. Surgical.

Fig. 27.2. Positioning of the forearm and wrist on the hand table. (Courtesy of AM Surgical)

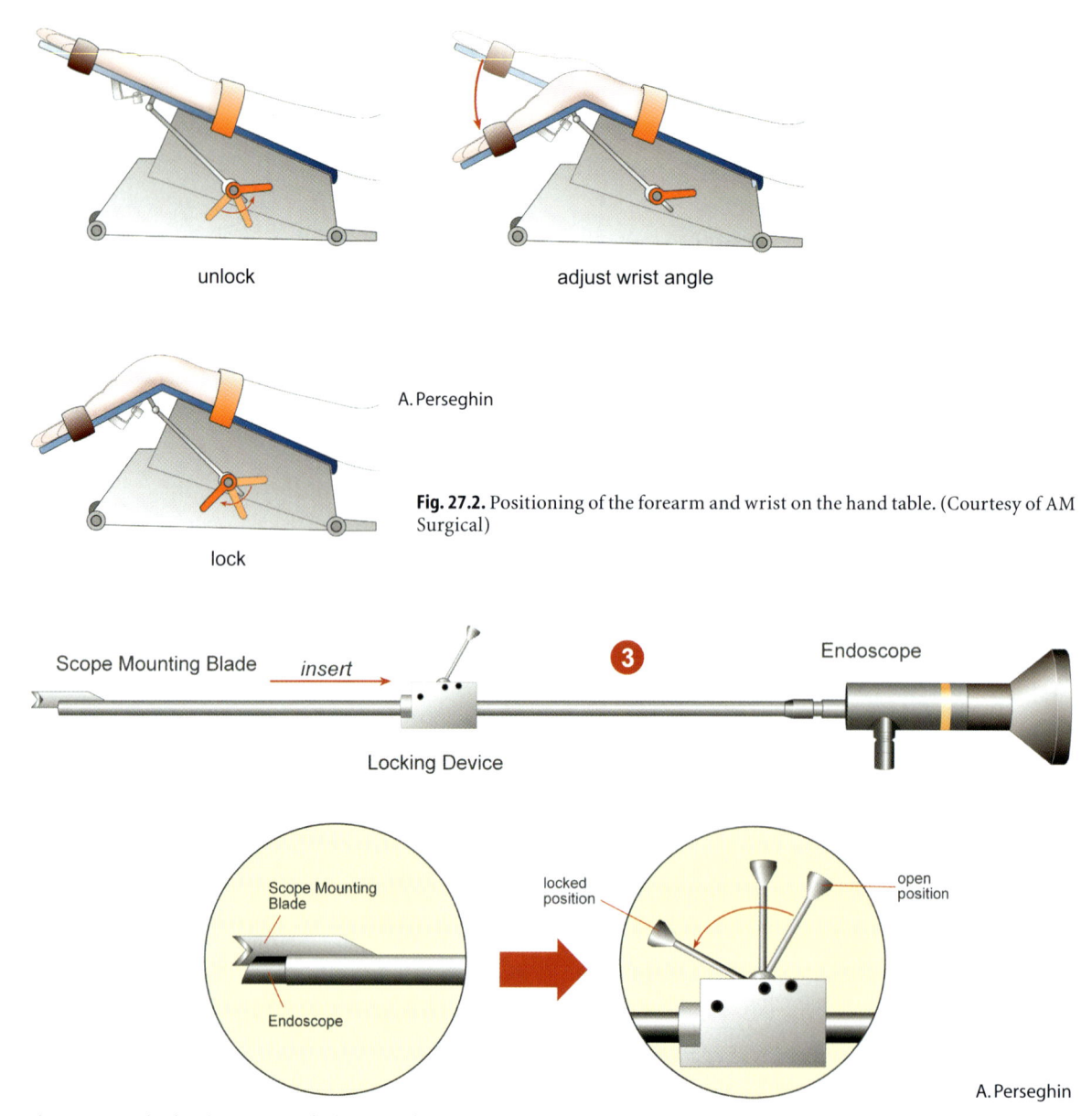

Fig. 27.3. Standard arthroscope with sleeve/knife assembly and locking device. (Courtesy of AM Surgical)

sector assembly, then, remove the obturator and insert the scope. The cannula can be rotated toward the radial side to visualize the median nerve, and then rotated toward the ulnar side to visualize the flexor tendon. This maneuver is very important for beginners because it allows the surgeon to ascertain the position of the median nerve and the flexor tendon. No attempt at endoscopic release should be made unless the transverse fibers of the TCL are clearly seen through the endoscope with no other structures obstructing the view. If this cannot be achieved, convert to an open carpal tunnel release procedure at this time.

Once the transverse fibers are identified, the endoscope is withdrawn from the slotted cannula. The sleeve/knife device is then slid over the endoscope and locked into place by depressing the lever on the locking device (Fig. 27.3). Next, the sleeve-knife-scope assembly is introduced into the cannula, dividing the TCL along a distal-to-proximal direction by means of gently pushing the knife/scope assembly proximally under endoscopic visualization (Fig. 27.4). The design of the instrument allows one to continuously visualize the knife and TCL during the division (Fig. 27.5). When the division of the TCL is complete, the knife can be palpat-

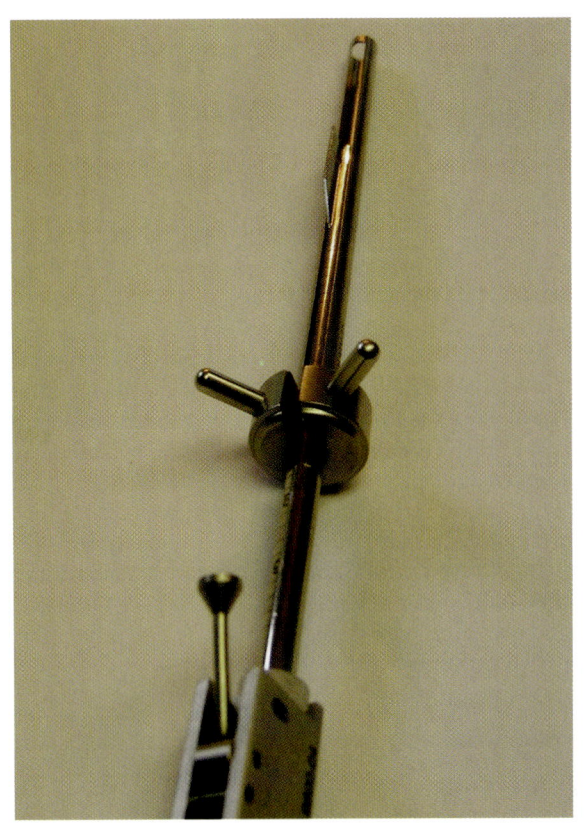

Fig. 27.4. Knife/scope unit dividing the flexor retinaculum (FR) while preserving the interthenar fascia (IF) [15] (reprinted with permission from the Arthroscopy Association of North America)

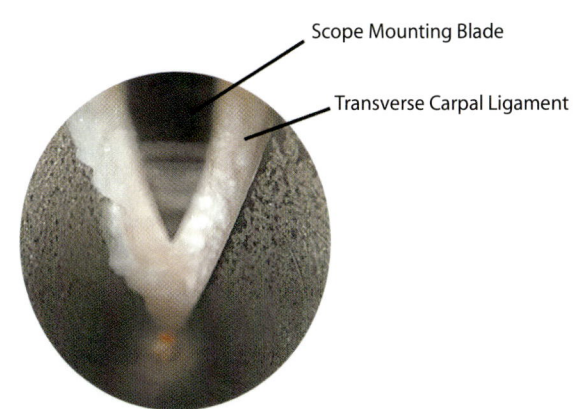

Fig. 27.5. Endoscopic photograph of knife/scope assembly dividing flexor retinaculum. (Courtesy of AM Surgical)

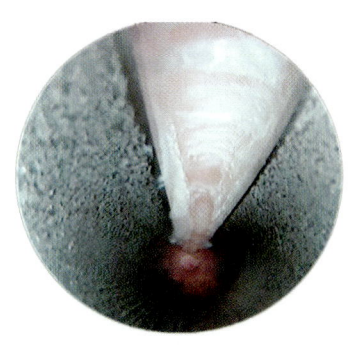

Fig. 27.6. Endoscopic photograph showing division of the TCL with herniation of adipose tissue. (Courtesy of AM Surgical)

ed through the skin with the surgeon's opposite hand, at a point proximal to the wrist flexion crease. This will ascertain the proximal-most portion of the division of the TCL, which should be proximal to the wrist crease. The knife/scope assembly is then removed from the cannula and the knife/sleeve device is detached from the endoscope. The scope is reintroduced into the slotted cannula to ascertain the complete division of the TCL. By rotating the cannula, the cut edges of the TCL, as well as the median nerve and flexor tendons, are visualized. The cut edges of the TCL segment are notably thicker when compared with the cut edges of the thinner antebrachial fascia located in the distal forearm. The transverse fibers of the "interthenar fascia" are preserved in some patients and are seen superficial to the divided TCL. These fibers are less densely arranged than those of the TCL and herniation of palmar adipose tissue is often noted proximal to them (Fig. 27.6).

Upon completion of the surgery, the wound is irrigated and then closed with a running subcuticular closure consisting of 4-0 Prolene sutures. Steristrips are then applied, 5–8 ml of 0.5% bupivacaine is infiltrated subcutaneously, and the hand is wrapped in a soft bulky dressing; the tourniquet is then deflated.

Results

Demographics

One thousand eight hundred seventy-seven cases of CTS were evaluated for this study. Electromyographic and nerve conduction studies were performed to confirm the diagnosis in those patients with questionable clinical findings. Five hundred seventy-three cases were excluded from this study. The majority were excluded because the endoscopic carpal tunnel release was accompanied by other procedures or the patient had a history of wrist instability. Additional patients were excluded because the endoscopic procedure was converted to a modified open carpal tunnel release, or because the patient had a prior carpal tunnel release by a different surgeon, and due to continued symptoms, open carpal tunnel release was indicated. Thus, the following results are reported on 1,304 unaccompanied cases, of whom 877 were female and 427 were male. Among the 1,304 patients for whom data were available, the mean age was 52.4 years (n = 1,279).

Patient-Reported Symptoms

Table 27.1 demonstrates the relative frequency (%) distribution of the patient-reported symptoms of pain, tingling, numbness, burning, and swelling, over time. These symptoms are reported prior to surgery, 10 days postsurgery, 4 weeks postsurgery, 8 weeks postsurgery, 6 months postsurgery, and 1 year postsurgery. In Table 1 we note that the percentage of patients reporting the absence of the symptoms (the category "None") increased steadily after surgery. By 1 year, a minimum of 90% of the patients for whom data are reported exhibited no symptoms. This trend is apparent across all reported symptoms.

Hand Strength

Table 27.2 presents the median percent change in grip strength, lateral pinch strength, and precision pinch strength at the indicated time points postsurgery. The median values are reported because the distribution of the data set is asymmetric.

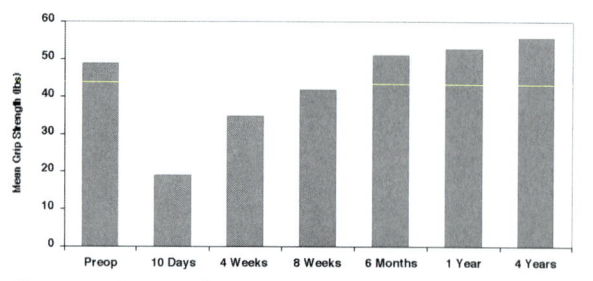

Fig. 27.7. Grip strength

The median grip strength approached a preoperative level after 8 weeks and was greater than the preoperative value by 6 months (Table 27.2). The overall mean grip strength for the reported data is shown in Fig. 27.7. By 8 weeks, median lateral and precision pinch strengths increased 10% and 14%, respectively, over preoperative values (Table 27.2). Figure 27.8 illustrates the overall mean pinch strength findings for the lateral and precision pinch data reported. By 1 year postsurgery, lateral pinch strength was twice that reported at

Table 27.1. Patient-reported symptoms. Relative frequency (%) distribution

Symptom		Pre-op	10 days	4 weeks	8 weeks	6 months	1 year
Pain	None	16.5	61.9	78.5	87.9	97.3	97.1
	Slight	13.6	26.6	17.5	9.5	1.6	1.4
	Moderate	33.3	10.3	3.2	2.3	0.5	1.4
	Severe	36.6	1.2	0.7	0.2	0.5	0
	Total (n)	982	929	713	472	188	70
Tingling	None	2.3	54.7	72.4	80.5	88.3	95.7
	Slight	9.2	32.7	23.1	15.8	10.1	4.3
	Moderate	33.5	10.3	4.2	3.6	1.1	0
	Severe	54.9	2.3	0.4	0.2	0.5	0
	Total (n)	990	945	720	476	188	70
Numbness	None	1.4	46.2	61.4	69.6	80.2	90
	Slight	7.8	34.8	30.4	24.1	16	8.6
	Moderate	31.6	14.9	6.8	5.1	2.7	1.4
	Severe	59.2	4	1.4	1.3	1.1	0
	Total (n)	990	945	718	474	187	70
Burning	None	67.5	84	93.7	94.7	98.9	100
	Slight	10	12.1	4.5	4.7	1.1	0
	Moderate	12.1	3	1.7	0.4	0	0
	Severe	10.4	1	0.1	0.2	0	0
	Total (n)	972	935	712	473	185	70
Swelling	None	58.9	79.5	92.4	94.6	96.7	98.6
	Slight	12	15	6.5	4.9	3.3	1.4
	Moderate	18.6	4.8	1	0.2	0	0
	Severe	10.5	0.6	0.1	0.2	0	0
	Total (n)	966	928	711	465	184	70

Table 27.2. Strength by time since surgery

Strength measurement	Median percent change from preoperative value				
	10 days	4 weeks	8 weeks	6 months	1 year
	n=925	n=1077	n=913	n=527	n=302
Grip	−66.7	−33.3	−15.6	4.4	8.9
Lateral pinch	−40	0	10	20	20
Precision pinch	−28.6	0	14.3	14.3	14.3

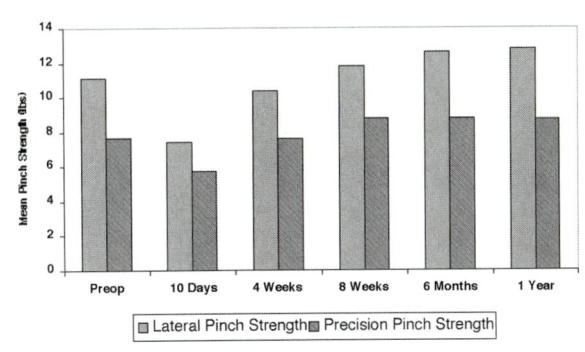

Fig. 27.8. Pinch strength

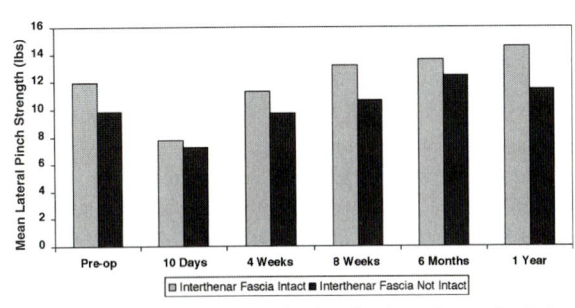

Fig. 27.9. Lateral pinch strength related to interthenar fascia integrity

8 weeks, with the precision pinch strength level remaining at the 8-week level (Table 27.2). Lateral pinch strengths were significantly higher at 8 weeks in patients whose interthenar fascia was left intact, and remained so through the 1-year time point (Fig. 27.9, $p = .009$).

Tenderness Postsurgery

At 8 weeks, tenderness to palpation along the postoperative scar, as well as the radial pillar and ulnar pillar was minimal. At 10 days postsurgery, all but 4 patients of the 903 reporting incisional tenderness exhibited, at most, moderate symptoms. By 6 months, all reporting patients exhibited either slight or no tenderness at the incision. Symptom changes were similar for those who reported radial pillar and/or ulnar pillar tenderness as well (Table 27.3).

Return to Work and Normal Function

Table 27.4 presents the mean and median time to return to work or normal activity as a function of insurance type. For this analysis insurance is either workman's compensation or some other insurance type (including no insurance). The results of applying a t-test (equal variances not assumed) indicate that the difference in the mean values of 14.5 days is statistically significant ($t = 7.9$, df $= 261.3$, $p < .001$).

Where available, the patient's occupation was classified as "White Collar" or "Other." Table 27.5 presents the mean time to return to work or normal activity as a function of occupation. The results of applying a t-test indicate that the difference in the mean values of 15 days is statistically significant as well ($t = 8.5$, $p < .0001$).

Table 27.4. Return to work and normal function. comparison of workman's compensation to other types of payment

Workman's compensation	Mean (days)	Median (days)	Standard deviation (days)	n
Yes	30.0	28	20.47	164
No	15.5	12	14.07	256
Difference	14.5	16	24.84	

Table 27.5. Return to work and function – by occupation. comparison of white collar workers to other types of workers

Occupation	Mean (days)	Standard deviation (days)	n
White collar	11.3	9.8	118
Other	26.1	19.1	165
Difference	14.8		

Table 27.3. Resolution of tenderness to palpation

		10 days	4 weeks	8 weeks	6 months	1 year
Incision	None	557	528	466	223	78
	Slight	257	154	56	5	0
	Moderate	85	38	14	0	0
	Severe	4	3	2	0	0
	Total (*n*)	903	723	538	228	78
Radial pillar	None	645	516	426	218	77
	Slight	200	167	84	9	1
	Moderate	55	39	24	0	0
	Severe	6	3	0	0	0
	Total (*n*)	906	725	534	227	78
Ulnar pillar	None	622	460	412	216	78
	Slight	216	200	96	9	0
	Moderate	61	55	26	2	0
	Severe	6	5	2	0	0
	Total (*n*)	905	720	536	288	78

The overall mean time for return to work and full function was 21 days. Patients not on worker's compensation returned to work sooner than the worker's compensation patients (Table 27.4).

Statistical Analyses

The database used for the analyses in this report contains 1,304 cases. Data for a number of the symptoms and findings are missing on many of these cases. No attempt to impute values for missing data was made. The number of cases containing values for each variable is reported in each table as appropriate. These numbers change from table to table because of missing values. Data collected from the patient questionnaires were converted to an SPSS for Windows file (SPSS, Inc., Chicago, IL) by using DBMSCOPY V7.05 (Conceptual Software Inc.). Differences between data sets were evaluated by performing a t-test. A level of $p < .05$ was accepted as statistically significant.

Complications

Data on pain management were available for 785 of the 1,304 patients studied. Among these 785 individuals, 27% required no analgesic therapy. For those requiring analgesia, the majority (60%) required the use of an analgesic, such as hydrocodone. The remaining patients (13%) alleviated their surgical discomfort with acetaminophen or NSAIDs.

Due to continued complaints of numbness and tingling, five patients underwent a second procedure. Median nerve compression was found in one of these five patients. An open release was performed in this case, and improvement was noted in two-point discrimination as well as all other reported symptoms. Other complications consisted of two cases of mild reflex sympathetic dystrophy (RSD), one common digital nerve injury, and three cases of persistent numbness to the middle and ring fingers. The RSD improved with conservative management in one patient and one patient was lost to follow-up. These three cases of persistent numbness were previously reported as injury to the communicating branch of the ulnar nerve, which we characterized as neurapraxia [14]. This condition resolved in the affected patients. We now conclude that this was likely due to neurapraxia of the median nerve and not injury to the communicating branch. No injuries occurred to the median nerve or its motor branch, or the palmar arch.

Discussion

The identification of key anatomic structures in the midpalm is important when performing a CTR [3]. The small, longitudinal incision in the palm described with the distal, single incision, scope-assisted carpal tunnel release provides identification of the palmar arch, the median nerve and its branches, as well as the distal edge of the TCL. This exposure has been shown to minimize complications previously reported, such as the inadvertent release of Guyon's canal, injury to the palmar arch, or injury to the median nerve or its motor branches [7, 8, 10, 11, 25].

The knife was designed to accomplish transection of the flexor retinaculum simply, in one pass, while providing good endoscopic visualization and control. The knife mounts on a standard 4-mm arthroscope, avoiding the purchase of costly new equipment. The endoscopic release described here divides the TCL as well as the most distal portion of the anterior brachial fascia.

Since Rotman and Manske [24] further clarified the anatomic relationships surrounding the carpal canal, we now have a better understanding of the superficial fascia, which is palmar to the TCL. We refer to this layer as the "interthenar fascia" because it receives most of its contribution from the thenar muscle fascia and lesser contributions from the hypothenar and palmaris brevis muscle fascia [5, 24]. The interthenar fascia is usually left intact in some patients after dividing the flexor retinaculum with one pass of the knife/scope assembly. It appears as intact transverse fibers not as densely arranged as the fibers of the divided TCL (Fig. 27.6). Less widening of the transverse carpal arch has been seen when comparing ECTR with open CTR [26]. Keeping the interthenar fascia intact may contribute to less pillar migration, with an associated decrease in postsurgical loss of strength and pillar tenderness, resulting in an early return to work. We, as well as many others, elect to leave the fascial layer superficial to the TCL intact. If one chooses to divide it, a second pass of the knife/scope assembly will accomplish this. Preserving the interthenar fascia appears to significantly increase the return of strength postoperatively.

The incision is small, usually concealed in the thenar crease, resulting in a cosmetically appealing scar. The one palmar incision avoids the transverse incision at the wrist. Thus, using the single distal incision technique may account for the absence of ulnar nerve neurapraxia, compared with a 10%–13% incidence of transient postoperative ulnar nerve neurapraxia reported with other techniques that use a transverse skin incision at the wrist with retraction near the ulnar neurovascular structures [19].

Overall, we observed good postoperative relief of symptoms and an early return of strength with little use of pain medication. Of the 1,304 patients analyzed in our study, 1.7% (22 cases) were converted to a modified open CTR because of inadequate visualization, usually due to excessive tenosynovitis. Most of these conversions were done earlier in the series and such conversions became less frequent as proficiency with the endoscopic technique increased. Conversion to the open technique is simply accomplished by extending the incision proximally in the usual fashion [20, 21].

This report summarizes findings gathered over a 13-year period of clinical practice. Data collection and analysis methods begun at the outset of the study have been refined over time and although we have attempted to present our findings as clearly as possible, gaps in the patient-reported symptoms exist. Regardless of this shortcoming, we have observed that the trends in the data remained consistent throughout our study.

Conclusion

Our 13-year experience with this technique has demonstrated good short-term as well as consistent long-term results. The safety of the technique is ascribed to the ability of the surgeon to see the pertinent anatomy with both direct and endoscopic vision. The authors feel this technique combines the safety of the open CTR with the rapid recovery and patient satisfaction of the endoscopic CTR.

Acknowledgements. Special thanks to Beth Porco for her help with data collection and analysis. Editorial assistance was provided by Dominic De Bellis, Ph.D., with statistical analyses by Robert P. Thiel, Ph.D.

References

1. Agee JM, McCarroll HR Jr et al. (1992) Endoscopic release of the carpal tunnel: a randomized prospective multicenter study. J Hand Surg [Am] 17(6):987–95
2. Brown MG, Keyser B et al. (1992) Endoscopic carpal tunnel release. J Hand Surg [Am] 17(6):1009–11
3. Brown RA, Gelberman RH et al. (1993) Carpal tunnel release. A prospective, randomized assessment of open and endoscopic methods. J Bone Joint Surg Am 75(9):1265–75
4. Chow JC (1989) Endoscopic release of the carpal ligament: a new technique for carpal tunnel syndrome. Arthroscopy 5(1):19–24
5. Cobb TK, Dalley BK et al. (1993) Anatomy of the flexor retinaculum. J Hand Surg [Am] 18(1):91–9
6. Dawson DM, Hallet M et al. (1990). Entrapment neuropathies. Little, Brown. Boston, pp 25–92
7. Feinstein PA (1993) Endoscopic carpal tunnel release in a community-based series. J Hand Surg [Am] 18(3):451–4
8. Lanz U (1977) Anatomical variations of the median nerve in the carpal tunnel. J Hand Surg [Am] 2(1):44–53
9. Learmonth J (1933) The principle of decompression in the treatment of certain diseases of peripheral nerves. Surg Clin North Am 13:905–913
10. Lee DH, Masear VR et al. (1992) Endoscopic carpal tunnel release: a cadaveric study. J Hand Surg [Am] 17(6):1003–8
11. Luallin SR, Toby EB (1993) Incidental Guyon's canal release during attempted endoscopic carpal tunnel release: an anatomical study and report of two cases. Arthroscopy 9(4):382–6; discussion 381
12. Menon J (1994) Endoscopic carpal tunnel release: preliminary report. Arthroscopy 10(1):31–8
13. Mirza MA, King ET Jr (1993) Palmar uniportal extrabursal endoscopic carpal tunnel release. 23rd Meeting of the American Association of Hand Surgery, Cancun, Mexico
14. Mirza MA, King ET Jr (1996) Newer techniques of carpal tunnel release. Orthop Clin North Am 27(2):355–71
15. Mirza MA, King ET Jr et al. (1995) Palmar uniportal extrabursal endoscopic carpal tunnel release. Arthroscopy 11(1):82–90
16. National Institute for Occupational Safety and Health (1997) Carpal Tunnel Syndrome. (http://www.cdc.gov/niosh/ctsfs.html, Accessed October 27, 2004)
17. Okutsu I, Ninomiya S et al. (1989) Endoscopic management of carpal tunnel syndrome. Arthroscopy 5(1):11–8
18. Paget J (1900) Lectures on surgical pathology. Lindsay & Bakiston. Philadelphia, pp 1842–1854
19. Palmer DH, Paulson JC et al. (1993) Endoscopic carpal tunnel release: a comparison of two techniques with open release. Arthroscopy 9(5):498–508
20. Phalen GS (1951) Spontaneous compression of the median nerve at the wrist. J Am Med Assoc 145(15):1128–33
21. Phalen GS (1972) The carpal-tunnel syndrome. Clinical evaluation of 598 hands. Clin Orthop 83:29–40
22. Praemer A, Furner S et al. (1992) Occupational Injuries. Musculoskeletal conditions in the United States. AAOS, Park Ridge, IL, pp 98–104
23. Resnick CT, Miller BW (1991) Endoscopic carpal tunnel release using the subligamentous two-portal technique. Contemp Orthop 22(3):269–77
24. Rotman MB, Manske PR (1993) Anatomic relationships of an endoscopic carpal tunnel device to surrounding structures. J Hand Surg [Am] 18(3):442–50
25. Seiler JG, 3rd, Barnes K et al. (1992) Endoscopic carpal tunnel release: an anatomic study of the two-incision method in human cadavers. J Hand Surg [Am] 17(6):996–1002
26. Viegas SF, Pollard A et al. (1992) Carpal arch alteration and related clinical status after endoscopic carpal tunnel release. J Hand Surg [Am] 17(6):1012–6

28 Carpal Tunnel Release with Limited Visualization

C. Panciera, P. Panciera

Introduction and History

We are presently using a median nerve surgical neurolysis technique that has been developed to reduce, as much as possible, the anatomical damage that can be incurred to the hand during carpal tunnel syndrome surgery. This technique is both reliable and efficient and renders more than satisfactory results. Our cutaneous incision is a modification and simplification of the incision that has been proposed by Kuhlman-Tubiana-Lisfranc [1] (Fig. 28.1) in 1978, which ran in a zig-zag direction for about 11 cm (7 cm proximally to the distal transverse wrist crease and 4 cm distally). We have used this type of incision for some years; and progressively have shortened it both distally and proximally.

We have been constantly supported in our "experimental surgical evolution," by positive experiences and results from both a clinical and patient satisfaction point of view [2].

The actual incision is about 2 cm in length and is located at the wrist but does not invade the palmar skin (the incision is only lengthened in cases of synovectomy).

In the last 15 years, we have treated over 20,000 cases.

Technique Description

Presurgical Preparation

This surgical technique is habitually performed in a day-surgery setting and only by one surgeon. The surgeon is also the one who administers the local anesthesia, except in rare cases such as children, or noncollaborating patients. Ischemia is obtained by positioning a tourniquet around the patient's surgical upper arm and inflating it until the pressure is about 50 mmHg higher than patient's systolic blood pressure.

The instruments that are necessary for performing this surgical procedure are: scalpel, straight scissors with blunt points, surgical tweezers, a Farabeuf retractor, an autostatic retractor, surgical needles, and cutaneous suture material.

The patient enters the preoperating area and their head and shoes are covered. Once they have thoroughly washed their hands and lie down on the operating table, the surgeon traces the sign of the cutaneous incision on their wrist with a surgical pen.

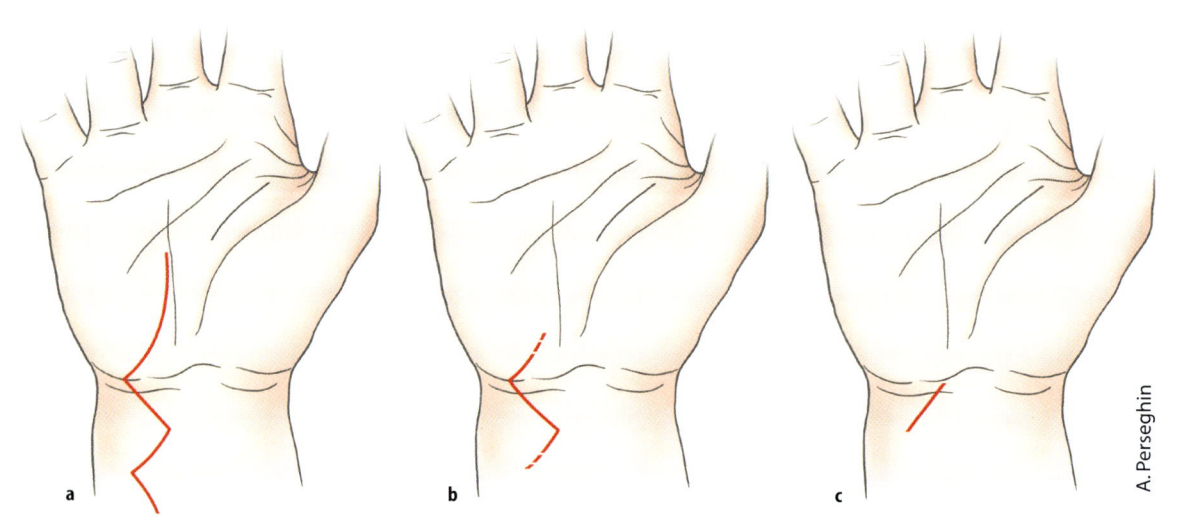

Fig. 28.1 a Cutaneous incision proposed by Kuhlmann-Tubiana-Lisfranc (KTL). **b** Progressive simplification of the incision proposed by KTL. **c** Actual cutaneous incision (see text)

Anesthesia

The surgery is performed under local-regional anesthesia. Ten milliliters of Mepivacaine at 1% is infiltrated into the wrist and palm in the zone that corresponds to the pretraced skin incision and distally, at the same level of the transverse volar carpal ligament (Fig. 28.2a, b). The incision is made 2 cm long, beginning at the angle that is formed by the intersection of the forearm's median line and the distal transverse wrist crease and moves in a ulno-proximal direction (Fig. 28.3).

Surgical Technique

The skin is incised (Fig. 28.4) and using the autostatic retractor its borders are separated so the superficial fascia is seen. Next, the palmaris longus or gracilis is located (about 20% of cases do not have this muscle); it is found immediately under the skin and extrafascia (Fig. 28.5). The surgeon is at a very important anatomical landmark, since at the ulnar border of this tendon there is the fascia zone that must be incised for accessing the tunnel. The radial border's margin is where the median nerve's palmar cutaneous branch is located so this area must be respected and protected.

At the ulnar border of the palmaris longus tendon the superficial fascial sheath is lifted up by using the surgical tweezers (Fig. 28.6). A hood is made with the scissors by carefully separating this sheath from its underlying tissue in a longitudinal manner. The change of tissue color from a pearly white to a clear yellow lets the

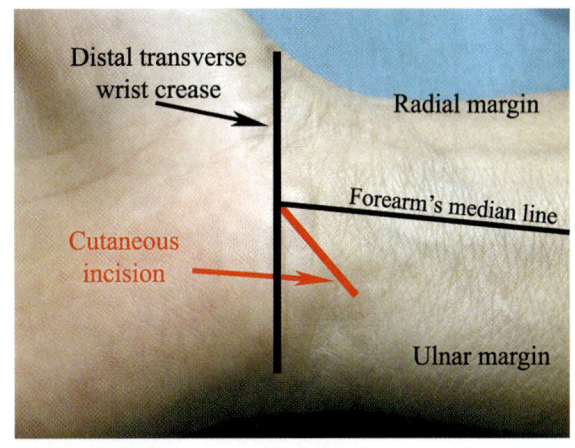

Fig. 28.3. Design of cutaneous incision

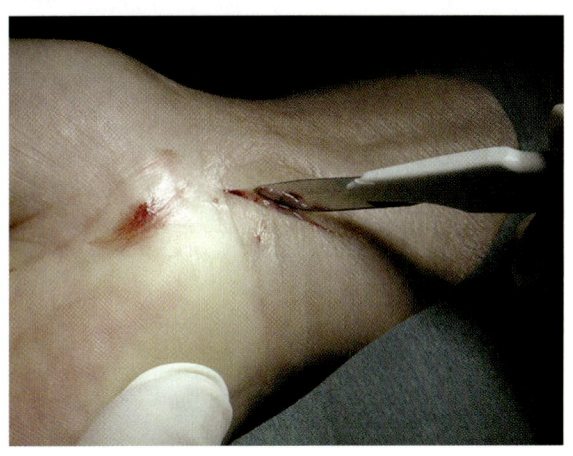

Fig. 28.4. Skin incision

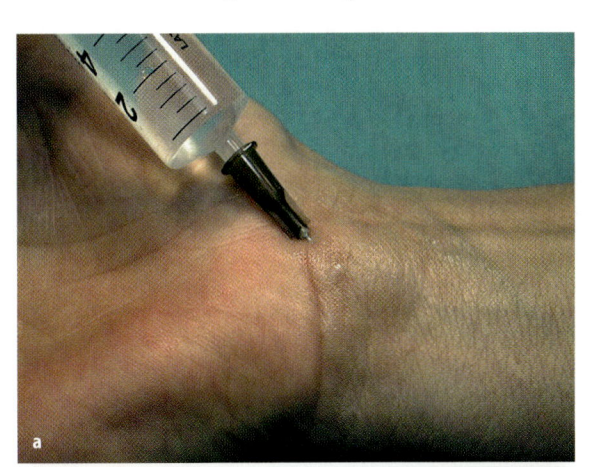

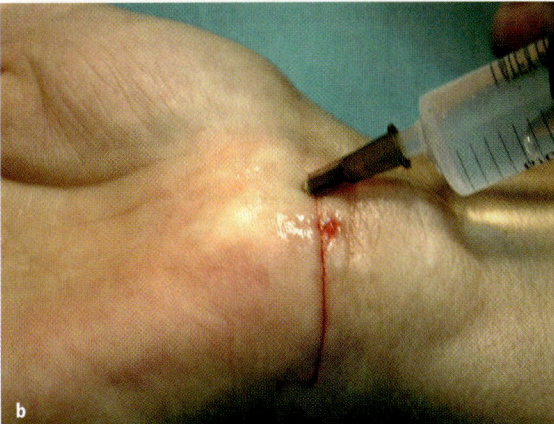

Fig. 28.2. Injection of local anesthesia

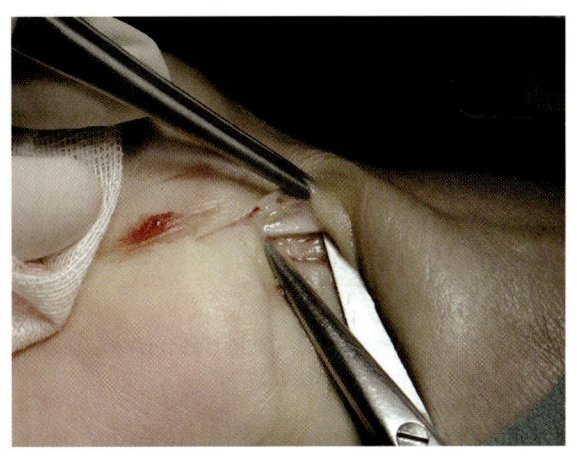

Fig. 28.5. Location of palmaris gracilis (or longus) tendon

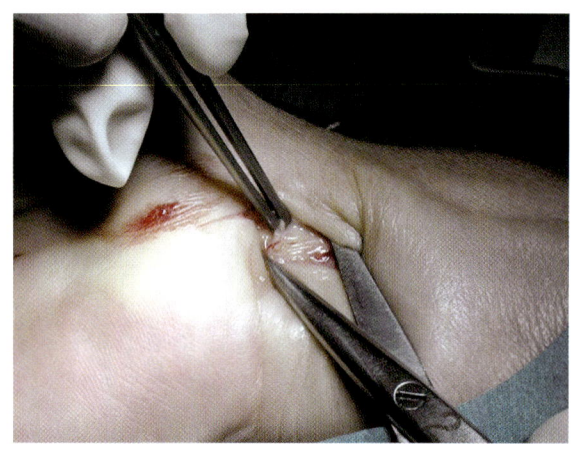

Fig. 28.6. A hood is made in the superficial fascial sheath by lifting it up

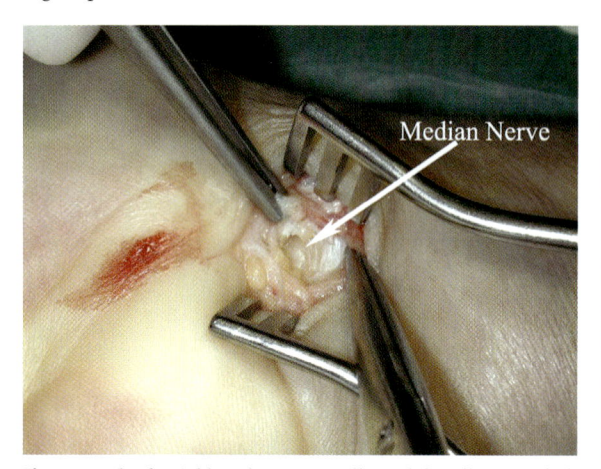

Fig. 28.7. The fascial hood is proximally and distally extended

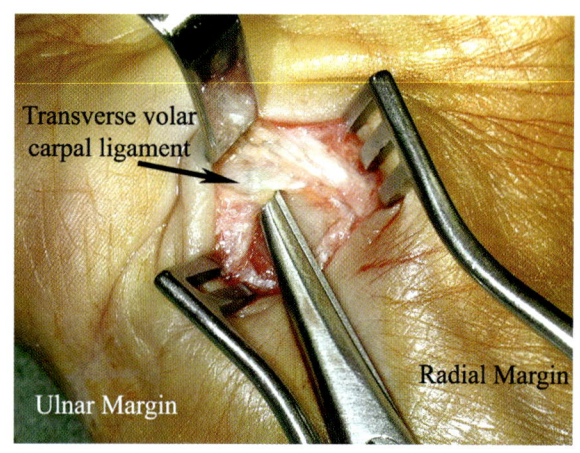

Fig. 28.8. The Farabeuf retractor has been inserted at the wrist's distal transverse crease, in a space between the superficial and the fascia, created by using the blunt points of the scissors. The proximal margin of the transverse volar carpal ligament and the median nerve can be easily seen

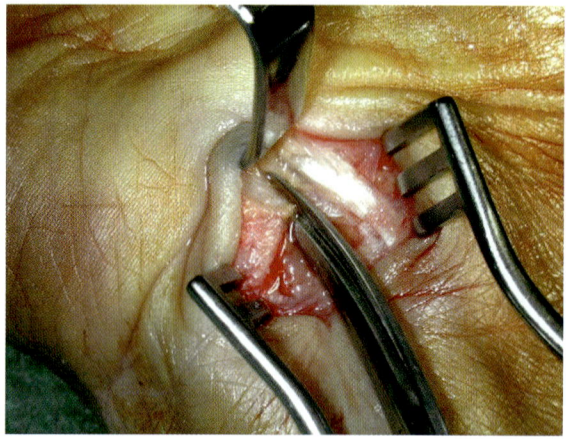

Fig. 28.9. By using the blunt point scissors, the section of the transverse carpal ligament is begun

surgeon know that they have surpassed the fascia and are entering into the carpal canal. The surgical opening is proximally and distally extended for some millimeters along the fascia, always separating it from above and below the hood using the blunt scissors (Fig. 28.7).

It is necessary to complete a few successive surgical maneuvers before proceeding with the surgery:

1. The surgeon must check, through the fascial opening, the presence and location of the median nerve, which normally appears as the most superficial structure, and of a yellowish color.
2. With the point of the scissors, the surgeon must create a space at the wrist's distal transverse crease between the superficial and the fascia so that the Farabeuf retractor can be inserted.
3. The patient's wrist is positioned in light hyperextension, and it is maintained in this position by placing a rolled-up sterile drape under the dorsum of the wrist.
4. By using the Farabeuf retractor, the skin and subcutaneous layers can be elevated and separated from the underlying fascia (Fig. 28.8). At this point, the last few millimeters of the fascia is dissected, as is the transverse volar carpal ligament (Fig. 28.9). This is the most fundamental part of the surgery. The sectioning of the transverse carpal ligament must be performed in the most delicate manner in graded steps.
5. The ligament is sectioned along a line that lies ulnar and parallel to the median nerve. Before beginning to cut, it is fundamental to precisely locate the nerve's margins, which should correspond to a straight line along the radial border of the hand's fourth ray, about 1 cm ulnar to the wrist's and hand's median line.

As has been noted, the carpal tunnel, seen from a sagittal section, has the form of an hour glass, with its narrowest zone in correspondence to the central part of the transverse volar ligament. It is evident that when the patient is symptomatic, the soft tissue structures and the median nerve that are contained in the narrowest part of the canal are compressed. The constriction can be so severe that it does not allow for a rigid surgical structure to be inserted under the ligament. In these severest compression cases, which actually occur quite frequently, (as we have seen in our experience) we feel it is too risky to section the ligament with techniques that require the insertion of any type of rigid instrument (for example: dilators, cannula, or trocar) *before* cutting the ligament. In fact, in such cases, we feel that when the surgeon insists on introducing a rigid instrument into this area, they could cause a crush injury, with an elevated risk of further damaging the median nerve.

We use a system that allows us *to cut the ligament in all cases*, even when it is severely constricted, without risking damage to the median nerve. In order to do this we utilize some studied surgical tricks.

1. Both at the beginning and during each successive step of the ligament dissection (see number 2) prior to "cutting," we delicately undermine and separate the ligament from its surrounding anterior and posterior structures by using the blunt point scissors. They are inserted inside the opening for only very short tracts (about 1 or 2 mm) in front of and behind the ligament. This maneuver is always possible even if the ligament is extremely tight and narrow.
2. By using the same scissors, we cut the ligament, not all in one go but in many successive steps, "inching" through progressively, each time delicately moving forward and cutting only 1–2 mm of the undermined ligament at a time.
3. It is necessary to enlarge the surgical visual field inside the tunnel and to obtain constant visual field control of the median nerve. A step by step sectioning of the ligament is done by using the Farabeuf retractor. It is moved in a distal direction. The area is "explored" by separating the fascial margins opening the points of the blunt scissors (Fig. 28.10). The use of an autostatic retractor is precious, especially in cases in which the patient has an abundance of underlying adipose tissue. The ligament is dissected until the tunnel is completely open (Fig. 28.11) and the scissors can enter the tunnel without encountering any obstacle (Fig. 28.12). The dissection should never surpass the transverse ligament's distal margin because immediately on the other side of this border lies the superficial palmar arch which must absolutely be respected.
4. Actually the sectioning of the ligament is only under visual control for its proximal two thirds; the last part of its tract is "blindly" sectioned or better, using one's "tactile perception" through the scissor

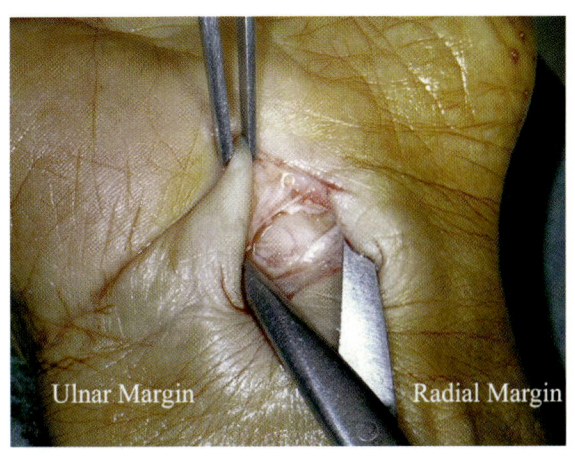

Fig. 28.10. At every moment of surgery, the opened points of the scissors can help in exploring the surgical area

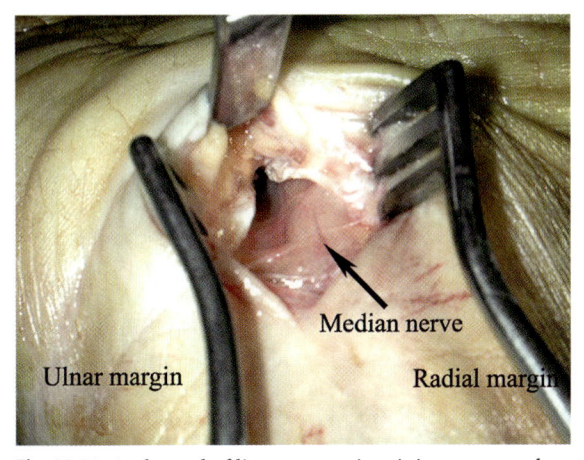

Fig. 28.11. At the end of ligament section, it is easy to explore the median nerve

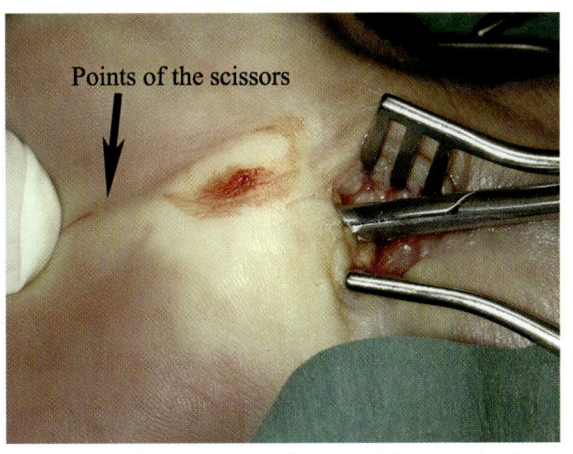

Fig. 28.12. If the transverse volar carpal ligament has been completely cut, the points of the scissors could be easily discerned by the surgeon's fingertip under palmar skin

end's resistance. Obviously, when one is sectioning this area, they must be extremely prudent and proceed in very short tracts.

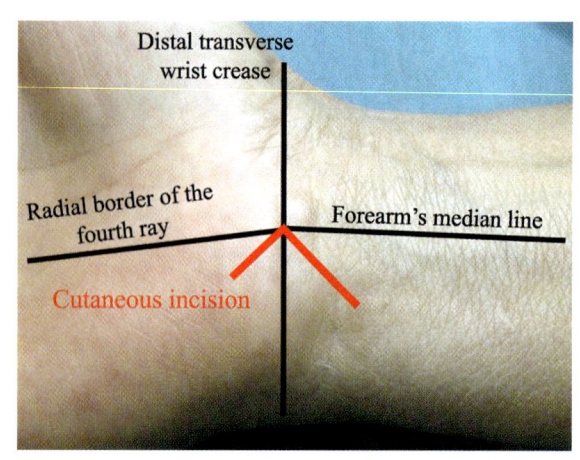

Fig. 28.13. The L-shaped skin incision, suggested in particular cases (see text)

Attention: *A very important fact to remember*, it is possible, even in expert hands, that if you do not check yourself each time you proceed distally and open the fascial tract, you may end up in a wrong way when sectioning the ligament. If the surgeon is not scrupulous in checking their dissection, they can "believe" that they are in the carpal tunnel but instead they are in the Guyon canal, which is adjacent to it by only a 1- to 2-mm distance. If the surgeon does not realize this immediately, they run the risk of damaging the ulnar nerve. Therefore, it is indispensable that, before proceeding with the dissection, the median nerve must be identified and verified that it is in its correct anatomical space.

One should suspect that they are in the wrong tract if they see a bluish structure (ulnar artery) rather than a yellowish structure (median nerve) at the bottom of the fascial opening. However, if in doubt, we suggest that the palmar incision is lengthened by 1 cm, transforming it from a straight line incision into an L-shaped incision (Fig. 28.13). We suggest this "surgical maneuver" when using our technique, at least for the first time surgical procedures, so that the surgeon proceeds through the tunnel safely and their learning curve is favorable.

Indications – Contraindications

We base our CTS diagnosis on clinical and scientific objective and subjective data: a positive electromyography report is not indispensable for the diagnosis. A surgical candidate is chosen according to the severity of their symptoms (nerve irritation, paresthesia or paralysis, and/or functional deficit), the duration of their symptoms, patient's age, and their physiological (pregnancy) or pathological conditions, (dialysis, diabetes, rheumatoid arthritis, etc.). In the initial stages of this pathology (nerve irritation) we first treat the patient by using conservative therapy such as: rest, application of a local anesthetic/cortisone infiltrations, anti-inflammatory drugs and/or physical therapy. If the patient's symptoms do not decrease in severity within 1–2 months, we suggest surgical intervention, especially if the patient reports that they are awakened during the night by painful and paresthesia-like symptoms (in our opinion, these symptoms indicate surgical treatment).

We opt for immediate surgery in the severest of cases (in cases in which functional hand deficits are present or the patient has hand paralysis) independent of the patient's age (we have operated on patients ages ranging from 14 to 96 years and a 6-year-old child who was afflicted with Weil-Marchesani syndrome).

We feel that there are no contraindications for this type of surgery when using our technique. This technique can be used even in cases where the patient has a generally compromised health situation since the type and quantity of anesthesia used is quite minimal (5–10 ml of mepivacaine to 1%). Obviously, in particular cases, we practice extreme caution when administering the anesthesia and an anesthesiologist is present in the operating room for only these specific cases.

Complications

We have followed-up on various patient groups that comprise our 20,000 operated cases. In summary, we have re-evaluated 1,802 patients of which 1,577 were females and 225 males with the average age being 52 years; they were evaluated at an average distance of 65 months from surgery (24–126 months).

We separated out the cases with general and local complications with both immediate and late symptom onset. Apart from rare cases, in which patients had a vagal crisis, which was immediately resolved with an endovenous infiltration of atropine, no other general complications have to be enumerated.

Immediate local complications, included *vascular injuries*, which were taken care of immediately and *nerve injuries*. In the cases of nerve injury, the patient immediately reported feeling an electric shock and we therefore enlarged the incision and repaired any eventual damage.

- *Vascular injuries*: we had three cases where there was a partial ulnar artery injury (0.016%), and 48 cases of injury to the superficial palmar arch (2.7%). These events manifest themselves by producing bleeding when the brachial tourniquet is deflated and a light hematoma. In these cases we performed a "watertight" suture of the cutaneous incision, advised the patient that there would be a

progressive disappearance of the hematoma and or bruise from the hand and wrist within weeks. The hematomas always resolved within 2–3 weeks without causing residual complications. These patients were instructed to mobilize their fingers immediately postoperatively.
- *Nerve injuries*: the median nerve was partially injured in one of our cases by a surgeon in training. The nerve was repaired immediately along its ulnar border. We have had two cases (0.11%) where there was a presumable injury to the median nerve's thenar motor branch, in which the patient reported a functional deficit in thumb opposition. More frequently, (27 cases out of 1,800 patients followed-up, equal to 1.5% of the cases) injury to the common and proper digital sensitive branch of the fingers (22 cases) and the thumb (5 cases) occurs. These injuries were immediately repaired in 23 patients (equal to 85.2% of the cases). All these cases healed with a residual light hypoparesthesia.

Results

In 1,710 cases (95%) this surgical technique quickly and completely resolved the patient's hand paresthesia and pain. In 1,620 cases (90%) functional hand strength, endurance and dexterity deficit was resolved. Hand sensibility was perfectly regained in 973 cases (54%); but in 793 cases (44%) a light amount of hypoesthesia and in 36 cases hyperesthesia (2%) was reported. Probably it is due to the gravity of cases and the duration of the disease before surgery. Thenar eminence hypotrophy improved in nearly half of the operated cases but was never fully recuperated. Thumb opposition remained invariable in all the operated cases. Only in 23 cases (1%), was the surgery unsuccessful for resolving persistent residual wrist and hand pain and paresthesia. In 1,715 cases (95%) the patients reported that they obtained complete satisfactory results from the surgical procedure.

Conclusions

We think that this surgical technique is:

- *Simple*: it can be performed under local anesthesia, in 5–10 min, by one only surgeon.
- *Economic*: no expensive instruments are needed; back to work in 3 weeks.
- *Nontraumatic and safe*: complications are rare.
- *Effective*: it gives very good results in a high percentage of cases.

References

1. Kuhlmann N, Tubiana R, Lisfranc R (1978) Apport de l'anatomie dans la compréhension des syndromes de compression du canal carpien et des séqueles des interventions décompressives. Rev Chir Orthop 64:(1);59–70
2. Panciera C, Pasquon P, Rocchetto F (1990) Neurolisi esterna del mediano attraverso mini incisione nella sindrome del tunnel carpale. Presentazione di 550 casi. In Atti Second World week of professional updating in Surgery. Università di Milano, 15–21 luglio 1990. Monduzzi Ed. S.P.A. Bologna, pp 221–226

29 Closed Technique With Paine Retinaculotome and Modified Retinaculotome MDC

A. Mantovani, L. De Cristofaro, A. Ciaraldi

Introduction

It has been proven that flexor tenosynovectomy and median neurolysis are practically not useful in the treatment of "essential" carpal tunnel syndrome and should be reserved for specific indications [13, 19, 36]. The fact that the improvement in function following surgery has to be attributed completely to the division of the transverse carpal ligament [36] has been recognized only recently. Closed techniques for decompression of the median nerve at the wrist in carpal tunnel syndrome, along with endoscopic methods, have received particular attention towards the end of the 1980s. Yet, Paine had already designed and presented the use of his retinaculotome [31] in 1955. It is really evidence of genius as only a few dozen cases of carpal tunnel syndrome had been recognized and treated by open decompression up to 1950 [3]! In his series published in 1983 [32], Paine reported remarkable results with a minimal rate of recurrence, early resumption of use of the operated hand and, above all, absence of iatrogenic lesions. We were among the first few surgeons in Italy to adopt this technique since 1990. We presented our initial results [22] in 1991, certain modifications in the procedure [23] in 1994, a videocassette recording [21] in 1995, and a larger series of cases [24] in 1997.

Other significant reports of this method include the series presented by Pagnanelli [33] in 1991 and that of Grangie [14] who compared it with results obtained using the traditional open technique of carpal tunnel release in 1992. In 1995, Carneiro [4] presented his results at the 6th Congress of the International Federation of Societies for the Surgery of the Hand (IFSSH) at Helsinki. He described the use of the retinaculotome in the disto-proximal direction, i.e., with an incision in the palm. However, this entails identification and isolation of the structures in the palm before division of the flexor retinaculum and cannot be considered an example of the original Paine technique, which involves an approach at the wrist.

We have examined this approach and studied a series of 100 patients, operated upon by the same surgeon, 50 of which were treated by the original Paine technique and the remaining 50 by the palmar approach. The results of this study were analyzed and presented in the 33rd Congress of the Italian Hand Society at Brescia in 1995 [20]. This was part of a multicentric study with a common protocol for evaluation of various techniques in the surgical treatment of carpal tunnel syndrome. We prefer to use the retinaculotome in the proximo-distal direction with an approach at the wrist.

Technique

The retinaculotome (Fig. 29.1) consists of a spatula made of stainless steel with rounded edges. It is 1.5 mm thick, 7 mm wide, and 4.4 cm long. The handle of the instrument is angled at 30°. A 3.3-mm-high vertical blade emerges at the center of the spatula. Its superior border is rounded and protrudes 1.5 mm beyond the cutting edge of the blade. This peculiar shape enables us to perform a true "closed" section of the transverse carpal ligament as long as we strictly adhere to the sequence of steps of the procedure. For surgeons beginning to use this instrument, we would recommend performing an open release for the first few cases. This would allow the surgeon to visualize the relationship between the passage of the retinaculotome and the surrounding anatomical structures and to become familiar with the "feel" of complete division of the transverse carpal ligament.

Proper knowledge of the local anatomy is essential. Some authors [15, 16] consider the transverse carpal ligament to be synonymous with the flexor retinaculum. Despite being a localized thickening of the central segment of the flexor retinaculum, the transverse carpal ligament is a discrete anatomical structure with specific bony attachments [6]. The flexor retinaculum, in its turn, is just a distal prolongation of the deep fascia of the forearm that ends as the interthenar fascia in the palm [6] (Fig. 29.2).

As we proceed in the proximo-distal direction, one can distinguish three segments of the flexor retinaculum: the first segment is a thickening of the deep fascia of the forearm, the central segment constitutes the true transverse carpal ligament, while the third segment is the interthenar fascia [6].

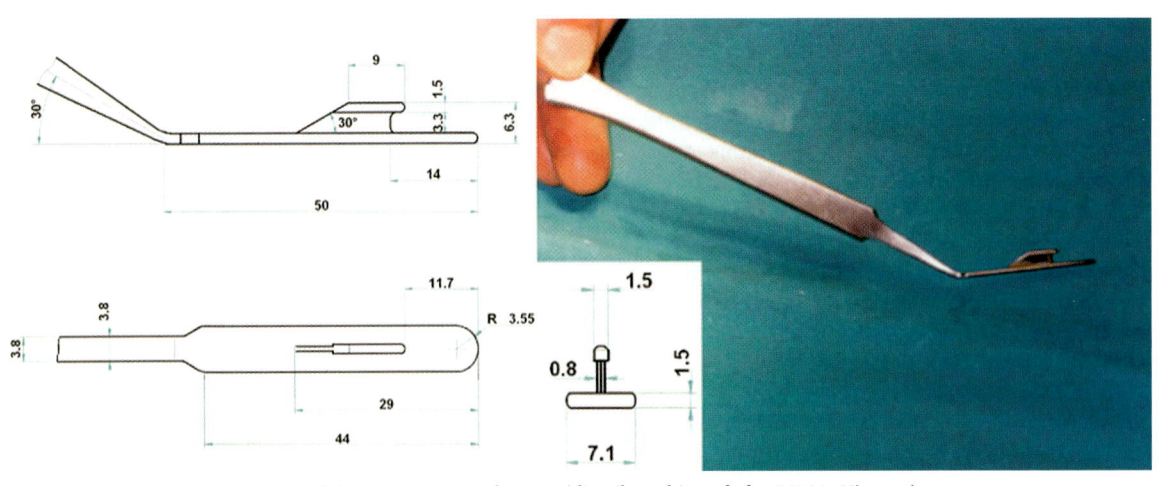

Fig. 29.1. Photograph and design of the Paine retinaculotome (distributed in Italy by DIMA, Vicenza)

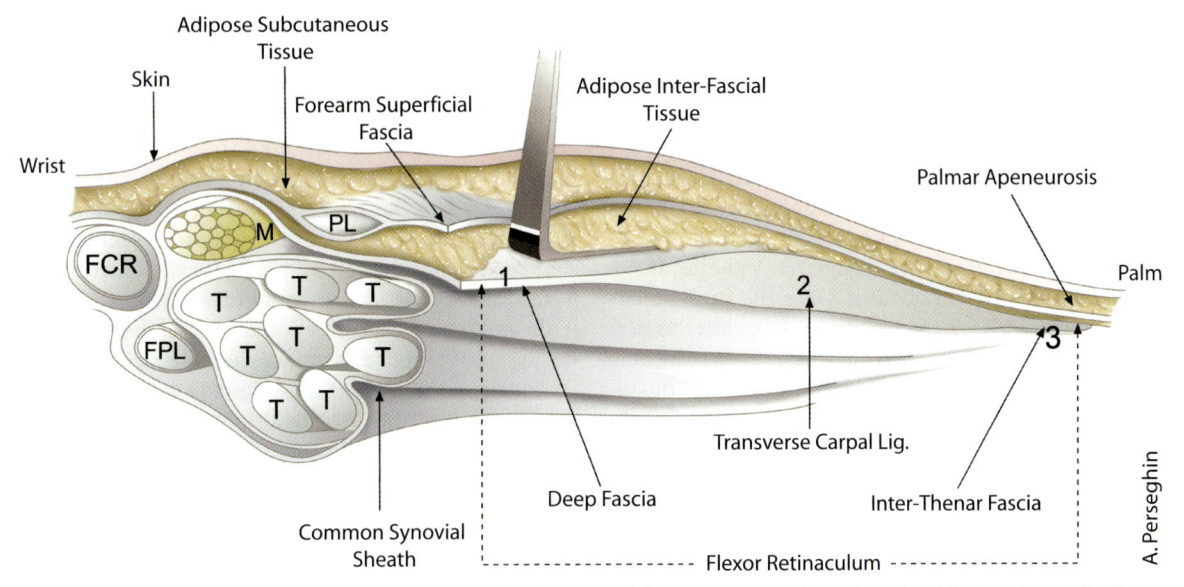

Fig. 29.2. A transverse section at the wrist and longitudinal section of the carpal tunnel along the axis of the fourth ray. The flexor retinaculum consists of three consecutive segments: the localized thickening of the deep fascia of the forearm (*1*), the transverse carpal ligament (*2*) and the interthenar fascia (*3*) in the proximo-distal direction. The superficial fascia of the forearm continues distally as the palmar aponeurosis and is separated from the flexor retinaculum by adipose interfascial tissue. *FCR*: tendon of flexor carpi radialis; *FPL*: tendon of flexor pollicis longus; *PL*: tendon of palmaris longus; *T*: flexor tendons of the fingers; *M*: median nerve

The flexor retinaculum represents the first pulley that helps transmit and amplify the force exerted by the flexor tendons on the phalanges of the fingers and, at the same time, the roof of the carpal tunnel. In three-dimensional terms, the carpal tunnel is not a true cylinder but resembles a clepsydra with the point of maximal narrowing at the level of the hook of the hamate [6].

The tendon of the palmaris longus provides the guide to the operation of carpal tunnel release using the closed technique of Paine. It passes superficially to the flexor retinaculum and continues as the palmar aponeurosis. This overlies the transverse carpal ligament and the interthenar fascia and is separated from them by a layer of fatty tissue [29] (Fig. 29.2).

According to some authors [12, 27], the palmar aponeurosis is separated from the flexor retinaculum by another interthenar fascia in addition to the layer of fatty tissue described above. However, this fascia is closely adherent to the transverse carpal ligament and cannot be isolated and protected during the surgery for carpal tunnel release using the retinaculotome in the proximo-distal direction. The contents of the carpal tunnel include the eight flexor tendons of the fingers enveloped by the folds of their common synovial lining while the flexor pollicis longus has its separate synovial sheath. These synovial folds do not surround the median nerve, while lies "extrabursal" with respect to the flexor tendons [2] (Fig. 29.2). The carpal tunnel is completely filled with the flexor tendons and their sheaths so that the extrabursal space within the canal is only potential.

The median nerve always occupies a radial position along its course proximal to as well as within the carpal tunnel: proximally, it lies between the tendons of the palmaris longus and that of the flexor carpi radialis while, within the carpal tunnel, it courses between the tendon of the flexor digitorum superficialis to the middle finger and that of the flexor pollicis longus [2], i.e., towards the radial side of the carpal tunnel (Fig. 29.2). In addition, the palmar cutaneous branch of the median nerve, which emerges in the subcutaneous plane proximal to the flexor retinaculum, runs radially close to the tendon of the flexor carpi radialis [37]. It is obvious, then, that the approach for closed section of the transverse carpal ligament should lay ulnar and deep to the palmaris longus tendon. The ulnar nerve and vessels are retracted medially. The Guyon's canal lies superficial and ulnar to the carpal tunnel and the contents of the Guyon's canal are involved only partially in the proximal portion of the Paine technique.

We recommend use of regional anesthesia and a tourniquet for the initial cases. Once the surgeon has become familiar with the technique, it is better to perform the surgery under local anesthesia (1 % Lidocaine with adrenaline) and without application of a tourniquet, as recommended by other authors [35, 38]. In fact, the reflex perfusion following the release of the tourniquet could result in the formation of local hematomas.

The limb is prepared and draped. The local anesthetic agent is injected with a thin needle (no. 26G or finer). It is first injected in the subcutaneous tissue at the site of incision, i.e., at the distal wrist flexion crease. In practice, the lidocaine is not injected within the carpal tunnel or towards the median nerve as the surgical approach courses in a plane superficial to the nerve. The wrist is held in the neutral position and not in hyperextension so that the contents of the carpal tunnel are not compressed against the transverse carpal ligament.

The surgeon sits in a position that would allow him to operate using his dominant hand, i.e., a right-handed surgeon would sit on the ulnar side of the patient's hand while operating upon the right carpal tunnel and on the radial side for surgery for the left carpal tunnel.

The incision lies along the distal wrist flexion crease, close to the palmaris longus tendon and extending ulnarward for 2 cm up to the palpable border of the pisiform bone (Fig. 29.3). Hence, the approach passes in the space between the palmaris longus and the ulnar neuro-vascular bundle and between the superficial and deep fasciae of the forearm (Fig. 29.2).

There are no major anatomical structures at this site apart from small vessels and terminal cutaneous branches of the median and ulnar nerves, which can be easily retracted along with the local fatty tissue to expose the underlying edge of the flexor retinaculum. This can be isolated well by careful retraction of the interfascial fatty tissue, already infiltrated with lidocaine, in the proximo-distal direction following the tendon of the palmaris longus as a guide. The superficial fascia of the forearm is thickened at this level to form the roof of the Guyon's canal. It is called the palmar carpal ligament [8] (Fig. 29.4). Division of this ligament helps open the Guyon's canal superficially.

A flat retractor is inserted to retract the tendon of the palmaris longus and another helps retract the ulnar neurovascular pedicle medially. Instruments of a size

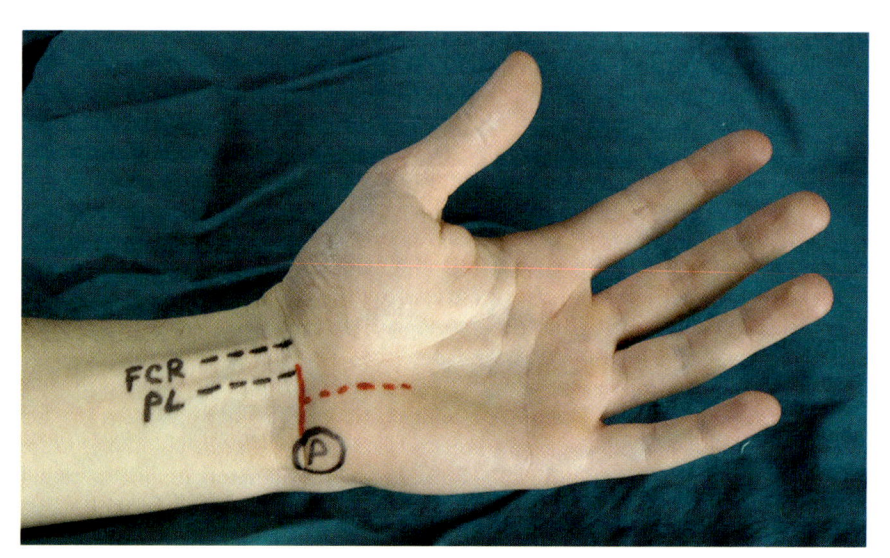

Fig. 29.3. Essential surface markings for decompression of the median nerve using the Paine technique. The *continuous red line* indicates the site of the skin incision. The *dotted red line* indicates the line of action of the retinaculotome (explained in text). *FCR*: tendon of the flexor carpi radialis; *PL*: tendon of the palmaris longus; *P*: cutaneous projection of the site of the pisiform bone

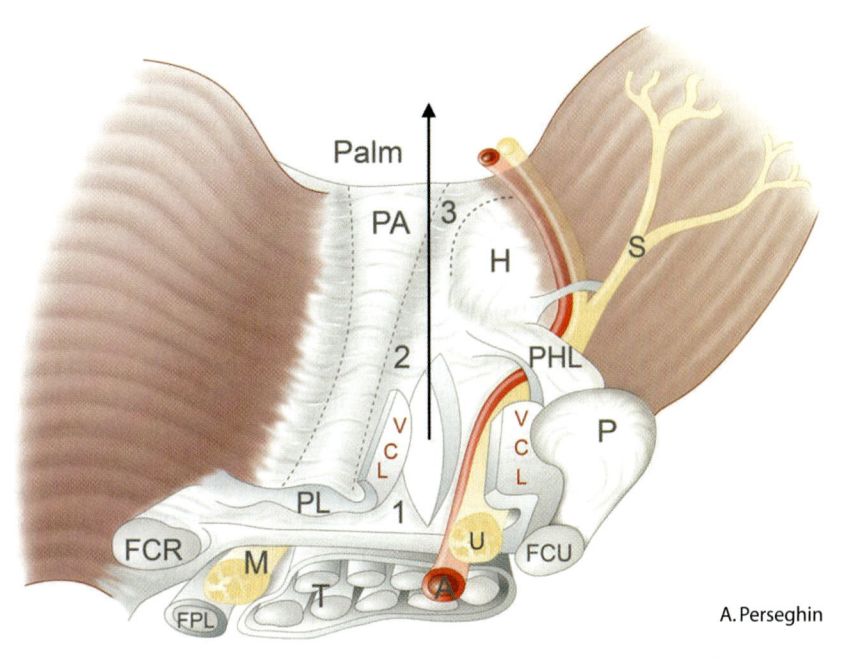

Fig. 29.4. The flexor retinaculum in relation to the neuro-vascular bundle in the Guyon's canal during the surgical approach by the Paine technique. Division of the volar carpal ligament opens the mouth of the Guyon's canal superficially. It is opened on its deep aspect when a buttonhole is made under vision in the proximal portion of the flexor retinaculum. The Paine retinaculotome is introduced into the carpal tunnel through this buttonhole and the remaining portion of the flexor retinaculum is divided by a closed technique along the direction of the *arrow* shown, which corresponds to the axis of the fourth ray. The instrument rests on the hook of the hamate in its passage along this course. *A:* ulnar artery; *M:* median nerve; *U:* ulnar nerve; *S:* sensory branch of the ulnar nerve; *T:* flexor tendons of the fingers; *P:* pisiform bone; *H:* hook of the hamate; *PL:* tendon of palmaris longus; *PA:* palmar aponeurosis; *VCL:* divided volar carpal ligament; *PHL:* piso-hamate ligament; *FCR:* tendon of flexor carpi radialis; *FCU:* tendon of flexor carpi ulnaris; *1-2-3:* 3 consecutive segments of the flexor retinaculum

suitable for this surgery are essential. The blades of each of these right-angled retractors should be 5 mm wide and 1 mm thick. The retractor placed under the palmaris longus tendon should be 2 cm long while that used to retract the ulnar nerve and vessels should be 2.5 cm long. Both these retractors should be applied in the proximo-distal direction. Proper retraction of the interfascial fat using the two retractors exposes the proximal two thirds of the flexor retinaculum. A longitudinal incision is made over the ulnar aspect of the flexor retinaculum using a no. 15 blade. This incision should be extended distally for 1.5–2 cm under complete visual control. Thus the division of the transverse carpal ligament is started under vision, taking care to avoid injury to the underlying synovial sheath of the flexor tendons. At this stage, the assistant plays a vital role by proper retraction of the fatty tissue superficially so that the plane of the transverse carpal ligament is lifted off the synovium, which is then visible through the buttonhole made in the flexor retinaculum (Figs. 29.4. 29.5).

One must mention that the beginning of the release of the transverse carpal ligament also implies release of the proximal part of the Guyon's canal. The roof of the Guyon's canal is opened by division of the superficial forearm fascia and the palmar carpal ligament before placement of the retractors during the exposure of the flexor retinaculum while division of the portion of the transverse carpal ligament that lies between the pisiform and the hook of the hamate produces a release of the floor of the Guyon's canal (Fig. 29.4).

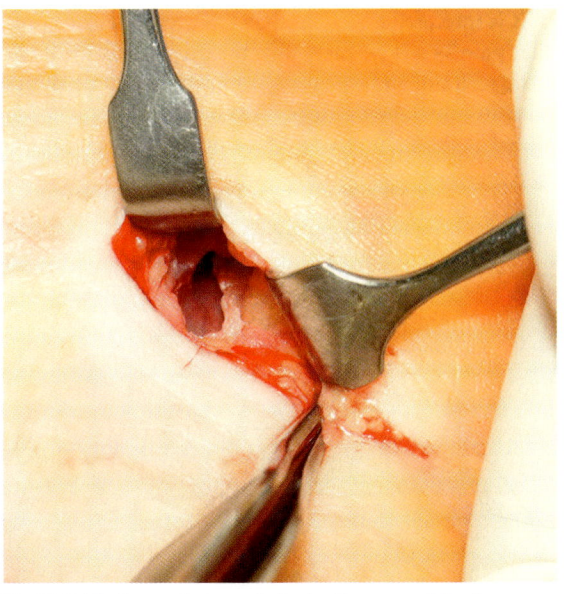

Fig. 29.5. The buttonhole made in the first part of the flexor retinaculum is visible through the wound in the skin. The Paine retinaculotome is inserted through this buttonhole

At this stage, one has to inject a further dose of local anesthetic agent into the interfascial fatty tissue towards the palm. The insulin needle is directed along the fourth ray and is placed superficial to the plane of the transverse carpal ligament. An additional dose of lidocaine is allowed to drip through the buttonhole in the ligament while the patient is instructed to execute movements of complete flexion and extension of the fingers repeatedly. Throughout this procedure, care is taken to maintain retraction to expose the rent made in the transverse carpal ligament.

Additional anesthetic is allowed to drip through the buttonhole in the flexor retinaculum and the patient is instructed to flex and extend his fingers repeatedly while the traction on the retractors is maintained. Thus the synovial sheath is bathed in anesthetic fluid without being infiltrated with it. The active movements facilitate diffusion of the fluid. Infiltration of local anesthetic would produce swelling and compromise the space in the canal that is already limited.

One can now introduce a thin and smooth retractor with a handle angulated at 30° (similar to the retinaculotome) under the flexor retinaculum in order to separate the synovial sheaths from it. This, too, is passed in the direction of the fourth ray. The passage of this instrument serves three objectives: the local anesthetic fluid is pushed deeper and toward the median nerve; it prepares the path for the passage of the retinaculotome subsequently; the surgeon gets a "feel" of the degree of stenosis he will encounter while attempting division of the retinaculotome.

It is interesting to note that this step does not produce pain as it is performed in the presence of local anesthetic fluid and because the instrument does not come in contact with the median nerve, which gets displaced radially. In practice, one does not look for the median nerve as the transverse carpal ligament is divided along its ulnar portion (Fig. 29.6).

Finally, after these indispensable steps, one can introduce the retinaculotome into the buttonhole in the flexor retinaculum. The vertical blade immediately encounters the distal angle of the buttonhole. Before proceeding with the division of the ligament, one must ensure that the flat portion of the instrument rests on the ulnar bony insertion of the flexor retinaculum, i.e., the hook of the hamate (Fig. 29.6) and, having confirmed this, one can push the retinaculum distally along the axis of the ring finger and complete the division of the transverse carpal ligament. The force applied on the instrument will depend upon the sharpness of the blade and the resistance encountered, which varies from one patient to the next. This step requires the same degree of attention as one applies while incising through different types of skin (one must avoid excessive pressure). Hence, it is advisable to acquire a "feel" of complete section of the transverse carpal ligament by doing it with an open technique initially. One will learn, thus, to stop pushing the retinaculotome as soon as there is a sudden decrease in the resistance to the passage.

The edges of the transverse carpal ligament remain visible after this selective division, even in the distal part if the traction on the retractors is maintained. The edges are pulled apart approximately 1 cm and one can confirm the increase in space within the canal and that the nerve is decompressed. One can introduce any smooth instrument, with its end turned towards the

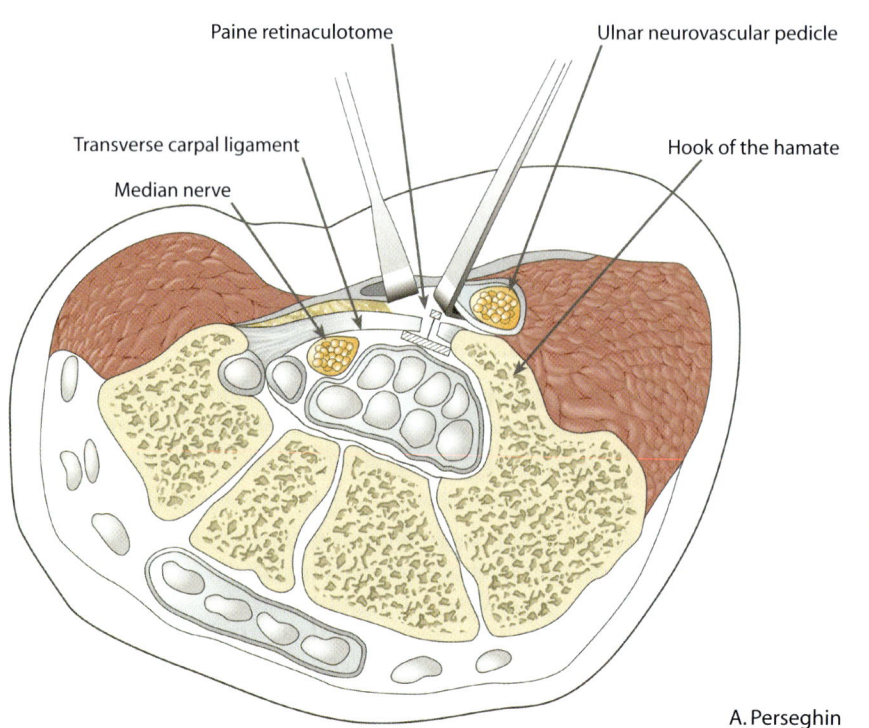

Fig. 29.6. Transverse section of the wrist at the level of the hamate during carpal tunnel decompression by the Paine technique. Placement of the retinaculotome on the hook of the hamate ensures that the transverse carpal ligament is divided at a site away from the median nerve so that the resultant scar does not cover it. In addition, the instrument occupies minimal space within the carpal tunnel that is already tight. Advancement of the retinaculotome progressively enlarges the canal

A. Perseghin

palm, in order to confirm complete division of the ligament in the portion distal to that visible in the wound. This step becomes superfluous once the surgeon has developed confidence with this technique. One can also visualize the median nerve but this would be futile as no further procedures on the nerve are planned.

The surgeon can wash the wound with saline and antibiotics according to his or her choice. The wound is then closed with three interrupted everting sutures or with an intradermal suture using absorbable material. A simple local adhesive dressing usually suffices. Use of lidocaine with adrenaline results in minimal bleeding during surgery and postoperative hematomas are rare. Hence, we have abandoned application of compressive dressings immediately after surgery, which was our practice earlier and which was recommended by Paine. In addition, use of antibiotics following the operation was found to be futile [22] as the surgery is performed in a proper operation theatre under strict aseptic conditions. It is preferable to obtain access to a vein on the opposite upper limb for administration of intravenous medications, if necessary, before the patient is wheeled into the operation theatre. The patient usually does not need hospitalization and the surgery is performed as a "day surgery" procedure.

Finally, we recommend maintenance of the sharpness of the blade of the retinaculotome by rubbing along its cutting edge with fine sandpaper wrapped around a Kirschner wire after every 10 operations.

Indications and Contraindications

The Paine technique implies closed division of the transverse carpal ligament without exploration of the carpal tunnel or visualization of the median nerve. Hence, it is essential to avoid demeaning this operation by adhering to strict indications and by proper selection of the patients. One must be certain that the condition is "essential" carpal tunnel syndrome and not "secondary" to space-occupying lesions within the carpal tunnel. For this reason, we evaluate each of our patients according to a standardized pre- and postoperative protocol [25], which includes all the data derived from clinical examination and investigations that are aimed at identification of other pathology as well as other levels of nerve compression.

Thus, we consider the Paine technique to be contraindicated in the following conditions:

1. Polyarticular rheumatoid arthritis: here complete flexor tenosynovectomy is essential in addition to division of the transverse carpal ligament.
2. Gout and tuberculous tenosynovitis: here one needs to excise the inflamed tenosynovium and to send a sample for histopathological evaluation.
3. Suspected cases of nerve tumors or tumors of other tissues within the carpal tunnel.
4. Recurrent carpal tunnel syndrome: here exposure of the median nerve is essential as the regional anatomy may be altered following the earlier surgery.
5. The rare cases of acute carpal tunnel syndrome in which open exploration of the median nerve would be necessary.

On the other hand, the selective and minimally invasive technique using the retinaculotome makes it the method of choice in diabetics and in patients undergoing hemodialysis following renal failure. However, open tenosynovectomy is preferred for dialyzed patients with hypertrophied flexor tenosynovium. In addition, the Paine retinaculotome can be utilized in cases of posttraumatic carpal tunnel syndrome with displaced carpal fractures or intercarpal dislocations. However, the closed technique is contraindicated if there exist posttraumatic bony deformities that need to be corrected.

Double-level compression of the median nerve, at the wrist as well as at the elbow or in the neck, is not a contraindication for the Paine technique. However, the patient must be warned about the possibility of incomplete relief from his symptoms following surgery.

Use of the Paine technique is also justified in elderly patients with long-standing symptoms and persistent pain, even if the thenar muscles are already atrophied. In fact, it has been shown that some clinical and electromyographic improvement does occur even following such delayed decompression of the carpal tunnel [28]. We feel that use of a minimally invasive technique is more important than exploration and neurolysis of the median nerve.

Finally, we strongly advise against doing the surgery on both hands during the same operation, even though the simplicity of the procedure makes it feasible. Disappearance of the symptoms in the opposite hand following surgery on one side is well known [26]. We call this phenomenon the "reset" effect, which enables the patient to resume normal activities very quickly and to rehabilitate the operated hand.

Surgery on the opposite hand can be considered later if the "reset" effect proves transitory and the symptoms recur or become disconcerting.

In a recent study of 362 operated cases [26], we noted that the "reset" effect persisted until 20 days after the operation in 120 cases (33%) and at 7 months in 160 cases (44%). However, the same study revealed worsening of symptoms on the opposite side following unilateral surgery in 47 patients (13%) at 20 days and in 111 cases (31%) at 7 months.

Finally, an interesting and practical suggestion would be to exclude all cases of unilateral carpal tunnel syndrome if it cannot be conclusively proved to be "primary" or due to repetitive stress to that hand at work.

In fact, one must look for conditions other than primary carpal tunnel syndrome in all cases with unilateral symptoms. To this end, one can utilize investigations such as radiographs, ultrasonography, MRI, and/or hematological tests necessary to determine any secondary cause of median nerve compression.

Apart from carpal tunnel syndrome due to excessive use of one hand, unilateral cases are extremely uncommon. In fact, the large majority of cases of carpal tunnel syndrome are "primary" in origin, i.e., due to a constitutional stenosis of the carpal tunnel. The symptoms occur mainly in the dominant hand or the hand that is more involved at work. This is supported by a recent observation [30] that 87% of patients with symptoms of carpal tunnel syndrome present with bilateral affection while the remaining 13% of cases with unilateral symptoms show evidence of median nerve compression on electrophysiological tests in the opposite hand, indicating subclinical involvement. Other authors [1, 9, 34] have shown with CT scan measurements that patients with carpal tunnel syndrome have a significantly narrower canal as compared to normal controls. In this context, one must emphasize that the retinaculotome divides the transverse carpal ligament progressively in its passage along the carpal tunnel so that an additional instrument does not compromise the narrow space within the canal at any stage of the procedure. It differs from other closed techniques in this respect; all other procedures involve insertion of an instrument (although smooth) within the restricted space of the canal prior to decompression. In practice, the use of the retinaculotome is truly atraumatic for the median nerve as well as the other adjacent structures.

Complications and Results

The safety of the Paine technique is due to the qualities of the instrument as well as the care taken in each step of the procedure. The smooth and blunt superior border above the blade pushes aside structures superficial to the transverse carpal ligament and helps protect even anomalous tissues such as a communicating branch between the median and ulnar nerves [10, 11] (Fig. 29.7). Such a branch and all its variant forms would be more susceptible to injury in carpal tunnel release by the open or by an endoscopic technique [10] rather than with the Paine method.

The flattened spatula below the blade retracts and protects the underlying flexor tendons and their synovial sheaths (Fig. 29.7). Resting the base on the ulnar aspect of the carpal tunnel allows us to run the instrument along the hook of the hamate so that the transverse carpal ligament is divided close to its ulnar insertions. This provides protection to the median nerve, which lies radially, as well as its motor branch (in all its varia-

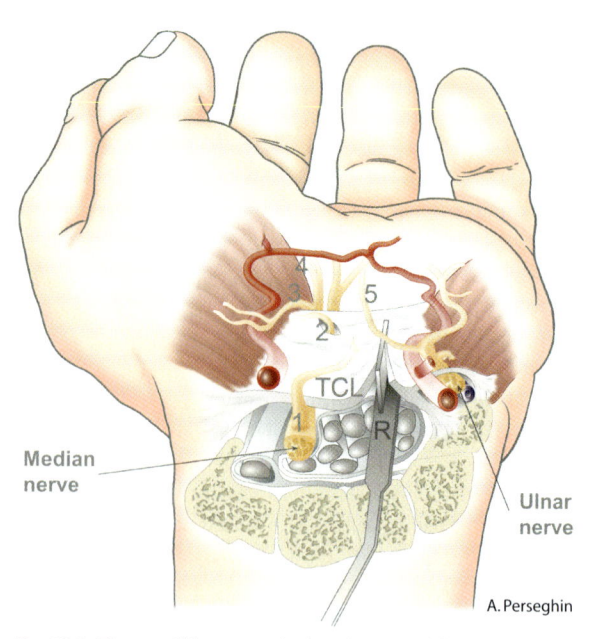

Fig. 29.7. The possible anatomical variations of the median and ulnar nerves [33–35] with respect to the division of the transverse carpal ligament using the Paine retinaculotome. *TCL*: transverse carpal ligament; *R*: Paine retinaculotome; *1*: palmar cutaneous branch of the median nerve; *2*: transligamentous variant of the motor branch (23%); *3*: subligamentous variant of the motor branch (31%); *4*: extraligamentous variant of the motor branch (46%); *5*: communicating branch in the palm between the median and the ulnar nerves

tions) [18] and the palmar cutaneous branch [37] (Fig. 29.7). In addition, the defect in the transverse carpal ligament and the consequent scarring does not overlie the median nerve. This could explain the low incidence of recurrent symptoms as well as the minimal loss of grip strength following this procedure. Finally, the superficial palmar arch lies 2–26 mm beyond the distal edge of the flexor retinaculum [7] and there is no risk of injury from the blade of the retinaculotome.

We presented a large series of cases in 1997 [24] in which we found that there were no complications such as iatrogenic lesions (of any type), hematomas, postoperative sepsis or reflex sympathetic dystrophy in 853 patients operated upon by five different surgeons between 1990 and 1996. There were 28 failures (3%) of which 8 had incomplete relief. Two of these eight patients suffered from diabetes mellitus while the remaining six had median nerve compression at two levels (double-crush).

There were 16 cases of early recurrence of symptoms (2%) that appeared within 3 months following surgery. In each of them, the cause of failure was found to be incomplete division of the transverse carpal ligament, which was revealed during secondary decompression by the open technique. These incidents of incomplete release could be attributed to the inexperience of the operating surgeon as the rate of failure progressively decreases when the surgeon has performed a large number of such procedures.

Late recurrence of symptoms (appearing beyond a year from the operation) was noted in 4 cases (0.5%). The cause of the recurrence was not evident during the second operation, which, in each case, produced complete and permanent relief from the symptoms.

We could hypothesize that the cause could be a defect in the technique employed in the first operation. If the site of section of the transverse carpal ligament was not adequately ulnar, the resulting scar could overlie the median nerve and produce perineural fibrosis and constriction. This, in turn, could be responsible for the recurrent symptoms. We have never found it necessary to convert the closed procedure to an open technique due to intraoperative problems. This indicates the simplicity of the Paine technique.

The so-called pillar syndrome [5] was a minor complication that we noted in 145 (17%) operated patients [26]. This refers to painful swelling in the interthenar region slightly toward the ulnar side, i.e., along the course of the blade of the retinaculotome. This complication occurred gradually after 15–30 days following the operation with complete absence of paresthesias. There was painful induration of the scar deep to the skin, apparently arising from the interfascial plane in which the retractors were placed. This is an irritating condition, at times alarming to the patient, especially as it is a new symptom that has appeared after surgery. However, it is always transitory and disappears gradually over a few months without compromising the result of surgery. Hence, it has been considered as a minor complication.

Another minor complication is a slight decrease in grip strength due to the division of the first and most important pulley for the flexor tendons. It occurs following carpal tunnel release by any technique and the patient must be warned in advance about its occurrence. In addition, it is always temporary. In our study [26], using the Jamar dynamometer, we constantly noted an average loss of grip strength of 1.6 kg for the right hand and 1.3 kg for the left hand at 20 days following surgery. However, at 7 months from the operation, we found an average increase in grip strength of 1.8 kg for the right hand and 2.2 kg for the left hand with respect to the values noted before surgery. Other authors [17] have shown a progressive increase in grip strength up to 2 years after the operation.

Even the thumb-index pinch grip decreases in the immediate postoperative period and, then, recovers to a level higher than the preoperative value. However, these variations are over a few grams and the patient is usually not informed about them [26].

The patient usually resumes work around 1–3 weeks after the operation with the Paine technique and the delay depends upon the type of work. It is very important to encourage the patients to resume some light work with the wrist in extension in order to prevent adhesions around the tendons and the median nerve. The patient is encouraged to resume normal activities of daily living with respect to the operated hand from the day of surgery itself and to take care to keep the wrist extended in all movements.

Thus, occupational rehabilitation is started very early taking care to instruct the patients to increase their activities gradually in order to avoid evoking a reactive tenosynovitis.

In patients who have been properly informed, we have noted excellent compliance with respect to the surgery and postoperative therapy. This occurs despite the fact that most of these patients are operated upon in "day surgery" and drive home the same day. In addition, we feel that it is very important to re-evaluate these patients clinically at periodic intervals. We review our patients on the day following surgery, after 8–10 days and at a month after the operation. We advise the patients to come back for review if any new symptoms occur or, in any case, at a year with an electromyogram of the opposite hand.

We also warn the patients about the possibility of flexor tenosynovitis in all the fingers due to the overloading of the pulleys following division of the flexor retinaculum. If such tenosynovitis is noted, with or without triggering of the finger, we infiltrate a locally acting steroid solution into the tendon sheath and this usually provides relief without recourse to surgery. We found this problem in 11% of our cases operated upon by the Paine technique [26].

In conclusion, we are convinced that the excellent results obtained following carpal tunnel release using the Paine retinaculotome depend upon the qualities of the instrument itself, application of precise indications, and rigorous adherence to the details of the surgical procedure. Thus, the procedure becomes safer, selective, and can be performed at very low cost.

The Modified Retinaculotome MDC

In April, 2003, when Dr. Luchetti requested us to provide a translation of our chapter in English, we had recently started using a modified version of the retinaculotome. It was designed for patients whose hands were of a smaller size than the average. We decided to call it the MDC after the initials of the names of the authors. We would now like to elaborate the modifications made in the version of the retinaculotome described earlier.

We had already noted that the Paine retinaculotome enabled us to operate upon any patient with carpal tunnel syndrome. However, in patients with very small wrists, particularly in women of short stature, we felt that the original retinaculotome occupied too much space in the canal with respect to the size of the wrist.

For this reason, we decided to modify the instrument in order to adapt to the smaller size of the canal in such patients. The new design is represented in Fig. 29.8. It is slightly smaller than the Paine retinaculotome but the height of the blade remains the same. The broad base of the blade, too, is tapered. In addition, we have introduced a curve in this base and increased the angulation of the handle of the instrument. These simple modifications help adapt the retinaculotome to the altered conditions in smaller wrists so that the instrument follows the course of the flexor retinaculum. In fact, the tapered base of the blade allows the instrument, which rests on the hook of the hamate, to constantly maintain the course of section of the flexor retinaculum along its ulnar aspect even as it widens distally (Fig. 29.9). The curved form of the instrument enables it to follow the inclination of the flexor retinaculum (Fig. 29.10). Finally, the greater vertical angulation of the handle improves the execution of the operation as it ensures that the surgeon's hand does not impinge on the patient's forearm.

In the 73 cases operated upon using the MDC during 2003, with, however, a short follow-up, we have obtained results similar to those seen using the classical Paine retinaculotome. Thus, we maintain that the MDC is a refined instrument more adapted to suit surgery for patients with smaller wrists. In such cases, the modifications have proved to be very important in facilitating the execution of this operation, which has often been termed as minor surgery or as surgery of well-being. Although this operation does not save lives, it does, however, improve the quality of life for the patients and, hence, cannot be trivialized. In fact, partial improvement is not acceptable in such cases and modifications in the described surgical techniques are necessary and justified.

Acknowledgements. The authors thank Dr. Anil Bhatia for his help in translating this article into English, Andrea Bozzetti for the technical designs and Francesco Mantovani for his help with the computer.

References

1. Bleecker ML, Bohlma M, Moreland R et al. (1985) Carpal tunnel syndrome: role of carpal canal size. Neurology 37: 1599.
2. Bonola A, Caroli A, Celli L (1981) La mano. Piccin ed. Padova, pp 257–259

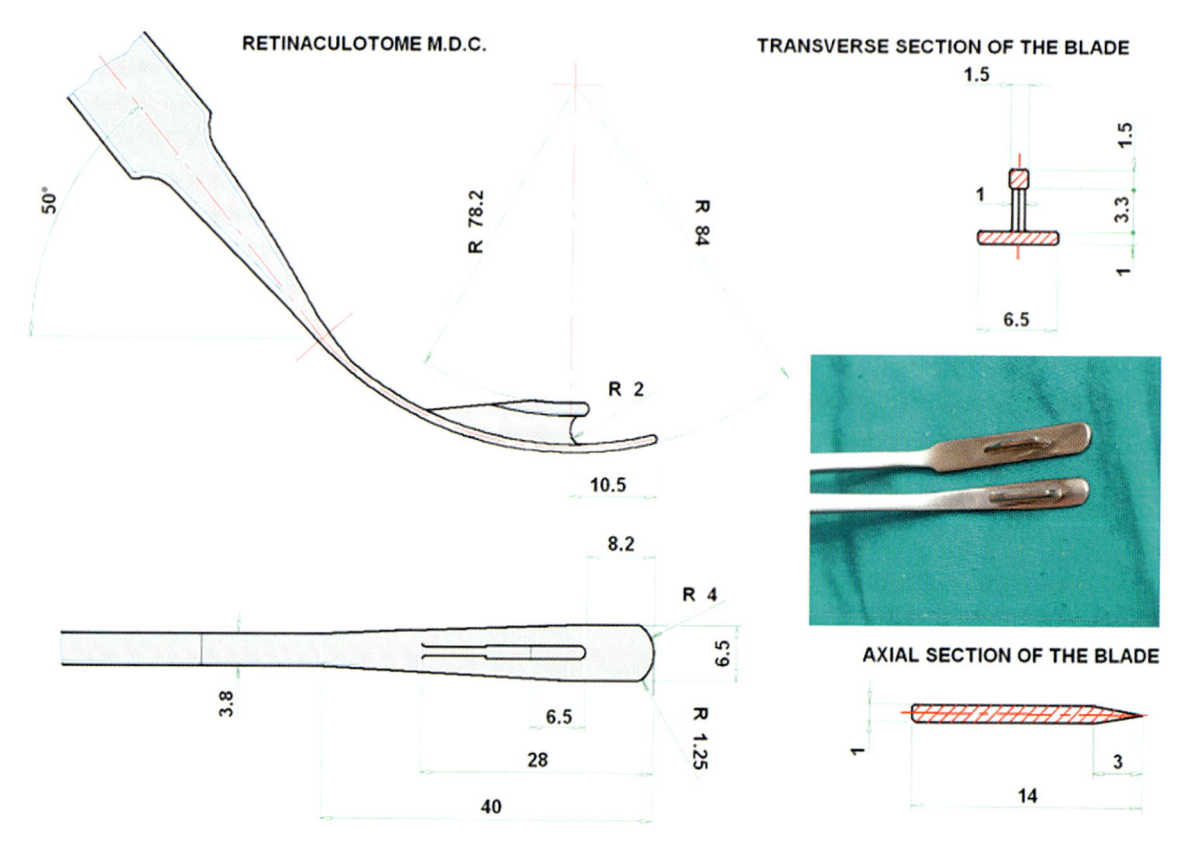

Fig. 29.8. Comparative photograph of the Paine retinaculotome and retinaculotome MDC technical design (distributed in Italy by DIMA)

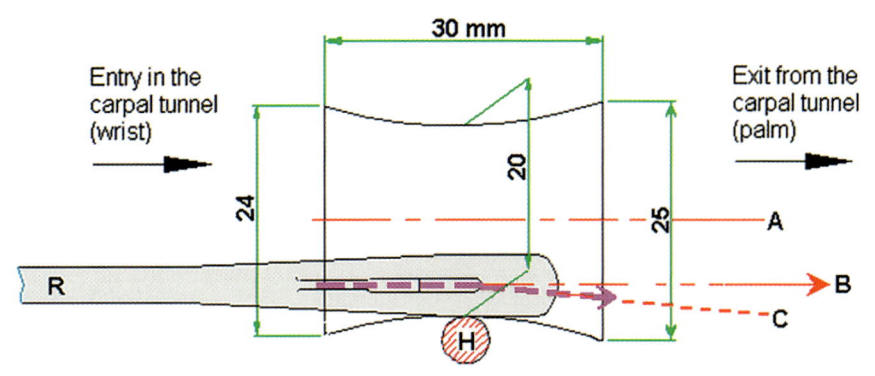

Fig. 29.9. A central coronal section of the left carpal tunnel containing the retinaculotome MDC (*R*) and its line of action (*C*). Due to the shape of the canal, the narrowest part lies at the level of the hook of the hamate (*H*) [17]. The figures in millimeters refer to the average values for the dimensions of the carpal tunnel [17]. The instrument is pushed in the proximo-distal direction along the axis of the fourth digital ray (*B*), resting on the hook of the hamate. The tapering base of the blade ensures that the flexor retinaculum is divided along a course that occupies the most ulnar portion of the retinaculum, i.e., along the *line C* while the instrument is directed along the *axis B*. A: central axis of the carpal tunnel. B: axis of the retinaculotome MDC and of the fourth digital ray. C: line of section of the flexor retinaculum

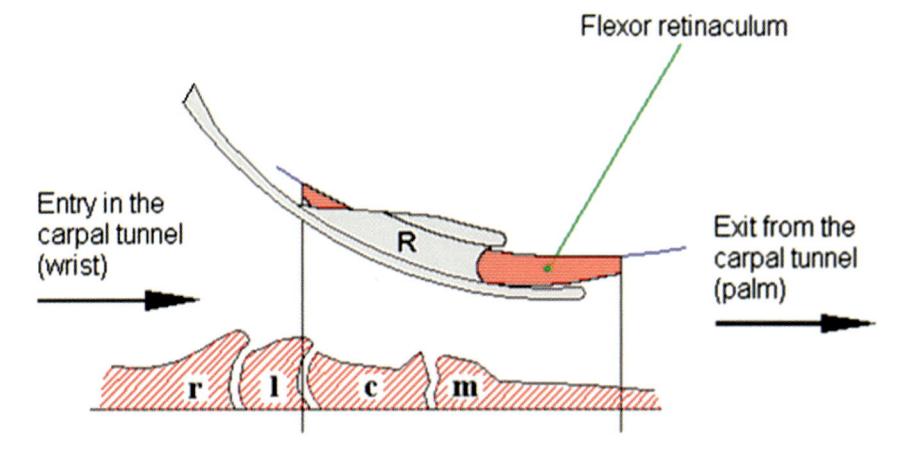

Fig. 29.10. The sagittal section of the carpal tunnel along the axis of the fourth digital ray with the passage of the retinaculotome MDC (*R*) as it divides the flexor retinaculum. The retinaculum is inclined in the proximo-distal direction and in the dorso-palmar plane [17] and the curved form of the instrument enables it to follow this inclination. r: radius; l: lunate; c: capitate; m: fourth metacarpal

3. Cadot B, Le Corre N, Michaud Y (1996) Syndrome dit idiopathique du canal carpien: techniques chirurgicales. In: 17eme Cours de chirurgie de la main e du membre supérieur de l'Hopital Bichat, Paris, Faculté Xavier Bichat 25–26 janvier 1996, pp 204–211
4. Carneiro RS, James K (1995) Release of carpal tunnel syndrome with the retinaculatome. In proceedings of the 6th Congress of the International Federation of Societies for Surgery of the hand. Helsinki, Finland. 3–7 july 1995, abstract book, 0–490
5. Clayton ML, Linsheid RL (1988) Carpal tunnel surgery: should the incision be above or below the wrist? Point-counterpoint in Orthopedics 11–5:819
6. Cobb TK, Dalley BK, Posteraro Rh et al. (1993) Anatomy of the flexor retinaculum. J Hand Surg 18A:91
7. Cobb TK. Knudson GA, Coony (1995) The use of topographical landmarks to improve the outcome of Agee endoscopic carpal tunnel release. Arthroscopy 11:165
8. Cobb TK, Carmichael SW, Cooney WP (1996) Guyon's canal rivisited: An anatomy study of the carpal ulnar neurovascular space. J Hand Surg 21A: 861
9. Dekel S, Papaioannou T, Rushworth G et al. (1980) Idiopathic carpal tunnel syndrome caused by carpal stenosis. Br Med J 280:1297
10. Don Griot JPW, Zuidam JM, Van Kooten OE et al. (2000) Anatomic study of the ramus communicans between the ulnar and median nerves. J Hand Surg 25 A: 948
11. Ferrari GP, Gilbert A (1991) The superficial anastomosis on the palm of the hand between the ulnar and median nerve. J Hand Surg 16B:511
12. Foucher G (1994) Chirurgie des sindromes canalaires du poignet. Encycl Med Chir- Tecniques Chirurgicales. Orthopedie Traumatologie 44–362
13. Gelberman RH, Pfefer GB, Galbraith RT et al. (1987) Results of treatment of severe carpal tunnel syndrome without internal neurolysis of the median nerve. J Bone Joint Surg 69A:896
14. Grangié S, Ciaraldi A, Baietta D et al. (1992) La sindrome del tunnel carpale. Valutazione a confronto di due metodiche chirurgiche. Lo scalpello 6:345
15. Gray H, Clemente CD (Eds.) Anatomy of the Human Body. 13th ed. Philadelfia (1985) Lea & Febiger, pp 531, 542, 551
16. Hoppenfeld S, deBoer P (1984) Surgical exposures in orthopedics: the anatomic approach. Philadelfia: JB Lippincott, pp 162–165
17. Katz JN, Fossel KK, Simmons BP et al. (1995) Symptoms, functional status and neuromuscular impairment following carpal tunnel release. J Hand Surg 20A:549
18. Lanz U (1977) Anatomical variations of the median nerve in the carpal tunnel. JHand Surg 2:44
19. Lowry W Jr, Follender AB (1988) Interfascicular neurolysis in severe carpal tunnel syndrome. Clin Orthop 227: 252
20. Luchetti R, Catalano F, Cugola L et al. (1995) La sindrome del Tunnel carpale. Confronto fra decompressione endoscopica, a cielo aperto, mediante mini incisione ed a cielo chiuso. Studio Pluricentrico. Riv Chir Riab Mano Arto Sup 32:151

21. Mantovani A (1995) La sindrome del tunnel carpale: tecnica chirurgica con il retinacolotomo di Paine. In Video Giornale di Ortopedia Ed. Pfizer Italiana spa, Roma, 1995 Vol. 2
22. Mantovani A, Zambelli P, Pecori G (1991) L'uso del retinacololomo di Paine nella sindrome del tunnel carpale: primi risultati. Riv Chir Mano 28 – 3:213
23. Mantovani A, De Cristofaro L (1994) I.a decompressione del tunnel carpale con il retinacolotmo di Paine: aspetti innovativi della metodica. Riv Chir Riab Mano Arto Sup 31 – 33:264
24. Mantovani A, De Cristofaro L, Zambelli P (1997) Il trattamento in day surgery della sindrome del tunnel carpale con la tecnica di Paine e il protocollo valutativo di Nogara. In Atti 2° Congresso Nazionale Società Italiana di Chirurgia Ambulatoriale e day Surgery. Napoli. Italia, 26 – 28 giugno1997, Casa Ed. Mattioli. Fidenza 1997, pp 169
25. Mantovani A, De Cristofaro L, Zambelli P (1997) Protocollo valutativo informatizzato di Nogara per la sindrome del tunnel carpale. Riv Chir Riab Mano Arto Sup 34:19
26. Mantovani A, De Cristofaro L (1998) Analisi di un protocollo valutativo per la sindrome del tunnel carpale. http://www.aulsslegnago.it/pagina_convegni.htm
27. Mirza MA, King ET (1996) Newer techniques of carpal tunnel release. Orthopedic Clinics of North America 27 – 2: 355
28. Nolan WB, Alkaitis D, Glickel SZ et al. (1992) Results of treatments of severe carpal tunnei syndrome. J Hand Surg 17A:1020
29. Okutsu I, Hamanaka I, Tanabe T et al. (1996) Complete endoscopic carpal tunnel release in long term hemodialisis patients. J Hand Surg 21B:668
30. Padua L, Padua R, Nazaro M et al. (1998) Incidence of bilateral symptoms in carpal tunnel syndrome. J Hand Surg 23B:603
31. Paine KWE (1955) Instrument for dividing flexor retinaculum. Lancet 1:654
32. Paine KWE, Polyzoidis KS (1983) Carpal tunnel syndrome. Decompression using the Paine retinaculotome. J Neurosurg 59:1031
33. Pagnanelli DM, Barrer SJ (1991) Carpal tunnel syndrome: surgical treatment using the Paine retinaculotome. J Neurosurg 75:77
34. Papaioannou T, Rushworth G, Atar D et al. (1992) Carpal canal stenosis in man with idiopatich syndrome. Clin Orthop 285: 210
35. Srinivasan H (1995) Letters to editors. J Hand Surg 20A: 698
36. Szabo RM, Madison M (1992) Carpal tunnel syndrome. Orthopedic Clinics of North America 23 – 1: 103
37. Taleisnik J (1973) The palmar cutaneus branch of the median nerve and the approach of the carpal tunnel. J Bone Joint Surg 55A: 1212
38. Tzarnas CD (1993) Carpal tunnel release without a tourniquet. J Hand Surg 18A:1041

Closed Carpal Tunnel Release Technique with GRS 30

A. Atzei, M.D. Putnam, S. Tognon, L. Cugola

Introduction

The GRS (Guided Release System) consists of a disposable kit plus two resterilizable elements: an anatomic guide (right and left) (Fig. 30.1), that follows the physiological biplanar curve of the ulnar side of the carpal tunnel, and a probe with two ends: one smooth to be used as a dilator for the soft tissues of the carpal tunnel, the other one "spoon-shaped," to be used as a lift for the tip of the guide.

The disposable kit includes an elevator for the transverse carpal ligament (TCL) and a half-moon-shaped blade for the cut (Fig. 30.2), and a table of tests to evaluate the correct positioning of the guide during surgery (Fig. 30.3).

The GRS is electively indicated in idiopathic carpal tunnel syndrome (CTS), while clinical evidence of flexor tendons synovitis or a reduction in normal wrist range of motion (ROM) are only limited indications. The absolute contraindications to the use of this system are infections, failure of previous surgical treatment, or incomplete completion of the intraoperative functionality table of tests.

Surgical Anatomy and Skin Incision Landmarks

The mandatory condition for a correct surgery with this technique is an accurate knowledge of district anatomy, particularly identifying the so-called safe canal into the CT (Fig. 30.4), into which the guide has to be directed to correctly slide the blade for sectioning the TCL, maintaining a safe distance from the median nerve and the ulnar neuro-vascular bundle. The proxi-

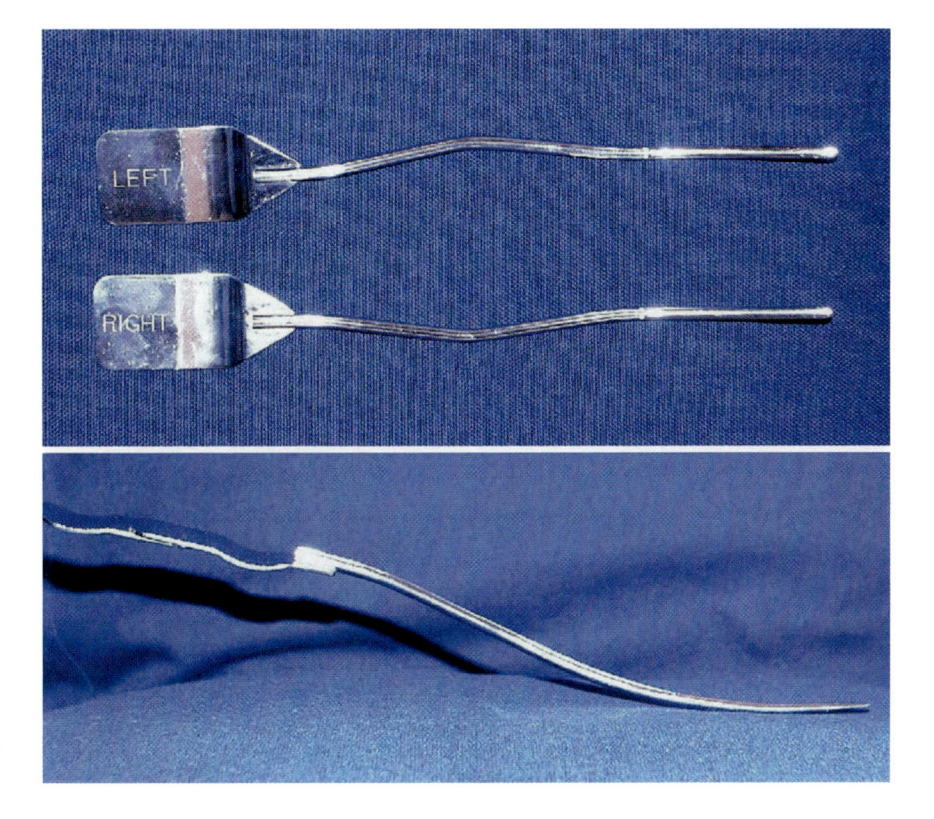

Fig. 30.1. Anatomic grooved guide

212 III Treatment

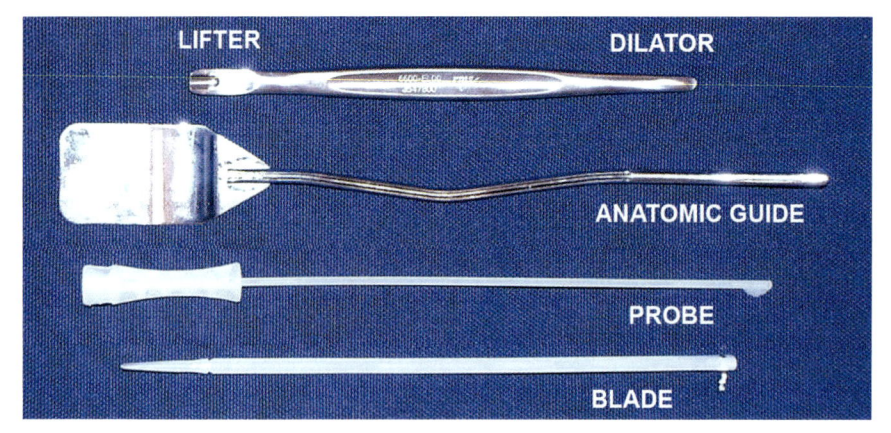

Fig. 30.2. GRS instrumentarium

Fig. 30.3. Functional intraoperative table: the three rows indicate the tests to be performed before and after guide positioning and after TCL incision

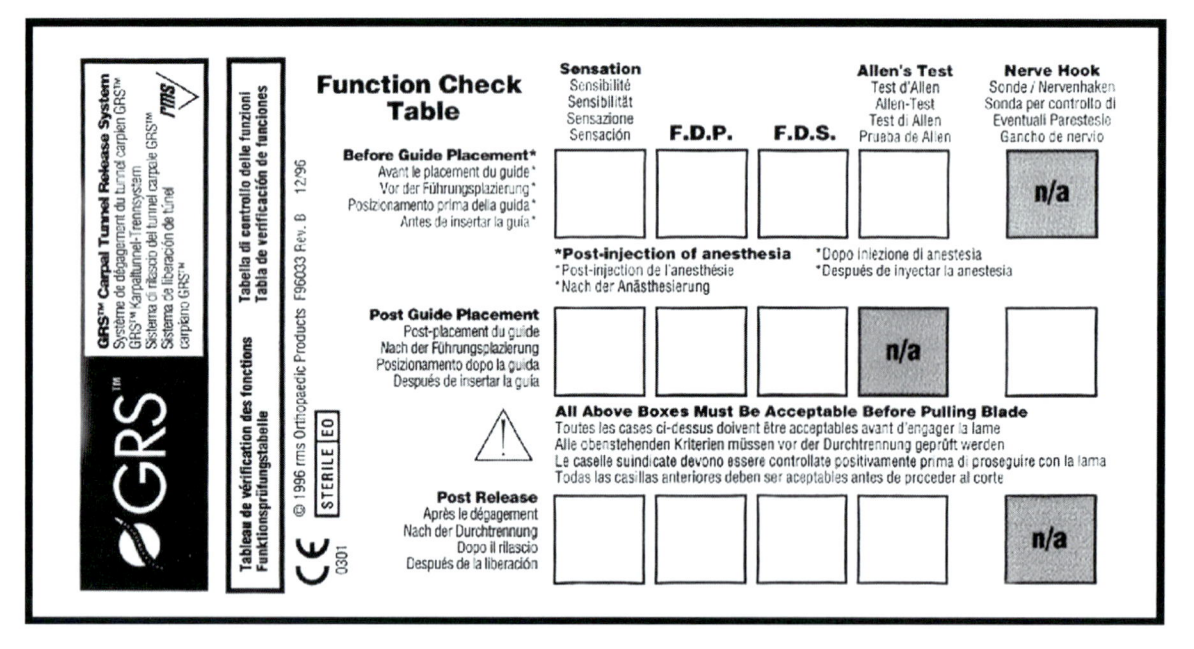

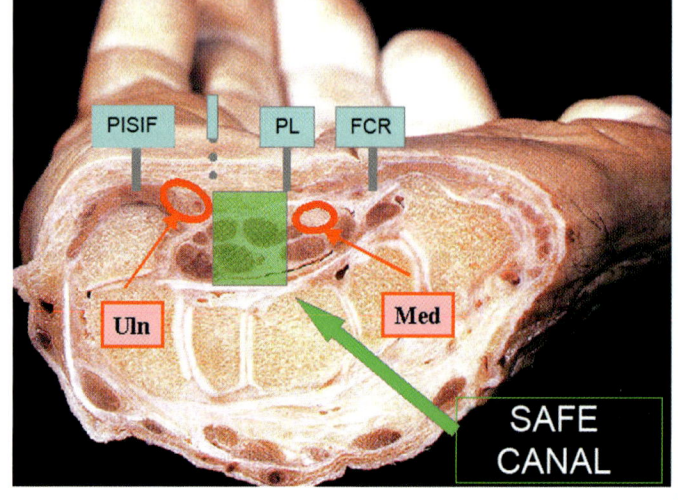

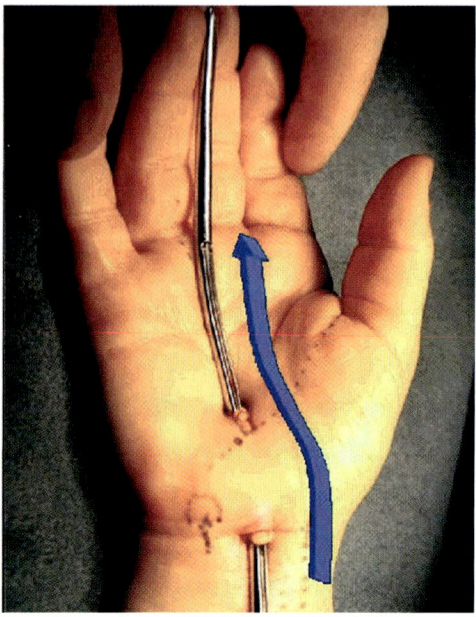

Fig. 30.4. Surgical anatomy of carpal tunnel: the safe canal is indicated in the section and in its winding development from the distal part of the forearm into the palm

mal margin of this canal is at the distal flexion crease of the wrist and corresponds to the middle third of the segment joining the skin projection of the flexor carpi radialis (FCR) tendon with the one of the center of the pisiform, or the radial-half of the segment joining the center of the pisiform with the palmaris longus (PL) tendon (in subjects in which this tendon is present). The safe canal has a specific spatial shape: aiming distally from the skin access in the distal forearm, it goes deep under the dorsal TCL surface, parallel to the longitudinal forearm axis for about 2 cm, just to reach the hook of the hamate around which it curves smoothly to exit in the palm, distally to the line of Kaplan, in line again with its proximal part.

The positioning of the anatomical guide into the safe canal is obtained by two skin incisions to be localized considering the following anatomic landmarks (Fig. 30.5):

1. Flexion distal crease of the wrist.
2. FCR tendon.
3. PL tendon.
4. Center of the pisiform: particular attention has to be given to finding the skin projection exactly perpendicular to the center of this bone, the surgeon being by the axillary side of the hand could draw the point too ulnarly, thereby entering the Guyon canal.
5. Cardinal line of Kaplan: distally to it one can draw the skin projection of the superficial palmar arch.
6. A line uniting the center of the second metacarpal head and the center of the pisiform: its intersection with the Line of Kaplan indicates the skin projection of the hook of the hamate [1].
7. A line running from the center of the fourth ray and the radial side of the PL tendon: it represents the interval between the terminal branches of the median nerve and those of the ulnar. In patients without the PL tendon it could be drawn from the radial side of the middle third of the segment joining the skin projection of the FCR tendon and the center of the pisiform on the distal flexion crease of the wrist.

The *proximal incision* is drawn on the diagonal of the square that has its base on the middle third of the segment joining the skin projection of the FCR tendon with the one of the center of the pisiform, or the radial half of the segment joining the center of the pisiform with the PL tendon (when present). The oblique direction is more convenient in order to avoid possible complications during surgery that would require conversion to an open release.

The *distal incision* is in the palm, just distally to the Kaplan line, often within 1 cm on the ulnar or radial side of the line passing from the center of the fourth ray and the radial side of the PL tendon. It is advisable to cut the skin after checking the exact positioning of the tip of the guide, palpating it through the skin.

Control of Correct Position of the Guide

Considering the cutaneous landmarks we just described, the guide can be easily introduced into the safe canal of the carpal tunnel, just near the deep surface of the TCL, without interfering with the flexor tendons and lying at a safe distance from adjacent vascular and nervous structures.

Since the GRS does not include any video-assisted tools, the control of the correct positioning of the device depends on the completion of the tests indicated in the functional table that comes with the sterile kit (Fig. 30.3). It consists of a series of common clinical tests to evaluate sensitivity of the median and ulnar nerves distally to the carpal tunnel, the function of superficial and deep flexors tendons for the fingers, Allen test for the superficial palmar arch integrity, and for eventual interposition of the median nerve or its ulnar nerve communicating branch between the TCL and the guide itself (palpatory test).

These tests must be performed after each of the following steps of the operative procedure:

Before the guide insertion, except for the palpator test, (test in the first row of the table); with the guide in

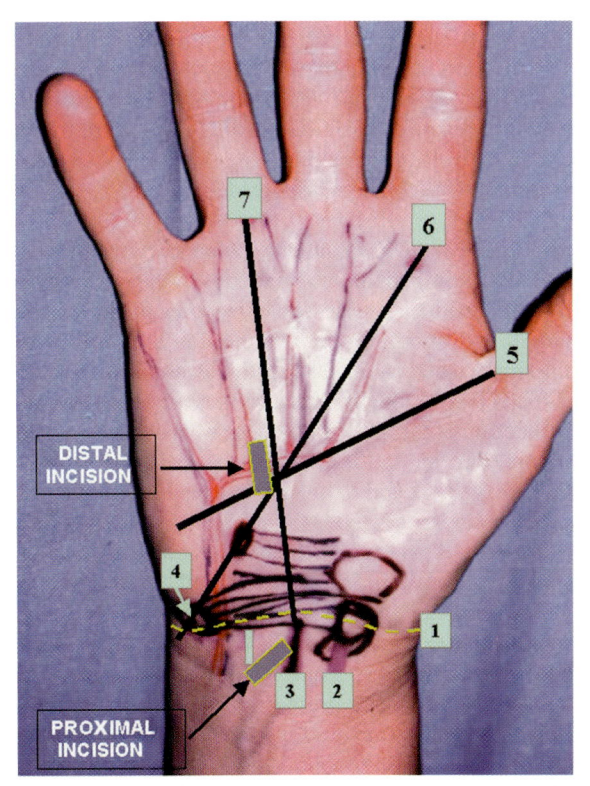

Fig. 30.5. Anatomical landmarks to set the skin incisions: for numbers see text

place, except for the Allen test (test in the second row of the table); after TCL sectioning, except for the palpator test (test in the third row of the table).

When registering digital sensitivity disturbance (paresthesia) and deep and superficial flexor tendons functional deficit (reduced excursion) during guide positioning, it is probable that the median/ulnar nerves (or their terminal branches) are compressed or contused, or that the impingement of a tendon between the TCL and the guide is produced; in these cases the guide has to be removed and repositioned as appropriate. If some test abnormalities after TCL sectioning (with an anesthetic area or a loss of digital flexion) are experienced, a nerve or flexor tendon lesion is probable, and has to be explored and repaired.

A failure of the Allen test after TCL sectioning indicates the compression of the superficial palmar arch or its damage (accompanied by significant bleeding) and will have to be explored and repaired.

The introduction of the palpator along the groove of the guide before the TCL sectioning enables the surgeon to feel the classical "railway sign" transmitted to the palpator handle. In order to find the railway sign, it is recommended to repeat the gliding of the instrument a few times, to find the railway sign and to position the guide again in the presence of one of the following circumstances:

- An abnormal digital movement (which indicates interposition of a tendon between the TCL and the guide)
- The patient reports the appearance of a significant Tinel sign (which indicates interposition of a nerve between the guide and the TCL)

In such cases (a sensation of "blocking" or some pressure the patient feels in the center of the wrist or hand are the only acceptable disturbances), it is advisable to extract and reposition the guide in an appropriate position. When symptoms are still present after guide reposition, mainly when the neurological signs are persistent, it is preferable to convert to open carpel tunnel release (OCTR).

Surgical Technique

The technique of surgical carpal tunnel release with the GRS makes provision for eight surgical steps as follows:

Anesthesia and Carrying Out of the Intraoperative Tests (First Row): With a solution of carbocaine and marcaine in equal doses, without epinephrine, infiltrate only the skin and subcutaneous tissues just to the fascial plane, in the areas corresponding to the skin incisions and the tract the blade has to follow to section the TCL, as described in Fig. 30.6. When administering

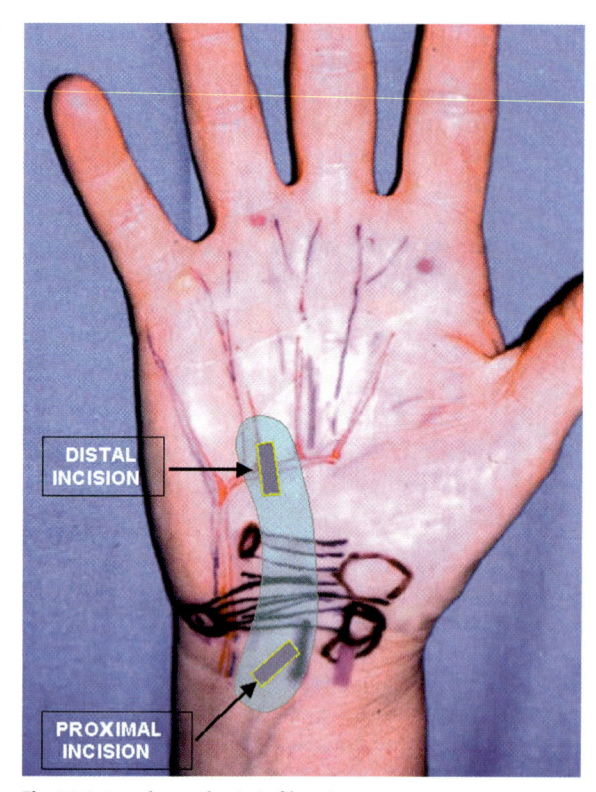

Fig. 30.6. Local anesthesia infiltration area

the anesthesia the tests of the first row have to be checked. It is essential that the anesthetic reaches only the skin and subcutaneous tissues, because if it went down to a deeper plane evaluation of distal sensitivity would become impossible, exposing the patient to the risk of neurological complications: in such a case conversion to OCTR has to be considered.

Proximal Portal Assessment: After cutting the skin and descending to the subcutaneous tissue one reaches the antebrachial fascia. The dissection plane for the handle of the blade for the TCL incision is superficial to the antebrachial fascia. Deeper to the fascia, an incision is made longitudinally which creates a path for the introduction of the guide into the safe canal of the carpal tunnel (Fig. 30.7). It is advisable to use a little Freer to palpate the TCL and to be sure to free the antebrachial fascia from subcutaneous tissue and the synovium. It is also essential to avoid entering the Guyon canal: in this case the patient could report a violent Tinel at the ulnar nerve territory and it will not be possible to palpate the wrinkled deep surface of the TCL or feel the hook of the hamate with the Freer or the guide itself. When neurological symptoms are present a new, accurate evaluation of guide position and/or a re-evaluation of the dissection planes is advisable.

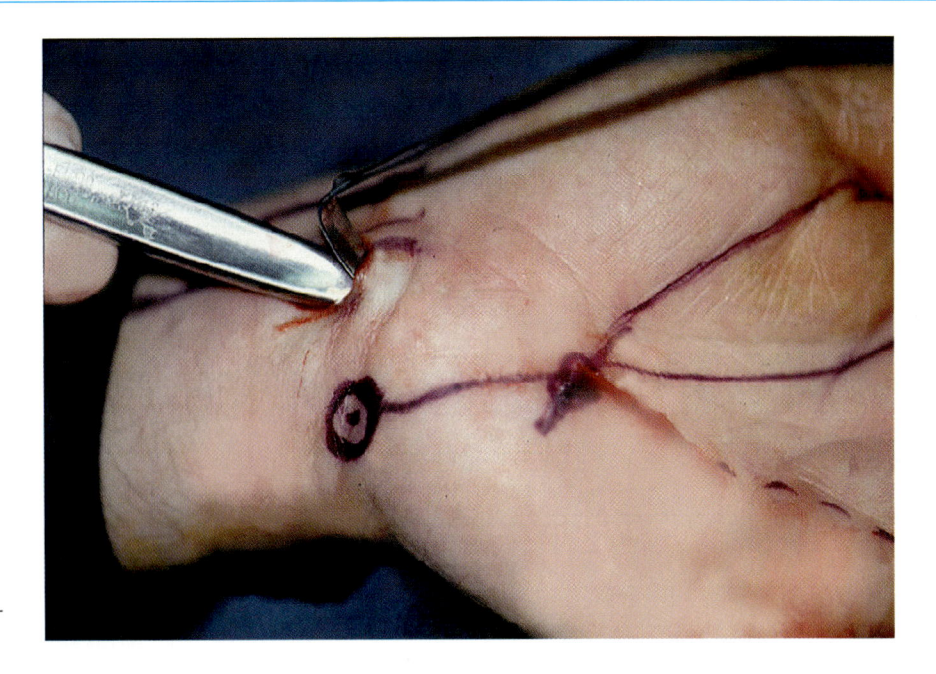

Fig. 30.7. Spreader introduction

Introduction of the Dilator: The dilator has to be used to widen the tracts through which the guide and the handle of the blade have to be inserted for the TCL incision. Initially, the instrument has to be inserted under the antebrachial fascia, into the carpal tunnel, aiming distally towards the exit area in the palm, to make it ready for the passage of the grooved guide. During instrument introduction one has to feel the railway sign given by the deep surface of the TCL and the touching of the hook of the hamate. The lack of these findings or the appearance of neurological troubles indicate a possible misposition of the instrument into the Guyon canal, and it is advisable to repeat the procedure. A feeling of "blocking" or of pressure in the center of the wrist represents the only acceptable disturbances during this phase. Following this, the dilator is introduced into the subcutaneous tissue, over the antebrachial fascia and the TCL towards the exit area in the palm to get the way ready for the handle of the blade for the dissection of the TCL itself.

Distal Portal Assessment: Once the dilator is inserted, its tip could be palpated into the palm, over the distal border of the TCL, in the area in which the line between the center of the fourth ray and the radial border of the PL tendon crosses the Kaplan line. The ideal incision stays on the cutaneous projection of the superficial palmar arch, distally to the carpal tunnel and slightly radially to the hook of the hamate. After cutting the skin, much attention has to be given to dissecting the deep planes. It is advisable to proceed as follows:

- Expose the palmar aponeurosis
- Separate its longitudinal fibers and cut the transverse ones
- Locate the distal margin of the TCL and possibly make a short longitudinal incision (2–3 mm,)
- Avoid being too distal with the exit of the guide.

Proceeding deeply one can isolate the common digital nerves and vessels and the superficial palmar arch that have to be protected during the subsequent phase of guide positioning.

Guide Positioning: First, select the anatomical guide appropriate for the side then proceed by introducing the guide from the proximal portal under the antebrachial fascia. The guide is aimed distally at a 45° angle with respect to the antebrachial plane. Push the guide slightly with only two fingers (to avoid creating an incorrect path instead of the one created by the dilator) just under the TCL (it is possible to feel the railway sign, which confirms the exact positioning of the guide) (Fig. 30.8). During its progression distally along the ulnar border of the carpal tunnel, the tip of the guide reaches the hook of the hamate, which can be avoided by tilting the handle slightly ulnar. After surpassing the distal border of the TCL, the tip of the instrument can be felt in the area in which the distal portal had been previously localized. After cutting the skin and separating the subcutaneous tissues, the palmar arch and the vascular and nervous structures have to be moved away from the exit trajectory of the guide with the elevator. When the guide exits the skin it is possible to divaricate the edges of the distal incision to visualize the distal margin of the TCL and verify that the superficial palmar arch is not over the guide. For an easier insertion, it is possible to slightly extend the wrist on a rolled-up towel and to insert the guide rotated at a 90° angle with

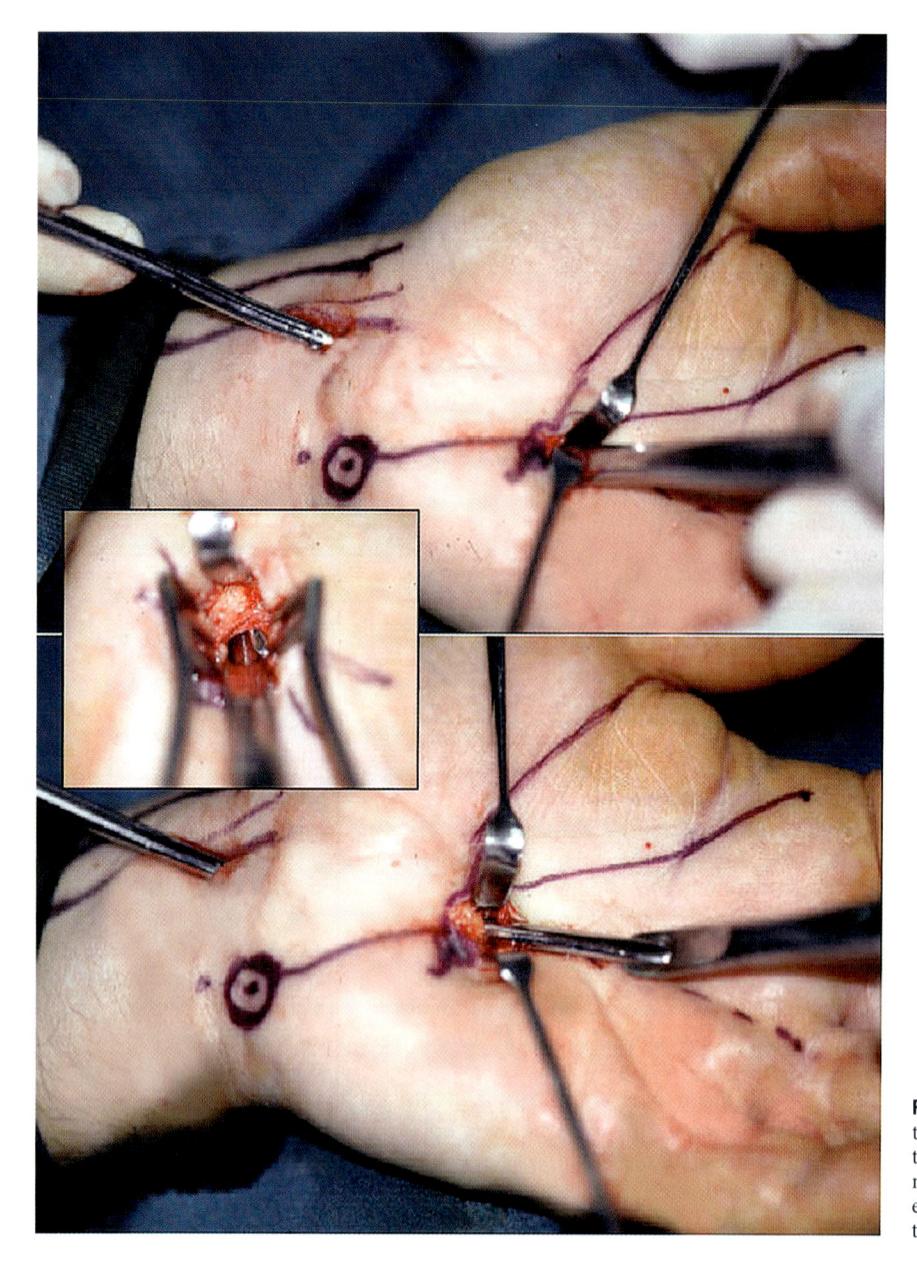

Fig. 30.8. Guide positioning: the *insert* shows the distal tip coming out from the palmar incision, under the CTL, elevated from the "spoon" tip of the spreader

respect to the table (with the flat part of the handle on the previously indicated side and facing the ulnar side of the patient) just to reach the hook of the hamate, then rerotate on a horizontal plane (with the flat part of the handle parallel to the table) when exiting the distal portal. Thusly the guide "spontaneously" adapts to the anatomic shape of the carpal tunnel, near the hook of the hamate, and its extremity stays in the space between third and fourth fingers.

Use of the Palpator and Intraoperative Tests (Second Row): With the guide in place into the carpal tunnel, the surgeon performs the tests of the second row of the intraoperative functional table to verify the position of the instrument into the safe canal. The palpator for the TCL is inserted into the groove of the guide and pulled back and forth a few times to call attention to possible disturbances (Fig. 30.9): only when the surgeon can confirm the negativity of the tests will he or she start with the following phases of the GRS technique, otherwise it is advisable to convert to an OCTR.

One additional key point: The surgeon is able to look at the distal margin of the transverse carpal ligament and verify that the superficial palmar arch is not visible distal to the ligament and is thus "protected" by the guide.

Cutting of the TCL: With the guide lying in the carpal tunnel, the handle of the blade is inserted into the prox-

30 Closed Carpal Tunnel Release Technique with GRS   217

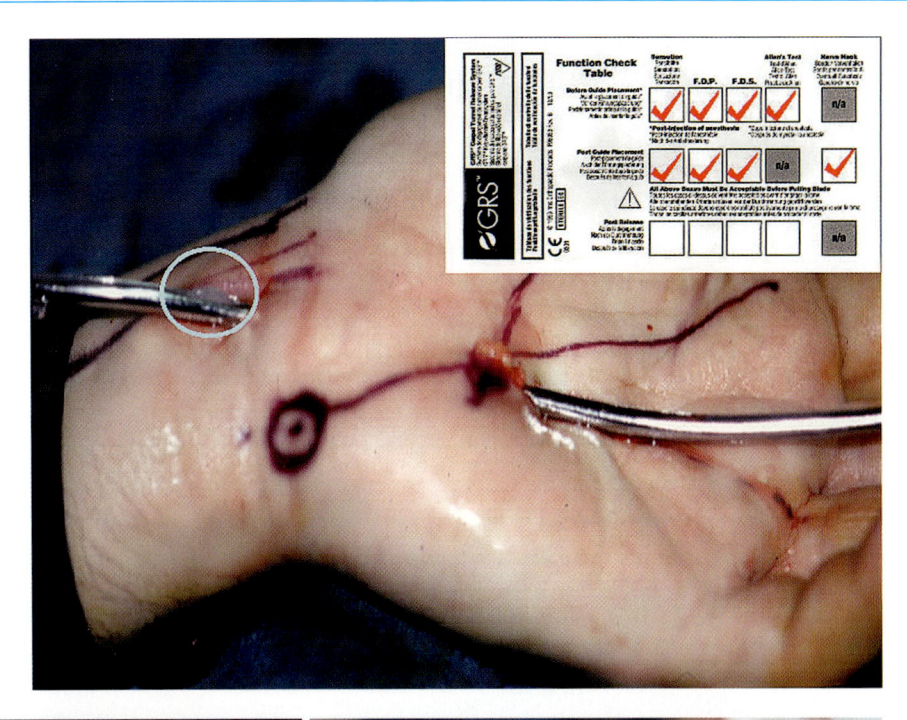

Fig. 30.9. Introduction of the elevator into the grooved guide and performance of the second intraoperative test series

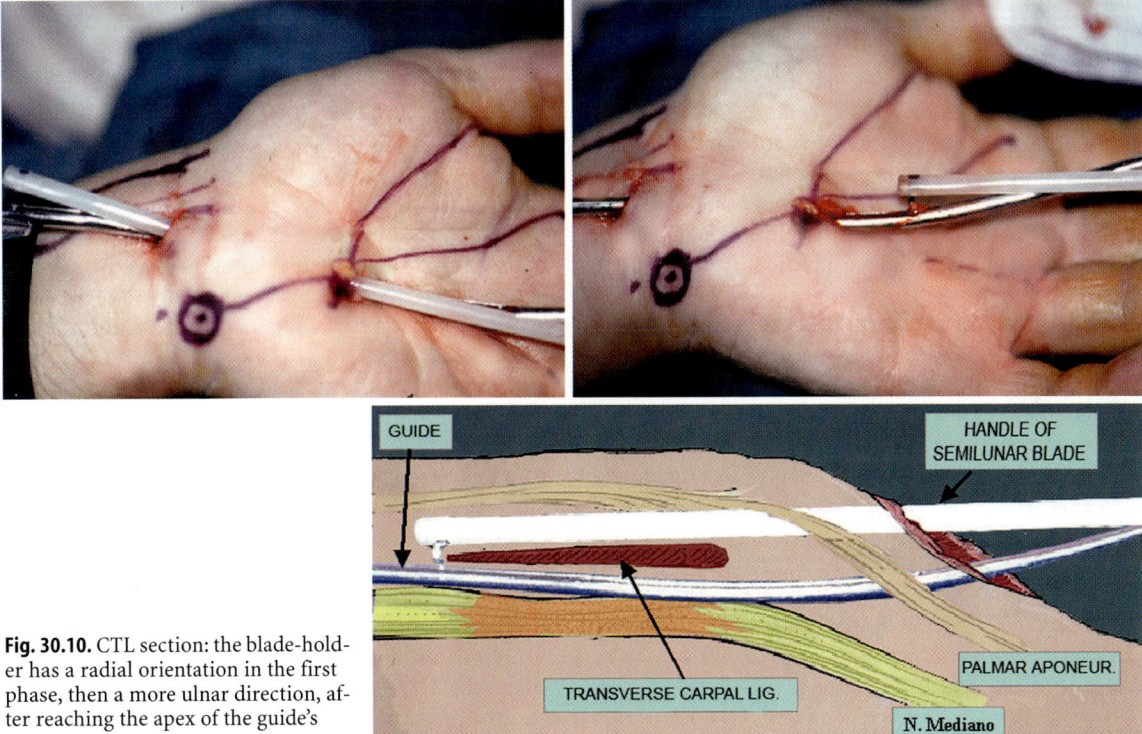

Fig. 30.10. CTL section: the blade-holder has a radial orientation in the first phase, then a more ulnar direction, after reaching the apex of the guide's curve

imal portal over the antebrachial fascia and the TCL and is pushed distally along the tract previously created with the dilator, exiting at the distal portal, parallel to the guide. To firmly grasp the blade for the traction maneuvers it is possible to insert the tip of the handle of the blade into the proximal side of the palpator. Then, the blade has to be released from its protection and the sphere on its tip is introduced into the groove of the guide. The proximal edge of the guide is stabilized by having the groove facing upwards during this maneuver. It is useful to divide this maneuver into two phases: during the first phase, the handle is maintained radial to the guide, then, when the blade has reached the apex of the curve of the guide; the second phase starts when the

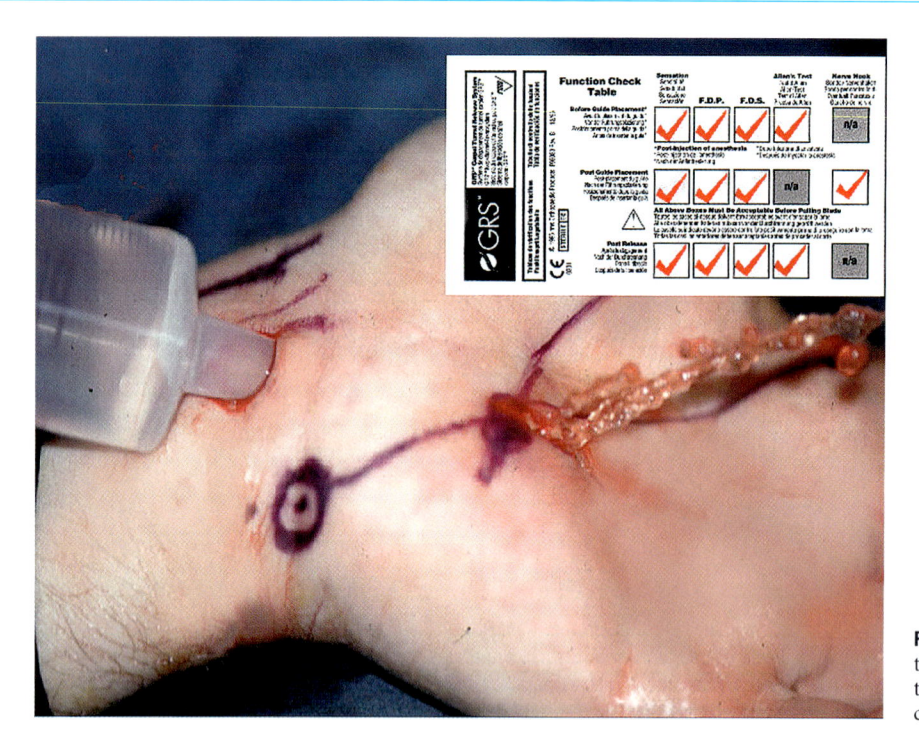

Fig. 30.11. Yellowstone-sign: the typical gush exits from the distal portal to confirm complete CTL release

traction maneuver is completed with the handle held in a more ulnar direction, with a constant and progressive pull (Fig. 30.10). If a sudden stop is encountered or the blade is stopped during its gliding into the guide, converting to an OCTR is advisable. In no case should the handle of the blade be pulled vertically since the instrument could break at the metal-plastic junction.

Intraoperative Tests (Third Row) and TCL Section Confirmation: Before removing the guide, the tests corresponding to the third row of the intraoperative evaluation table are performed. After the TCL is cut, the migration of the anesthetic could limit the results of the tests, possibly rendering them useless. The irrigation of the canal with some saline from the proximal portal typically produces a gush from the distal portal, indicating a complete TCL release (Yellowstone-sign) (Fig. 30.11).

Postoperative Treatment

A light bandage, allowing finger movement, is applied for about 2 weeks, during which time it is advisable to avoid flexing the wrist. Manual activities are gradually reintroduced during the third week, except hard hold with the wrist flexed, which must be postponed for 3 more weeks.

Discussion

A few endoscopic (ECTR) techniques were proposed during the second half of the 1980s, to allow carpal tunnel decompression preserving the palmar fascia, the subcutaneous connective tissue, and the skin of the proximal part pf the palm. Many perspective studies demonstrated that the advantages of these techniques consist of a reduced incidence of scar pain, a faster functional recovery, and an early return to work [2–5]. However, the need to use video-assisted instrumentation and a long learning curve represent limits to the diffusion of these techniques.

As an alternative to the ECTR techniques other researchers developed "percutaneous" TCL release techniques with the same simplicity and safety of execution of the OCTR classic technique, and into which a procedure could be converted in case of risk of intraoperative complications.

Having this target, M.D. Putnam of the University of Minnesota (USA) developed the GRS, based on the use of a grooved anatomical guide along which a blade is pulled to section the TCL in a "closed" manner, without video assistance.

The characteristics of being a minimally invasive technique and the chance to have an early functional recovery are the best advantages offered by the GRS technique. Moreover, another positive characteristic compared to other similar instrumentation is represented by the shape of the guide which, free from dimensional limits due to video-assisted tools, is able to anatomically adapt to the winding profile of the carpal tunnel and is of smaller dimension compared to the video-assisted instruments, in a way that permits the use of the GRS in so-called little or narrow wrists. In particular, not having excessive filling of the carpal canal, only anesthesia of the overlying skin is required, with good compliance from the patient, allowingclinical flexor tendon and sensitivity testing. So, even though a contusion of the tendinous or neuro-vascular structures is always possible during incorrect maneuvers, an accurate performing of the intraoperative tests reduces the risk of their injury or even partial section considerably.

The evaluation of a correct positioning of the guide thanks to the clinical tests represents the crucial phase of this operation, and guarantees the ability to work safely without video assistance. For this reason the surgeon must be completely sure of their effectiveness before sectioning the ligament. On the other hand, when the surgeon is not sure of the correct performing of the tests, as with anxious patients, it is advisable to convert to a traditional open technique, leaving the probe in the canal and exploring the nearby structures to check for possible lesions.

If, even though the technical help has been used during the various surgical steps, a tendinous or neuro-vascular lesion occurs, the changes in the clinical tests or conspicuous, pulsating bleeding will indicate such a complication and will prompt immediate treatment, thereby avoiding an unpleasant surprise for the surgeon and the patient, upon waking up, of a more extensive anesthetic block.

Injuries in clinical use with this method/tool have been rare. In the second author's (MDP) experience, collected in a training center, no nerve or tendon injuries have occurred in over 500 documented cases. In this same group of cases, one superficial palmar arch laceration occurred (arterial flow was not impaired and ends were ligated without sequelae) and 5 patients underwent an extended open release at a second setting for management of incomplete symptom resolution (less than 1% failure to achieve acceptable symptom improvement).

At least one anatomic study has reported on the relative safety of the approach employed by this method [6]. In this study, Abousahr, Patsis, and Chiu report on their experience using the same pathway for release in conjunction with a guided speculum and note their ability to isolate and accurately divide the ligament with a similar approach.

In sum, release of the transverse carpal ligament with a guide and captured knife appears to afford the same advantages of minimal incision methods with reduced equipment requirements and cost and may also lend safety because of the ability to carefully control the path of the knife and avoid Guyon's canal.

References

1. Cobb TK, Dalley BK, Posteraro RH et al. (1993) Anatomy of the Flexor retinaculum. J Hand Surg 18A: 91
2. Agee JM, McCarrol HR, Tortosa RD et al. (1992) Endoscopic release of the carpal tunnel: a randomized prospective multicenter study. J Hans Surg 17A: 987
3. Brown RA, Gelberman JH, Seiler JB III et al. (1993) Carpal tunnel release: A prospective randomized assessment for open and endoscopic methods. J Bone Joint Surg 75A: 1256
4. Chow JCY (1989) Endoscopic release of the carpal ligament: A new technique for carpal tunnel syndrome. Arthroscopy 5:19
5. Okutsu I, Ninomya M et al. (1987) Subcutaneous operation and examination under Universal Endoscope. J Jap Orthop Ass. 61: 491
6. Abouzahr MK, Patsis MC, Chiu DT (1995) Carpal tunnel release using limited direct vision. Plast Reconst Surg 95(3): 534–538

31 Carpal Tunnel Syndrome Release Using the Chiena Technique

V.P. De Tullio

Introduction

In recent years one of the most important concerns of surgeons is not to disrupt the biological homeostasis of the local soft tissue when performing surgery. Therefore, the trend is to develop the least invasive surgical methods possible. This work describes a new method that has been conceived following this guideline.

Surgical Technique

The tools are a retractor and scissors, congruent (Figs. 31.1, 31.2).

Surgery is performed under local anesthesia: 3–4 cc of 1% carbocaine are injected in between the subcutaneous spaces at the distal wrist crease (in the area between the flexor carpis radialis and flexor carpis ulnaris tendons) and in the subcutaneous space over the transverse carpal ligament (TCL) (Figs. 31.3, 31.4).

The arm is abducted at about 90°, the hand is supinated on the operative table, and the wrist is extended at about 45°. The skin is incised transversally through

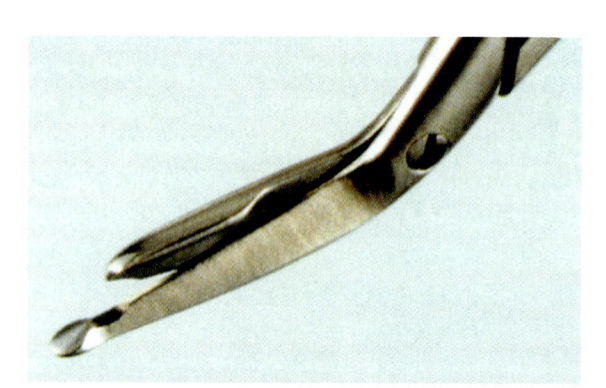

Fig. 31.1. The scissors

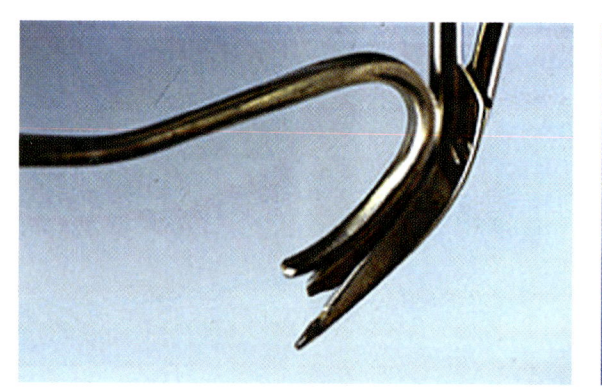

Fig. 31.2 Comparison between scissors and retractor

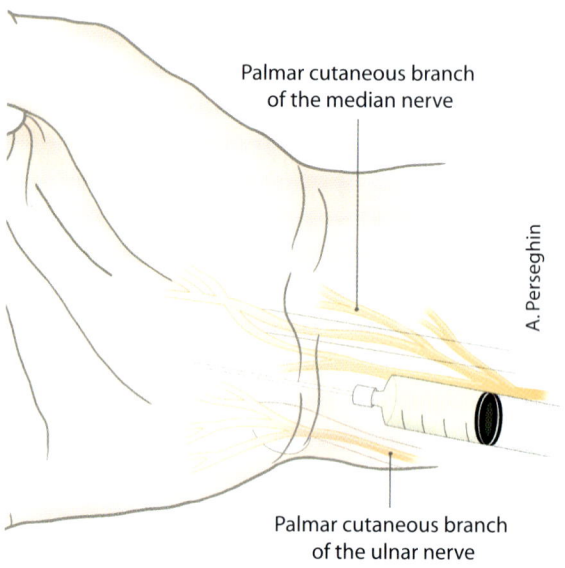

Fig. 31.3. Local anesthesia

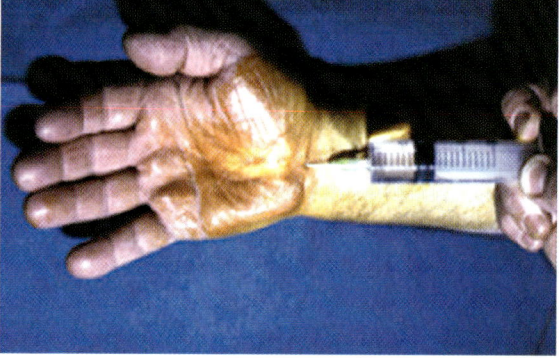

Fig. 31.4. Local anesthesia

about 1.5–2 cm in the central area of the distal wrist crease (Figs. 31.5, 31.6); afterward the deeper layers are bluntly dissected by the scissors in order to reach the fascia and the proximal border of the TCL; the tissues are dissected longitudinally in order to avoid the cutaneous branches of the ulnar and median nerves. If the cutaneous palmaris nerve runs through the radial area of the incision, it can be isolated and gently protected.

The antebrachial fascia is identified and the scissors bluntly enters through a 3-cm subcutaneous space over the TCL in order to create a passage for the insertion of the retractor (Figs. 31.7, 31.8).

A transverse 1-cm incision of the antebrachial fascia is performed at the level of the proximal border of the flexors retinaculum, starting on the ulnar side of the palmaris longus tendon when present. Performing gentle maneuvers, a plane is created between the deep surface of the transverse carpal ligament and the synovial membrane of the flexor tendons and the ulnar margin of the median nerve (Figs. 31.9, 31.10).

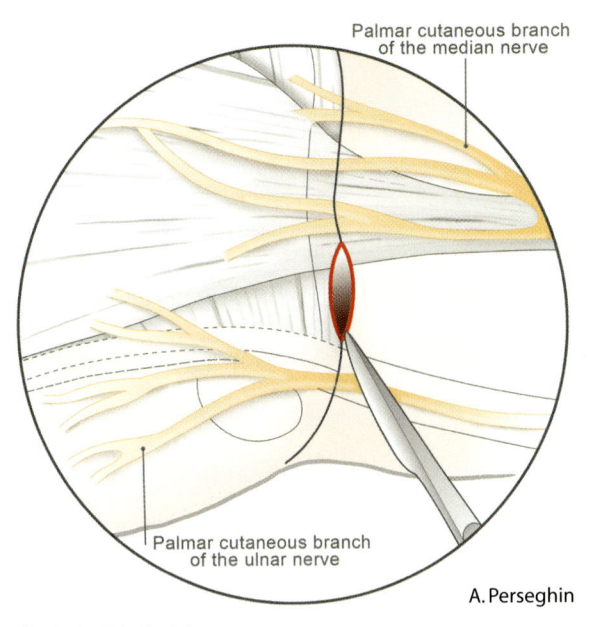

Fig. 31.5. Skin incision

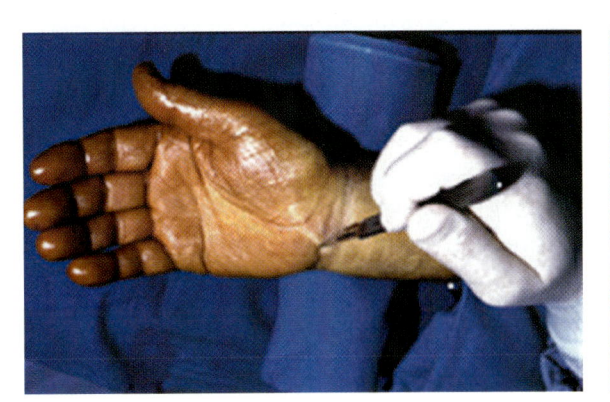

Fig. 31.6. Skin incision

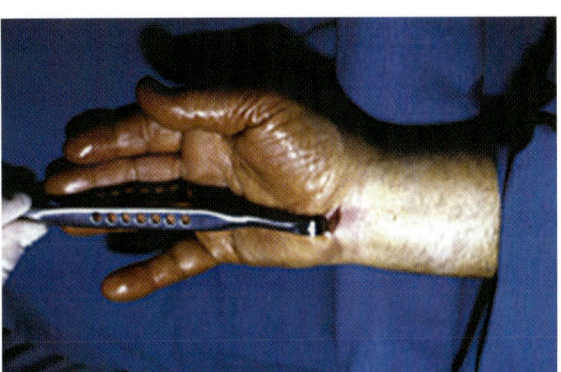

Fig. 31.8. Site of retractor introduction

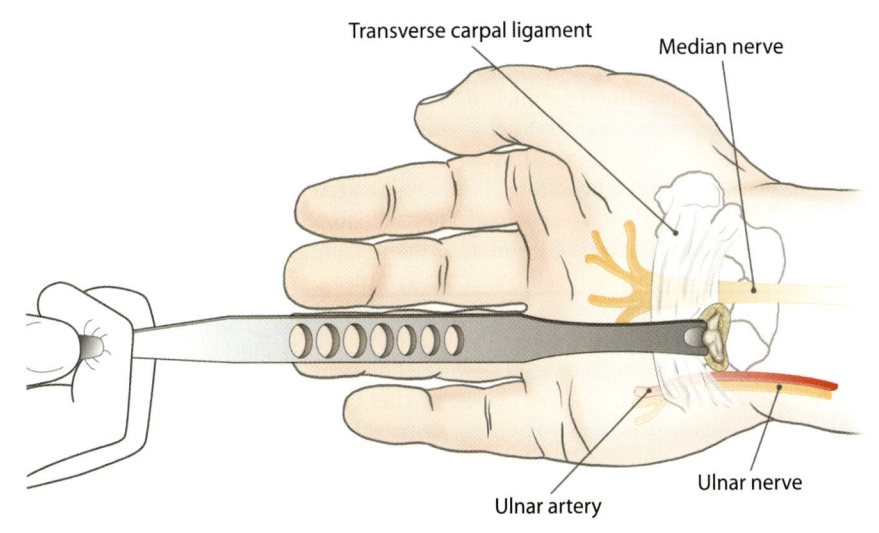

Fig. 31.7. Site of retractor introduction

222 III Treatment

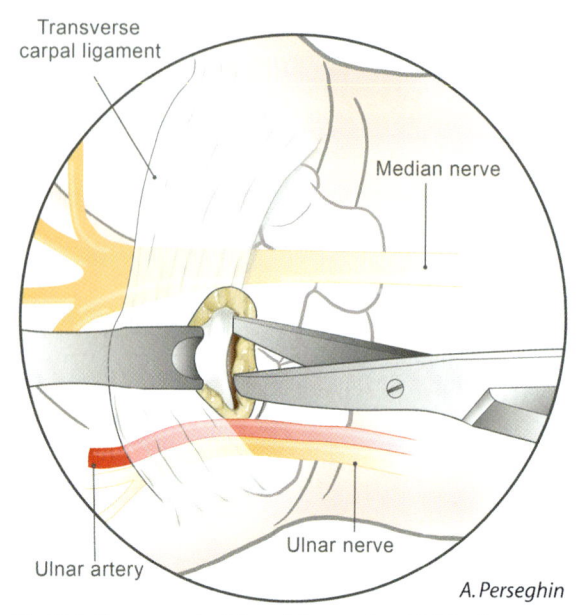

Fig. 31.9. Transverse incision of the antebrachial fascia

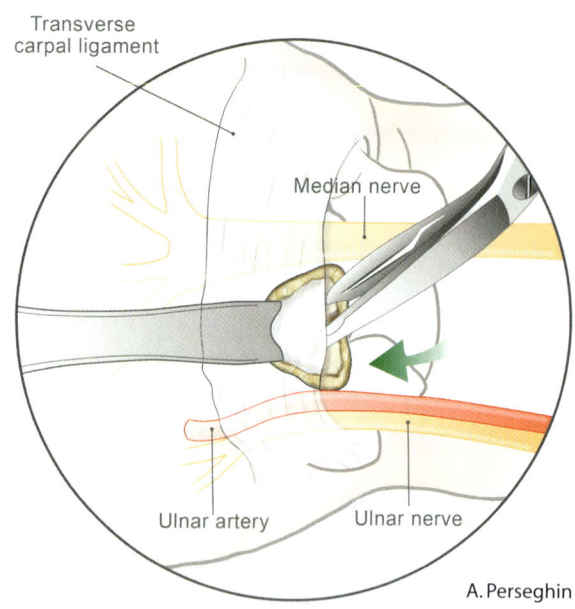

Fig. 31.11. Scissors introduction

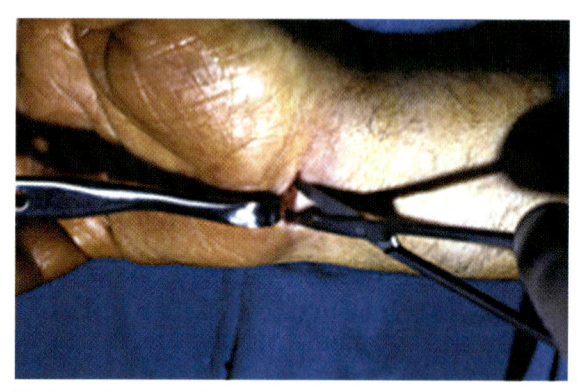

Fig. 31.10. Transversal incision of the antebrachial fascia

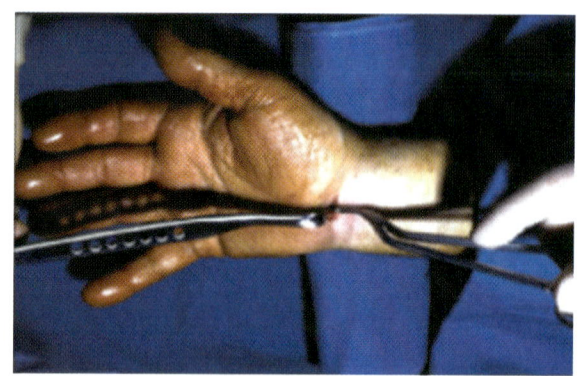

Fig. 31.12. Scissors introduction

The rounded jaw of the scissors is introduced into the distal edge of the incision and the scissors are opened according to the thickness of the TCL, so that the shorter jaw engages along the groove of the retractor. The groove must be maintained parallel to the cutaneous plane of the palm, whereas the retractor must be parallel to the ring finger axes (Figs. 31.11, 31.12). The scissors are pushed distally only after it has been assured that their direction of entry is correct. They will stop against the retractor when the ligament is completely resected (Figs. 31.13, 31.14). As the surgeon is cutting, the advancement of the scissors will feel smoother at about 1–2 mm before it encounters the spatula of the retractor: this confirms that the transverse ligament has been totally resected. This can also be further verified by palpating the rounded tip of the scissors subcutaneously in the palm (distally to the distal border of the tunnel).

It is possible to verify both the TCL sectioned (whose margins are about 1 cm apart) and part of the

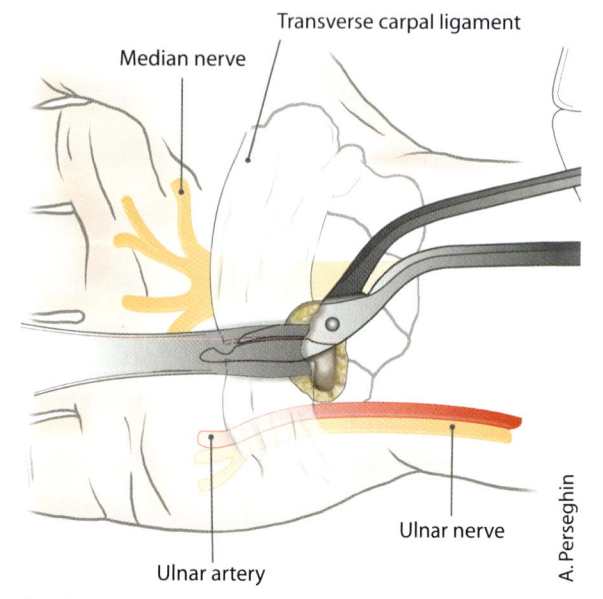

Fig. 31.13. The stop of scissors against retractor

31 Carpal Tunnel Syndrome Release Using the Chiena Technique

be sectioned by introducing the closed scissors into the space. The sharp groove proximally to the rounded jaw of the scissors can cut them during a retracting maneuver of the scissors themselves (Figs. 31.17, 31.18).

The proximal part of the antebrachial fascia must be sectioned by using the same scissors: the proximal edge of the fascia is raised through the same skin incision, then the rounded jaw is introduced into the proximal edge of the loop previously made in the antebrachial fascia and a 2-cm longitudinal incision is performed in a proximal direction. This will prevent proximal compression of the median nerve (Figs. 31.19, 31.20).

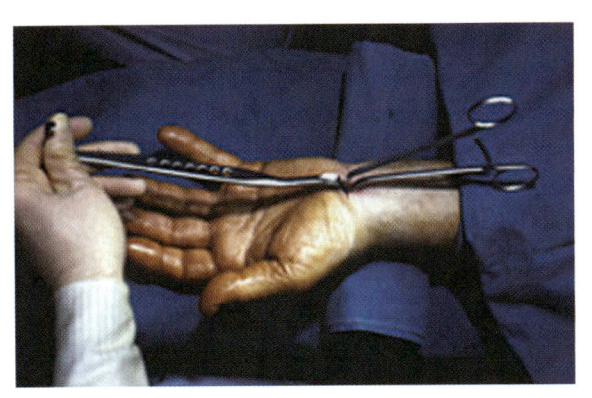

Fig. 31.14. Scissors against retractor

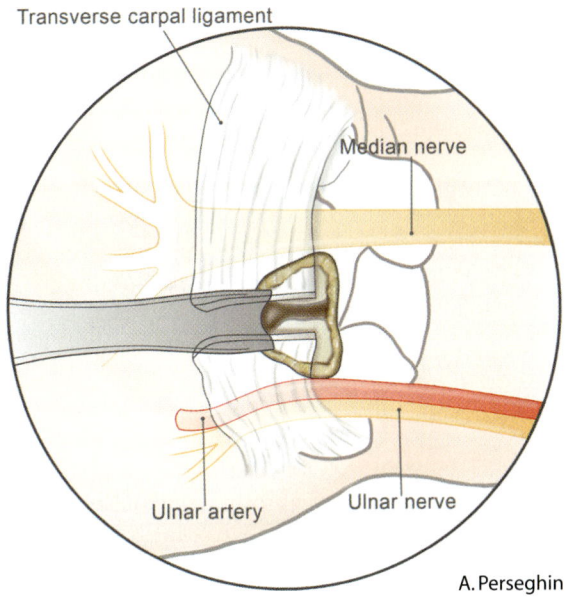

Fig. 31.15. The inspection of the carpal tunnel content

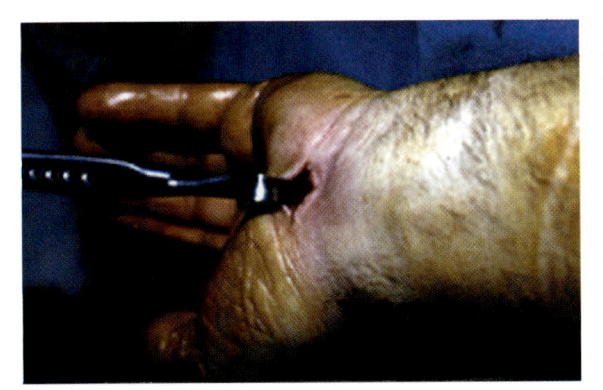

Fig. 31.16. Inspection of the carpal tunnel content

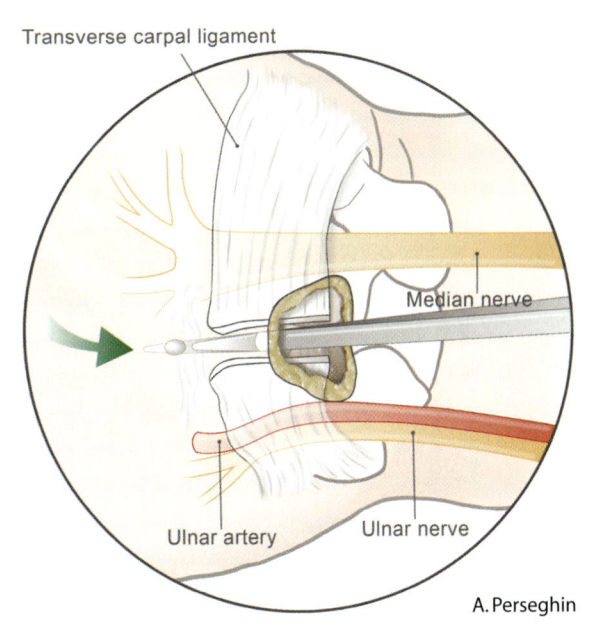

Fig. 31.17. The remnant fibers of the distal part of the TCL can be resected by the closed scissors

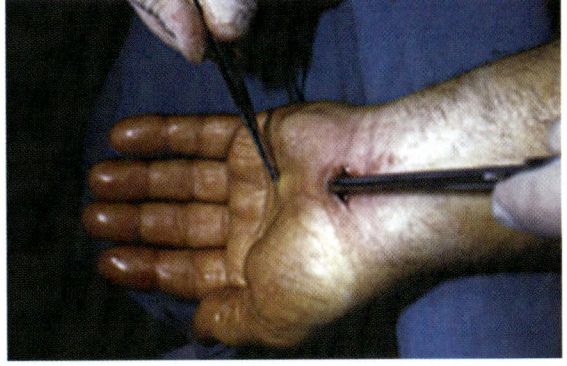

Fig. 31.18. The remnant fibers of the distal part of the TCL can be resected by the closed scissors

carpal tunnel content (Figs. 31.15, 31.16), by removing the scissors and raising the retractor while it is still in situ.

Sometimes, overstretched transverse fibers of the palmar fascia can remain attached at the palm level: they can

The skin is sutured with 3–4 reabsorbable stitches and the wound is dressed with cotton, a gel pack, and an elastic bandage, all to be replaced with a simple plaster after 6 h (Figs. 31.21, 31.22).

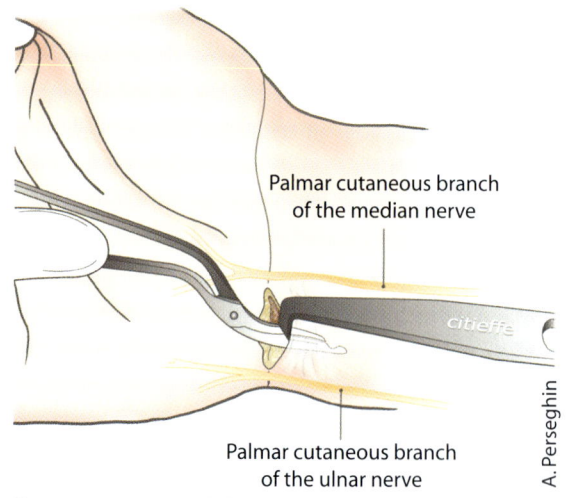

Fig. 31.19. Incision of the proximal edge in the antebrachial fascia

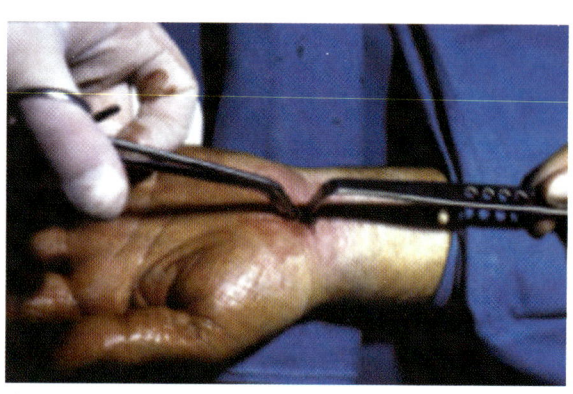

Fig. 31.20. Incision of the proximal edge in the antebrachial fascia

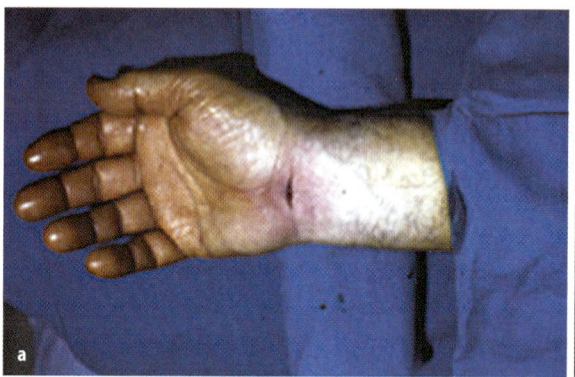

Fig. 31.21. a, b Suture and medication

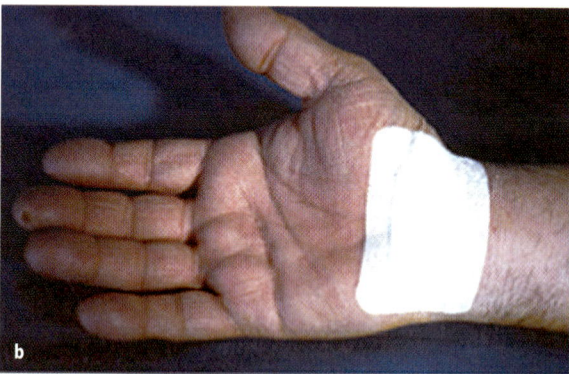

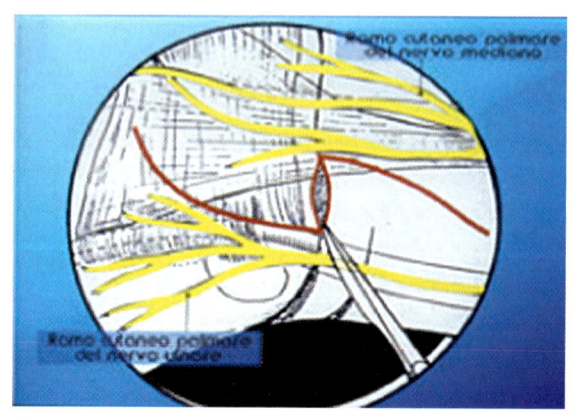

Fig. 31.22. Sometimes the incision can be longitudinally widened and surgery performed as an open technique

Material and Method

Between June 1992 and December 2003, 612 patients were operated on, 55 bilaterally, for a total of 667 cases (475 were females, 137 males). The age of the patients ranged between 25 and 90 years. The right wrist was affected in 395 cases.

At mean follow-up of 24 months (ranged from 3 to 30 months) 565 patients, for a total amount of 620 cases operated, were evaluated. The overall outcome, according to the patients' evaluation, was excellent in 599 cases, very good in 14, good in 3, sufficient in 2, and poor in 2. Patients returned to previous work after an average of 4 days.

Conclusions

The most important advantages of the Chiena technique seem to be the following:

1. Surgery can be performed using a very small amount of local anesthetic, with no limb ischemia even on outpatients.
2. Fast and simple execution (4–7 min).
3. The operation is safe: the tools are calibrated and simple to use, if properly placed and used. Retractor and scissors are congruent, decreasing the possibility of nerve insult. Furthermore, they allow a direct view of the nerve, once the carpal tunnel is opened.
4. The instruments are cheap and they can be used repeatedly.
5. Versatility of the equipment, which is suitable for different operations in other areas.
6. Good and quick functional recovery with possibility to return to previous work 24 h after surgery.

Contraindications are:

- Reoperations.
- Compression of the median nerve due to cysts, tumors, rheumatoid arthritis, nervous or vascular abnormalities.
- Wrist deformities and/or stiffness due to defects from old fractures: in such cases the incision can be longitudinally widened and surgery performed by an open technique (Fig. 31.22).

For the above-mentioned reasons this technique is a surgical advancement compared to the traditional surgical methods. Its reliability is proportional to the experience and skill of the surgeon, which of course improves with practice: in fact, the outcome of the last 497 operations was always estimated as excellent.

References

1. De Tullio VP (1995) A new technique for the release of the median nerve at the carpal tunnel. Abstract Book 6th Congress of the International Federation of Societies for Surgery of the Hand. Helsinki 0. 478
2. De Tullio VP (1995) Una nuova tecnica per la decompressione del nervo mediano al tunnel carpale. Rivista di Chirurgia e Riabilitazione della mano e dell'arto superiore. Vol. XXXII, Fascicolo 2–3, pag. 153
3. De Tullio VP (1998) The Carpal Tunnel Syndrome: a review of 277 surgeries through Chiena technique. Abstract Book 7th Congress of the International Federation of Societies for Surgery of the Hand. Vancouver, Canada, P- MO -82

32 Reconstruction of the Flexor Retinaculum

A. Lluch

Division of the flexor retinaculum (FR) is generally accepted as the most effective method for treating median nerve compression at the carpal tunnel. However, the main drawbacks from surgery are a decrease of grip strength and prolonged palmar scar pain.

Most authors attribute the loss of grip strength to the loss of the pulley effect of the flexor retinaculum on the finger flexor tendons. The cause of the palmar incisional pain, also known as "pillar pain" is more controversial.

Reconstruction of the FR tends to diminish the incidence of both of these complications.

Morphological Changes of the Carpal Tunnel After Division of the Flexor Retinaculum

The morphological changes of the carpal tunnel in patients who underwent division of the flexor retinaculum (FR) for the treatment of carpal tunnel syndrome (CTS) was examined with a CAT scan [1]. These are the first reported results in the medical literature [2]. We measured the transverse diameter of the carpal canal at the level of both the proximal and distal carpal rows. The transverse diameter at the level of the distal carpal row was chosen for the study because the measurements are more reliable at this level, and also because this is the level where the main compression of the median nerve occurs. We measured the distance between the radial corner of hook of the hamate bone and the ulnar corner of the trapezium. Measurements at the level of the proximal carpal row could be altered by an ulnar displacement of the pisiform bone, which was observed in some cases. Piso-triquetral subluxation has also been observed by other authors, and considered as a cause of continued hypothenar pain, called "piso-triquetral pain syndrome" [3].

Our examinations were done in 13 patients [1]. In 4 of them, the measurements were taken both before and after FR release. In the remaining 9 patients, the measurements were done after FR release, and the opposite nonoperated hand was used as a control. The transverse dimension of the carpal canal at the distal carpal row measured an average of 20.2 mm, with a minimum of 18 mm and a maximum of 23 mm. After division of the FR the transverse diameter increased only 1 mm. It was evident that the increase of volume of the carpal tunnel occurred mainly in the antero-posterior diameter as the FR was seen displaced anteriorly. No measurements were done of the anterior displacement of the FR, as a CAT scan is not as precise as an MRI examination, which was not available at that time.

The first published results in the English literature measuring carpal arch widening after carpal tunnel release using a plain radiographic technique were those of Gartsman et al. [4]. They measured the distance between the anterior ridge of the trapezium and the hook of the hamate in 50 patients on standard "carpal tunnel views" with the wrist at 50° of extension. In 6 of them, measurements were taken before and after open carpal tunnel release, while in the remaining 44, the contralateral unoperated wrist was used as a control. The amount of widening ranged from 0 to 8.5 mm with an average widening of 2.9 mm. They found an average increase of 13.6% in the transverse diameter of the carpal canal, ranging from 0% to 52%.

Viegas et al. [5] also measured the transverse dimension of the carpal canal on x-ray films using a "carpal tunnel view" with the wrist at 50° of extension. The measurements were done in 87 wrists, before surgery and on an average of 10 days following endoscopic carpal tunnel release using Chow's technique [6]. They observed an average widening of 1.7 mm (from 0.0 to 5 mm). This represents a 7% average increase in the transverse diameter of the carpal canal, ranging from 0% to 25%.

The first published studies in the English literature measuring carpal arch widening after carpal tunnel release using MRI were those of Richman et al. [7]. They measured the transverse diameter of 15 hands in 14 patients with CTS, before and 6 weeks after division of the FR. Preoperatively, the carpal width averaged 24.0 ± 2.4 mm. Six weeks after surgery, the carpal width averaged 25.5 ± 1.8 mm, representing an average increase of 1.5 mm.

Kato et al. [8] measured the transverse diameter of the carpal canal by MRI in 10 hands treated for CTS using the Universal Subcutaneous Endoscope system designed by Okutsu [9]. The transverse diameter increased from 22.1 mm ± 2.2 mm to 23.8 mm ± 1.0 mm after the procedure, an average increase of 1.7 mm.

During surgery, Garcia-Elias et al. [10] measured the width of the carpal canal in 21 wrists before and after division of the FR. The distance between 2 Kirschner wires perpendicularly inserted into the trapezium and the hook of the hamate increased an average of 11%.

Chaise et al. [11] measured carpal volume with a CAT scan in 22 wrists before and after open FR release. They observed an increase from 7% to 44% in the antero-posterior diameter, with a negligible widening of the carpal canal.

Richman et al. [7] were the first to measure both carpal volume and anterior displacement of the carpal contents using MRI. They found that the carpal volume increased from 6.3 ± 1.0 ml to 7.8 ± 1.5 ml after the operation, representing a 22% ± 14% increase in volume. The median nerve was found to have displaced anteriorly on average of 3.5 ± 1.9 mm in relation to its original position.

Kato et al. [8] observed that the cross-sectional area of the carpal tunnel increased from 232 mm^2 to 320 mm^2 after endoscopic carpal tunnel release, with a significant postoperative palmar displacement of the flexor tendons from their original position.

Ablove et al. [12], by MRI measured the morphologic changes following endoscopic release in 11 wrists and two-portal subcutaneous carpal tunnel release in 7 wrists on an average of 24 weeks after surgery. The transverse carpal arch dimension increased an average of 1.0 ± 1.5 mm in the endoscopic group using the Agee Carpal Tunnel Release System [13], and 0.6 ± 0.3 mm in the subcutaneous group. The carpal volume increased 23 ± 12% in the endoscopic treated group and 26 ± 13% in the subcutaneous group.

Although from the anatomical point of view, the FR seems to provide transverse stability of the carpal arch [14], laboratory studies using cadaveric specimens concluded that very little difference was encountered in the carpal arch structure under a dorsal-palmar compression load after the FR has been divided [15]. Therefore, the FR has not proven to be an important factor in maintaining the stability of the carpal arch.

Earlier intraoperative and postoperative radiological measurements of the carpal width reported an increase of an average from 7% to 13.6%, but more accurate measurements using CAT scan and MRI examinations have proven that the carpal canal just widens from 0.6 mm to 1.5 mm.

In conclusion, all reported studies demonstrated that the postoperative increase in carpal volume is obtained by a slight widening of the carpal arch, but mainly secondary to an anterior displacement of the divided flexor retinaculum, allowing for anterior displacement of the median nerve and flexor tendons. The carpal canal becomes more rounded postoperatively, and Guyon's compartment cross section changes from triangular to round [7].

Function of the Flexor Retinaculum as a Flexor Tendon Pulley

The FR is a very strong anatomical structure that contributes minimally to maintenance of the transverse carpal arch. Its main function seems to be that of a pulley to maintain the strong flexor tendons close to the center of rotation of the wrist. If the flexor tendons are allowed to displace anteriorly during wrist flexion, the muscle-tendon unit will become relatively longer from its points of origin and insertion, thus decreasing its maximum contractility. This is known as the Blix curve [16], and it explains why there is a decreased grip strength and increased difficulty to touch the finger tips to the distal palmar crease as flexion of the wrist is increased.

After division of the FR, most surgeons have observed an anterior displacement of the flexor tendons. If the FR is divided on its ulnar side, the flexor tendons to the ring and small fingers will have a tendency to dislocate over the hook of the hamate bone, particularly if the wrist is flexed [17, 18]. It is quite evident that the FR has lost its function as a pulley, allowing the flexor tendons to displace anteriorly, mainly when the wrist is flexed [19].

The moment arm (distance to the center of rotation of the wrist) and the excursion of the finger flexor tendons was measured by Kline and Moore [20] in four fresh frozen specimens before and after sectioning the FR. They observed that after sectioning of the FR, the flexor digitorum superficialis (FDS) tendons were allowed to move 5.8 mm farther away from the center of rotation of the wrist, and the flexor digitorum profundus (FDP) tendons 6.2 mm. In these circumstances, flexion of the wrist consumes 25% more excursion of the FDP tendons and 20% more excursion of the FDS tendons, decreasing the force transmitted to the fingers by the muscle contraction.

Studies by Brown et al. [21] and Netscher et al. [22] on cadaveric specimens confirmed the importance of the FR as a flexor tendon pulley, demonstrating that with either open or endoscopic techniques, flexor tendon excursion was equally altered. The studies done by Netscher et al. [23] on 10 fresh cadaver upper extremities demonstrated that transverse carpal ligament reconstruction conferred a mechanical advantage, so that postoperative differences from presurgical measurements were not significant.

Loss of Grip Strength After Carpal Tunnel Release

Subjective loss of grip strength after CTS release has been brought to the attention of surgeons in the past years, and was reported by Fissette and Onkelinx [24] to be present in 25% of their operated hands. In 1987 [25], we first demonstrated loss of grip strength after division of the FR for the treatment of CTS. We measured the grip strength in 220 hands from 120 women and 25 men at an average of 3 years and 10 months after surgery (minimum 2 years and maximum of 8 years and 9 months). The grip strength was measured with a JAMAR dynamometer with the wrist at 20° of extension and at 20° of flexion. The average grip strength with the wrist in extension was 20.6 Kg and decreased to 13.5 Kg when the measurement was taken with the wrist at 20° of flexion. These measurements proved that the operated hands lost an average 16% of their grip strength as compared with the contralateral nonoperated hand when the measurement was taken with the wrist in extension. If the measurement was taken with the wrist in flexion, the loss grip strength increased to 24% as compared to the opposite wrist in the same position of wrist flexion.

The loss of grip strength and bow-stringing of the flexor tendons was measured by Kiritsis and Kline [26] after open and endoscopic sectioning of the FR, as well as after repair of the FR. The study was done on 10 fresh-frozen forearm specimens. They used the repair technique described by Jakab [27], and the two-portal endoscopic technique described by Chow [6]. Sectioning of the FR using either the open or the endoscopic techniques resulted in a significant increase in the amount of excursion of the flexor tendons that was consumed by motion of the wrist. Reconstruction of the FR resulted in a smaller increase.

Netscher et al. [28] measured the grip strength and performed MRI examinations on patients after CTS release, with and without FR reconstruction. They observed a 3.3 mm anterior displacement of the median nerve after open carpal tunnel release, and 2.5 mm anterior displacement after transposition flap repair. The difference is not significant, as MRI studies are static measurements done with the wrist in neutral position; but when grip strength was measured, they observed that the group in which the FR retinaculum was repaired maximal grip and pinch strengths were regained 12 weeks after surgery, surpassing the other group of patients.

Gellman et al. [29] measured grip strength in 24 wrists after CTS release, observing that it was at 28% of their preoperative level by 3 weeks, and at 73% by 6 weeks, and returning to preoperative levels by 3 months. However, these measurements were done with wrist extension. The postoperative results were reported as a percentage of the preoperative value in the ipsilateral extremity, as their patient population was not homogeneous, showing a wide variation in preoperative grip strength, varying from 5 to 75 pounds.

Karlson et al. [30] compared the grip strength in patients whose FR was simply divided and others in which it was repaired. With the wrist at 45° of extension, the group with FR reconstruction had an average grip strength of 106.8 (27.6–248.0) kPa as compared to just 82.7 (20.7–296.0) kPa in the FR section only. Surprisingly, when grip strength was measured with the wrist at 45° of flexion, the FR reconstruction group had a lower grip strength [72.3 (13.8–137.8) kPa] than the group with FR section only [124.0 (13.8–186.0) kPa]. Perhaps these paradoxical results are influenced by the fact that the measurements were taken early after the procedure and the group with reconstruction of the FR underwent a more lengthy and extensive surgical exposure leading to a longer period of local inflammation.

Netscher et al. [23] measured the grip strength in 3 groups of 17 patients each, at 6 and 12 weeks after CTS release. In one group the FR was longitudinally divided without reconstruction. In another group the FR was reconstructed with the two-flap technique described by Jakab [27]. In the third group the FR was reconstructed by suturing the ulnar cut edge of the palmar aponeurosis to the radial cut edge of the FR. The transposition flap repair group was significantly stronger than the other 2 groups at 6 weeks, although the differences decreased slightly by 12 weeks.

In conclusion, all published studies demonstrate that division of the FR results in loss of grip strength, which is more evident when it is measured with the wrist in moderate flexion. Repair of the FR seems to diminish the loss of grip strength.

Palmar Scar Pain

Most patients treated for CTS experience palmar scar pain for several weeks and even months after surgery. At first, this was thought to be secondary to the division of the palmar cutaneous branches of the median nerve, and in order to avoid this complication Taleisnik [31] proposed to place the longitudinal palmar incision at the ulnar side of the axis of the ring finger. Anatomical studies done by Engberg and Gmeiner [32] demonstrated that by using this incision there was the risk of injuring the less common palmar cutaneous branch of the ulnar nerve. Taking into consideration the above studies and others [33, 34], most authors agree that placing the incision along the longitudinal midaxis of the ring finger has the least chance of injuring the palmar cutaneous branches of either the median or ulnar nerves. However, Martin et al. [35] observed that there may not be a true "internervous plane" in the palm, as in many cases they have observed transverse cutaneous nerve fibers connecting the ulnar and median cutaneous branches at the palm. Seradge and Seradge [36] suggested that the pain was secondary to ulnar displacement of the pisiform in relation to the triquetrum and named it "piso-triquetral pain syndrome" or "pillar pain."

It is our impression that palmar scar pain after CTS surgical release is secondary to excessive fibrous tissue formation between the divided ends of the flexor retinaculum. All patients complaining of persistent palmar scar pain present with an increased collagenoblastic activity at the palmar scar. The intensity of pain may fluctuate, which is always directly related to hand activity and the amount of fibrosis noted on palpation of the scar. Pain secondary to neuroma formation is completely different. In these cases, the pain is felt just at the point of nerve transection, rather than along the entire surgical scar, as observed after CTS release. Symptoms related to a nerve division are felt as an electric shock just at the point where the nerve has been severed, as described by Tinel [37]. Pain secondary to a neuroma is localized to the anatomical site of nerve transection, is not directly related to the amount of fibrosis, and usually persists after the fibrotic process resolves.

Patients undergoing CTS release by endoscopy, in which palmar skin nerve branches are not transected, also experience palmar scar pain. A prospective randomized study on 169 hands done by Brown et al. [38] found that 61% of the hands treated by open release and also 46% of the hands treated by endoscopy, experienced palmar scar pain 84 days after the procedures.

We performed a clinical study of 15 patients undergoing palmar fasciectomy for the treatment of Dupuytren's contracture. In these patients, the proximal part of the palmar incision was continued proximally, following the midaxial line of the ring finger until it reached the distal wrist flexion crease. This incision was the same used for the open release of CTS. None of the above patients experienced palmar scar pain as seen in patients treated for CTS.

From all above observations, we hypothesized that palmar scar pain is secondary to excessive fibrosis formed between the divided edges of the flexor retinaculum, which will be stretched from the pressure of the underlying flexor tendons during hand activities. Palmar scar pain was absent in most of our patients in which the FR retinaculum was repaired in an elongated position.

Methods of Reconstructing the Flexor Retinaculum

Because division of the FR for the treatment of CTS causes loss of grip strength, some authors have proposed its repair in a lengthened position.

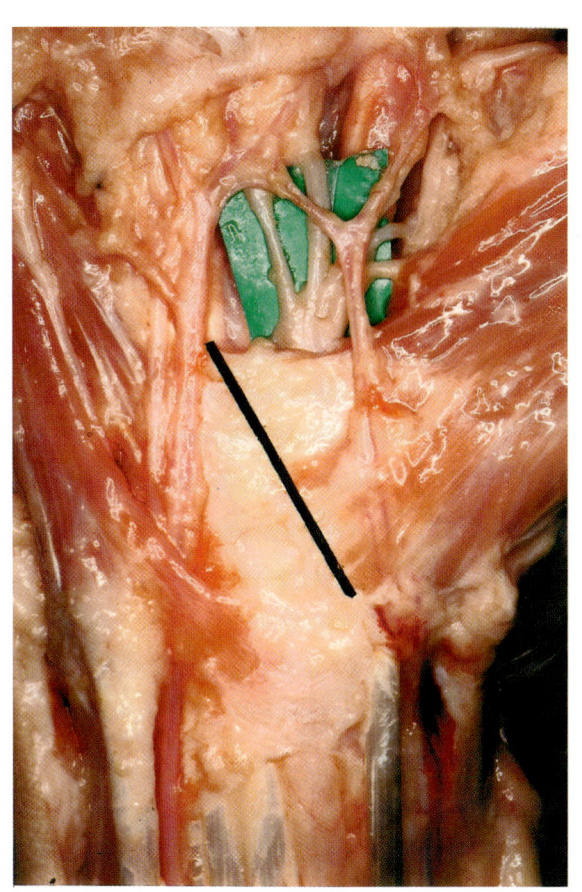

Fig. 32.1. Anatomical preparation demonstrating the oblique incision of the flexor retinaculum. The sensory and motor branches of the median nerve can be seen emerging under the distal edge of the FR. The roof of Guyon's compartment has been removed to show the ulnar nerve and artery emerging at the radial side of the pisiform bone. The ulnar artery and the anterior branch of the radial artery form the superficial palmar arterial arch

Lluch in 1984 [1, 39] published the first known description for reconstructing the FR for the treatment of carpal tunnel syndrome. The FR was sectioned in an oblique direction, from the ulnar side of its distal edge to the radial side of its proximal edge (Fig. 32.1). The division at the distal edge was done on the ulnar side to avoid a possible injury to the motor branch of the median nerve, as some anomalies can be observed [40]. The divided edges of the FR are sutured together after slight sliding in opposite directions of the radial and ulnar oblique flaps, enlarging the carpal volume (Figs. 32.2, 32.3).

Kapandji in 1990 [41] described a lengthening technique after division of the FR in a zig-zag fashion using two triangular flaps sutured in the middle. This technique was done in 46 hands, without any immediate postoperative complications, but no long-term clinical follow-up or grip strength measurement were provided in his publication.

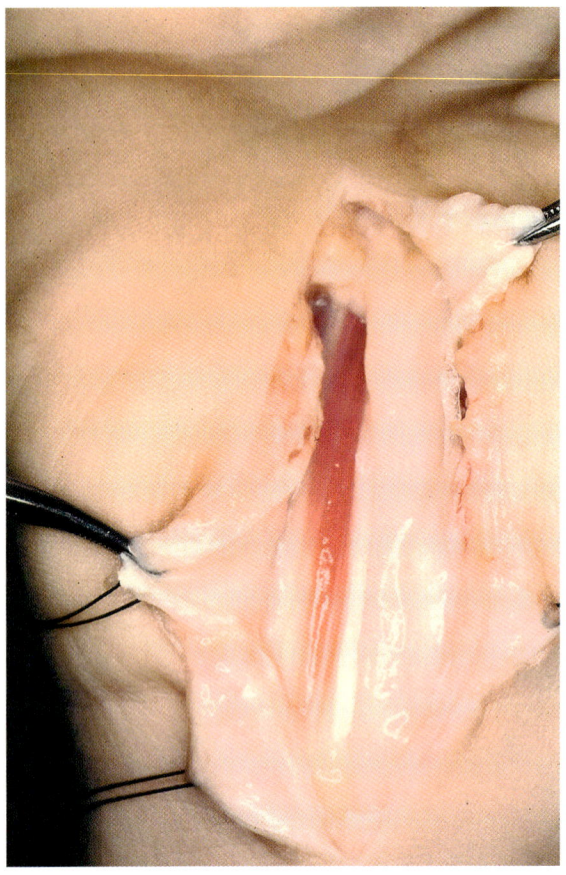

Fig. 32.2. The oblique division of the FR results in two flaps. The radial flap is longer distally and the ulnar flap is longer proximally. The design of a distal radial flap avoids injury to a possible transretinacular motor branch of the median nerve. An extended palmar incision needs to be used for this method of FR reconstruction

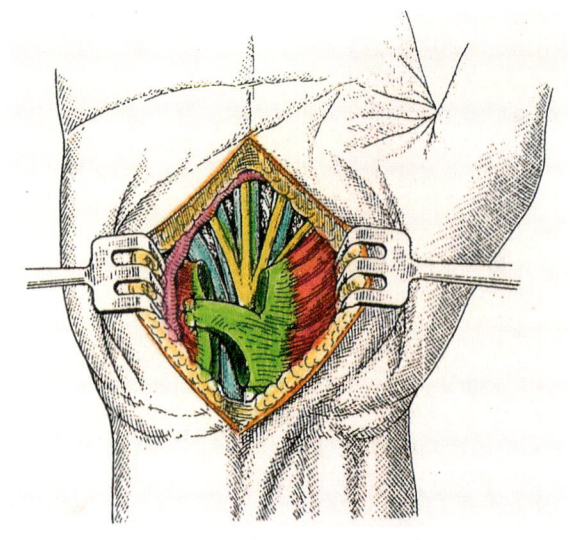

Fig. 32.4. Tubiana-proposed reconstruction of the FR with a 1-cm slip obtained from the distal end of the radial flap of the divided FR, and suturing it to the hook of the hamate

The same year, Tubiana [18] described another technique for repairing the FR, consisting of creating a 1-cm slip from the distal end of the radial side of the divided FR and suturing it to the hook of the hamate (Fig. 32.4). He does not routinely use this technique, except in cases where there is a clear subluxation of the flexor tendons outside the carpal canal.

Jakab at al. [27] used a distal radially based flap and a proximal ulnarly based flap to reconstruct the FR. The surgery is done through a 4- to 5-cm palmar incision, as recommended by Taleisnik [31], beginning at the distal wrist crease and continuing distally in line with the axis of the ring finger (Fig. 32.5).

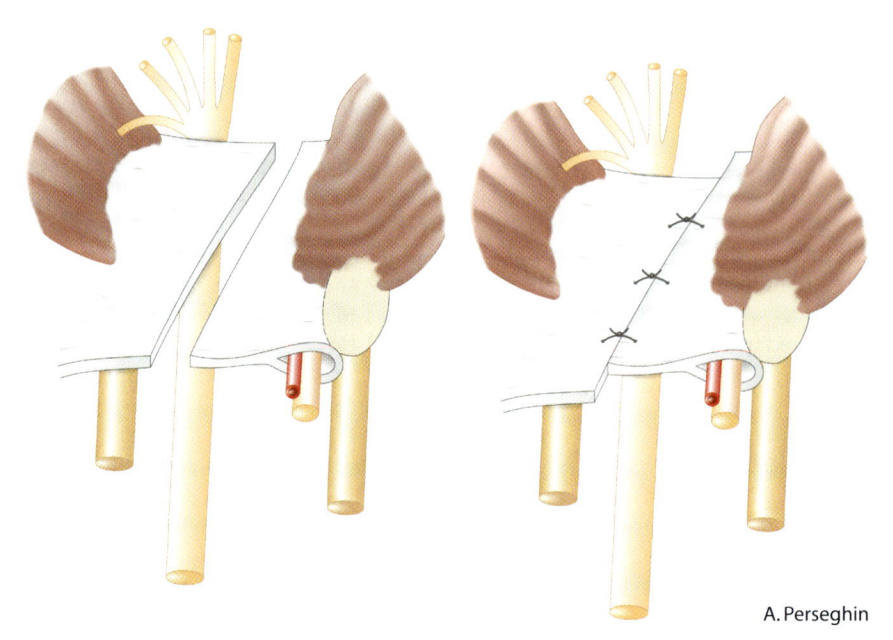

A. Perseghin

Fig. 32.3. The sliding flap technique first used by the author in the reconstruction of the FR

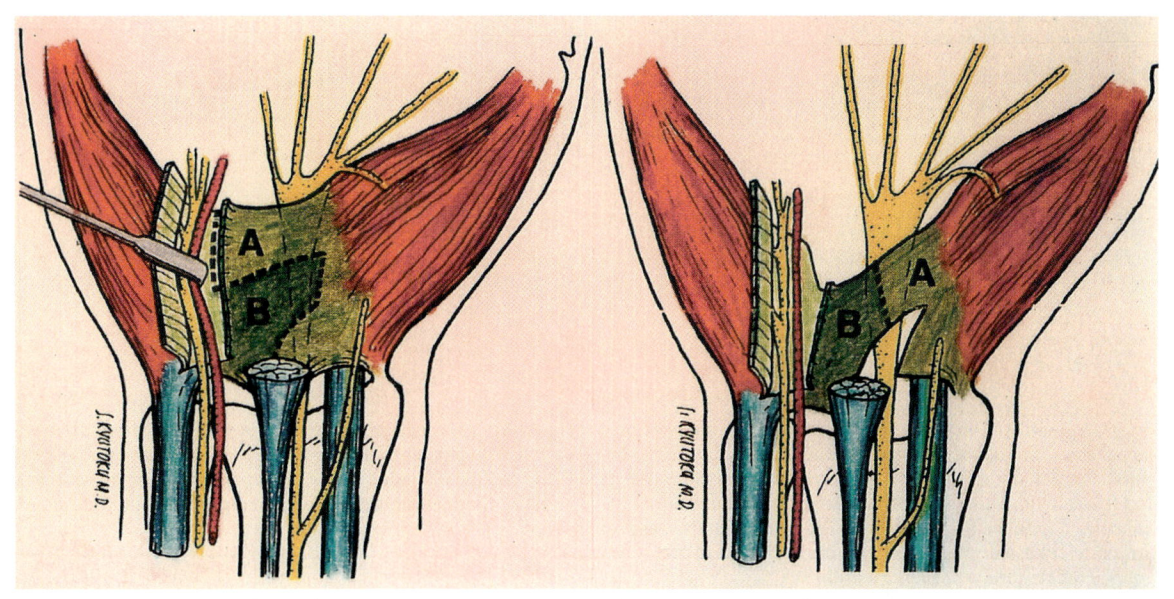

Fig. 32.5. Jakab used a two-flap technique to reconstruct the FR. The distally based radial flap is sutured in the midline to the proximal ulnarly based flap

Hunter [42] recommended a lengthening technique using an oblique incision of the FR, as we did for our first cases, while using an extended palmar incision measuring from 8 to 10 cm in length.

Personal Technique for Reconstruction of the Flexor Retinaculum

After observing that all patients treated for CTS had a loss of grip strength [1, 25], it was decided to reconstruct the FR in young working men.

Since 1975 we have routinely use a 4- to 5-cm long palmar incision in line with the long axis of the ring finger, as suggested by Taleisnik [31] (Fig. 32.6). The FR is then longitudinally divided near its ulnar side insertion, thus preserving a radially based flap of uninjured FR that gives support to the flexor tendons and the median nerve, without danger of later entrapment of the nerve from scar tissue (Fig. 32.7). We are very pleased with the postoperative results, as we never had a recurrence of median nerve entrapment. The oblique division of the FR first done by us required a longitudinal skin incision slightly longer and more radially placed, which could cause injury to palmar cutaneous branches of the median nerve. However, the major concern was the section of the FR over the median nerve, as in all cases of recurrences of CTS, the nerve has been found to be englobed by the fibrous tissue originated from the divided edges of the FR [17, 18, 42] (Fig. 32.8). For this reason, this technique of FR repair was only used in the first 6 patients [43], as we preferred to use a more ulnar and shorter skin incision.

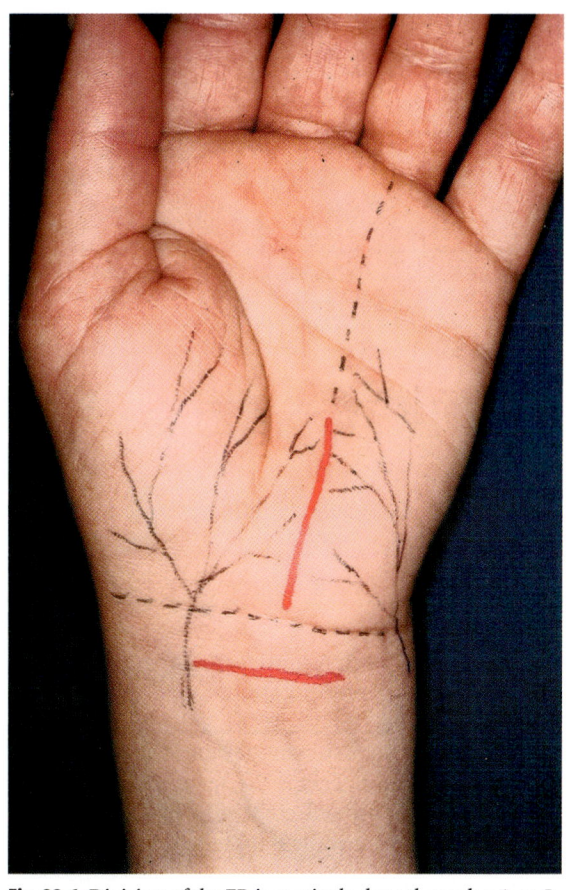

Fig. 32.6. Division of the FR is routinely done through a 4- to 5-cm long palmar incision, just distal to the wrist flexion crease. This incision is in line with the longitudinal axis of the ring finger, and follows the theoretical boundary between median and ulnar innervation in the hand

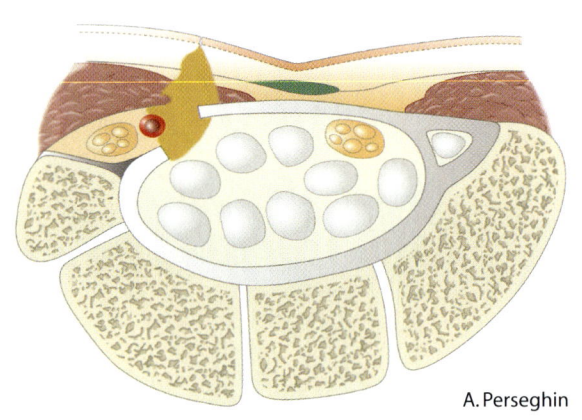

Fig. 32.7. Cross section of the wrist at the level of the proximal carpal row. The roof of Guyon's compartment is divided to facilitate section of the FR at its ulnar insertion into the pisiform and triquetrum. This will preserve a smooth and uninjured retinacular flap to facilitate gliding of the flexor tendons, and at the same time will prevent englobing the median nerve by postoperative fibrous tissue formation

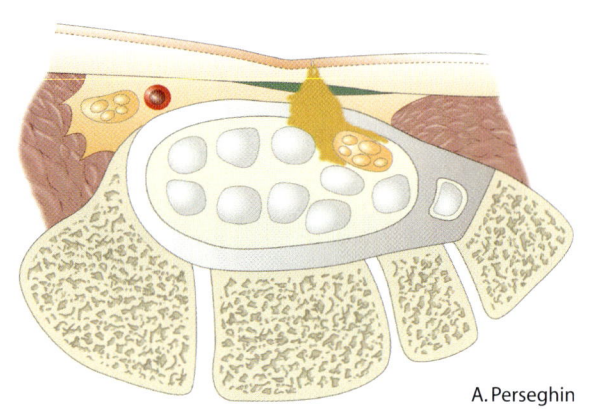

Fig. 32.8. Cross section of the wrist at the level of the proximal carpal row. Division of the FR in the midline or on its radial side should be avoided as the postoperative fibrous tissue will englobe the median nerve and be responsible for CTS recurrence

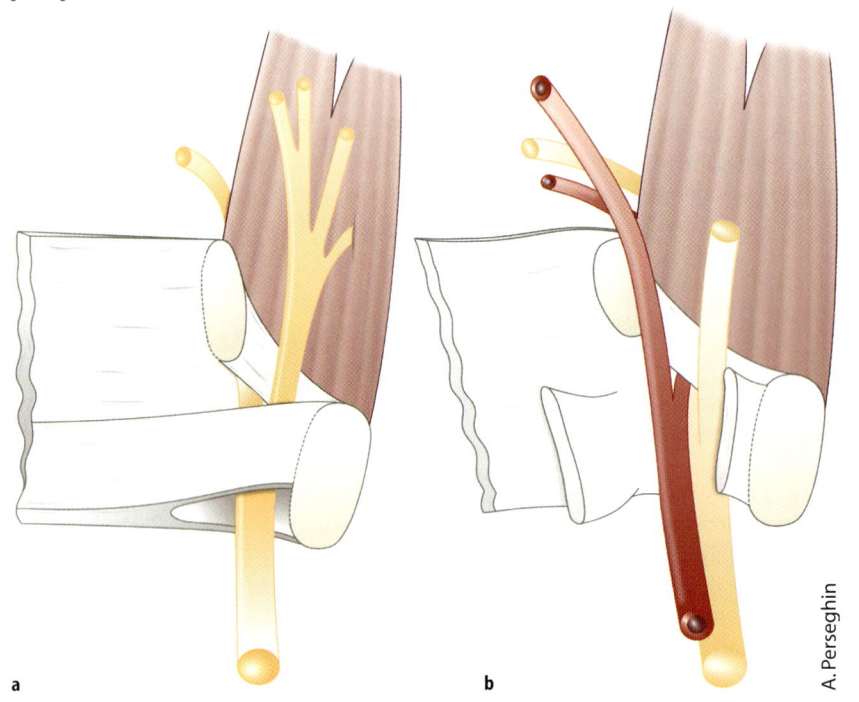

Fig. 32.9 a The ulnar boundaries of the FR. The hook of the hamate and the pisiform are colored in *green*. The hook of the hamate is in line with the longitudinal axis of the ring finger, while the pisiform is more ulnarly located. The ulnar artery and nerve cross the wrist inside Guyon's compartment. **b** The ulnar artery and nerve can clearly be seen after dividing the roof of Guyon's compartment. The ulnar artery is more superficial and radial than the ulnar nerve as it has to travel distally in a superficial and radial direction to form the superficial palmar arterial arch

Since 1985 we've been reconstructing the FR in all patients, even in the revision cases for recurrence of CTS, using the following technique [44, 45]. Surgery is done through a 4-cm palmar skin incision just distal to the wrist flexion crease. This is the theoretical boundary between the median and ulnar skin innervation, and therefore it is theoretically impossible to divide a sensory palmar nerve branch (Fig. 32.6). After the skin, subcutaneous fat tissue, and frequently the radial insertion of the palmaris brevis muscle are divided, the roof of Guyon's compartment is longitudinally incised (Fig. 32.9a, b). The ulnar nerve and artery are next retracted towards the ulnar side with a blunt retractor. The FR is divided just radial to the hook of the hamate bone, by pushing the knife blade down until the finger flexor tendons are visualized. The division is then continued distally up to the distal edge of the FR (Fig. 32.10). The ulnar artery and the superficial palmar arch are found and should be distally and ulnarly retracted in order to avoid injury. The FR is then proximally divided in an ulnar direction of about 45° towards the pisiform bone. This results in the proximal part of the radially based flap of the FR being longer than the distal part (Figs. 32.11 – 32.14). The radial and

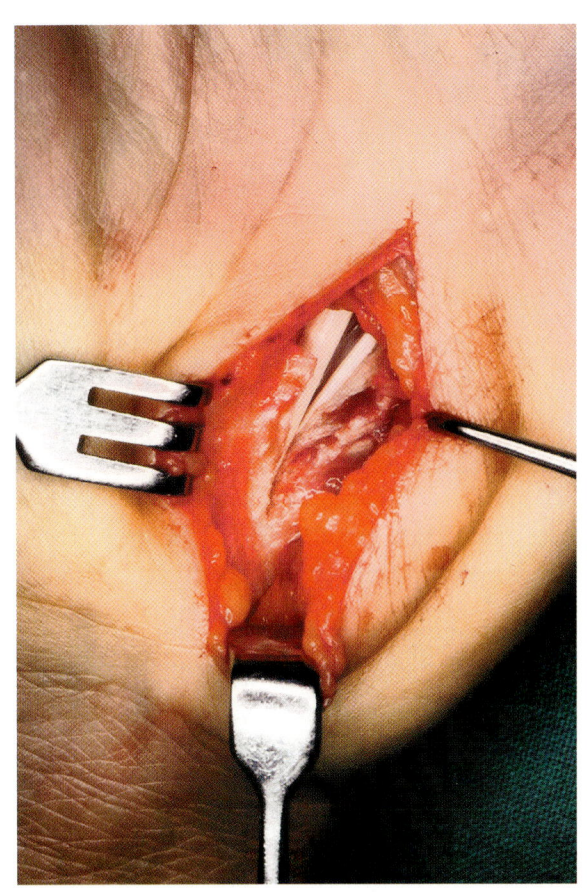

Fig. 32.10. The ulnar artery and nerve are retracted ulnarly after division of the roof of Guyon's compartment. The FR is then divided at its distal end close to the hook of the hamate. The distal edge of the FR and the superficial palmar arterial arch can be clearly seen, facilitating complete release of the distal FR and thus avoiding inadvertent injury to the artery

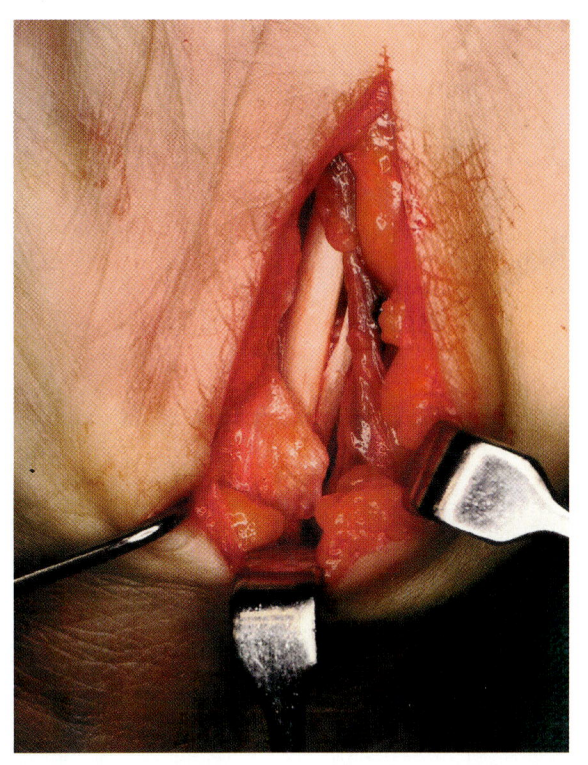

Fig. 32.11. The FR is then divided obliquely towards the ulnar side, thus creating a longer proximal flap. In this intraoperative picture, the flexor tendons of the ring and small finger, the ulnar artery and the divided flexor retinaculum with a larger proximal radial flap are shown

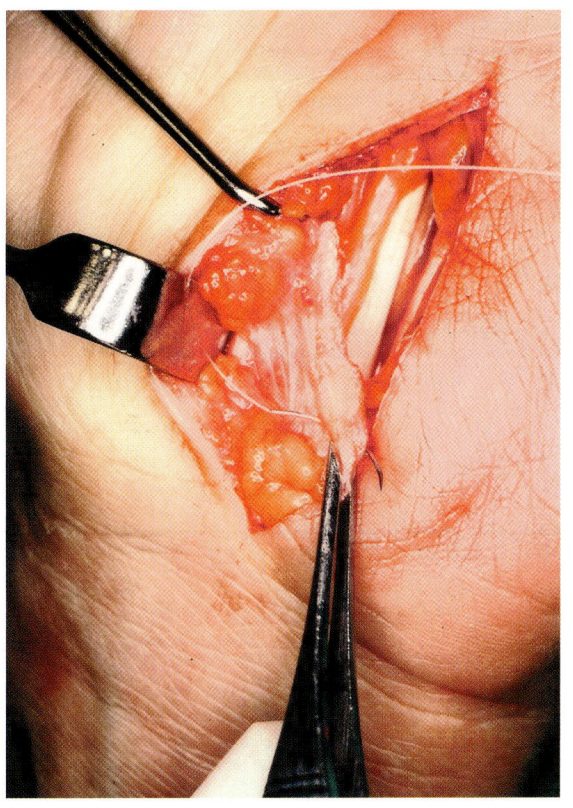

proximal cut edge of the FR is then sutured to the ulnar edge of the FR, just proximal to the hook of the hamate, with a number 1 metric (5-0 USP) suture (Fig. 32.12). By doing so the FR is repaired in a lengthened position at the level of the hook of the hamate, which is the point where tendon subluxations occur (Figs. 32.13–32.15).

The median nerve is never disturbed, as neurolysis is unnecessary and even harmful in many cases [46, 47]. The fibrous tissue around the flexor tendons does not need to be excised, as it is not a true synovitis, and not the cause but the consequence of the increased carpal tunnel pressure [48, 49].

After removing the five skin sutures of 0.7 metric (6-0 USP) nonabsorbable monofilament material, the wrist is immobilized in moderate extension for a total of 3 weeks to allow for healing of the repaired FR.

▷
Fig. 32.12. A suture is placed trough the edge of the proximal radial flap of FR

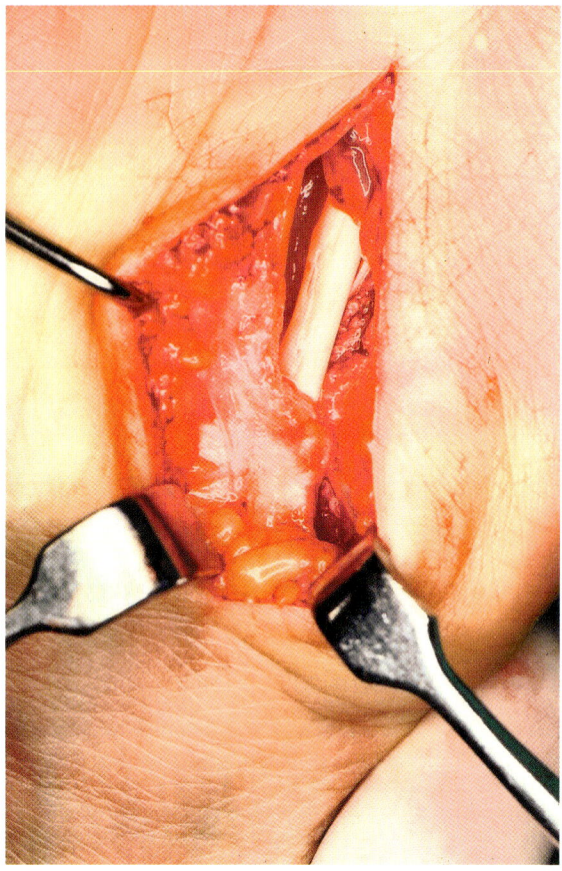

Fig. 32.13. Later, the radial flap is sutured to the ulnar edge of the FR at the level, or just proximal, to the hook of the hamate. By doing so, the FR is reconstructed in a lengthened position, and the subluxation of the flexor tendons observed in Figs. 32.11 and 32.12 is prevented

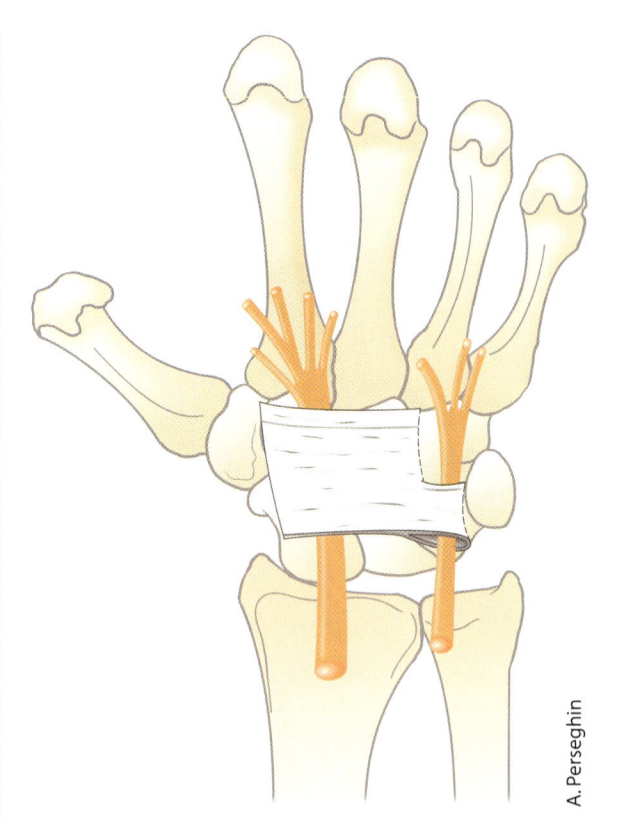

Fig. 32.14. The FR in relation to the median and ulnar nerves. The median nerve travels through the carpal tunnel on its radial side. The ulnar nerve travels through Guyon's compartment, located just superficial to the proximal part of the carpal tunnel. The ulnar side of the FR is longer proximally than distally

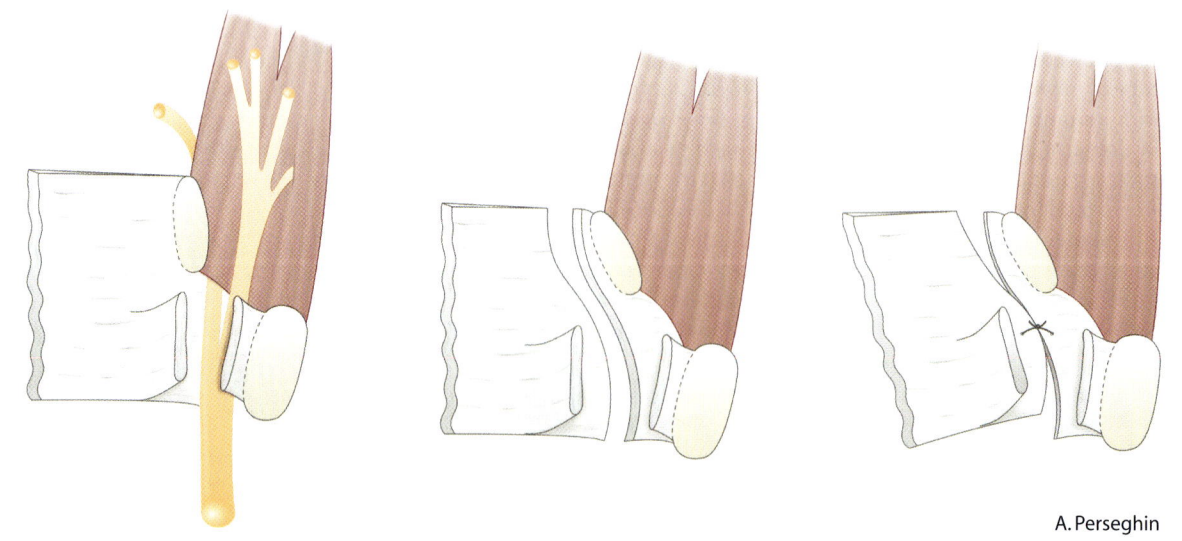

Fig. 32.15. The surgical technique used to reconstruct the FR. On the *left*, the roof of Guyon's compartment is divided, exposing the ulnar nerve and artery. In the *center drawing*, the FR has been divided obliquely near its ulnar insertion, in order to create a longer proximal radial flap. On the *right*, the longer proximal radial flap is sutured to the ulnar edge of the divided FR next to the hook of the hamate bone

Results After the Reconstruction of the Flexor Retinaculum

Kapandji [41], Tubiana [18], and Hunter [42] have not reported the results on grip strength after use of their techniques.

Jakab et al. [27] reviewed the results of their technique in 104 hands with a minimum follow-up of 2 years after the procedure and could not find any appreciable diminution of postoperative grip strength.

Karlson et al. [30] compared the results of simple FR division and FR lengthening and did not find any significant differences in the postoperative grip strength. They used a technique similar to the one described by Kapandji [41], creating two triangular flaps on each side of the FR. They observed that the patients in the lengthening group had a longer postoperative sick leave, probably secondary to longer surgical time and tissue trauma.

One hundred forty-five patients, in which the FR was divided at its ulnar border and later reconstructed using the flap lengthening technique, suturing it to the hook of the hamate, have been examined at an average of 4 years and 3 months after surgery, ranging from 6 months to 12.5 years. There were 89 women and 28 men with an average age of 52 years, ranging from 18 to 82 years of age. In 14 patients, bilateral CTS was treated at different times. Grip strength measured with the wrist in extension decreased 4%, while in flexion decreased 7%, demonstrating a much lesser loss of grip strength than observed in patients in which the FR was not reconstructed. After the same postoperative follow-up, the latter group of 210 patients had a 16% and 24% loss of grip strength, measured with their wrists in extension and flexion respectively.

In 1995 we started a prospective study measuring the grip strength of our patients before and after the operation, at 3-month intervals up to 1 year, and have observed a slight decrease in grip strength in most of them. We abandoned the prospective study of grip strength as we found that the main benefit of the procedure was a definite decrease of the so-called pillar pain. A painful, inflamed, and fibrotic palmar scar was present for several weeks and up to 6 months in some patients in the group without FR reconstruction [50]. Some patients had so much pain upon pressure at the palmar incision that they required a short period of immobilization with a plaster bandage for comfort. After FR reconstruction, the period of palmar pain was much shorter, averaging 1–3 weeks after cast removal.

Most patients who had CTS surgical release complained of excessive fibrosis, which causes discomfort and pain when applying pressure over the palmar skin incision, and which can last for several months [51–59]. It is our impression that the palmar pain observed in these patients is secondary to excessive fibrous tissue formation bridging the severed edges of the FR. In a separate clinical study, we performed an identical palmar skin incision on patients undergoing palmar fasciectomy for the treatment of a Dupuytren's contracture. None of these patients complained of prolonged palmar pain as seen in those who had FR release. This observation made us believe that palmar pain is not just secondary to the skin incision, but mainly related to the divided edges of the flexor retinaculum. If the flexor retinaculum is repaired in a lengthened position, the incidence of postoperative fibrosis is greatly reduced.

At present, we think that the main benefit of FR reconstruction is a considerable decrease of postoperative scar pain both in intensity and duration. Maintenance of grip strength is a secondary benefit of the procedure.

Secondary Reconstruction of the Flexor Retinaculum

The FR can also be reconstructed secondarily in those patients complaining of severe bow-stringing of the flexor tendons and grip weakness when manipulating objects with the wrist in flexion. These problems are usually seen in those patients in whom the FR had been excised. Surprisingly, most patients are not willing to undergo another surgical procedure as they adapt to the new situation.

Grip strength testing is commonly used to evaluate the results of some surgical procedures. It is a common misconception that as grip testing is expressed in numbers it should be considered to be an objective test. This test relies heavily on subject motivation, clearly observed in patients looking for some secondary gain. Furthermore, Young et al. [60] have demonstrated fluctuations of grip strength between 5.1 and 8.4 Kg, or between 19.2% and 23.7% in a group of 95 healthy subjects after 12 separate measurements during a 3-month period. Like any other human performance, it may be conditioned by various factors such as mood, motivation, and energy level. Patients with decreased grip strength after FR release can adapt to the situation by limiting wrist flexion, as most activities can be done with just 5° of flexion [61], although other studies claim that up to 40° of wrist flexion is needed [62].

We performed secondary FR reconstruction only in 2 patients suffering from focal dystonia, and in whom bow-stringing of the flexor tendons after CTS release worsened considerably their symptoms of focal dystonia. Loss of grip strength was a minor complaint next to the great disability in the manipulation of objects for the activities of daily living. One of the patients was unable to write after CTS release because the bow-stringing of the flexor tendons further increased the preoperative

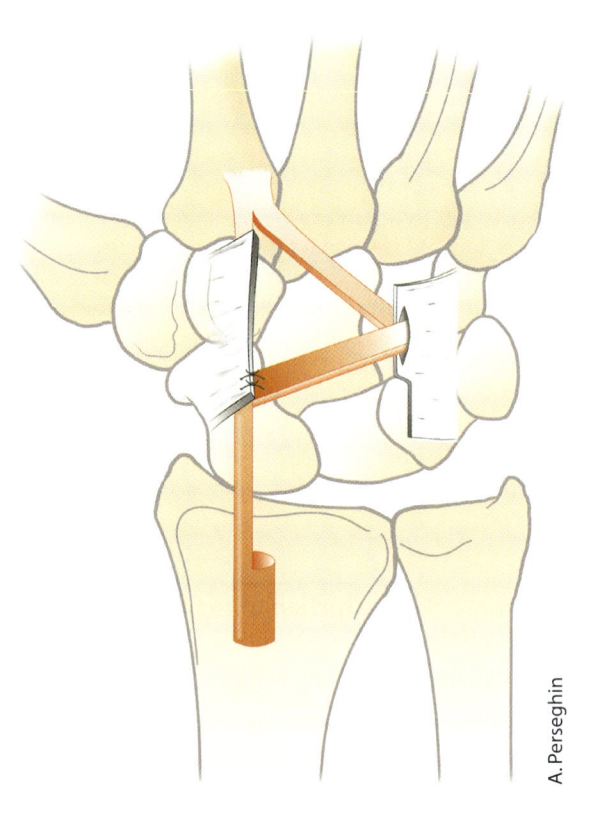

Fig. 32.16. The technique for secondary reconstruction of the FR used by the author. A slip of half the thickness of the flexor carpi radialis tendon is left attached distally and then passed through a slit in the remains of the FR next to the hook of the hamate. The tendon slip is then sutured under tension to the radial edge of the FR at the level of the tubercle of the scaphoid

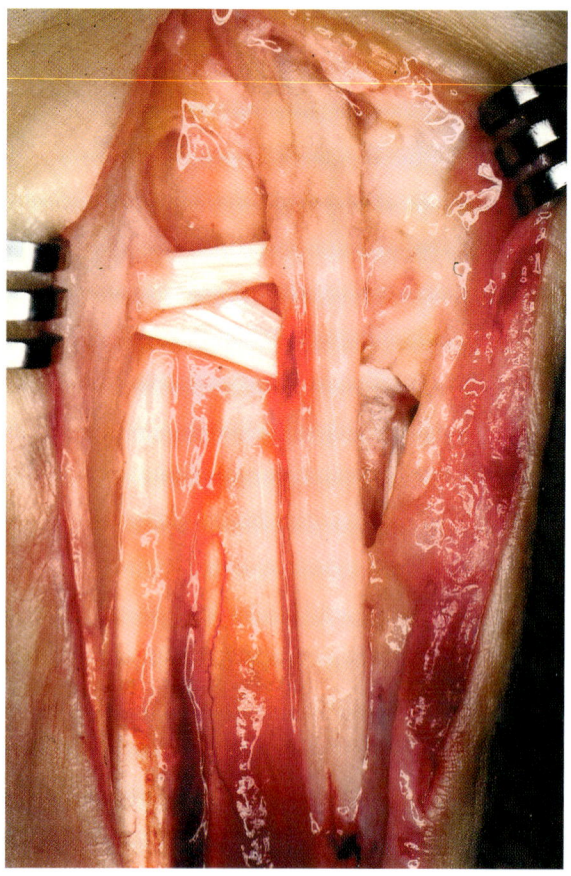

Fig. 32.17. An intraoperative photograph showing the reconstructed FR with a slip of the flexor carpi radialis tendon. All flexor tendons are securely maintained inside the carpal canal under this double pulley sutured to the radial and ulnar bony boundaries of the carpal canal. The median nerve is left in an area of unscarred subcutaneous fat tissue to avoid secondary nerve compression

tendency to flex the wrist during hand writing. Both were satisfied with the secondary reconstruction of the FR, and did not have any neurological symptoms due to having the median nerve in the subcutaneous tissue.

The FR can not be used for secondary repair of the FR as it either has been excised or is severely scarred. In those cases, we use a tendon slip from the flexor carpi radialis (FCR) tendon to reconstruct the FR. A tendon slip of half of the thickness of the FCR tendon is dissected distally from the main tendon starting approximately 5 cm proximal to the wrist crease. The dissection is carried down to the distal part of its compartment at the level of the trapezium. The free end is then passed through a hole made in the remaining FR at the level of the hook of the hamate. The tendon slip is then sutured under tension to the radial side of the carpal canal at the level of tubercle of the scaphoid (Fig. 32.16). This provides for a strong pulley which will maintain the flexor tendons within the boundaries of the carpal canal. The median nerve is left in a subcutaneous position, to avoid a secondary compression inside the carpal tunnel (Fig. 32.17).

Conclusions

Sectioning of the FR allows for anterior displacement of the finger flexor tendons away from the center of rotation of the wrist joint. The magnitude of this displacement is dependent on wrist position. When the wrist is flexed there is an increasing bow-stringing of the flexor tendons causing a relative lengthening of the muscle-tendon unit and, in consequence, decreasing its maximum contractility. This explains why, in normal circumstances, there is decreased grip strength and increased difficulty to flex the fingers as flexion of the wrist is increased.

Most biomechanical cadaveric works demonstrated that there is little difference between open and endoscopic techniques as to the amount of flexor tendon bow-stringing, as the palmar fascia is not an equally effective pulley as the FR to prevent anterior displacement of the flexor tendons. Anterior displacement of the flexor tendons can only be prevented by reconstruction of the FR.

The technique previously described has several advantages over other techniques. It only minimally increases surgical time, as it requires only one suture, and it is easy to perform. It can be done through a limited palmar incision under local anesthesia. The FR is divided on its ulnar side, as far away from the median nerve as possible, thus avoiding a postoperative entrapment by scar tissue. The median nerve is found at a distance of only 10.7 ± 2.2 mm from the radial margin of the hook of hamate [63]. Other techniques for reconstructing the FR require a longer operative time and cause scarring of the FR in the vicinity of the median nerve, which has been described as the main cause of recurrence of symptoms [64–71].

The only disadvantage of FR reconstruction is the fact that it requires a 3-week period of immobilization. However, all patients are very satisfied from the procedure, as the incidence and intensity of postoperative palmar scar pain is greatly decreased. Probably both the repair of the FR and the period of plaster immobilization are responsible for the reduced palmar fibrosis. Most important however, is the fact that patients treated this way never complain of loss of grip strength or recurrence of CTS.

References

1. Lluch A (1984) Abordaje palmar en el tratamiento del síndrome del túnel carpiano. Revisión personal a largo plazo de 147 manos. Rev Esp Cir Mano 12: 7–32
2. Lluch A (1992) Carpal tunnel syndrome: Morphological changes after the release of the transverse carpal ligament (letter) J Hand Surg 17A: 379
3. Seradge H, Seradge E (1989) Piso-triquetral pain syndrome after carpal tunnel release. J Hand Surg 14A: 858–862
4. Gartsman GM, Kovach JC, Crouch CC et al. (1986) Carpal arch alteration after carpal tunnel release. J Hand Surg 11A: 372–374
5. Viegas SF, Pollard A, Kaminski K (1992) Carpal arch alteration and related clinical status after endoscopic carpal tunnel release. J Hand Surg 17A: 1012–1016
6. Chow JCY (1989) Endoscopic release of the carpal ligament: a new technique for carpal tunnel syndrome. Arthroscopy 5: 19–24
7. Richman JA, Gelberman RH, Rydevik BL et al. (1989) Carpal tunnel syndrome: Morphologic changes after release of the transverse carpal ligament. J Hand Surg 14A: 852–857
8. Kato T, Kuroshima N, Nimomiya S, Okutsu I (1994) Effects of Endoscopic Release of the Transverse Carpal Ligament on Carpal Canal Volume. J Hand Surg 19A: 416–419
9. Okutsu I, Ninomiya S, Natsuyama M et al. (1987) Subcutaneous operation and examination under Universal Endoscope. J Jpn Orthop Assoc 61: 491–498
10. Garcia-Elias M, Sanchez-Freijo JM, Salo JM, Lluch A (1992) Dynamic changes of the transverse carpal arch during flexion-extension of the wrist: Effects of sectioning the transverse carpal ligament. J Hand Surg 17A: 1017–1019
11. Chaise F, Roger B, Laval-Jeantet M, Alhomme Ph (1986) Exploration tomodensitométrique des modifications anatomiques du poignet entraînées par la section du ligament annulaire antérieur. Rev Chir Orthop 72: 297–302
12. Ablove RH, Peimar CA, Diao E et al. (1994) Morphologic changes following endoscopic and two-portal subcutaneous carpal tunnel release. J Hand Surg 19A: 821–826
13. Agee JM, McCarrol RH, Tortosa R et al. (1992) Endoscopic release of the carpal tunnel: a randomized prospective multicenter study. J Hand Surg 17A: 987–995
14. Kaplan EB (1965) Functional and surgical anatomy of the hand. Philadelphia: JB Lippincott pp 188
15. Garcia-Elias M, Kai-Nan A, Cooney WP et al. (1989) Stability of the transverse carpal arch: An experimental study. J Hand Surg 14A: 277–282
16. Blix M (1891) Die Länge und die Spannung des Muskels. Skandinavisches Arch Physiol 3: 295–318
17. Hagen JK, Sennwald D, Das KTS (1990) Ursache einer ungenügenden Operationstechnik? Helv Chir Acta 57: 125–128
18. Tubiana R (1990) Carpal tunnel syndrome: some views on its management. Ann Hand Surg 9: 325–330
19. Braun RM, Rechnic M, Fowler E (2002) Complications related to carpal tunnel release. Hand Clinics 18: 347–357
20. Kline SC, Moore JR (1992) The transverse carpal ligament. An important component of the digital flexor pulley system. J Bone Joint Surg 74A: 1478–1485
21. Brown RA, Gelberman RH, Seiler JG et al. (1993) Carpal tunnel release: A prospective randomized assesment of open and endoscopic methods. J Bone Joint Surg 75A: 1265–1275
22. Netscher D, Dinh T, Cohen V, Thornby J (1998) Division of the transverse carpal ligament and flexor tendon excursion: Open and endoscopic carpal tunnel release. Plast Rec Surg 102: 773–778
23. Netscher D, Steadman AK, Thornby J, Cohen V (1998) Temporal changes in grip and pinch strength after open carpal tunnel release and the effect of ligament reconstruction. J Hand Surg 23A: 48–54
24. Fissette J, Onkelinx A (1979) Treatment of carpal tunnel syndrome. Comparative study with and without neurolysis. Hand 11: 206–210
25. Lluch A (1987) El síndrome del túnel carpiano. Barcelona: Editorial Mitre. pp: 137–140
26. Kiritsis PG, Kline SC (1995) Biomechanical Changes after Carpal Tunnel Release: A Cadaveric Model for Comparing Open, Endoscopic, and Step-Cut Lengthening Techniques. J Hand Surg 20A: 173–180
27. Jakab E, Ganos D, Cook FW (1991) Transverse carpal ligament reconstruction in surgery for carpal tunnel syndrome: A new technique. J Hand Surg 16A: 202–206
28. Netscher D, Mosharrafa A, Lee M et al. (1997) Transverse carpal ligament: Its effect on flexor tendon excursion, morphologic changes of the carpal canal, and on pinch and grip strengths after open carpal tunnel release. Plast Rec Surg 100: 636–642
29. Gellman H, Kan D, Gee V et al. (1989) Analysis of pinch and grip strength after carpal tunnel release. J Hand Surg 14A: 863–864
30. Karlsson M K, Lindau T, Hagberg L (1997) Ligament lengthening compared with simple division of the transverse carpal ligament in the open treatment of carpal tunnel syndrome. Scand J Plast Reconstr Hand Surg 31: 65–69
31. Taleisnik J (1993) The palmar cutaneous branch of the median nerve and the approach to the carpal tunnel. J Bone Joint Surg 55A: 1212–1217
32. Engberg WD, Gmeiner JG (1980) Palmar cutaneous branch of the ulnar nerve. J Hand Surg 5: 2629
33. DaSilva MF, Moore DC, Weiss A-P C et al. (1996) Anatomy

of the palmar cutaneous branch of the median nerve: Clinical significance. J Hand Surg 21A: 639–643
34. Watchmaker GP, Weber D, Mckinnon SE (1996) Avoidance of transaction of the palmar cutaneous branch of the median nerve in carpal tunnel release. J Hand Surg 21A: 644–650
35. Martin CH, Seiler III JG, Lesesne JS (1996) The cutaneous innervation of the palm: An anatomic study of the ulnar and median nerves. J Hand Surg 21A: 634–638
36. Seradge H, Seradge E (1989) Piso-triquetral pain syndrome after carpal tunnel release. J Hand Surg 14A. 858–862
37. Tinel J (1915) Le signe du "fourmillement" dans les lesions des nerfs périphériques. Press Med 47: 388–389
38. Brown RA, Gelberman RH, Seiler JG et al. (1993) Carpal tunnel release. A prospective, randomised assessment of open and endoscopic methods. J Bone Joint Surg 75A: 1265–1275
39. Lluch A (1993) Transverse carpal ligament reconstruction for carpal tunnel syndrome. (letter) J Hand Surg 18A: 170–171
40. Lanz U (1977) Anatomical variations of the median nerve in the carpal tunnel. J Hand Surg 2: 44–53
41. Kapandji AI (1990) La plastie d'agrandissement du ligament annulaire antérieur du carpe dans le traitement du syndrome du canal carpien. Ann Chir Main 9: 305–313
42. Hunter JM (1996) Reconstruction of the transverse carpal ligament to restore median nerve gliding. The rationale of a new technique for revision of recurrent median nerve neuropathy. Hand Clin 12: 365–378
43. Lluch A (1987) El síndrome del túnel carpiano. Barcelona: Editorial Mitre. pp: 118–120
44. Lluch A (1989) Carpal tunnel-ligament reconstruction. Corresp Newsletter Am Soc Surg Hand
45. Lluch A (1994) Carpal tunnel surgery. In: Technical tips for hand surgery (Eds: Kasdan ML, Amadio PC, Bowers WH). Philadelphia: Hanley & Belfus, Inc. pp: 168–170
46. Lluch A (1987) El síndrome del túnel carpiano. Barcelona: Editorial Mitre. pp: 177
47. Mackinnon SE, McCabe S, Murray JF et al. (1991) Internal neurolysis fails to improve the results of primary carpal tunnel decompression. J Hand Surg 16A: 211–218
48. Lluch A (1992) Thickening of the synovium of the digital flexor tendons: cause or consequence of the carpal tunnel syndrome? J Hand Surg 17B: 209–212
49. Nakamichi K, Tachibana S (1998) Histology of the transverse carpal ligament and flexor tenosynovium in idiopathic carpal tunnel syndrome. J Hand Surg 23A: 1015–1024
50. Lluch A (1987) El síndrome del túnel carpiano. Barcelona: Editorial Mitre. pp: 132–133
51. Cseutz KA, Thomas JE, Lambert EH et al. (1966) Long term results of operation for carpal tunnel syndrome. Mayo Clinic Proc 41: 232–241
52. Hybinette CH, Mannerfelt L (1975) The carpal tunnel syndrome. A retrospective study of 400 operated patients. Acta Orth Scand 46: 610–620
53. Das SK, Brown HG (1976) In search of complications in carpal tunnel decompression. Hand 8: 243–249
54. MacDonald RI, Lichtman DM, Hanlon JJ, Wilson JN (1978) Complications of surgical release for carpal tunnel syndrome. J Hand Surg 3: 70–76
55. Erdman MWH (1994) Endoscopic carpal tunnel decompression. J Hand Surg 19B: 5–13
56. Bande S, DeSmet L, Fabry G (1994) The results of carpal tunnel release: open versus endoscopic technique. J Hand Surg 19B: 14–17
57. Shinya K, Lanzetta M, Conolly B (1995) Risk and complications in endoscopic carpal tunnel release. J Hand Surg 20B: 222–227
58. Kluge W, Simpson RG, Nicol AC (1996) Late complications after open carpal tunnel decompression. J Hand Surg 21B: 205–207
59. Karlsson M K, Lindau T (1999) Complications and outcome in open carpal tunnel release. Ann Chir Main 18: 115–121
60. Young VL, Pin P, Kraemer BA et al. (1989) Fluctuation in grip and pinch strength among normal subjects. J Hand Surg 14A: 125–129
61. Palmer AK, Werner FW, Murphy D, Glisson R (1985) Functional wrist motion: a biomechanical study. J Hand Surg 10A: 39–46
62. Ryu J, Cooney WP, Askew LJ et al. (1991) Functional ranges of motion of the wrist joint. J Hand Surg 16A: 409–419
63. Omokawa S, Tanaka Y, Ryu J et al. (2002) Anatomy of the ulnar artery as it relates to the transverse carpal ligament. J Hand Surg 27A: 101–104
64. Inglis AE (1980) Two unusual operative complications in the carpal-tunnel syndrome. J Bone Joint Surg 62A: 1208–1209
65. Langloh ND, Linscheid RL (1972) Recurrent and unrelieved carpal tunnel syndrome. Clin Orthop Rel Res 83: 41–47
66. Paine KWE (1963) The carpal-tunnel syndrome. Can J Surg 6: 4467
67. Phalen GS (1966) The carpal tunnel syndrome 17 years' experience in diagnosis and treatment of 654 hands. J Bone Joint Surg 48A: 211–228
68. Phalen GS (1972) The carpal tunnel syndrome: Clinical evaluation of 598 hands. Clin Orthop Rel Res 83: 29–40
69. Rose EH, Norris MS, Kowalske TA et al. (1991) Palmaris brevis turover flap as an adjunt to internal neurolysis of the chronically scarred median nerve in recurrent carpal tunnel syndrome. J Hand Surg 16A: 191–201
70. Wadstroen J, Nigst H (1986) Reoperation for carpal tunnel syndrome. Ann Chir Main 5: 54–58
71. Botte MJ, von Schroeder HP, Abrams RA, Gellman H (1996) Recurrent carpal tunnel syndrome. Hand Clin 12: 731–743

Critical Appraisal of Transverse Carpal Ligament Reconstruction. Theoretical, Experimental, and Clinical Considerations

M. ALTISSIMI

Introduction

Changes in grip strength following section of the transverse carpal ligament (TCL) for carpal tunnel syndrome (CTS) have been evaluated in several experimental and clinical studies because return to working activities is strictly related to postoperative weakening and timing of grip strength recovery. Even endoscopic techniques have been developed to obtain a more rapid recovery of grip strength and a quick return to work.

TCL lengthening and reconstruction has been suggested [6, 7] to maintain a pulley for flexor tendons and to preserve their mechanical *efficiency*. However the efficacy of ligamentoplasty to improve postoperative variation of grip strength after carpal tunnel release is still debated and experimental and clinical data are so far controversial.

In this chapter the rationale for a ligamentoplasty, Jakab's technique of ligament lengthening and reconstruction and clinical results found in the literature will be discussed.

Postoperative Variations of Grip Strength

Open carpal tunnel release is usually followed by reduction of grip strength for several weeks [1–3, 6–8]. The lowest values are recorded 3–4 weeks after surgery; preoperative values are then restored at 3 months and subsequently a significant increase in grip strength occurs, reaching a plateau between 6 and 12 months postoperatively. Gellman [2], in 24 patients, recorded a 72% decrease in grip strength at 3 weeks, recovery of preoperative values at 3 months, and a 16% increase at 6 months. Azzarà [1], in 50 patients, found a 37% decrease in grip strength 4 weeks after surgery, a 14% increase at 3 months followed by a progressive further increase up to 36% after 6–12 months as compared to the preoperative values. Foucher [7], in 66 patients reviewed at 1 month, recorded a 27% decrease in grip strength, recovery of preoperative values after 3 months in the 29 patients available at the follow-up, and no significant increase (-7%) in the 6 patients reviewed at 6 months.

The significant decrease in grip strength following carpal tunnel release is *attributed* to the section of the TCL [3] and to the subsequent changes in volume and shape of carpal tunnel [5]. The integrity of the TCL is in fact important for the maintenance of the transverse carpal arch and of mechanical *properties* of flexor tendons that during wrist flexion are not allowed to move anteriorly by an intact TCL.

Section of the TCL produces considerable changes in volume and shape of the carpal tunnel. A 13.6% widening of the transverse diameter of the carpal tunnel after surgery has been measured by a radiological study by Gartsman [3] in 50 patients. Richman [5] with pre- and postoperative MRI showed, in 12 patients, a 24.2% increase in volume and an anterior shift of the content of the carpal tunnel of 3.5 mm.

These anatomical variations are able to modify the biomechanics of flexor tendons that loosen an important pulley. Kline and Moore [10] have demonstrated a 20%–25% loss of tendon excursion with wrist flexion following section of the TCL. This can explain the reduction in grip strength experienced by patients operated for CTS.

Gartsman [3] believes that grip strength postoperative decrease is proportional to the widening of the carpal tunnel and that it is clinically relevant for widening greater than 20%.

Transverse Carpal Ligament Reconstruction

Based on these experimental and clinical studies, the need for TCL reconstruction in carpal tunnel release to restore a pulley for flexor tendons has been suggested by some authors [6, 8, 9].

The technique described by Jakab [8] is probably the most popular one and it has been used in the few perspective randomized studies that compare results after simple section and after section and reconstruction of the ligament.

Jakab's ligamentoplasty is performed through a 4-cm skin incision. The incision of the TCL is started in the distal and ulnar portion and carried longitudinally in a proximal direction to the level of the hook of the hamate. At this point the incision is directed in a transverse direction for about 2 cm and then again longitudinally in the radial portion of the ligament. This Z-shaped incision creates two flaps that are sutured together, obtaining lengthening of the ligament. Jakab reported that, of 110 patients operated with this technique, all had recovered a grip strength described as normal after 2 years.

Evaluation of Results of Ligament Reconstruction

The effectiveness of ligament reconstruction to prevent a significant postoperative decrease in grip strength, although suggested by anatomical considerations, is scarcely supported by clinical evidence in published studies. There are only a few perspective randomized studies that compare simple ligament section and reconstruction, and their results are controversial.

The studies of Foucher et al. (1996) and Azzarà et al. (1997) can be compared for case selection, method, and surgical techniques.

In Foucher's study [7] simple ligament section (77 patients), ligament reconstruction (133 patients, 55 by Jakab's technique), and endoscopic release (99 patients) are compared. Patients were reviewed every month for 6 months. In patients of the simple section group and in those of the Jakab's reconstruction group a similar reduction in grip strength after 1 month (−27% and −24%, respectively) and recovery of preoperative values after 3 months (+1% and +4.5%, respectively) was observed. At the 6-month follow-up very few patients could be reviewed in both groups (6 and 4, respectively) and the 7% reduction of the preoperative values after simple section and the 24% increase after ligament reconstruction cannot be considered therefore as significant.

In a perspective randomized study Azzarà [1] has compared the results in 50 patients after simple section of the TCL and in 50 patients after Jakab's ligament lengthening and reconstruction. Patient were reviewed at 1, 3, 6, and 12 months postoperatively. Three of the 100 patients were excluded from further evaluation, 1 for reflex sympathetic dystrophy, 2 for flexor tenosynovitis, leaving 49 hands in the section group and 48 in the reconstruction group.

Resolution of pain and paraesthesia as well as recovery of sensibility was comparable in both groups. Postoperative change in grip strength was also similar in the two groups of patients. More specifically, grip strength 1 month postoperatively showed a 37% decrease in the section group and a 46% decrease in the reconstruction group (no statistical difference). At 3 months there was an initial increase (respectively 14% and 15%) as compared to preoperative values. A further progressive increase was then observed up to 36% between 6 and 12 months. At 12 months grip strength had increase from 38.69 kPa to 52.66 kPa in the section group and from 38.96 kPa to 53.02 in the reconstruction group, with no statistical difference in the two groups.

These two clinical studies seem to support the results of Kiritsis and Kline's [11] cadaver study that shows very similar biomechanical changes after simple TCL section and after step-cut lengthening and reconstruction. Karlsson [4] in a clinical retrospective study found no difference in the results after simple ligament section and after ligament reconstruction and believes that there is no advantage in TCL reconstruction.

In conclusion, both the French and the Italian perspective, randomized studies do not support the idea that reconstruction of the TCL is able to give a more rapid and greater recovery of grip strength after open carpal tunnel release.

References

1. Azzarà A, Altissimi M, Mancini GB, Romeo F (1997) Variazioni di forza dopo semplice sezione e dopo allungamento e ricostruzione del legamento trasverso del carpo nella sindrome del tunnel carpale. Riv Chir Riab Mano Arto Sup, 34 (3): 343–346
2. Gellman H, Kan D, Gee V et al. (1989) Analysis of pinch and grip strength after carpal tunnel release. J Hand Surg 14A: 863–864
3. Gartsman GM, Kovach JC, Crouch CC et al. (1986) Carpal arch alteration after carpal tunnel release. J Hand Surg 11A: 372–373
4. Karlsson MK, Lindau T, Hagberg L (1997) Ligament lengthening compared with simple division of the transverse carpal ligament in the open treatment of carpal tunnel syndrome. Scand J plast Reconstr Surg 31: 65–69
5. Richman JA, Gelberman RH, Rydevik BL et al. (1989) Morphologic changes after release of the transverse carpal ligament. J Hand Surg 14A: 852–857
6. Foucher G (1994) Chirurgie des syndromes canalaires du poignet. Téchniques Chirurgicales, Orthopédie-Traumatologie, 44–362, 8, p.1944. Editions Téchniques. Encycl Méd Chir (Paris-France)
7. Foucher G, Van Overstraeten L, Braga da Silva J, Nolens D (1996) Changes in grip strength in a randomized study of carpal tunnel release by three different techniques. European Journal of Orthopaedic Surgery and Traumatology 6: 185–189
8. Jakab E, Ganos D, Cook FW (1991) Transverse carpal ligament reconstruction in surgery for carpal tunnel syndrome: a new technique. J Hand Surg 16A:202–206
9. Kapandji AL (1990) La plastie d'agrandissement du ligament annulaire anterieur du carpe dans le traitement du syndrome du canal carpien. Ann Chir Main Memb Super 9: 305–313
10. Kline SC, MooreRJ (1992) The transverse carpal ligament: an important component of the digital flexor pulley system. J Bone Joint Surg 74A: 1478–1485
11. Kiritsis PG, Kline SC (1995) Biomechanical changes after carpal tunnel release: a cadaveric model for comparing open, endoscopic and step-cut lengthening techniques. J Hand Surg 20A:173–180

Comparison of Grip Strength Evolution After Carpal Tunnel Release by Three Different Techniques

G. Foucher, G. Pajardi, L. Van Overstraeten, J. Braga Da Silva

Introduction

Carpal tunnel syndrome (CTS) secondary to compression of the median nerve in the palm is the most frequent nerve entrapment of the upper extremity. Some forms are accessible to medical treatment, others need surgical treatment. The simple section of the transverse carpal ligament has been successfully used with predictable relief of distal paresthesia. However, diminished grip strength and/or palmar soreness are frequently an issue, resulting in a delayed return to work and recreational activities. The recent introduction of endoscopic release of CTS bolstered by commercial benefits has led us to set up a randomized prospective study to compare evolution of grip strength after three methods of carpal tunnel release (CTR) performed by the same surgeon: simple open section of the ligament, open section with ligament reconstruction, and endoscopic release (Agee procedure).

Material and Methods

During the period September 1990 to December 1992, 303 CTRs corresponding to the inclusion criteria have been randomized to compare grip strength recovery after three techniques. Inclusion criteria were CTS diagnosed on clinical grounds confirmed by EMG study without associated pathology. Cases with rheumatoid arthritis, associated neuropathy, diabetes or recurrent CTS were excluded. The technique was randomly assigned at consultation with special attention for the endoscopic group. In cases of strictly unilateral involvement in young patients, if endoscopic technique was assigned, CT scan or MRI was performed to exclude any local tumor or abnormal muscles. Out of 277 patients, 26 were operated bilaterally. Two hundred forty were females and 37 male patients. Among them, 223 were right-handed, 54 left-handed, and 187 times, the dominant hand was operated on. Twenty-four patients (30%) were manual workers, 35 (13%) white-collar, and 160 (59%) had no job or were retired.

Preoperative symptoms were nocturnal paresthesia in 58%, permanent paresthesia in 25%, and 3% had clinical amyotrophy. All patients were submitted to an EMG study with recording at constant temperature of sensory conduction and motor velocity to confirm the clinical diagnosis, exclude associated pathology, and justify a surgical indication. Fourteen percent had electromyographic signs of muscular atrophy.

Four different techniques were randomly assigned by drawing lots. In group I, a simple open section of ligament was performed in 77 cases (25.4%): 44 on the dominant hand, and 33 on the nondominant hand. Skin incision was in the axis of the fourth finger. The section of the ligament was closed to the hook of the hamate (Fig. 34.1a) to avoid the median nerve being trapped into the ligament or cutaneous scar. Neurolysis was sometimes followed by a tendon synovectomy (65%) with exploration for accessory tendons or abnormal muscles.

In group II (133 cases), a reconstruction of the flexor retinaculum was performed. Skin incision was identical to group I, but in group IIa (68 cases) a reconstruction was performed according to a technique used for the last 15 years in our unit, with a rotation retinaculum flap cut at the expense of the proximal radial rim (Fig. 34.1b) and fixed with a nonresorbable stitch to the ulnar edge. In group IIb (55 cases, 21.5%), the opening of the ligament was Z-shaped with the first longitudinal cut closed to the ulnar border of the canal (away from the motor branch) according to the technique described by Jakab et al. [21] and Kapandji [25] (Fig. 34.1c). Closure allowed a lengthening of the ligament an average of 0.7 cm.

The endoscopic release was performed through a single portal extra-bursal technique with slight modifications (group III, 99 cases). A 1-cm horizontal incision in the proximal wrist flexor crease was performed on the ulnar rim of the palmaris longus. After freeing the deep aspect of the ligament, close to the hook of the hamate, dilatation preceded the introduction of the second generation Agee blade. Lubrication was performed to avoid shear friction on the median nerve. The ligament was cut under permanent coaxial vision. The intermuscular fascia between the thenar and hypothenar muscles superficial to the ligament itself was saved to avoid tendon bow stringing and to limit the separation

During the open procedures, 25 abnormal tendons or muscles (8%) were found: eight deep palmaris longus, seven abnormal lumbricals, and ten accessory bands for flexor tendons profundus. In nine cases, anatomical median nerve variations were found (4%): one high division of median nerve and four transligamentous motor branches of the median nerve. In three cases, a thrombosis of the median artery was noticed and treated by arterial resection. In six of the nine cases of clinical thenar atrophy, lack of opposition was corrected by a Camitz transfer protected postoperatively by an immobilization for 21 days. Being the only immobilized patients, they will be analyzed separately. In all other cases, unrestricted use of the hand was authorized the day following the intervention. Full manual activity without formal rehabilitation was encouraged at 10 days.

Before each operation, grip strength was measured for each hand with a Jamar dynamometer; the patient being seated, the elbow flexed at 90° along the trunk. Three successive measurements led to a calculated mean value. Postoperative strength was controlled monthly by the same team, in the same conditions. In order to correct for dominance, the strength of the nondominant hand was multiplied by a 10/9 factor.

Results

Complications

Except one moderate reflex sympathetic dystrophy (RSD) without final impairment of function, diagnosed on a three-phase scintigraphy, due to persistent edema at the 10th postoperative day, no other major complication was noticed. In six cases of group III, the endoscopic release was converted into an open procedure. In one case it was due to the presence of an abnormal muscular belly, and in the other cases during the endoscopic procedure due to a too-narrow canal after a wrist fracture (1 case), an interposed synovial fringe (2 cases), a neural interposition (2 cases), a vascular anomaly (1 case), all confirmed during the formal opening by a separated distal incision. In groups I to III, respectively, 86%, 87%, and 91% of patients were eventually entirely relieved from preoperative clinical symptoms. All patients not entirely relieved in group III had postoperative EMG to exclude incomplete release and to validate our technical modifications. None of the patients in the whole series needed reoperation.

Grip Strength Evolution

The mean preoperative strength values deviated very little. The mean extremes were 22 kgf and 27 kgf. Of relevance is a frequently diminished preoperative grip strength on the side of the symptomatic CTS. The mean

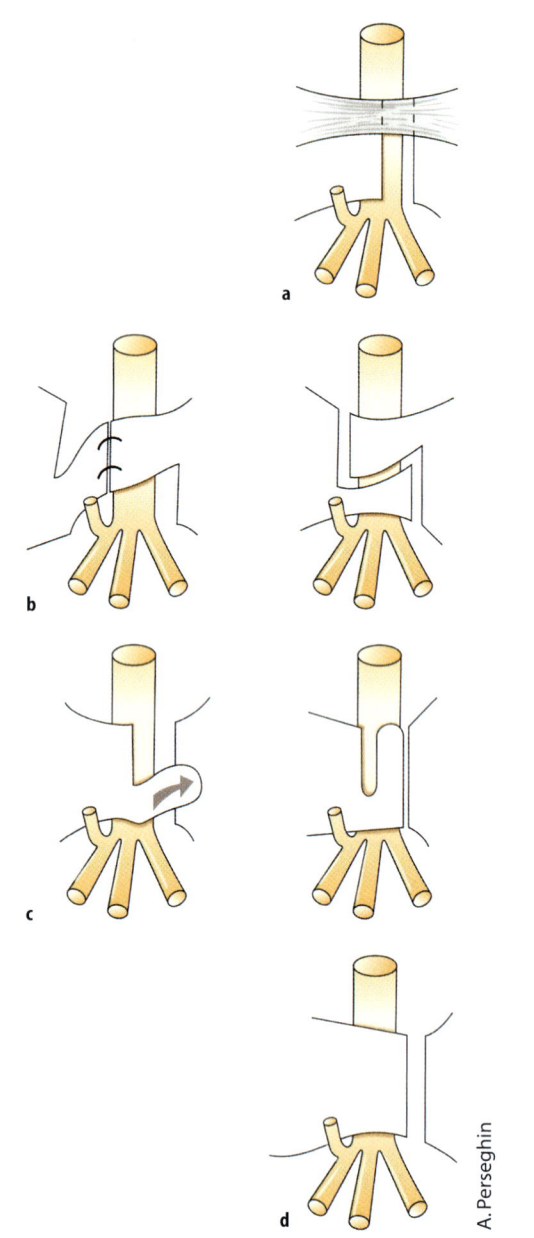

Fig. 34.1. Drawing of the different techniques used in the different groups. **a** Classical open ligament release on the ulnar side of the median nerve. **b** Personal ligamentoplasty with a flap taken from the radial border of the ligament. **c** Jakab ligamentoplasty with a "Z" lengthening. **d** Endoscopic release of the ligament with preservation of the intermuscular distal fascia (between thenar and hypothenar muscles)

of the two edges (Fig. 34.1d). To ascertain the total section of the ligaments, the blade must be introduced between the two edges of the ligament with control of the rims by tilting the blade to allow them to snap inside the lumen of the device. All these cases were part of the "learning series," including our first case of endoscopic release.

strength loss (compared to the contralateral side) was an average of 18%. There was no significant difference with the group of nine clinical atrophy cases with a mean deficiency of 24%. We have not been able to establish any correlation between strength and electromyographic motor latency. The postoperative evolution of strength on the nonoperated hand showed a constant increase of 2%–12.5%, this being independent of the technique and followed, at a lower scale, the improvement of the operated hand.

For each patient, the postoperative deficiency was calculated by dividing the pre- and postoperative difference by the preoperative strength.

(F POST-OP – F PRE-OP) / F PRE-OP

The postoperative loss of strength and its recovery according to time elapsed is illustrated in Tables 34.1–34.3, according to job (Table 34.1), to each separated hand (Table 34.2), and to bilateral cases (Table 34.3). Table 34.4 illustrates the number of patients regaining strength identical or superior to preoperative values for each period of control.

Comments on Grip Strength Evolution

Postoperative grip strength improved constantly whatever technique was used. The progression took 3–6 months. Unrelated to technique, in all cases, at a certain stage a transitional drop of strength appeared between the third and the 5th month. Fifty percent of patients from group I stopped progressing at 3 months, and 25% even had a drop in their recovery curve. In group II, improvement was faster with recovery at 2 months (36% of group IIa and 40% of group IIb). Patients from group III were characterized by a very limited initial drop compared to all other techniques (mean 5% compared to 27%), followed by a recovery identical to group II.

The comparative figures, according to technique, demonstrated the most frequent (Table 34.4), the more

Table 34.1. Evolution of grasp according to job

	Section (G I)	Endoscopy (G III)	Plasty (G IIa)	Plasty (G IIb)
Manual workers				
1 month	−28.15% [21]	−8.54% [11]	−36.69% [14]	−23.98% [14]
2 months	−15.68% [14]	−8.73% [11]	−14.01% [14]	+0.01% [9]
3 months	+5.37% [12]	−0.56% [5]	+15.49% [9]	−1.03% [4]
4 months	+1.09% [5]	+2.93% [4]	−22.14% [5]	−6.98% [1]
5 months	−19.11% [3]			+18.62% [2]
6 months	−9.90% [2]		−18.22% [5]	
White collars				
1 month	−32.52% [7]	−15.63% [9]	−23.43% [6]	−42.28% [5]
2 months	−16.41% [4]	−9.65% [6]	−3.84% [6]	−17.58% [3]
3 months	−32.84% [3]	+1.43% [4]	+12.39% [4]	−26.23% [1]
4 months	−0.56% [4]	−5.44% [1]	−0.00% [1]	+23.81% [1]
5 months	+18.37% [1]			−20.00% [1]
6 months	+2.38% [1]		+44.19% [1]	+22.50% [1]

Table 34.2. Mean strength recuperation for each technique (all sides)

	Section (G I)	Endoscopy (G III)	Plasty (G IIa)	Plasty (G IIb)
1 month	−26.66% [66]	−4.82% [64]	−27.00% [44]	−24.33% [51]
2 months	−12.79% [46]	−6.20% [35]	−7.95% [42]	+0.43% [31]
3 months	+1.00% [29]	+9.89% [19]	+9.02% [33]	+4.52% [23]
4 months	+3.41% [13]	+0.34% [9]	−16.78% [9]	+10.28% [4]
5 months	−7.17% [7]	−3.45% [1]	−1.85% [1]	+4.70% [7]
6 months	−6.97% [6]		+3.67% [20]	+23.63% [4]

Table 34.3. Mean strength loss for each technique according to dominance in bilateral cases (22)

	Section (G I) [10]	Plasty (G IIa) [10]	Section (G I) [12]	Plasty (G IIb) [12]
All hands				
1 month	−28.47% [7]	−26.06% [8]	−26.16% [12]	−20.50% [10]
2 months	−11.95% [4]	+9.51% [8]	−11.23% [9]	−9.05% [6]
3 months	−1.83% [3]	+12.90% [6]	+3.49% [5]	−0.04% [5]
4 months	−4.37% [4]	−42.62% [1]	−5.35% [4]	
5 months	+18.37% [1]	+15.37% [2]	−8.65% [4]	+4.88% [1]
6 months		+23.13% [8]	−10.93% [4]	+22.54% [2]

NB: Endoscopy excluded for reason of not significant number

Table 34.4. Number of patients regaining a strength superior to preoperative data

	Section (G I) Def>0 Tot	Endoscopy (G III) Def>0 Tot	Plasty (G IIa) Def>0 Tot	Plasty (G IIb) Def>0 Tot
1 month	8/56 (14.3%)	22/64 (34.4%)	8/44 (18.2%)	8/49 (16.3%)
2 months	11/46 (23.9%)	10/35 (28.6%)	15/42 (35.7%)	13/32 (40.6%)
3 months	11/29 (37.9%)	11/19 (57.9%)	17/33 (51.5%)	13/24 (54.2%)
4 months	8/16 (50.0%)	4/9 (44.4%)	3/9 (33.3%)	2/4
5 months	2/8 (25.0%)	0/1	0/1	3/7 (42.8%)
6 months	1/5		9/20 (45.0%)	3/4

relevant and quickest recovery in group IIb and III, and the slowest and most incomplete in group I. For the bilaterally operated patients, with simple section on one side and ligamentoplasty on the other, the data are even more obvious (Table 34.3). Professional occupation played an important role, the strength recovery being slowest in white-collars, and the type b plasty being especially gainful for manual workers. The low 25% men representation excludes any statistical conclusion related to gender.

Finally, we did study postoperative palmar soreness and pillar pain to try to find a correlation with diminished strength. Soreness was less frequent in groups IIa, IIb, and III (3%) than in group I (28%).

Discussion

The majority of operated CTS series review a variable amount of complications, although a decreased grip strength is frequently mentioned. A frequent explanation concerns flexor tendon bow stringing after simple ligamentous section. In a biomechanical cadaver study, Kiritsis and Kline [26] measured flexor tendon course after CTR. After open release, an increase in tendon excursion consumed by wrist motion was demonstrated for flexor digitorum profundus (26%) and flexor digitorum superficialis (18%) tendons. A 21% and 15% increase in tendon excursion was also demonstrated after endoscopic CTR and step-cut lengthening of the transverse carpal ligament. Increased excursion was noted after 20–30° of wrist flexion as tendon bow stringing occurred.

An anterior migration of the flexor tendons has been confirmed by postoperative tomography and MRI and was reduced in case of ligament reconstruction. Even after 3 weeks of immobilization, values of 3.5 mm could be seen according to Richmann et al. [33], and persisted 8 months after intervention, being even higher without immobilization. Meanwhile, what is good for strength might be detrimental for the nerve, as was recently stressed by Dellon [10], who stated that an immobilization for more than 1 week after a neurolysis can be followed by nerve adhesion with subsequent traction lesions. Cook et al. [8], in a prospective randomized study, assessed the role of postoperative splintage for 2 weeks following surgery compared to range-of-motion exercises on the first postoperative day. Splinted patients had significant delays in recovery of grip strength and return to activities (daily living, return to work at light and full duty). They also experienced increased pain and scar tenderness during the first postoperative month. In a similar study, Bury was not able to show any difference but also concluded there was no beneficial aspect for postoperative splinting.

However, the bow stringing of the flexor tendon is not the only factor explaining the loss of strength after CTR, and Fuss and Wagner [17] have demonstrated the partial disinsertion (10%–20%) of the intrinsic muscles of the hand.

The more recent endoscopic techniques have shown similar clinical signs of improvement compared to open CTR, even on a long-term basis, and the majority of authors claim better strength recovery. We conducted a randomized study to assess grip strength progression after three surgical methods of CTR: classic open release (group I), ligamentoplasty reconstruction (group II), and endoscopic release (group III). Endoscopic release can be conducted through a double portal (wrist and palmar incisions) or through a single forearm portal, using a special device (Agee). In 1992, Chow mentioned at the meeting of the American Society for Surgery of the Hand a complication rate of 0.3% in his own series, but figures as high as 22% for surgeons not having been trained in his workshops. We selected the Agee technique for this series. Except one case of RSD, without sequel, no other complications were noticed. Moreover, during the learning curve of endoscopic CTR, six cases were converted into a classical open release (with no other opening in the consecutive 965 cases). In our experience, temporary postoperative paresthesia has disappeared with lubrication of all material introduced in the canal to avoid any shear friction on the median nerve; these paresthesia were also mentioned by Arner et al. [2] in more than 10% of their short series with the Chow approach, where hyperextension of the wrist could be another mechanism.

We limited our study to the evolution of grip strength as our first 45 patients did not show any difference for pinch strength. This was also mentioned by Sennwald and Benedetti [35] in their randomized prospective study of 47 patients operated either by Agee or open release. If the improvement of grip strength was significantly better after endoscopic release, the key-pinch showed a similar pattern of improvement in both groups.

In our study, evolution of grip strength was characterized by a constant postoperative drop around 25% in open techniques (with or without ligament plasty), less severe after endoscopic release (5%), followed by a steady recovery. Surprisingly, a temporary secondary drop was frequently noticed between the 3ird and the 5th postoperative month. Except in group I, the final strength exceeds preoperative figures (+24%) which means a "normal" strength due to the 18% preoperative loss in relationship to CTS. Our study showed a better and faster recovery of strength after Agee endoscopic release and ligamentoplasty. A similar conclusion was drawn in a study by Palmer [31] comparing the open technique and two endoscopic approaches (Agee and Chow). Endoscopically treated patients achieved faster recovery (for grip and pinch strength and wrist range of motion) and had less midpalm tenderness. Tenderness and time off were even less with the Agee procedure compared to the two other techniques.

We could hardly find any study in the literature describing a randomized prospective comparison of these three different techniques performed by the same surgeon with the same postoperative protocol and a 6-month follow up. Multicenter series, small cohorts, variable postoperative protocol (immobilization), retrospective review, short postoperative control and sometimes absence of preoperative grip strength measurement bias the majority of the studies. Our study has demonstrated that comparison with the contralateral side is not valid for three reasons: the bilaterality of CTS (electromyographically presented in 56%), a significant drop in preoperative strength in the CTS (mean 18%), and a constant postoperative increased strength (2%–12.5%) on the contralateral side.

Each of the three different techniques have been studied in the literature. Jakab et al. [21] described a series of 110 hands with normal strength 2 years after ligamentoplasty. Gellmann in a prospective study of 24 patients with preoperative measurement, showed after classic open release a 72% drop after 3 weeks (with postoperative immobilization) with a return to normal after 3 months. At final review, the strength was 116% compared with preoperative values but still 29% down compared with the "healthy" side. Chow [7] mentioned in a series of 149 endoscopic CTR normal value at 3 weeks in 32% of patients, and 100% at 4 weeks. These brilliant and surprising results could not be duplicated. In Agee's multicentric study [1], a 33% drop of strength after 2 weeks was noticed (55% in the control group with classical opening). At 3 months, the drop did not exceed 5% (15% in the control group). No measurement was done before 6 months, when strength returned to normal in both groups. Superior endoscopic results in the literature have not provided any clear explanation, but absence of postoperative immobilization and early use of the hand could be relevant factors.

Our results are superior to those published by Agee and we could hypothesize some anatomical reasons. In his study, Viegas et al. [38] found a mean widening of the transverse carpal arch of 0.17 cm (7%), ranging from 0 to 0.5 cm. Seventy percent of the patients remained in the 0%–10% margin but 26% showed 10%–20% widening, and 4% showed even more than that. This widening could be controlled and limited by preservation of the intermediate fascia between the superficial palmar aponeurosis and the carpal ligament in the distal part of the tunnel. This fascia has transverse fibers extending between the thenar and hypothenar muscles. Contrary to the classical description, we saved these fibers, thus limiting the final distance between the two edges of the ligaments. This space was close to the lengthening obtained by the Jakab ligamentoplasty. Our figures of 5% drop compared to the Agee's 30% could be explained by their postoperative splinting but also by the section of the fibers mentioned above. More recently, Mirza et al. [28] developed another device for endoscopic CTR to save also these transverse fibers and claimed earlier return to work, better strength, and decreased palmar tenderness. The only drawback of this preservation is a more limited drop in the intracanal pressure (G. Foucher, unpublished data, 1995), a fact confirmed by the study of Nakao et al. [29]. However a long-term study (L. Erhardt et al., in press) did not demonstrate any clinical consequence.

Conclusion

With the three techniques of CTR, ligamentoplasty and Agee's endoscopic technique scored better on strength recovery than simple open section. One of these two techniques should be offered to manual workers and sports professional athletes.

References

1. Agee J, Tortosa R, Berry D, Peimer C (1990) Endoscopic release of the carpal tunnel: a randomized prospective multicenter study. 45th Annual Meeting of American Society for Surgery of the Hand, Toronto
2. Arner M, Hagberg L, Rosen B (1994) Sensory disturbances after two-portal endoscopic carpal tunnel release: a preliminary report. J Hand Surg. Am. 19, 548–51
3. Buch-Jaeger N, Foucher G (1994) Correlation of clinical signs with nerve conduction tests in the diagnosis of carpal tunnel syndrome. Journal of Hand Surgery 19B, 720-724
4. Buch-Jaeger N, Stutzmann-Simon S, Jesel M, Foucher G (1998) Efficacité clinique à moyen et long terme du traite-

ment chirurgical du syndrome du canal carpien. La Main 3, 195–201
5. Bury TF, Akelman E, Weiss AP (1995) Prospective, randomized trial of splinting after carpal tunnel release. Ann Plast Surg 35, 19–22
6. Chaise F, Roger B, Laval-Jeantet M, Alhomme Ph (1986) Exploration tomodensitométrique des modifications anatomiques du poignet entraînées par la section du ligament annulaire antérieur. Revue de Chirurgie Orthopédique 72, 297–302.
7. Chow J (1990) Endoscopic release of the carpal ligament: a new technique for carpal tunnel syndrome. Arthroscopy 6, 289–296
8. Cook AC, Szabo RM, Birkholz SW, King EF (1995) Early mobilization following carpal tunnel release. A prospective randomized study. J Hand Surg Br 20, 228–30
9. Das SK, Brown HG (1976) In search of complications in carpal tunnel decompression. The hand 8, 243–249
10. Dellon AL (1992) Patient evaluation and management considerations in nerve compression. Hands Clinics 8, 229–239.
11. Duncan KH, Lewis RC, Foreman KA, Nordyke MD (1987) Treatment of carpal tunnel syndrome by members of the American Society for Surgery of the Hand: Results of a questionnaire. J Hand Surg 12A, 384–391
12. Foucher G, Malizos C, Sammut D et al. (1991) Primary palmaris longus transfer as an opponensplasty in carpal tunnel release. A series of 73 cases. J Hand Surg Br 16, 56–60
13. Foucher G (1994) Chirurgie des syndromes canalaires du poignet. Encyclopédie médico-chirurgicale (Paris-France), Techniques chirurgicales, Orthopédie Traumatologie 44–362
14. Foucher G, Braga Da Silva J (1995) Ouverture endoscopique du canal carpien. Chirurgie 120, 100–104.
15. Foucher G, Allieu Y, Buch N (1995) Bilan d'une expérience de libération endoscopique du canal carpien par la technique d'Agee. À propos de 280 cas. Rhumatologie 47, 2, 47–51
16. Foucher G, Van Overstraeten L, Braga Da Silva J, Nolens N (1996) Changes in grip strength in a randomized study of carpal tunnel release by three different techniques. Eur. J Orthop Surg Traumatol 6, 185–189
17. Fuss FK, Wagner TF (1996) Biomechanical alterations in the carpal arch and hand muscles after carpal tunnel release: a further approach toward understanding the function of the flexor retinaculum and the cause of postoperative grip weakness. Clin Anat 9, 100–8
18. Garstman GM, Kouach JC, Crouch CC et al. (1986) Carpal arcle alterations after carpal tunnel release. J Hand Surg 11A, 372–374
19. Gellmann H, Kan D, Gee V et al. (1989) Analysis of pinch and grip strength after carpal tunnel release. J Hand Surg 14A, 863–864
20. Gibbs KE, Rand W, Ruby LK (1996) Open vs endoscopic carpal tunnel release. Orthopedics 19, 1025–8
21. Jakab E, Ganos D, Cook FW (1991) Transverse carpal ligament reconstruction in surgery for carpal tunnel syndrome: a new technique. J Hand Surg 16A, 202–206

22. Jarit P (1991) Dominant-hand to non-dominant hand grip strength ratios of college baseball players. Journal of Hand Therapy 123–126
23. Jessurun W, Hillen B, Zonneveld F et al. (1987) Anatomical relation in the carpal tunnel: a computed tomographic study. J Hand Surg 12B, 64–67.
24. Jimenez DF, Gibbs SR, Clapper AT (1998) Endoscopic treatment of carpal tunnel syndrome: a critical review. J Neurosurg 88: 817–26
25. Kapandji AJ (1990) La plastie d'agrandissement du ligament annulaire antérieur du carpe dans le traitement du syndrome du canal carpien. Ann Chir Main 9, 305–314
26. Kiritsis PG, Kline SC (1995) Biomechanical changes after carpal tunnel release: a cadaveric model for comparing open, endoscopic, and step-cut lengthening techniques. J Hand Surg Am 20, 173–80
27. Langloh ND, Linscheid RL (1972) Recurrent and unrelieved carpal tunnel syndrome. Clinical Orthopaedics 41–47
28. Mirza MA, King ET Jr, Tanveer S (1995) Palmar uniportal extrabursal endoscopic carpal tunnel release. Arthroscopy 11, 82–90
29. Nakao E, Short WH, Werner FW et al. (1998) Changes in carpal tunnel pressures following endoscopic carpal tunnel release: a cadaveric study. J Hand Surg Am 23, 43–7
30. Netscher D, Mosharrafa A, Lee M et al. (1997) Transverse carpal ligament: its effect on flexor tendon excursion, morphologic changes of the carpal canal, and on pinch and grip strengths after open carpal tunnel release. Plast Reconstr Surg 100, 636–42
31. Palmer DH, Paulson JC, Lane Larsen CL et al. (1993) Endoscopic carpal tunnel release: a comparison of two techniques with open release. Arthroscopy 9, 498–508
32. Phalen GS (1966) The carpal tunnel syndrome. Seventeen years' experience in diagnosis and treatment of six hundred fifty-four hands. J Bone Joint Surg 48A, 211–228
33. Richmann JA, Gelberman RH, Rydevik BL et al. (1989) Carpal tunnel syndrome: morphology changes after release of the transverse carpal ligament. J Hand Surg 14A, 852–857
34. Rothan MB, Manske PR, Mirly AL (1993) Anatomical study of an endoscopic carpal tunnel device to surrounding structures. J Hand Surg 18A, 442–450
35. Sennwald GR, Benedetti R (1995) The value of one-portal endoscopic carpal tunnel release: a prospective randomized study. Knee Surg Sports Traumatol. Arthrosc 3, 113–6
36. Skorpik G, Landsiedl F (1996) Das Karpaltunnelsyndrom. Ein Vergleich der endoskopischen und offenen operativen Behandlung. Handchir Mikrochir Plast Chir 28, 133–7
37. Stutzmann S, Buch Jaeger N, Foucher G (1998) Syndrome du canal carpien. Résultats du traitement conservateur par orthèse de repos nocturne sur mesure. La Main 3, 203–210
38. Viegas SF, Pollard A, Kaminksi K (1992) Carpal arch alteration and related clinical status after endoscopic carpal tunnel release. J Hand Surg Am 17, 1012–6

Median Nerve Compression Secondary to Fractures of the Distal Radius

A. Badia

Fractures of the distal radius and carpal tunnel syndrome are both commonly occurring entities seen in the wrist. The latter condition is an occasional complication that should be well recognized as a result of the former traumatic condition. While treatment of distal radius fractures is currently undergoing a treatment revolution, the complication of carpal tunnel syndrome should be similarly recognized and given the respect that it deserves. Once significant median nerve injury or compression occurs as a result of a fracture of the distal radius, it can be much more difficult to treat, and the final outcome may be much less predictable than its idiopathic counterpart.

Abraham Colles first described the fracture of the distal radius in 1814 but maintained that functional deficiency or complications were surprisingly rare after this common traumatic injury [6]. Similarly, carpal tunnel syndrome associated with this fracture was given little attention and initially felt to be a rare sequela. Early textbooks discussing complications of Colles fractures rarely mentioned this nerve compression, and it was not until the classic paper by Abbott and Saunders in 1933 that this complication was clearly recognized as being not as rare as initially thought [1].

The first case report was actually a direct traumatic injury to the median nerve as recognized by Gensoul in 1836 where he had performed an autopsy on a young girl who died of tetanus following an open fracture of the distal forearm [12]. It was found that the median nerve was caught in the fracture site of the radius. Many of these early reports focused on the direct compression or contusion of the median nerve as a result of bony impalement or stretching of the nerve, rather than the more commonly seen secondary compression as a result of edema and swelling from this fracture.

It was not until the review by Abbott and Saunders that the popular Cotton-Loder position for immobilization of distal radius fractures was discredited. They first recognized the anatomical course of the median nerve at the wrist, noting that the flexed position of the wrist will lead to direct compression of the median nerve by the proximal edge of the transverse carpal ligament. They also recognized that the median nerve carries with it the majority of sympathetic nerve innervation to the hand and that this can cause the other commonly recognized complication of carpal tunnel syndrome: Complex Regional Pain Syndrome Type I. This was the first time it was recommended that conservative treatment of Colles fracture allow for immobilization of the wrist in a neutral position, mainly to avoid median nerve entrapment. However, despite elucidating this important concept, they went on to say that if median nerve symptoms persist even after 4 months of closed treatment, surgical exploration of the median nerve is warranted. This underscored the prevailing concept that median nerve compression should not be treated as aggressively as we now recognize. Hence, more aggressive treatment of displaced distal radius fractures should go hand-in-hand with decompression of the median nerve.

Meadoff wrote in 1949 that injuries of the median nerve in fractures about the wrist are not uncommon and that good reduction and immobilization of the wrist in the neutral position are the best means of preventing median nerve injury [17]. He also felt that the majority of patients with median nerve injury recover completely without surgery. In 1952, Mark Mason reviewed 100 cases of Colles fractures requiring closed reduction and found only one case developing a carpal tunnel syndrome [16]. However, his study had an average follow-up period of only 22 months since the time of the fracture, which this supports the notion that perhaps many carpal tunnel syndrome complications may occur years after the initial fracture event. Much like Abraham Colles, he found only five patients had any complications whatsoever and supported the existing belief that complications were exceedingly rare after this common fracture. Later studies countered this popular belief.

It was not until 1963 that Lynch and Lipscomb reported 3.3% of their patients with distal radius fractures developing carpal tunnel syndrome [14]. In a retrospective review of 600 distal radius fractures seen over 10 years at the Mayo Clinic, they found that 20 wrists developed this complication in 19 of their patients. Hence, they concluded that carpal tunnel syndrome is indeed frequently associated with a Colles fracture, and they supported the notion that this often occurs after immobilization in the Cotton-Loder position. They also emphasized that carpal tunnel syndrome following a Colles fracture can be classified as primary, when the median nerve is actually caught or directly contused between the fracture ends of the radius, and secondary when edema, hand position, and tenosynovitis lead to secondary compression within the carpal tunnel. Phalen himself noted in 1951 that a tardy median palsy might be associated with Colles fractures [22]. He stated that any condition which either increased the volume of structures within the tunnel or anatomic factors that decreased the diameter of the tunnel would lead to compression of the median nerve. Therefore, it is only logical that carpal tunnel syndrome would be a commonly seen complication after fracture of the distal radius, and it is an entity that should have a low threshold for consideration in postfracture management.

Smaill from New Zealand continued to reiterate Colles' belief that patients would regain full, painless function irrespective of how the fracture was treated [24]. He felt operative treatment or aggressive manipulation was unwarranted and only reported two complications in his series, both ruptures of the extensor pollicis longus, and no carpal tunnel syndrome. It is apparent in reviewing his treatise that many authors shared an acceptance of relatively poor outcomes after these fractures. Cole and Obletz in 1966 reviewed the end results of 33 cases of distal radius fractures treated by pins-and-plaster technique [5]. They found only one case of a transient median "neuritis," but the longest follow-up in their study was 5 years, with the shortest being only 18 months. They did recognize, however, that many of their patients had poor functional outcomes, and they agreed with Gartland and Werley, who determined that closed immobilization led to inadequate results in their 60 patients treated for Colles fractures [8].

During these years, carpal tunnel syndrome was frequently thought of as a chronic condition. It was not until 1970, when Adamson presented his paper, "The Acute Carpal Tunnel Syndrome," it was generally accepted that this condition can occur acutely [2]. They reported nine cases of acute carpal tunnel syndrome, of which one was after a severe Colles fracture from a fall on the wrist while ice skating. They concluded that acute carpal tunnel syndrome was much more common than ordinarily thought and, therefore, one can conclude that the Colles fractures would likely play a role in the etiology of this acute nerve compression. A similar report on acute carpal tunnel syndrome was written by McClain and Wissinger in 1976 [18]. They too presented nine different case reports; but in their study, four of the nine cases occurred from fractures of the distal radius. Two of these were classic, extra-articular Colles fractures; one was a Salter-Harris II fracture of the distal radius in an adolescent, and the last report involved an intra-articular fracture of the distal radius. They concluded that immediate surgical decompression was the most favored option. Bauman and Gelberman also published a paper entitled, "The Acute Carpal Tunnel Syndrome," and they presented five different cases of acute carpal tunnel syndrome in 1981 [3]. Of these, four cases involved distal radius fractures, and their review of the literature concluded that fractures of the distal radius were the leading cause of acute median nerve compression.

Gelberman went on to look at carpal tunnel pressures and wrist positions in patients with Colles fractures and stated that an awareness of the magnitude of increased interstitial fluid pressure should lead to an alternate method of treatment in many cases of distal radius fractures [4]. They found that intracarpal canal interstitial fluid pressures were highest in extreme flexion after Colles fractures. In contrast, similar studies in patients with no fractures have demonstrated that extreme extension actually produces the most intracarpal pressure [9, 15]. This underscores the importance of maintaining the wrist in a relatively neutral position during immobilization for this injury.

Besides causative factors such as hyperflexion of the wrist and direct entrapment of the median nerve at the time of fracture, a third cause of median nerve compression can occur by volarly displaced fragments. Paley and McMurtry first described compression of the median nerve against the proximal edge of the transverse carpal ligament by a volarly displaced fragment in this fracture pattern [21]. They concluded that not only was reduction of this fragment necessary, but that carpal tunnel decompression is also necessary. They presented nine patients with markedly displaced volar fragments in a distal radius fracture, with eight of these patients developing either acute or delayed carpal tunnel syndrome. They first described the concept that median neuropathy can occur acutely, subacutely, or late after Colles fractures. They further noted that compression from a volar displaced fragment was a much less common phenomenon but, nevertheless, should be recognized. Other authors have described late median nerve symptoms after displaced volar fragments with Lewis and Miller describing a case where a carpal tunnel syndrome developed 18 years after a Smith fracture [13]. Watson-Jones described a similar case [26], while Cooney reported that six out of 565 patients reviewed at the Mayo Clinic developed a late carpal tunnel syndrome directly attributed to a volar fragment compression [7]. Although this fracture pattern necessitates an open reduction, it should also be done for the reason of decompressing the median nerve since any attempt at closed reduction can cause further injury to the nerve due to the presence of this fragment against the nerve itself.

Secondary carpal tunnel syndrome is not limited to adults as Binfield from London described three cases of

Salter-Harris type II fractures of the distal radius leading to median nerve complaints [4]. As often done in children, the fractures were treated closed and once reduction was obtained, the symptoms quickly resolved. They were quick to conclude that adult management of a median nerve palsy associated with distal radius fracture usually necessitated exploration and decompression of the carpal canal. However, with children this decision is more controversial, and they supported the concept of closed reduction and close follow-up of the clinical symptoms over time.

Just as median nerve compression has been managed with increasing vigilance, we have also gradually come to a point where the distal radius fracture is treated much more aggressively. Due to the relative frequency of median nerve compression in these fractures, as we have seen with literature review, we might also conclude that perhaps median nerve compression should be implied once distal radius surgical management is undertaken. It is only in recent years that distal radius fractures are commonly being treated by open means due to the accepted notion that a more anatomic reduction will lead to a better clinical result [11]. Although there is still a role for the use of external fixation, it is becoming increasingly accepted that an open reduction with plates and screws is indicated. During this open reduction, it is often prudent to release the median nerve in that same sitting. This becomes even more intuitive when the approach for the fracture is performed in a volar fashion. Recent papers indicate that the distal radius anatomy and biomechanics dictate that a plate be placed on the volar side [19]. Consequently, this allows for a median nerve decompression since it can be done through the same volar side and perhaps even the same incision if it is approached in a more extensile manner.

Internal fixation of the distal radius through a volar approach is usually performed through a more distal Henry approach between the flexor carpi radialis (FCR) and the radial artery. In complex fractures, this approach can be extended more distally to better allow reduction of the articular surface, and the incision can be extended directly over the carpal tunnel to allow for open release of the transverse carpal ligament. This extension should be done in a zig-zag manner to avoid a longitudinal scar over the volar wrist creases. More complex fractures (Fig. 35.1) that require articular elevation may be approached through the extended FCR approach [20]. This was first described by Orbay and allows one to reduce the fracture through an intrafocal approach. This way the critical volar ligaments are not violated in reducing the articular surface. I also recommend arthroscopic assistance in many of these articular fractures in the younger, high-demand patient. Because of the amount of postoperative swelling that may occur after this aggressive approach, it may also be prudent to decompress the median nerve as a consequence of the surgical technique itself. It is my preference to perform the carpal tunnel release endoscopically. Hence, I make a separate, small, transverse incision in the midline to the wrist directly over or just ulnar to the palmaris longus tendon (Fig. 35.2). This tends to be several centimeters ulnar to the distal extent of the approach for distal radius volar open reduction. The endoscopic technique obviously results in less surgical trauma being a minimally invasive approach and is adequate in cases where reduction of associated fractures in the carpus are not necessary.

My personal preference is to decompress the median nerve first in fractures of mild-to-moderate displacement, and then perform the open reduction through

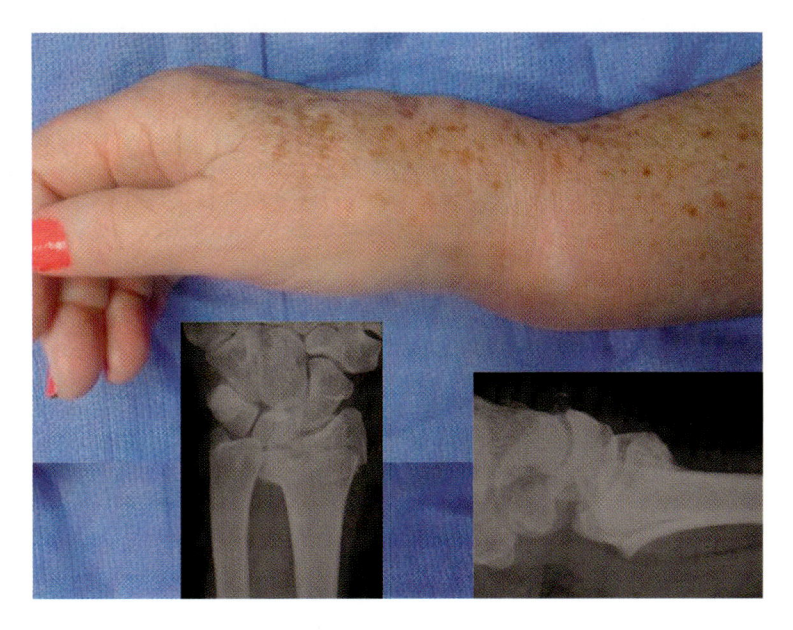

Fig. 35.1. Classic silver fork deformity of wrist with accompanying antero-posterior and lateral x-rays in severely displaced intra-articular fracture of distal radius. Note the location of direct compression on median nerve by the fractured end of the proximal fragment as indicated by the arrow

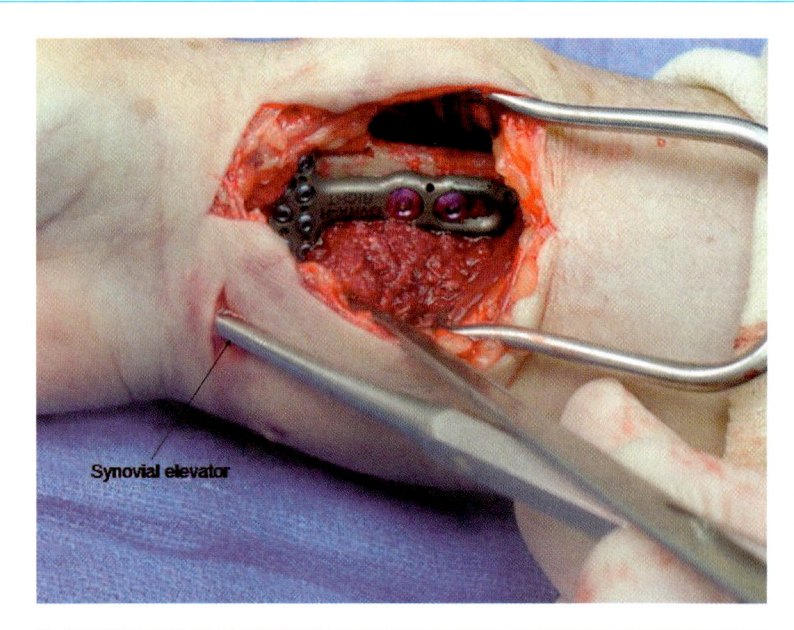

Fig. 35.2. Elevation of synovium from undersurface of transverse ligament via endoscopic approach incision next to volar approach illustrating reduction of fracture with volar plate fixation

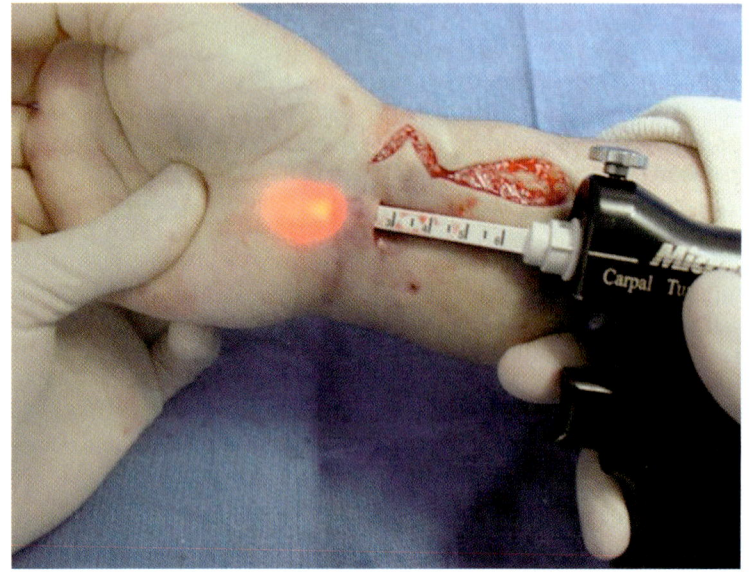

Fig. 35.3. Division of transverse carpal ligament by one portal endoscopic technique. Note the transillumination of the skin where the ligament has already been divided

the previously described volar approach through a separate longitudinal incision. More severely displaced fractures should be reduced first, prior to the median nerve decompression, since the severity of fracture displacement may place the median nerve in a much less predictable position, making endoscopic release more technically challenging. In these markedly displaced cases, I perform volar plating first, and then once the anatomy has been restored, it is much easier to release the transverse carpal ligament through the endoscopic approach (Fig. 35.3). I have frequently noted that the carpal tunnel is not tight once the fracture is reduced, although there is almost always blood within the carpal canal. Irrigating this out can also minimize neuritis from the effect of blood around the nerve. Despite the obvious advantages of decompressing the median nerve at the time of surgery, I have also found there to be other direct benefits. Besides preventing or reversing the effects of median nerve compression from the fracture, I also find that postoperative rehabilitation is much easier once the transverse carpal ligament is divided. This is because of the empiric observation that the patient can flex and extend the fingers much easier once the confines of the carpal tunnel are decompressed. We must realize that not only does the median nerve run within the carpal tunnel, but nine flexor tendons pass through this very narrow canal as well. Due to either anatomic variation in the carpal tunnel due to the fracture or the effects of swelling from interstitial edema or direct bleeding, the flexor tendons are narrowly constricted within the tunnel. Once the ligament is divided, the flexor tendons can glide free of relative

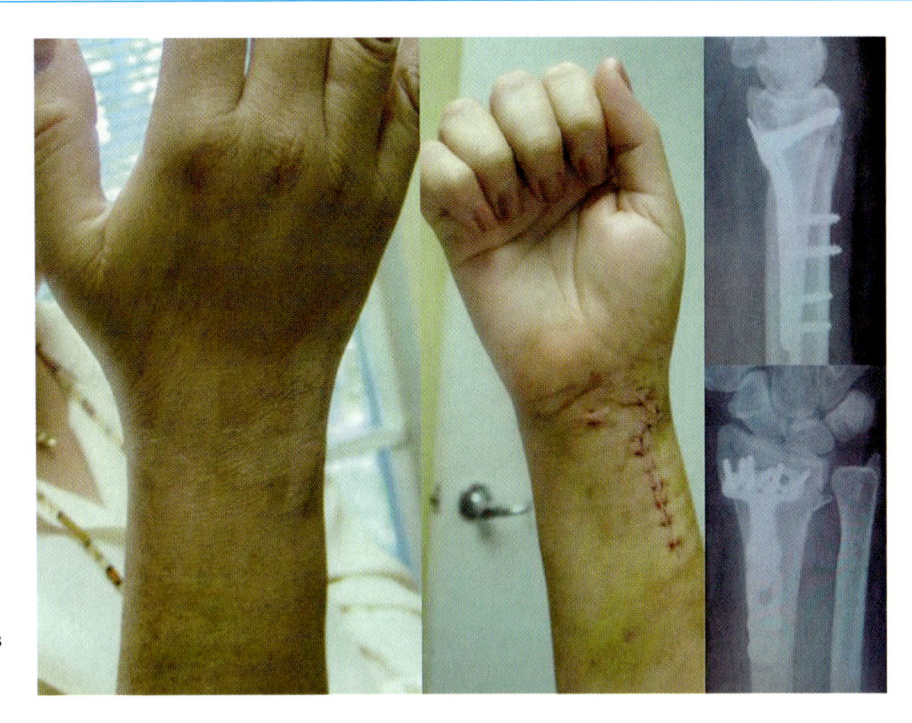

Fig. 35.4. Closed wounds illustrating the two-incision technique to stabilize the distal radius and decompress the carpal tunnel with concomitant reduction x-rays

restriction, and this allows for the patient to fully extend and flex the fingers immediately in the recovery room after open reduction/internal fixation. This has not only the advantage of allowing improved and less painful rehabilitation, but likely diminishes the possibility of developing a complex regional pain syndrome.

It is my current practice to perform an endoscopic carpal tunnel release in all patients who undergo open reduction/internal fixation for displaced distal radius fractures (Fig. 35.4). The vast majority of these patients undergo volar fixation using a subchondral peg support, but on rare occasions a shear articular fracture of the distal radius may require the application of an external fixator and concomitant arthroscopic reduction of the articular surface for management of this fracture. In these cases, once the external fixator is placed, a separate incision is made for endoscopic carpal tunnel release at that time. It has been my experience that these patients have much less pain and better digital function in the postoperative period as a direct result of median nerve decompression at the initial time of surgery.

In conclusion, it is now a well-accepted fact that carpal tunnel syndrome is a frequently seen complication of distal radius fractures, either in the acute period or delayed as a consequence of the swelling and deformity of the wrist. It might also be concluded that decompression of the median nerve should be done in conjunction with the ever-increasing operative treatment of displaced distal radius fractures. This has many benefits besides avoiding carpal tunnel syndrome which allows our patient with this common fracture to rehabilitate the hand in a more rapid and less painful fashion.

References

1. Abbott LC, Saunders JB de CM (1933) Injuries of the median nerve in fractures of the lower end of the radius. Surg Gynecol Obstet 57:517
2. Adamson JE, Srouji SJ, Horton CE, Mladick RA (1971) The acute carpal tunnel syndrome. Plast Reconstr Surg 47:322
3. Bauman TD, Gelberman RH, Mubarak SJ, Gardin SR (1981) The acute carpal tunnel syndrome. Clin Ortho 156: 151–156
4. Binfield PM, Sott-Miknas A, Good CJ (1998) Median nerve-compression associated with displaced Salter-Harris Type II distal radial epiphyseal fractures. Injury 29:93–94
5. Cole JM, Obletz BE (1966) Comminuted fracture of the distal end of the radius treated by skeletal traction in plaster cast. An end-result study of thirty-three cases. J Bone Joint Surg 48A:931–945
6. Colles A (1814) On the fracture of the carpal extremity of the radius. Edinburgh Medical and Surgical Journal 10:182
7. Cooney WP, Dobyns JH, Linscheid RL (1980) Complications of Colles' fractures. J Bone Joint Surg 62A:613–619
8. Gartland JJ, Werley CW (1951) Evaluation of healed Colles' fractures. J Bone Joint Surg 33A: 895–907
9. Gelberman RH, Hergenroeder PT, Hargens AR et al. (1981) The carpal tunnel syndrome. A study of carpal tunnel pressures. J Bone Joint Surg 63A, 380–383
10. Gelberman RH, Szabo RM, Mortensen WW (1984) Carpal Tunnel Pressures and Wrist Position in Patients with Colles Fractures. J Trauma 24:747–749
11. Knirk JL, Jupiter JB (1985) Late results of intra-articular distal radius fractures in young adults. Orthop Trans 9:456-457
12. Lobert M (1836) Observation et reflexions sure une complication grave des fractures. Arch Gen Med 41:198
13. Lewis D, Miller EM (1922) Peripheral nerve injuries associated with fractures. Trans Am Surg Assoc 40:489
14. Lynch AC, Lipscomb PR (1963) The carpal tunnel syndrome and Colles' fracture. JAMA 185:363–366

15. Luchetti R, Schoenhuber R, DeCicco G et al. (1989) Carpal túnnel pressure. Acta Orthop Scand 60: 397–399
16. Mason MC (1952) Colles' fracture. A study of end results. Br J Surg 40:340
17. Meadoff N (1949) Median nerve injuries in fractures in the region of the wrist. Calif Med 70:252
18. McClain EJ, Wissinger HA (1976) The Acute Carpal Tunnel Syndrome: Nine Case Reports. J Trauma 16:75–78
19. Orbay J, Fernandez D (2002) Volar fixation for dorsally displaced fractures of the distal radius: a preliminary report. J Hand Surg 27A:205-215
20. Orbay J, Badia A, Indriago I et al. (2001) The extended flexor carpi radialis approach: a new perspective for the distal radius fracture. Tech Hand Upper Extrem Surg 5:204-211
21. Paley D, McMurtry RY (1987) Median Nerve Compression by Volarly Displaced Fragments of the Distal Radius. Clin Ortho 215:139-147
22. Phalen GS (1951) Spontaneous compression of median nerve at wrist. JAMA 145:1128–1132
23. Pool C (1973) Colles' fracture. A prospective study of treatment. J Bone Joint Surg 55B:540–544
24. Smaill GB (1965) Long-term follow-up of Colles' fracture. J. Bone Joint Surg 47B:80–85
25. Sponsel KH, Palm ET (1965) Carpal tunnel syndrome following Colles' fracture. Surg Gynecol Obset 121:1252–1256
26. Watson-Jones R (1949) Leri's pleonosteosis, carpal tunnel compression of the median nerves and Morton's metatarsalgia. J Bone Joint Surg 31B:560

Part IV

Rehabilitation

IV

Postoperative Treatment of Carpal Tunnel Syndrome After Median Nerve Decompression (Open Field or Endoscopic Technique)

T. Fairplay, G. Urso

Introduction

The therapeutic treatment of a patient who has undergone a transverse carpal ligament release in the carpal tunnel varies broadly from patient to patient. The severity of the preoperative nerve compression, the patient's predisposition to systemic illness, scar length, the surgical techniques followed (internal or external neurolysis, open field or endoscopy approach) [2], the severity of thenar eminence atrophy and the patient's capacity to modify their activities of daily living are all fundamental factors which influence both the postsurgical rehabilitation time frame and the functional recovery prognosis of both the hand and wrist.

Some patients encounter postoperative complications such as: infections, neuromas, scar dehiscence, scar hypersensibility, keloids, or even reflex sympathetic dystrophy [3]. For this reason we have elaborated a therapeutic protocol for the treatment of these postoperative complications, as well as, for prevention of their onset. Obviously, it is impossible to apply the exact same protocol to each patient. Therefore, the following protocol is easily modified for its duration and timing, so that the individual patient can obtain optimal therapeutic effects for the decompression of the median nerve, whether or not they have been surgically treated in an open field or endoscopically.

The advantages of endoscopic treatment for carpal tunnel syndrome (CTS) have been greatly discussed among specialists of the medical community. In a clinical follow-up report of 22 months, on 149 cases of transverse carpal tunnel ligament release that have been performed endoscopically, it has been demonstrated that this technique renders similar results as those surgeries done using an open field approach, but with the advantage of producing a minute scar while maintaining hand grasp and pinch strength and a shorter recovery time [2, 4].

We feel that all patients should undergo rehabilitation sessions immediately after surgery, whether it be for a brief or long treatment program. At times the patient will need a complete re-education program for edema control, scar remodeling, sensory re-education, or work-hardening; at other times, it is sufficient enough to teach the patient median nerve and differential tendon gliding exercises that should be routinely performed to prevent scar adhesions. The duration and type of rehabilitation treatment depends however on the patient's physiologic recovery and the amount of hand and wrist strength that their work activities require of them.

Postoperative Treatment

The physical therapy treatment goals in the first 2 weeks are:

- Edema control
- Sensory evaluation
- Maintain complete finger range of motion
- Prevention of tendon adhesions
- Intermittent wrist immobilization and protection

The patient's wrist is immobilized in a neutral position using a dorsal resting splint.

During the first 2 weeks postoperatively, it is important that the wrist is not overly stressed with flexion and extension movements. If the patient is not able to hold their wrist in a neutral position autonomously, then a made-to-measure dorsal resting splint should be made using a lightweight thin thermoplastic material (1.6 mm thickness) that positions the wrist at 0° (Fig. 36.1).

The necessity, physiologic advantages, and the best position to posture the wrist after CTS surgery (whether open field or endoscopically) are arguments that are continually discussed between therapists and hand surgeons. Chaise studied grasp strength recovery time in two groups of patients where the variable, among these two groups, was whether or not the wrist was immobilized postoperatively. In one group the wrist was placed at 20° of wrist extension for 15–18 days; in the other group the wrist was not immobilized. The healing process was quicker in the group that was immobilized. Twelve months after surgery the group that was immobilized had recuperated 80% of their grasp strength with the wrist in a maximum wrist flexion position and 100% with the wrist in neutral. The group that was not

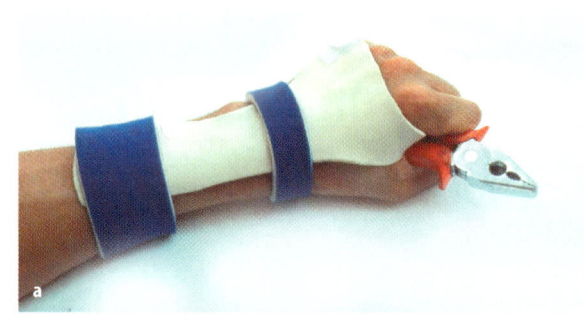

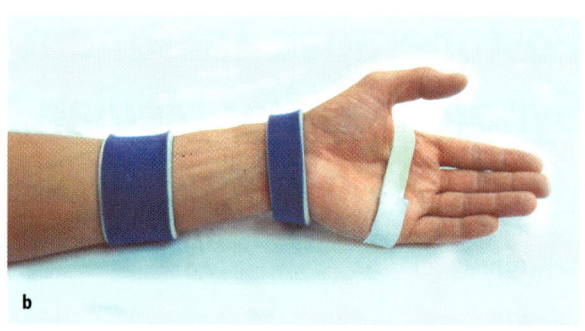

Fig. 36.1. a,b A dorsal resting wrist splint that the patient should wear continually for the first 14 days after surgery (only to be taken off to perform gentle wrist range of motion and flexor tendon gliding exercises at least four times a day) and for the following 3 weeks when performing moderate-to-heavy activities of daily living or when returning to work. **b** The splint is made of 1.6 mm light thermoplastic and allows for complete metacarpophalangeal flexion and thumb opposition

immobilized recovered 50% and 90% of their grasp strength respectively [5]. Weiss has demonstrated, in his studies on intracarpal canal pressure, that when the wrist is positioned at 20° of extension there is an increase in tunnel pressure in comparison to a neutral position [6, 7]. In 1993, at the annual American Society of Hand Therapists Congress, various standard protocol variations were reported regarding postoperative treatment of median nerve decompression in the carpal tunnel and the new standard protocol suggests that the patient's wrist is immobilized in a dorsal splint with the wrist at 0–15° of extension (Fig. 36.1b). Being that the splint is worn dorsally, it provides support to the wrist without interfering with hand grasping activities or compromising palmar sensibility [8]. Yoshida et al. have collected data on 58 subjects that have worn the dorsal splint; 37 of the 58 subjects in this study were diagnosed with CTS, 94.5% of these patients (55 patients) have correctly used the splint and 37 out of the 55 patients continued to wear the splint during manual labor [9].

The choice of using the dorsal rather than a volar splint is based on the following considerations:

1. The dorsal splint allows for complete gliding of finger flexor tendons and does not inhibit full grasp activities.
2. The thin palmar thermoplastic band, located just below the metacarpal articulations, does not impede thumb movement or completely remove palmar tactile sensation.
3. The splint allows the patient to perform both grasping and fine prehensile activities in a functional manner.
4. The same splint that is fabricated immediately after surgery can be easily modified and worn even when the patient returns to work.

The patient is instructed to wear the splint constantly for the first 14 days and only to remove it for medication changes and very carefully guided gentle wrist range of motion exercises that should be performed four times daily. The wrist is immobilized because strenuous or excessive range of motion could increase pressure on the median nerve leading to increased nerve irritability and hypersensibility. Wrist immobilization, for the first 14 days, also allows for complete remargination of the surgical scar and prevents dehiscence from occurring due to excessive overstretching of the scar borders. After 15 days, the patient is instructed to remove the splint during the day and only to wear it at night for the following 7 days or when performing moderate resistive repetitive activities of daily living. They are also instructed to avoid strenuous lifting of heavy objects in this time period and to avoid end-range wrist flexion or extension.

In only rare occasions do patients, who have undergone endoscopic median nerve decompression, require the wearing of a protective wrist splint. A standard protocol used by Chow, following endoscopic surgery, has been followed on 149 subjects, and the protocol requires that the subjects begin wrist range of motion exercises within 24 h from the time of surgery. For the first 2–3 weeks, the patient is instructed not to pick up heavy objects and not to resistively push objects with the palm of the hand [4].

Recovery of Finger Range of Motion and Differential Gliding Exercises for the Finger Flexor Tendons

These exercises are begun immediately. The patient is taught to raise their arm above their head and open and close the hand 10 times each hour. Each finger should be mobilized individually, as well as, in coordinated movements. The patient should be instructed by a hand therapist prior to surgery of the specific finger exercises that they should perform immediately after surgery. Studies have demonstrated that most patients are much more collaborative if they are given diagrammed exercises and a routine schedule to follow [10]. Differential finger gliding exercises are initiated in order to facilitate isolated excursion of each finger's two flexor tendons (flexor superficialis and flexor profundus), both which pass through the carpal tunnel. Each exercise is initiated with the fingers in complete extension and the wrist immobilized in a neutral position. In order to obtain differential gliding of the flexor profundus in respect to the flexor superficialis, the patient should make a hook fist in which the metacarpophalangeal joints are in extension but the proximal and distal interphalangeal joints are flexed. In order to obtain maximum flexor superficialis excursion the patient is taught to flex the metacarpophalangeal joints, as well as the proximal interphalanges but to extend the distal interphalanges. A closed fist is done to obtain maximum excursion of the flexor profundus [10]. The thumb must also be integrated into these exercises by flexing its metacarpophalangeal joint while extending its interphalanx and visa versa. All these exercises should be done in a series of 5 repetitions at least 10 times a day (Fig. 36.2a–e).

Retrograde Massage and Increasing Venous Return

Each patient is instructed on performing upper extremity exercises (raising the entire arm above the level of the heart) ten times each hour to aid in increasing venous return In addition, the patient is instructed on performing retrograde massage beginning at each finger and working in a distal-to-proximal direction to redirect distal edema, which eventually compromises full

Fig. 36.2. a–e Flexor tendon differential gliding exercises; these exercises are performed by the patient in order to obtain the maximum tendon excursion of the flexor superficialis. The patient is instructed to flex the metacarpophalanges and proximal interphalanges while the distal interphalanges remain in extension. A complete closed fist is performed in order to obtain maximum excursion of the flexor profundus

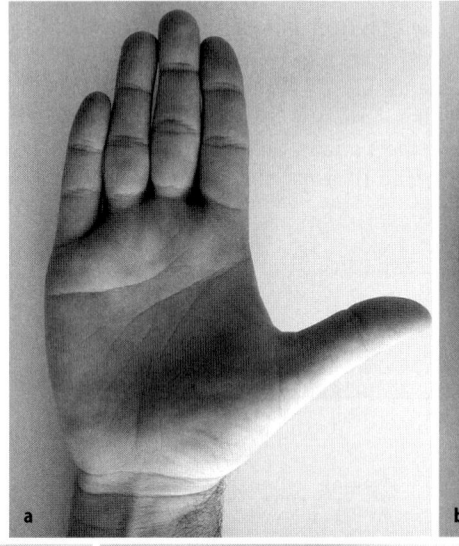

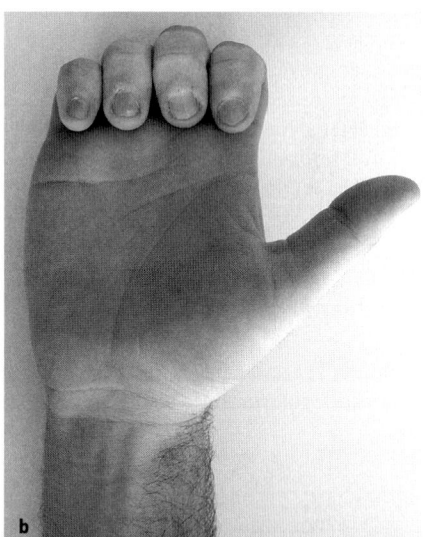

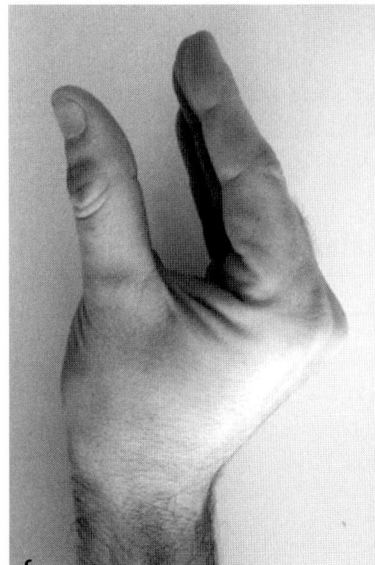

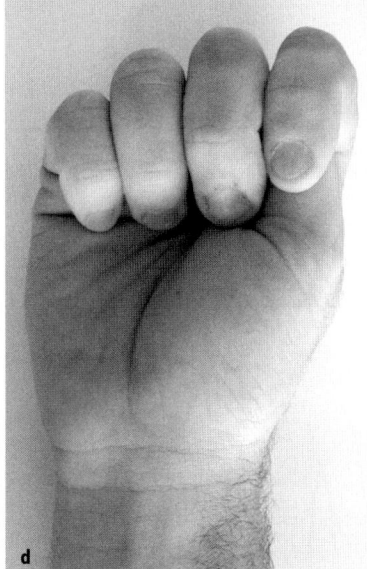

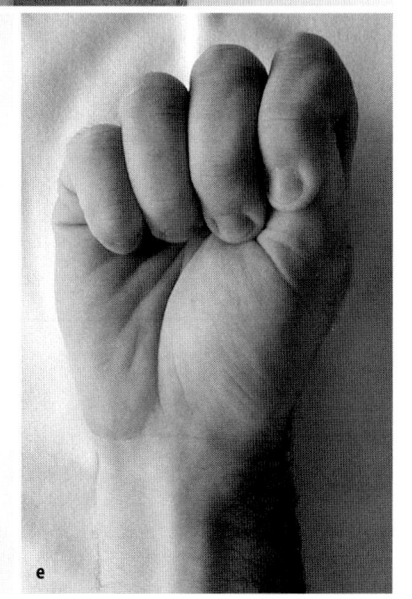

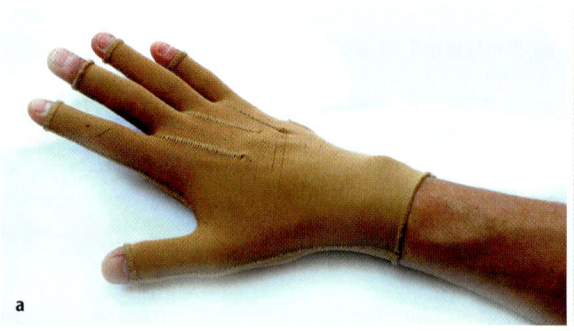

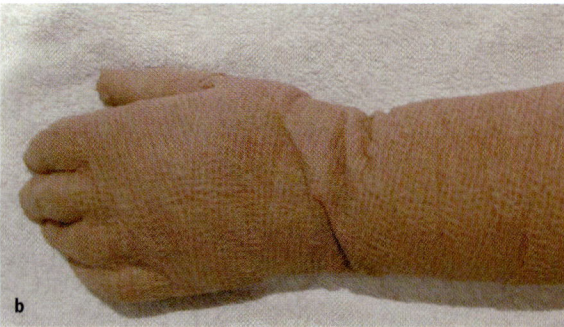

Fig. 36.3. a In cases in which the patient presents with a significant amount of hand and finger edema, a Jobst glove compression stocking used to control swelling of the fingers and hand. **b** COBAN wrapping is done to each finger and the entire hand up until the middle of the forearm when there is the presence of persistent finger and hand edema

finger flexion. When the patient presents with a moderate-to-severe amount of edema, the therapist should begin specific lymph drainage massage followed by wrapping the fingers, wrist, and forearm with a compression glove stocking (Fig. 36.3a), COBAN, or String Wrap in order to decrease the local edema [3, 10] (Fig. 36.3b). Ice application is a modality that is always helpful in decreasing severe edema and the patient should be instructed to use the ice no more than 10 min at a time.

Shoulder Exercises

Shoulder exercises that should be followed are: flexion, extension, internal and external rotation, adduction, and abduction. By moving the shoulder through all its movement planes the patient can maintain full shoulder mobility and prevent capsular adhesions from forming. All the shoulder exercises should be done at least three times a day and repeated each time for ten repetitions (Fig. 36.4a, b). These above-mentioned exercises should be performed for 14 days in addition to the physical therapy sessions that are scheduled with the hand therapist.

The goals of physical therapy in the third and fourth week from the time of surgery are:

- Complete finger range of motion
- Complete wrist range of motion
- Prevention of soft tissue scar adhesion formation
- Complete flexor tendon gliding freedom

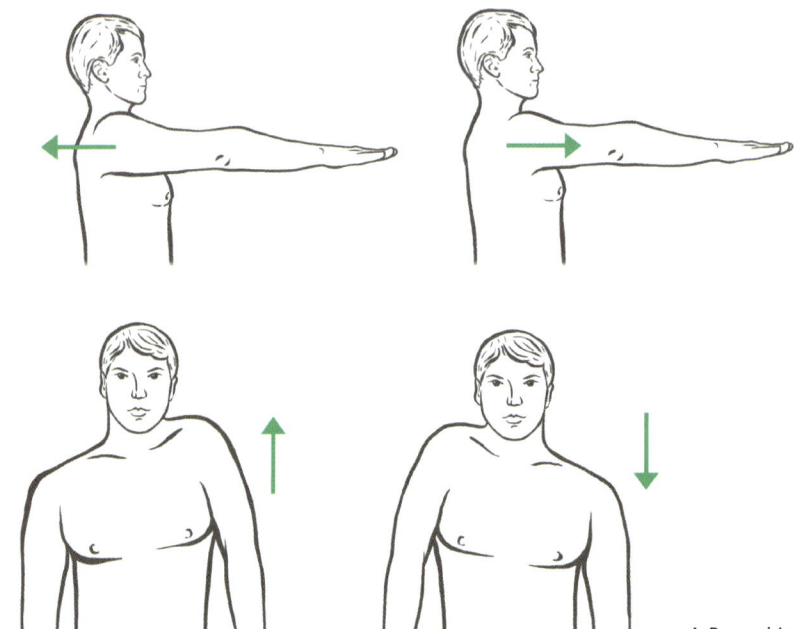

A. Perseghin **Fig. 36.4. a** Shoulder exercises

Fig. 36.4. b   b

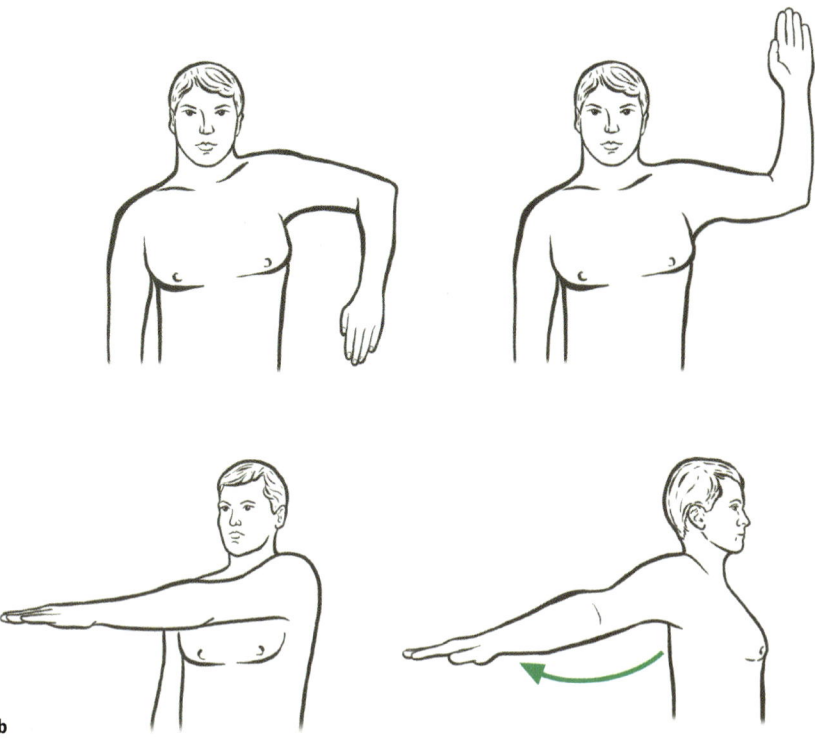

A. Perseghin

Splint Removal

The resting splint should be gradually abandoned and only used during the night or when the patient will be performing activities of daily living under effort or resistance.

Suture Removal

The patient's sutures are usually removed 14 days after surgery or when the scar has closed completely.

At this point, the therapist should begin to remodel the scar. Some patients will need to use an elastomer or silicone sheet [11] (Fig. 36.5), which is placed on top of the scar in order to prevent scar keloid formation. The patient is instructed on how to massage the scar and render it pliable by massaging it for a few minutes repetitively throughout the day, lifting up the epidermis and rolling it between the fingers between the two borders of the incision. This type of massage increases blood circulation (by the removal of local metabolites and catabolites) thus preventing the formation of adhesions between the skin and underlying soft tissue structures.

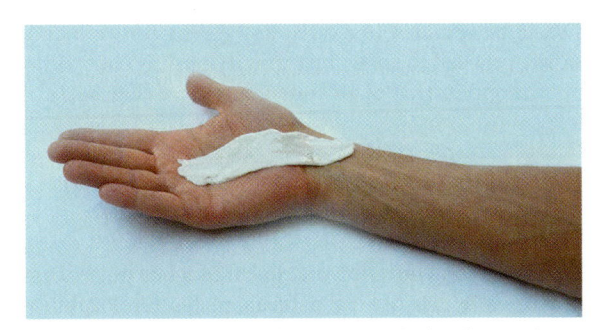

Fig. 36.5. "Elastomer" or "gel sheet" is applied to the scar in order to prevent a keloid formation

Scar Treatment; Remodeling, and Desensibilization (When Necessary)

A desensibilization program uses techniques that have been carefully studied and are known to reduce scar hypersensibility symptoms and gradually increase the patient's tactile tolerance to the area. The program consists of 5–10 min exercises 3–4 times a day. The patient is educated on how to perform these exercises first on the healthy hand. This vibration technique is based on an irritative stimulation application scale [12]. A manual vibrator can be used in proximity to the scar. The vibration is initially applied intermittently to the surrounding area of the scar and then gradually is placed on top of the scar itself. The vibration is then applied constantly rather than intermittently, directly to the

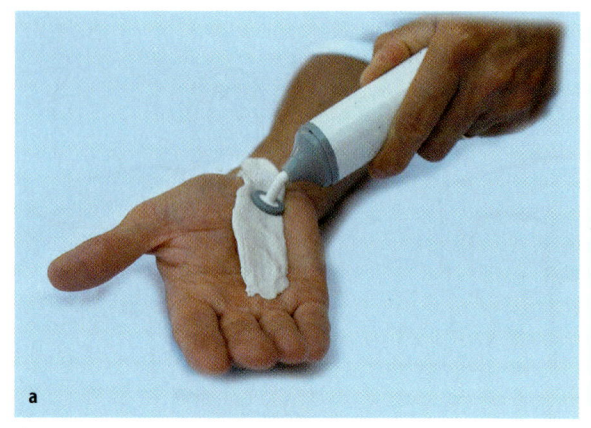

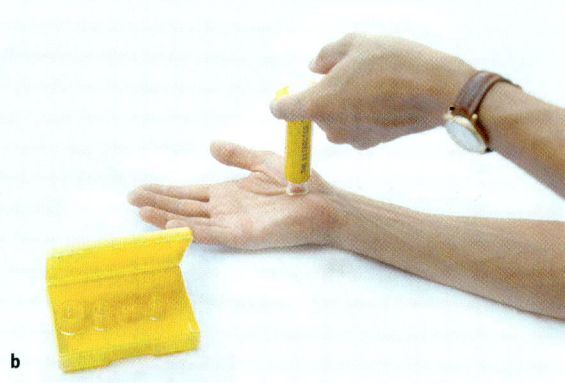

Fig. 36.6. a, b Scar desensibilization techniques

scar. It is also possible to apply an elastomer to the scar and use the vibration on top of the scar in order to dull the vibration sensation at first, thus favoring a gradual acceptance of this scar treatment by the patient. A scar suction pump, which creates a negative pressure on the scar site and its borders, can be used in the attempt to detach the epidermis from the underlying dermis in order to break up superficial scar adhesions; obviously this technique should only be performed once the scar has completely closed and healed (Fig. 36.6a, b).

Iontophoresis can be applied to the scar in cases in which the patient suffers from severe hypersensibility, edema, or adhesions. Iontophoresis consists of the direct administration of a pharmaceutical to the pathological site by means of a continual electric current appliance. Each type of substance such as acid, base, or salt that can be ionized, are adaptable for their use in iontophoresis. The pharmaceutical is prepared in its ionic form as a solution. This solution has a predisposed polarity and with the use of a direct current, a differential reaction is made between the positive electrode (pushes in only ions and positively charged radicals) and the negative electrode (pushes in only ions and negatively charged radicals). Therefore, the protocol changes depending on the pathology that is being treated and the substance that is being used [13]. For example: 2 cc lidocaine/1 cc dexamethasone sodium phosphate, by using a positive current of 4.0 mA, for about 20 min, reduces inflammation around the scar and leaves behind an analgesic effect where the electrode has been placed (Fig. 36.7); 3 cc of potassium iodide (solution of 10%) can be used with a negative current in order to soften the scar and prevent keloid formation from occurring in the epidermal and dermal layers [13].

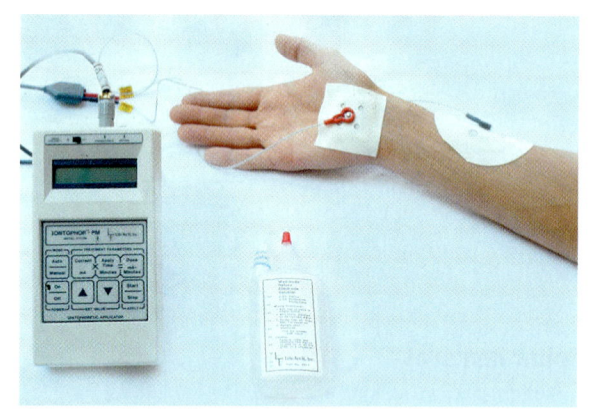

Fig. 36.7. The use of iontophoresis applied to the scar site, is effective in cases in which the patient is suffering from scar hypersensibility, edema, or subdermal adhesions

Wrist Range of Motion Exercises

The patient is instructed to perform both passive and active range of motion exercises three times a day. The exercises consist of having the patient arrive to their maximum range of motion in all the wrist planes of movement [3, 10] and slowly apply a constant but light pressure on the wrist to slowly stretch the scar without overloading the articulation or nerve. These exercises should be initiated in a wrist antigravity position and slowly proceed to an against-gravity position but without the application of an added resistance (Fig. 36.8).

Transcutaneous Electric Stimulation (T.E.N.S.) or Microcurrent Stimulation

The use of long duration and low frequency pulses can provoke a release of local natural opiates, (endorphin), and therefore, diminish pain perception [13]. The electrodes can be applied around the scar according to the

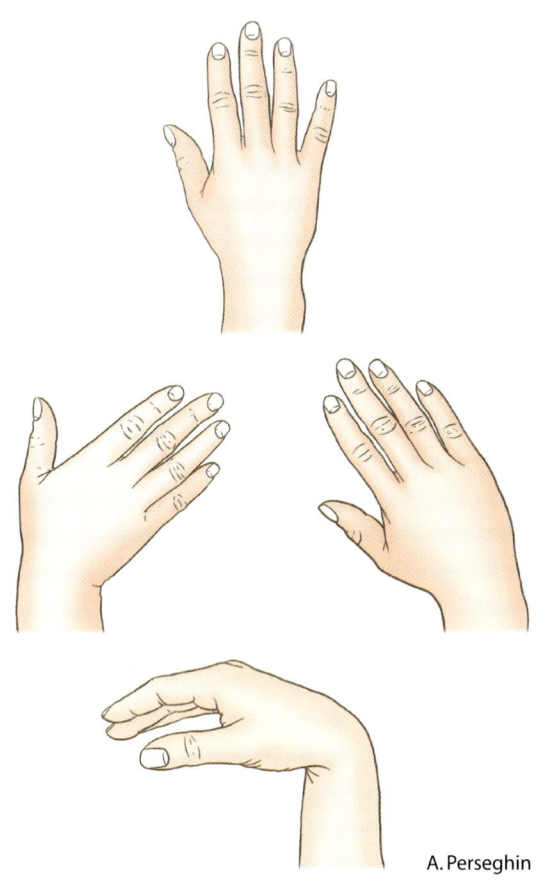

Fig. 36.8. Wrist range of motion exercises

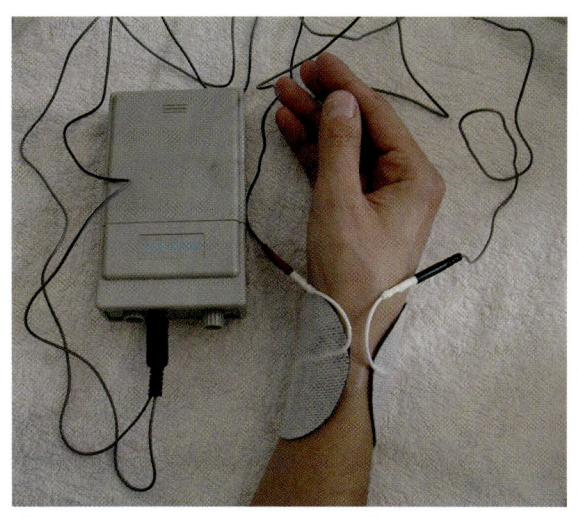

Fig. 36.9. Transcutaneous electric stimulation (TENS) or Microcurrent Stimulation: using long duration impulses and low frequency parameters provokes the release of local natural opiates (for example endorphins) and therefore, helps to decrease the patient's pain perception

Median Nerve Gliding Exercises

These exercises have the goal of facilitating the median nerve to glide through its tunnel and adjacent to the thenar eminence. When the wrist is in extension, the thumb can be passively stretched in order to prevent adhesions from forming between the skin and the median nerve's palmar cutaneous sensitive branch (Fig. 36.10). These patient's tolerance. T.E.N.S. should be applied at least 20 min every hour for the first few days and then decreased to 20 min every other hour thereafter, in order to have an analgesic effect. For this motive, a portable T.E.N.S. unit should be available for the patient to use at home. Microcurrent stimulation that has a relatively low voltage (60 V), has been demonstrated to be efficient for reducing pain. In addition, these appliances also enable the selection of treatment polarity. Research has demonstrated that the selection of a positive polarity can provoke an acidic reaction at the anode and it is efficient in reducing localized pain. The use of bipolar parameters at the end of the treatment is suggested in order to leave the soft tissue in a neutrally conductive state [13]. The advantage of using microcurrent stimulation is that it arrives to the brain at a subcortical level and therefore is well accepted by the patient who has a low pain threshold, or has reflex sympathetic dystrophy, since it does not provoke a fastidious sensation cortically (Fig. 36.9).

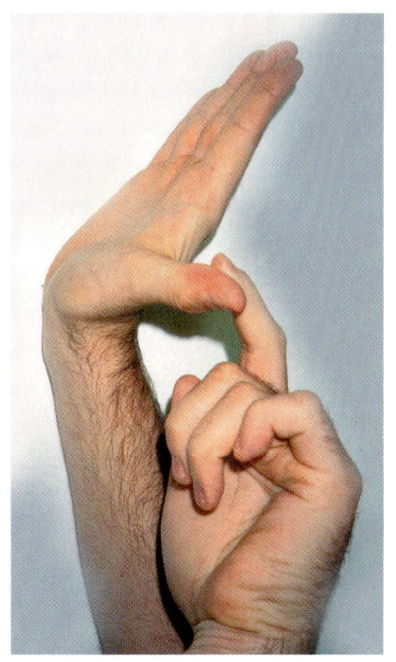

Fig. 36.10. Median nerve gliding exercises have the goal of facilitating the median nerve to glide through its tunnel and adjacent to the thenar eminence

exercises are done three times a day and each time for ten repetitions [3, 10].

The physical therapy goals in the fifth week are:

- Gradually recovery of hand and wrist strength
- Gradual recovery of hand and wrist endurance

Strengthening Exercises

A personalized hand strength recovery program should be set up for each patient according to their gender, profession, hand dominance, and habits. It is fundamental that this program is introduced into the entire rehabilitation program in a gradual fashion. The patient can begin by manipulating Thera-Putty of low resistance and gradually begin low-to-high level resistance exercises within a 1 month time frame. One should remember that, in order to obtain good postoperative results, the hand and wrist should not be overloaded (no lifting of more than 5 kg for the first 2 months from the time of surgery). Obviously, the patient is well instructed not to overstretch the muscle, tendons, or wrist articulation since they will run the risk of provoking a tenosynovitis. Hand and wrist exercises can be initiated by having the patient perform isometric exercises and then moving onto isotonic and isokinetic exercises, so that they obtain complete strength recovery throughout their wrist and hand range of motion (Fig. 36.11a–c). Isokinetic exercise is quite useful in the initial strength re-education phase since it provides the patient with instant biofeedback as to the force they are producing during the exercise. This type of biofeedback can also be used to limit the amount of force they are producing and remain within secure physiological limits. If the patient's profession requires heavy duty manual labor, it is advisable that the patient return to work only once they have fully recovered hand and wrist strength and that they wear a protective dorsal wrist splint which places the wrist in a neutral or in slight extension posture.

The goals six weeks after surgery are:

- Re-establish normal functional use of the entire upper extremity (sensibility, strength, resistance, and dexterity)

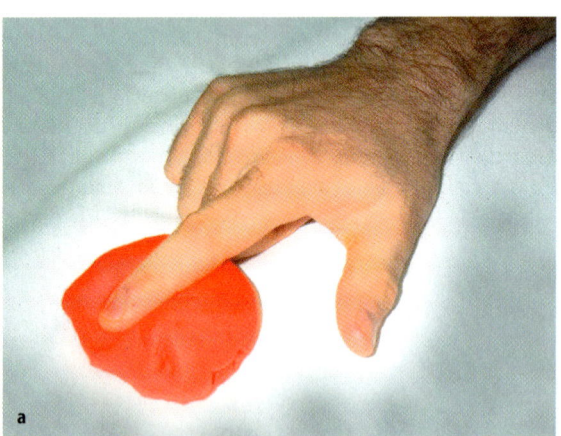

Sensory Evaluation and Re-education

There are many points of view regarding the most appropriate time to conduct a sensory evaluation in the entire hand rehabilitation program. If the hand is extremely swollen, a sensory evaluation renders quite unreliable results. Therefore, we advise that the sensory evaluation is conducted only once hand swelling is under control and during the initial days of hand exercise re-education. When there is a decrease in hand edema

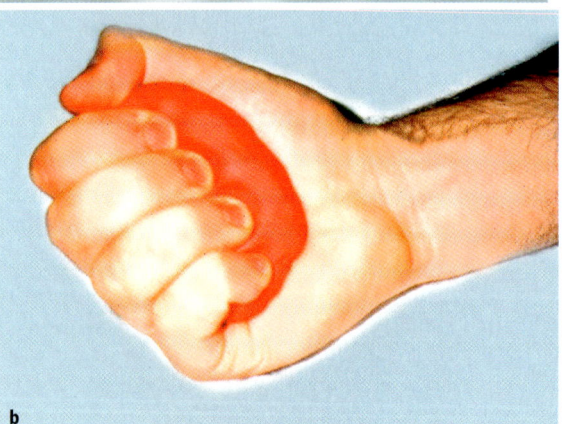

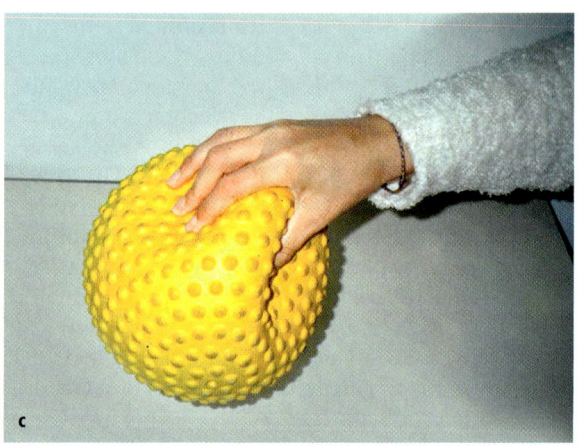

Fig. 36.11. a–c Functional hand and wrist strength recovery should be acquired gradually. The patient can begin resistive hand exercises by manipulating low-resistance Thera-Putty and gradually moving on to progressive resistive strengthening exercises that require increased strength and repetitions. These exercises should be introduced into the hand therapy protocol over a 2-month period

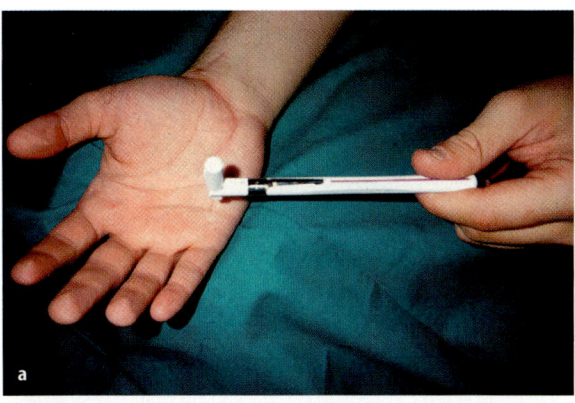

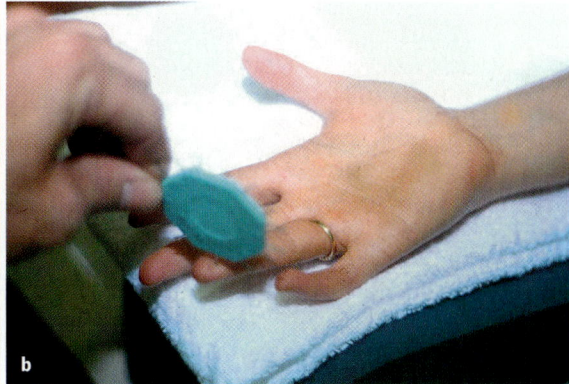

Fig. 36.12. a Semmes-Weinstein test. **b** Two-point discrimination test

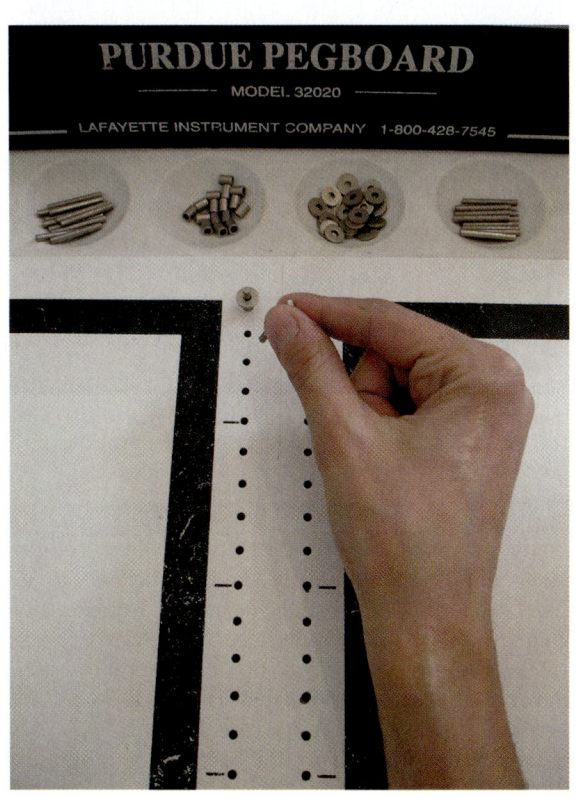

Fig. 36.13. Purdue Peg board test

there is a proportional increase in hand sensation. If a patient has had a prolonged median nerve compression, most likely a hand resensibilization program will be required for stimulating hand proprioception and sensibility return. The patient should initially undergo a Semmes-Weinstein test (Fig 12a), two-point discrimination test (Fig. 36.12b), Moberg pick-up test, and a Purdue pegboard test (Fig. 36.13) [14]. These hand sensory-dexterity evaluation tests provide baseline values as to the patient's tactile sensation capacity, as well as their hand proprioception capacity. These tests have standardized procedures which must be followed in order for them to render reliable data. They provide the therapist with quantitative baseline values which can be compared to successive re-evaluation values in order to monitor the patient's tactile return sensation and to check if the sensory re-education program is providing sufficient results or needs to be modified.

Ergonomic Therapy (Work Hardening)

One month from the time of surgery, the patient can begin a work hardening program. The patient is instructed to use their hand as much as possible in their activities of daily living without overloading the wrist articulation. Slowly they can begin to lift up weights against resistance but not over 5 kg for the first 2 months after surgery [10]. Only after 2 months can they begin to load and strengthen their involved wrist and upper extremity The therapist should include ergonomic training sessions in which the patient is educated on assuming a correct posture and combining that with articular energy conservation when lifting up or moving heavy objects, as well as when they are sitting or standing at work and performing repetitive movements with their hands. Many times this requires that the therapist does an on-site evaluation of the patient's work conditions (e.g., height of work table, evaluate the velocity and number of repetitions of certain movements per minute, unilateral or bilateral use of upper extremities, etc.) and develops a specific work hardening program for the patient to follow in order to reinforce both muscle strength and endurance before the patient is sent back to work [15]. Modern technology has made important improvements in the field of work simulation, therefore, the hand therapist has available instruments for specifically rehabilitating their patients to obtain optimal muscle performance. The DEXTER (Fig. 36.14a, b), the WorkSet (Fig. 36.14c), and the Lido Multi-active (Fig. 36.14d), are three different types of isokinetic rehabilitation machines and they allow the therapist to determine the patients muscle strength and endurance capacity, as well as rehabilitate

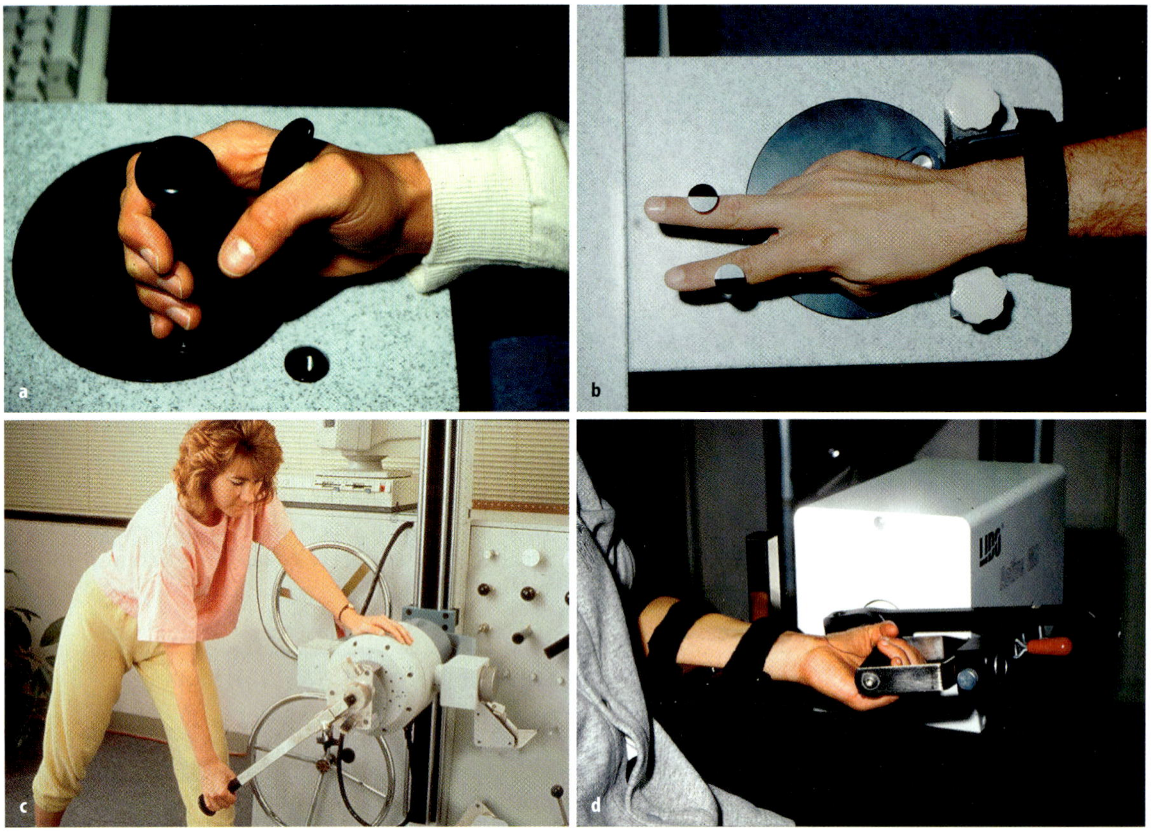

Fig. 36.14. a–d Examples of isokinetic machines that allow for functional hand evaluations and rehabilitation by reproducing specific hand and upper extremity movements that are performed by the patient during their work activities. These machines provide the therapist with quantitative data concerning the patient's hand strength and endurance capacity

and potentiate weakened muscles prior to sending the patient back to work in a compromised muscle potential situation. These machines permit the therapist to set-up specific protocols of isolated or complex movements and determine the amount of repetitions, velocity, and force that should be produced by the patient in order for the muscle to work at its maximum potential and mirror the same muscle potential requirements that are asked of them in their work activities. If the therapist has already done an on-site evaluation, they are well aware of the work requirements needed by the involved arm and can use this data to set-up isokinetic protocols, so that the patient can be rehabilitated in the most specific manner [15]. Often CTS is caused by the patient using their hand and wrist in an ergonomically incorrect manner. The patient can have hand muscle deficits that end up overloading the wrist muscles, thus placing excessive compression on the median nerve at the level of the carpal tunnel. If the therapist is knowledgeable of muscle physiology and hand muscle anatomy, they will be able to develop work-hardening programs, using the isokinetic machines, to recuperate a balanced equilibrium between muscle agonists and antagonists strength in the wrist and hand, thus reducing median nerve solicitation. The capacity of the isokinetic system to instantaneously adapt its resistance to the force produced by the patient determines a greater efficiency in the rehabilitation protocol since the patient is required to produce their maximum strength throughout all their range of motion [16]. Therefore, the patient can obtain a more precise and complete muscle recruitment at any point in their articular range of motion.

Conclusion

Research has demonstrated the importance of a global rehabilitation program after median nerve decompression in the carpal tunnel in order for a patient to return to their prior work. This is invariable whether the surgery has been performed endoscopically or in an open field [15, 16]. The therapist must be prepared to rehabilitate the patient from the initial phase through to a work-hardening phase prior to sending the patient back to work. An open line of communication is mandatory between the surgeon and therapist, in order to offer the patient a complete rehabilitation program that renders positive results.

References

1. Dawson et al. (1990) Entrapment Neuropathies. 2nd edition. Little Brown and Company, Boston pp. 83–85
2. Olsen, JD et al. (1994) Patient outcomes of Agee-3 M versus Chow-Dyonics endoscopic release of the carpal tunnel versus open release (Research Paper), The American Society of Hand Therapists XVI Annual Meeting, October 1993. Journal of Hand Therapy Vol.7/No.1, Hanley & Belfus, Inc.
3. Aiello B (1993) Carpal Tunnel Syndrome/Release. in: Clark GL, Wilgis EF, Aiello B, Eckhaus D, Eddington LV, Hand Rehabilitation: A Practical Guide. Churchill Livingstone, New York pp 199–204
4. Chow, James (1990) Endoscopic release of the carpal ligament for carpal tunnel syndrome: 22-month clinical result. Arthroscopy, Vol.6, No.4
5. Chaise F (1990) Immediate active mobilization or rigid postoperative immobilization of the wrist in carpal tunnel syndrome. Comparative analysis of a series of 50 patients. Rev Rhum Mal Osteoartic. May; 57 (5): 435–9
6. Weiss ND et al. (1992) Wrist position of lowest carpal tunnel pressure: A new method to measure intracarpal pressure as a function of wrist position. 47th annual meeting of ASSH, Phoenix
7. Luchetti R et al. (1994) Serial overnight recordings of intracarpal canal pressure in carpal tunnel syndrome patients with and without wrist splinting. J. Hand Surg 9 British and European Volume) 19B: 35–37
8. Garren K et al. (1994) Post-operative management of endoscopic carpal tunnel release (Clinical Papar). The American Society of Hand Therapists Sixteenth Annual Meeting, Journal of Hand Therapy Vol. 7/no.1 Jan/Mar
9. Yoshida T et al. (1993) A flexible dorsal wrist splint. Journal of Hand Therapy Vol. 6/No.4 323–325
10. Baxter-Petralia PL (1989) Therapist's Management of Carpal Tunnel Syndrome. In: Hunter JM, Schneider LH, Makkin EJ, Callahan AD (eds.): Rehabilitation of The Hand; Surgery and Therapy. 3rd edition. CV Mosby, St Louis pp. 640–646
11. Anthony, Mallory (1993) Wounds. In: Clark GL, Hand Rehabilitation, a practical guide. Churchill Livingstone, New York pp. 10–11
12. Anthony, Mallory (1993) Desensitization. In: Clark GL, Hand Rehabilitation, a practical guide. Churchill Livingstone, New York pp. 73–79
13. Kahn J (1993) Principles and Practice of Electrotherapy. 3rd Edition Churchill Livingstone, New York pp. 88–89, 112–113
14. Anthony, Mallory (1993) Sensory Re-education. In: Clark GL, Hand Rehabilitation, a practical guide. Churchill Livingstone, New York pp. 81–87
15. Travaglia TF (1993) Valutazione ergonomica dell'ambiente industriale e sua applicazione per screening di pre-assunzione e riabilitazione work-hardening. In: Bazzini G, Nuovi approcci alla riabilitazione industriale. Fondazione Clinica Del Lavoro Edizioni, Pavia pp. 33–48
16. Bombardi F (1993) Dinamometri isocinetici per la riabilitazione industriale. In: Bazzini G, Nuovi approcci alla riabilitazione industriale. Fondazione Clinica Del Lavoro Edizioni, Pavia pp. 103–111

Part V

Complications

Carpal Tunnel Syndrome Surgical Complications

P. Bedeschi

Introduction

Traditionally, there is a close correlation between the length of the skin incision and the breadth of the visual surgical field in carpal tunnel syndrome (CTS) surgery

The traditional surgical technique, known as "open field," responds to the need for the visual surgical field to be broad and deep. Only in this way can this surgical access adequately decompress the median nerve at the wrist level by providing large security margins, thus allowing for the complete sectioning of the transverse carpal ligament (TCL). By using the open field surgical technique, the surgeon can avoid running the risk of causing iatrogenic injuries to the superficial palmar vascular arch or the median nerve and its branches, even in the presence of anatomical anomalies. Using the open field technique also permits the surgeon to perform other complementary surgical procedures such as a flexor tendon tenosynovectomy or a median nerve neurolysis.

In the last 20–30 years, numerous statistical data have demonstrated that using the carpal tunnel open field technique may cause various complications.

A symptomatic cutaneous scar is one of the most frequently occurring complications that can arise from this surgical technique. Predominately, this occurs when a palmar perithenar incision has been made or when the palmar incision has been lengthened more proximal to the distal flexor crease of the wrist.

Other complications can occur due to secondary pathologies that arise from incorrect TCL healing. It has been noted [9] that after a CTS surgery correct TCL healing is necessary in order to allow for: increased carpal canal volume, proper alignment of the nine flexor tendons and the median nerve in the canal, functional recovery of the TLC pulley system, and the prevention of perinervous or peritendinous adhesions from occurring.

In order to avoid such complications, two proposals have been made; one is from a conservative point of view and the other, more radical.

The more conservative solution has been derived in order to avoid symptomatic cutaneous scars and consists of limiting the skin incision to the palm area in a more ulnar location, (that is at the demarcation line of the fourth digital ray), rather than making the incision in the traditional perithenar area.

In order to avoid incorrect TCL scar healing and perinervous and peritendinous adhesions, the TCL is sectioned on the ulnar side of the tunnel and the wrist is held postoperatively in a moderate amount of extension for 2 weeks, while the fingers are left free to move.

The more radical approach is aimed at drastically reducing the length of the cutaneous incision to 1–2 cm, making a mini-incision or transversal at the wrist's distal flexor crease, either longitudinal in the proximal palmar region.

This surgical technique is also known as a "closed field" technique. It must be taken into account that, with this mini-incision, the surgical access is performed without a direct visual field.

Recent scientific statistical revisions regarding this type of surgical approach have demonstrated that it produces a high rate of surgical complications, some even quite severe, and they are generally related to the incomplete sectioning of the TCL or an iatrogenic nerve or vascular injury.

The use of endoscopic instruments has reduced, but not completely resolved such complications, especially during the surgeon's training period when still trying to acquire dexterity and precision when using these instruments.

Classification of CTS Surgery Complications

The author has classified CTS surgical complications [8] by taking into consideration the proposals of various authors, and his own personal surgical experience. Langloh and Linscheid [67] distinguished specific surgical failures due to unrelieved or recurrent symptoms.

Das and Brown [31] divided CTS surgical complications into two groups, those with the presence of residual symptoms and those which developed secondary iatrogenic injuries.

Eason et al. [37] divided the complications into three groups: incomplete TCL resection, recurrent median nerve compression due to tenosynovitis or fibrotic proliferation, and iatrogenic injury to the median nerve or its branches.

Mackinnon [77] distinguished three symptomatic groups based on indications for secondary carpal tunnel surgery: persistent symptoms, recurrent symptoms, or new symptoms.

The author's classification system follows that of Mackinnon [77] in regards to the three principle groups: persistent symptoms, recurrent symptoms, and new symptoms.

This personal classification system includes new and more updated information, specifically regarding the third group of complications.

The author has not included in his classification the failures due to diagnostic error or an incomplete diagnosis, as in the double crush in nerve entrapment syndromes [104].

One must point out the importance of a correct CTS diagnosis, which is the primary condition for surgical success.

Possible surgical complications, both in open and closed field, have been analyzed and discussed according to the author's classification system in the Table 37.1.

Reference has also been made to complications correlated with the endoscopic technique.

It is important to evaluate and distinguish the complications that generally disappear spontaneously within a few weeks or months from those, generally more severe, which tend to be irreversible [10].

Finally, the prevention of the surgical complications is cited.

Table 37.1. Classification of CTS surgery complications

1	**Symptoms persistence**
1.1	Incomplete or complete lack of median nerve decompression
1.1.1	Incomplete sectioning of the distal part of the TCL
1.1.2	Incomplete sectioning of the distal part of the antebrachial fascia
1.1.3	Complete lack of TCL sectioning
2	**Symptoms recurrence**
2.1	Perinervous fibrotic scar proliferation
2.2	Hypertrophic tenosynovitis of the flexor tendons
3	**Onset of new symptoms**
3.1	Cutaneous scar pathology
3.2	Painful symptoms of nerve origin correlated to the cutaneous scar
3.2.1	Neuroma from the sectioning of the palmar cutaneous branch of the median nerve or of a sensitive branch of the radial nerve
3.2.2	Mini-neuromas from the sectioning of palmar cutaneous terminal endings of the median and/or ulnar nerve
3.2.3	Cutaneous scar adhesions to the median nerve
3.3	Painful symptoms that are not correlated to the cutaneous scar
3.3.1	Thenar and hypothenar pain (pillar pain)
3.3.2	Piso-triquetral pain
3.4	Nerve complications that are not correlated to the cutaneous scar
3.4.1	Total or partial injuries of the median or ulnar nerve and their branches
3.5	Vascular complications
3.5.1	Hematomas from nonsevere vascular injuries
3.5.2	Severe vascular injuries
3.6	Tendon complications
3.6.1	Adhesions between flexor tendons
3.6.2	Subcutaneous anterior subluxation of the flexor tendons
3.6.3	Non-pre-existing trigger finger
3.6.4	Ulnar subluxation of flexor tendons outside the carpal tunnel
3.6.5	Injuries of the flexor tendons
3.7	Reduction of hand grip strength
3.8	Infection
3.9	Reflex sympathetic dystrophy (algodystrophy)
3.10	Causalgia

Analysis of the Complications

Symptom Persistence

Postoperative CTS symptoms persistence is generally correlated to an incomplete or complete lack of median nerve decompression. The author, in accordance with Hunt and Osterman [51] and also with Strickland et al. [97], believes that it is possible to hypothesize that sometimes the persistence of specific neurological symptoms can depend on a partial irreversible damage of the median nerve caused by some nerve fiber bundles becoming ischemic and fibrotic.

Incomplete or Complete Lack of Median Nerve Decompression

The most common unsuccessful outcome of CTS surgery is due to the persistence of preoperative symptoms (Fig. 37.1). This surgical failure generally is caused by an incomplete or complete lack of median nerve decompression due to an incomplete sectioning of the TCL distal tract, or rarely, the distal part of the antebrachial fascia.

▷
Fig. 37.1. 59-year-old female. Operated elsewhere, 6 months prior to time of photo, for left wrist CTS. Complained of painful persistent symptoms after surgery. Reoperation was able to resolve symptoms. **a** Longitudinal proximal palmar scar along the third digital ray, 3 cm in length, and extended, for 1 cm, proximally to the wrist crease. **b** The surgical marker is used to draw a line indicating the location of the palmar scar. The *dots* indicate a zone of dysesthesia peri-scarring. The *asterisk* indicates the point where a Tinel sign is present and in correspondence to the proximal border of the entire distal part of the TCL. **c** The surgical marker line indicates the site of the reoperation palmar incision. It is made in a longitudinal direction along the fourth digital ray, 6 cm in length, and 1 cm ulnarly distanced from the initial scar. **d** The skin is incised and the cutaneous flaps are raised up from the fascial plane. One can view the entire palmar aponeurosis distal to a connective tissue scar. **e** Once the palmar aponeurosis is removed, one can observe a strip of the entire TCL, height 12 mm, that contin-

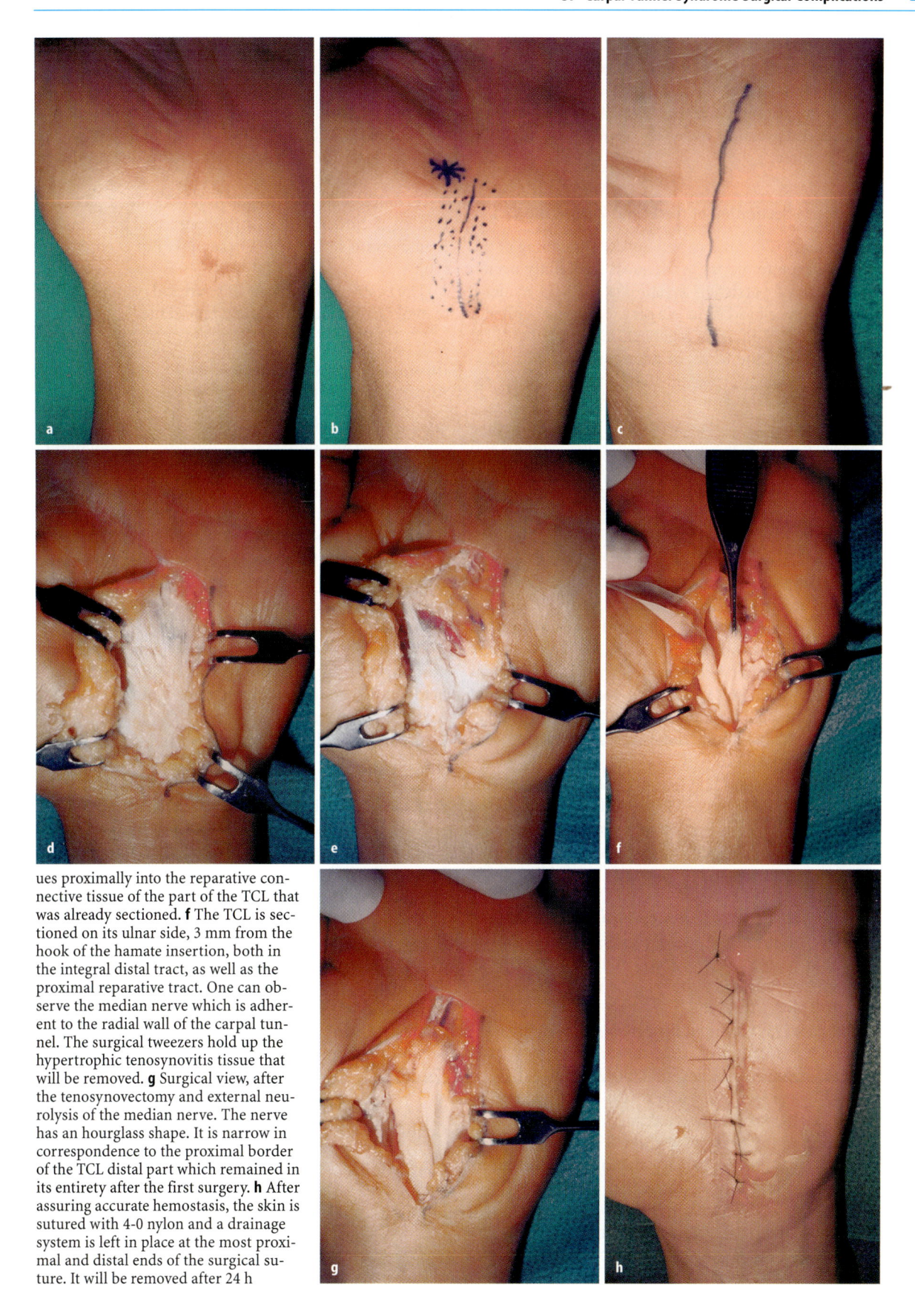

37 Carpal Tunnel Syndrome Surgical Complications 271

ues proximally into the reparative connective tissue of the part of the TCL that was already sectioned. **f** The TCL is sectioned on its ulnar side, 3 mm from the hook of the hamate insertion, both in the integral distal tract, as well as the proximal reparative tract. One can observe the median nerve which is adherent to the radial wall of the carpal tunnel. The surgical tweezers hold up the hypertrophic tenosynovitis tissue that will be removed. **g** Surgical view, after the tenosynovectomy and external neurolysis of the median nerve. The nerve has an hourglass shape. It is narrow in correspondence to the proximal border of the TCL distal part which remained in its entirety after the first surgery. **h** After assuring accurate hemostasis, the skin is sutured with 4-0 nylon and a drainage system is left in place at the most proximal and distal ends of the surgical suture. It will be removed after 24 h

According to Kuhlmann et al. [65] the flexor retinaculum must be divided from 4 to 5 cm at the palmar level and from 2 to 3 cm at the distal part of the forearm.

In very exceptional cases, complete lack of median nerve decompression has even been found with the TCL still intact.

Incomplete Sectioning of the Distal Part of the TCL

In secondary CTS surgery incomplete sectioning of the TCL has been found to be the most frequently occurring cause of persistent symptoms. This is evident, above all, in closed field surgery, in which either a transverse mini-incision has been made, at the distal flexor crease of the wrist, or a longitudinal mini-incision has been performed in the proximal palmar region.

Phalen [87] has cited a surgical case in which a transverse incision was made at the wrist. Langloh and Linscheid [67] have found this complication in 21 out of 34 reoperations that were associated with a perinervous fibrosis or a flexor tendon hypertrophic tenosynovitis. Hybbinette and Mannerfelt [53] found 4 out of 18 reoperated cases and Das and Brown [31] 4 out of 6 reoperated cases with a similar complication.

Eason et al. [37] found incomplete distal TCL sectioning in 4 cases out of 47 patients that were operated on reporting suboptimal results. In all the 4 cases, a transverse wrist incision was performed. Wadstroem and Nigst [106], in 13 out of 40 patients reoperated cases, observed incomplete distal TCL sectioning. O'Malley et al. [84] found these same findings in 10 out of 28 reoperated cases.

Chang and Dellon [21] found incomplete distal TCL sectioning in 1 case out of 35 reoperated, Luchetti et al. [74] 7 out of 15, Kern et al. [60] 10 out of 16, Strasberg et al. [96] 11 out of 50, Cobb and Amadio [25] 29 out of 131, Condamine et al. [28] 16 out of 18 and Bagatur [3] 23 out of 34.

Therefore, incomplete sectioning of the distal part of the TCL is a prime suspect for causing postoperative persistent symptoms that are similar to the patient's preoperative ones and these symptoms can also be present with objective signs.

De Smet [33] observed that, in these cases the Phalen test [87] is negative while the Gilliatt and Wilson test [48] is positive. A negative Phalen test [87] is explained by the sectioning of the TCL's proximal border which is responsible for median nerve compression when flexing the wrist. A positive Gilliatt and Wilson test [48] is justified by the fact that the nerve compression persists in the distal carpal tunnel tract.

On the basis of the author's personal experience, two additional signs have been found to be persistent. The Bedeschi sign [6], which evaluates the presence of anterior wrist region tension. In these cases, it is negative due to the proximal sectioning of the TCL which provokes a decrease in compartment pressure in the carpal tunnel's proximal part. The Tinel sign [100] is also negative in the wrist flexor region, at the entrance to the carpal tunnel and positive in the palm, which corresponds to the proximal border of the distal integral TCL.

A complete clinical diagnosis for the incomplete sectioning of the distal TCL can be confirmed by an instrumental exam such as a CAT scan [108] or even an MRI [80].

The best way to prevent this surgical complication is to avoid using the closed field technique.

Incomplete Sectioning of the Distal Part of the Antebrachial Fascia

It is rarely found that the persistence of CTS symptoms is due to the incomplete sectioning of the distal part of the antebrachial fascia. Louis et al. [72] reported 1 case out of 25 reoperations, Chang and Dellon [21] 1 out of 35, Strasberg et al. [96] 5 out of 50, Cobb and Amadio [25] 11 out of 131.

According to Mackinnon [77] such an occurrence could be favored by a previous trauma to the anterior portion of the wrist and forearm, which can lead to a thickening of the antebrachial fascia.

Incomplete sectioning of the distal part of the antebrachial fascia is possible when a palmar incision is made and has not been lengthened proximal to the wrist's distal flexor crease. From a diagnostic point of view, Phalen [87], Gilliatt and Wilson [48], and Bedeschi [6] signs are all positive. Even a Tinel [100] sign is positive at the classic carpal tunnel entrance site. CAT scan or MRI can be used to confirm these findings.

Special attention should be given to those surgeries which have been performed by a palmar incision which has not been extended proximal to the wrist's distal flexor crease. It is of utmost importance that the subcutaneous sectioning of the distal antebrachial fascia is approached with caution so that these complications do not occur. Fascial sectioning should be preceded by atraumatic separating of the subcutaneous plane from the fascia, so that subcutaneous vessels are not cut causing underlying hematomas (see p. 279). Fascial sectioning should extend proximal to the wrist's distal flexor crease for at least 2–3 cm.

Complete Lack of TCL Sectioning

Some authors have reported that they have found, in very exceptional cases, the persistence of CTS symptoms after surgery was due to the complete lack of TCL sectioning.

Two of such cases were reported by De Smet [33], 9 out of 50 reoperated patients were reported by Strasberg et al. [96], and 3 out of 34 reoperated cases, by Bagatur [3].

Such circumstances seem hard to believe, if one thinks that the surgeon, who is performing this type of surgical treatment, has a detailed knowledge of both wrist and hand anatomy.

One could also hypothesize, that in such cases, the TCL was only partially sectioned and that connective tissue healing formed in such a manner that during the reoperation the surgeon mistook this healed tissue as untouched tissue.

The prevention of this exceptional complication is correlated to a sufficient amount of surgical training in the treatment of CTS.

Symptoms Recurrence

After a postoperative regression phase, CTS symptoms can reoccur after a few weeks. Reoperatively, it has been found that the most frequent causes for these symptoms to reappear are the proliferation of a perinervous fibrotic scar and a hypertrophic tenosynovitis of the flexor tendons. Often these pathologies are variously associated.

Some authors [67, 96] have hypothesized that the TCL scar could be the cause of recurrent CTS symptoms. Actually, a correct scar healing, in the fascial plane, creates a positive anatomical situation [9] since it allows for a greater carpal canal volume and avoids median nerve and/or flexor tendon anterior subluxation (see pp. 276, 280). In addition, it can also be helpful towards gaining good TCL pulley system functional recovery (see p. 280).

The TCL scar can create recurrent symptoms only if it is associated with fibrotic adhesions of the median nerve.

Perinervous Fibrotic Scar Proliferation

This is quite a common finding during reinterventions for CTS recurrent symptoms. Phalen [87] has cited such a case. Langloh and Linscheid [67] found perinervous fibrotic proliferation alone or associated with an incomplete sectioning of the TCL or flexor tendons hypertrophic tenosynovitis, in 22 out of 34 reinterventions. In 13 of these cases, the scar adhesions were wrapped around the median nerve. Hybbinette and Mannerfelt [53] found a few cases of fibrotic tissue proliferation that presented alone or in association with flexor tendon hypertrophic tenosynovitis in 18 reinterventions. A perinervous fibrotic scar was observed by Wadstroem and Nigst [106] in 36 cases out of 40 reoperations, by O'Malley et al. [84] in 8 out of 20, and by Kern et al. [60] in 4 out of 16 reoperations.

Median nerve adhesions attached to the reparative TCL scar have been frequently reported on by Hunter [52], in 2 cases by Inglis [54], in 35 cases by Chang and Dellon[21], in 4 cases by Luchetti et al. [74], and a in various number of cases, not precisely specified, by Strasberg et al. [96].

There have also been reported findings in reoperative cases where scar adhesions were found between the median nerve and carpal tunnel radial wall [52, 93] or between the median nerve and the finger and thumb flexor tendons [52].

From the author's experience, perinervous fibrotic proliferation has been frequently found during reoperations. In particular, the author has observed, in various reoperated cases, scar adhesions between the median nerve and the reparative TCL scar, with the tunnel radial wall, with the finger flexor tendons or, in two cases, with the flexor pollicis longus tendon [10].

Perinervous scar proliferation is easily provoked by hematomas (see p. 279) and by a radical tenosynovectomy, above all, associated with a prolonged postoperative finger immobilization period [96].

From a diagnostic point of view, the reappearance of CTS symptoms is accompanied by objective signs. Tinel [100] sign and Gilliatt and Wilson [48] sign are generally positive, whereas Phalen [87] sign and Bedeschi [6] sign are negative.

It is important to observe if pain is provoked by wrist and finger extension since this clinical finding indicates a traction neuropathy [52]. Such symptoms are the clinical anatomical expression of median nerve fibrotic adhesions attached to the carpal tunnel wall or to the finger and thumb flexor tendons. In 2 reoperative cases, the author has found scar adhesions between the median nerve and the flexor pollicis longus tendon, which could provoke pain, when completely extending the second phalanx of the thumb.

The clinical diagnosis of perinervous fibrotic scar proliferation can be confirmed with instrumental exams such as CAT scan [109] or MRI [12, 80].

The prevention of this complication can be acquired by avoiding the formation of hematomas (see p. 279), and maintaining 15° of wrist extension [102], with a plaster volar valve or a dorsal thermoplastic splint [41] for 14 days. This modest extension of the wrist maintains the nine flexor tendons in place in the carpal canal [17], while the median nerve is sufficiently distanced from the TCL during the scar healing period, thus preventing the formation of scars between the nerve and the carpal tunnel anterior wall [10].

Postoperative wrist immobilization favors correct TCL scar healing [9] while the early and guided mobilization of the fingers avoids the formation of perinervous or peritendinous adhesions [41].

Hypertrophic Tenosynovitis of the Flexor Tendons

This complication is not infrequently found in reoperations due to CTS recurrent symptoms. Langloh and Linscheid [67] observed, during reintervention, in 14 cases out of 34, that there was the presence of flexor tendon tenosynovitis, either alone or also associated with a fibrotic tissue proliferation in the carpal canal, or an incomplete sectioning of the TCL. Hybbinette and Mannerfelt [53] found, during 18 reinterventions, a few cases where there was the presence of hypertrophic tenosynovitis of the flexor tendons, isolated or associated with a fibrotic proliferation. Eason et al. [37] reported two similar cases. Wadstroem and Nigst [106] observed 19 hypertrophic tenosynovitis cases out of 40 reoperations (1 case of rheumatoid arthritis and the other 18 of aspecific synovitis). O'Malley et al. [84] observed 5 cases of proliferative tenosynovitis out of 20 reoperations. Chang and Dellon [21] found hypertrophic tenosynovitis in all 35 cases that were reoperated on (6 cases of rheumatoid arthritis and 29 of aspecific synovitis). Zanlungo et al. [109] observed hypertrophic tenosynovitis of the flexor tendons in 11 out of 46 reinterventions, previously documented with a CAT scan.

Therefore, hypertrophic tenosynovitis of the flexor tendons represents, whether appearing on its own or in association with a proliferation of fibrotic perinervous scar tissue, an important cause of recurrent CTS symptoms.

Clinically, swelling in the anterior region of the wrist is visible and the patient presents with a positive Bedeschi [6] sign. Tinel [100] sign is generally positive, whereas Phalen [87] sign is negative.

The clinical diagnosis of flexor tendon hypertrophic tenosynovitis may be confirmed by ultrasound exam [82], or by CAT scan [109], or by MRI [12, 80].

From a preventative point of view, when there is the presence of a flexor tendon sheath proliferation, the author feels that it is opportune to perform a nonradical tenosynovectomy during the first surgery. This complementary surgical procedure must be done in an open field and not in a closed field technique or in endoscopic surgery. It must be kept in mind that when performing this procedure, accurate hemostasis must be performed and a drain set in place for 24 h.

Particular importance must be paid to the postoperative functional re-education of the fingers. The wrist should be immobilized for 14 days in 15° of extension.

Onset of New Symptoms

Another frequent cause of unsuccessful CTS surgery is the postoperative onset of new symptoms. These symptoms can be numerous and of various types, which are associated with different frequencies in occurrence in relation to the type of surgery performed: open field, closed field, or endoscopic technique.

Cutaneous Scar Pathology

Surgical scars which perpendicularly cross over the distal wrist flexor crease have the tendency to become hypertrophic or form a keloid and often tend to retract [61, 72, 76, 105].

In cases in which the incision correctly crosses over the distal wrist flexor crease, thanks to two angulations and an intermedial part that is based transversally along the fold, the palmar part of the scar does not tend to become hypertrophic, whereas the antebrachial part tends to become thick and keloid [53, 109]. Hybbinette and Mannerfelt [53] reported on 6 cases of keloid scars occurring on the incision's proximal part at the antebrachial level in 18 reoperated patients.

Keloid scars are more symptomatic than hypertrophic ones. Retracted scars provoke limited wrist extension range of motion.

From a preventative point of view, the best way to avoid these type of scars from forming is to perform an incision limited to the palm, without passing through the distal wrist flexor crease.

When there are situations in which there is an important hypertrophy of the flexor tendon sheath, as is found in rheumatoid arthritis, or in other cases, where it is necessary that the surgeon crosses the distal wrist flexor crease, it is necessary to make a short incision along the fold and change direction both proximally and distally with angles between 45° [84], 60° [65], and 90° [14].

Painful Symptoms of Nerve Origin Correlated to the Cutaneous Scar

The author has joined together three complication groups, characterized by painful cutaneous scar symptoms of nerve origin:

1. In the first group the scar is painful because it is in contact with a neuroma that has arisen from the sectioning of the palmar cutaneous branch of the median nerve or, more rarely, of a sensitive branch of the radial nerve.
2. In the second group, the scar is painful and there is the formation of minineuromas from the sectioning of the palmar cutaneous terminal endings of the median and/or ulnar nerve.
3. In the third group, the cutaneous scar is painful due to adhesions that have formed between the median nerve and the scar itself.

Neuroma from the Sectioning of the Palmar Cutaneous Branch of the Median Nerve or of a Sensitive Branch of the Radial Nerve

Sectioning of the palmar cutaneous branch (PCB) of the median nerve with the consequential formation of a neuroma, generally adherent to the cutaneous scar, is the main cause of a painful scar and often is quite debilitating. The pain is localized to the radial part of the distal wrist flexor crease, in the area of the scaphoid tubercle [19]. Percussing the scar, where the neuroma is located, elicits pain and often it radiates to the thenar region [105].

The anatomical tract of the median nerve which leads into the PCB and its palmar cutaneous terminal endings has been carefully studied by Carroll and Green [19], by Taleisnik [98] and, more recently, by Hobbs et al. [50], by Naff et al. [81], by Da Silva et al. [32], and by Watchmaker et al. [107].

The most dangerous incisions that could injure the PCB of the median nerve are those which pass transversally along the distal wrist flexor crease [19, 94, 98] and those around the thenar eminence that extend proximally [19, 98].

The occurrence PCB injury during CTS surgery has been documented by various authors [24, 29, 31, 37, 53, 66, 72].

Mac Donald et al. [76] found 11 neuromas of the PCB out of 186 surgical cases (5.9%), Lichtman et al. [69] 2 out of 100 surgical cases, and Wadstroem and Nigst [106] 2 out of 40 reinterventions.

Palmer and Toivonen [86] organized and published a questionnaire and its correlated responses that were received by 616 members of the American Society for Surgery of the Hand. In summary, it was noted that, following CTS surgery, in an open or closed field, but without the use of endoscopic instruments, there were 117 PCB injuries with consequential painful neuromas.

To prevent this nerve injury from occurring, Taleisnik [98] advises that the surgeon should avoid transverse incisions, as well as longitudinal ones, located on the radial aspect of the palm. He advises a palmar incision based on the ulnar side of the axis of the ray of the ring finger. Hobbs et al. [50] feel that in order to protect the PCB and its palmar cutaneous terminal endings, the incision should be based on the central axis of the fourth digital ray. In rare cases, which require a radially located incision that crosses the wrist's distal flexor crease, it is necessary to first identify and isolate the PCB of the median nerve [105]. This is also true when performing a volar approach in a proximal row carpectomy [7].

The development of a painful neuroma, due to the sectioning of a sensitive branch of the radial nerve after CTS surgery, is not a common occurrence. The author found two reported cases in the literature: one was reported by Louis et al. [72], the other by Strasberg et al. [96].

To prevent this nerve injury from occurring, it is sufficient to avoid making a very radially located incision at the level of the wrist.

In exceptional cases, which require this type of very radially placed incision, it is necessary to first identify and isolate the sensitive branches of the radial nerve.

Minineuromas from the Sectioning of Palmar Cutaneous Terminal Endings of the Median and/or Ulnar Nerve

The palm of the hand is innervated by the terminal endings of the median and ulnar nerve's palmar cutaneous branches. Both Taleisnik [98] and Watchmaker et al. [107] have described in detail the palmar zone which is covered by median nerve innervation and Engber and Gmeiner [38] regarding the palmar zone that is covered by ulnar nerve innervation. These authors think that there is a nervous demarcation line on the palm, that corresponds to the fourth digital ray axis. Therefore, a surgical palm incision, along this line, would avoid the sectioning of the terminal endings of both the median and ulnar nerve.

Ferrari and Gilbert [43] have done a detailed anatomical research on the hand and forearm and have demonstrated that frequently, in the palm of the hand, there is the presence of an anastomotic branch between the median and ulnar nerve. Another anatomical research performed by Martin et al. [78] demonstrated that there is a certain frequency of nervous palmar cutaneous terminal endings overlapping around this so-called demarcation line of the fourth digital ray.

According to more recent literature published by Matloub et al. [79], making an incision on the central axis of the fourth ray runs the risk of injuring the palmar cutaneous terminal endings of the median nerve by 25%, whereas an incision made ulnar to the central axis of the fourth ray, as suggested by Taleisnik [98], runs the risk of injuring the palmar cutaneous terminal endings of the ulnar nerve by 72%.

In summary, from a practical surgical point of view, an incision made on the central axis of the fourth ray will section a significantly lower number of cutaneous nerve branch endings than in the other parts of the palm.

Often, the scar can be painful and sensitive in the first months after surgery due to the sectioning of median or ulnar nerve's palmar cutaneous terminal endings.

Das and Brown [31] reported that out of 120 cases operated on (with a perithenar incision that was deviated ulnarly along the fourth ray in the proximal tract) the cutaneous scar was postoperatively frequently painful. At a 6-month follow-up, only 2 of the 120 cases continued to report having a painful scar (1.6%). Kulick et al. [66] reported on 130 patients who underwent a fourth ray incision and they found that the scar was painful after 1 month in only 6 cases (4.6%), and in none of the cases after 6 months. Seradge and Seradge [95] operated on 468 hands using the fourth ray incision and found 65% of their cases to report having painful cutaneous scars after 6 weeks, but in a 6-month follow-up, all cases reported that the painful scar had subsided.

Citron and Bendall [23] followed-up on 47 operated hands using two different techniques. The scar was frequently painful after 45 postoperative days, in the group of 21 cases that underwent the fourth ray palmar incision, but all the cases became asymptomatic within the 6-month follow-up. In the second group of 26 cases, which underwent a perithenar incision, the scar was even frequently painful after 45 days, but in 12 months there were some cases which continued to report having a painful scar.

From such numerous bibliographic documentation one can confirm that a scar located along the central axis of the fourth ray in the palm of the hand can be painful for some weeks but generally this pain subsides within 6 months.

From a preventative point of view, it is best to remember that although one can not avoid a painful scar immediately postoperatively, at least it is possible to prevent long-term scar pain by performing a fourth digital ray palmar incision. In this case, the location, not the length, of the incision is of importance. The duration of a painful scar can be greater in a small interthenar palmar incision located radially to the demarcation line of the fourth ray.

A possible prevention of postoperative scar pain consists of identifying and protecting the nerve terminal branches that cross over the surgical field determined by the palmar incision along the fourth ray [101]. In order to avoid postoperative scar pain, Biyani and Downes [13] proposed two separate small incisions. The proximal incision, 1 – 2 cm long, is made transversally along the wrist's distal flexor crease; the distal incision is 2 – 3 cm long and is longitudinal at the center of the palm. By doing so, the highly innervated skin of the proximal part of the palm is not incised. However, the author believes that this type of twin incision is quite risky since there is a high possibility of causing iatrogenic vascular or nerve damage, due to the reduced visual operative field.

Cutaneous Scar Adhesions to the Median Nerve

One of the worst complications of CTS surgery, especially with an open field approach, is the subluxation of the median nerve anterior to its fascial plane and the formation of cutaneous scar adhesions to the nerve.

This does occur rarely, but is a consequence when there is a lack of proper scar healing of the TCL and can be associated with an anterior subluxation of the finger flexor tendons (see p. 280). Conditions which tend to favor this complication to arise are: a perithenar cutaneous incision, sectioning of the TCL radially, removal of a part of the TCL, and improper wrist flexion posture postoperatively [9].

This complication is rarely documented in the literature. Wadstroem and Nigst [106] found 5 out of 40 reoperated cases in which this type of complication occurred, equal to 12.5%. Urbaniak [105], Omer [85], and Hunt and Osterman [51] have cited this complication to be a possible cause of palmar cutaneous scar pain.

The superficial location of the median nerve with adhesions to the cutaneous scar was demonstrated in one case by CT exam [109] and in another case by MRI [93].

This particular type of complication causes a very painful cutaneous scar. The pain can be accentuated not only with the application of pressure but even by the slightest touch, setting off a painful electric shock effect in the median nerve area of innervation of the hand. The pain can also be elicited by the simplest movement of the wrist, especially in the direction of wrist hyperextension.

Painful symptoms do not tend to heal themselves spontaneously but only worsen with repetitive surgeries, especially if the same scar is incised and an internal neurolysis is performed. In such cases one runs the risk of causing direct damage to the nerve, in the attempt to free-up the scar. In rare cases, the painful symptoms can evolve towards a causalgia (see p. 285).

In order to prevent this complication from occurring it is useful to perform a palmar incision located along the fourth digital ray, sectioning the TCL on the ulnar side of the tunnel thus avoiding, as complementary procedure, an internal neurolysis.

Postoperatively, the wrist must be immobilized for 14 days in slight extension with the fingers completely free. This is the appropriate way to ensure the correct healing of the TCL and to maintain the flexor tendons and median nerve inside the carpal canal, without producing perinervous or peritendinous adhesions.

Painful Symptoms That Are Not Correlated to the Cutaneous Scar

This paragraph will deal with thenar and hypothenar pain and piso-triquetral pain.

Thenar and Hypothenar Pain (Pillar Pain)

A kind of postoperative CTS pain has been described in both the thenar and hypothenar region, and it is accentuated with the application of localized pressure or when the patient performs a hand grasping gesture. This symptomatology has been coined "pillar pain" and usually resolves itself within a few months. [40].

There is quite a bit of controversy as to the direct cause of this pain. According to Eversmann [40] it is correlated to postoperative soft tissue edema in the proximal wrist region. The resolution of the pain is associated with the reabsorption of the edema. Kluge et al. [63], in a published revision of 89 CTS cases that were operated on using an incision placed along the ulnar longitudinal palmar skin crease, found 4% of their cases had postoperative pillar pain that resolved itself within 6 months.

According to Da Silva et al. [32], thenar and hypothenar pain should be related to the formation of mini-neuromas from the sectioning of the palmar cutaneous nerve branch endings. Brown et al. [18] contradict this hypothesis. These authors have not observed a difference in thenar and hypothenar pain in their patients' postoperative recovery period when comparing those patients operated on with open field technique as to those treated with endoscopic surgery. Even Citron and Bendall [23] contradict Da Silva et al.'s [32] hypothesis. These authors have not found a difference in their patients' postoperative recovery period when comparing those patients who underwent a perithenar incision as to those who underwent a fourth ray palmar incision. In all the cases, the patients reported resolution of thenar and hypothenar pain within 9 months.

Povlsen and Tegnell [90], in a revision of 51 CTS cases that were operated on, found thenar and hypothenar pain pressure in 21 cases (41%) after a month, in 13 cases (25%) after 3 months, and in 3 cases (6%) after 12 months. According to these authors, the complication should be correlated to reversible changes in the central processing of the low threshold mechano-receptive input from the skin.

Other authors [51, 56] feel that thenar and hypothenar pain is of muscle origin and depends on the temporary instability of the aponeurotic insertion of the thenar and hypothenar muscles after the sectioning of the TCL. According to anatomical research [26], the distal part of the TCL, which is called the "Flexor retinaculum," is made up of an aponeurotic tissue into which the thenar and hypothenar muscles insert.

This hypothesis, in which the author of this chapter is in agreement, upholds the spontaneous resolution of thenar and hypothenar pain that occurs parallel with aponeurotic scar healing and therefore the re-establishment of thenar and hypothenar insertion stability.

From a preventative point of view, it is useful to immobilize the wrist in slight extension for 14 days, leaving the fingers free to move. The wrist can be immobilized in a plaster volar valve, or a dorsal thermoplastic light-weight, for a quicker and correct healing of the TCL.

Piso-Triquetral Pain

Postoperative hypothenar pain usually resolves itself within 6 months (see p. 277); in few cases it may continue indefinitely, with notable repercussions regarding the patient's grip strength [95]. In a review of 468 CTS cases operated on using the palmar incision along the fourth digital ray, the authors Seradge and Seradge [95] found 56 cases (12%) that presented with pain at the base of the hypothenar region after 6 weeks and persisted in 5 cases (1.1%) for 6 months. They observed that in these 5 persistent pain cases, the pain was localized to the piso-triquetral joint. The pain increased in intensity with direct application of pressure on the pisiform and with resisted wrist flexion, extension, and ulnar deviation. The pain subsided temporarily with an intra-articular local anesthesia infiltration. Seradge and Seradge [95] suggest a radiographic lateral projection exam of the piso-triquetral joint in order to identify eventual signs of subluxation or articular arthrosis. The authors interpret the piso-triquetral pain as a secondary symptom due to an articular incongruency of the piso-triquetral joint in subjects that already have asymptomatic chondromalacia and/or articular instability. This symptomatic pathology can be caused by a poor and/or incorrect healing of the TCL. Indeed, the articular stability of the pisiform is determined by a dynamic equilibrium between the forces that traction it in an ulnar direction (flexor carpi ulnaris and abductor digiti minimi) and the forces which traction it radially, which is dependent upon establishing correct TCL tension [95]. The same authors suggest the removal of the pisiform when chronic piso-triquetral pain persists.

The hypothesis of Seradge and Seradge [95] has been confirmed by Rigoni [92] who published a study in which 600 CTS cases were operated on. Twenty-five of his cases (4.1%) had short term piso-triquetral pain and in 5 of these cases (0.8%.) the pain did not resolve itself. Rigoni [92] resolved these five cases by removing the pisiform.

To prevent this complication from occurring it is useful to immobilize the wrist in slight extension for 14 days leaving the fingers free to move. This postoperative procedure allows for quicker and correct TCL healing.

Nerve Complications That Are Not Correlated to the Cutaneous Scar

This paragraph includes both total or partial iatrogenic injuries of the median and/or ulnar nerve and their branches. These type of injuries have not frequently been documented in the medical literature. They are more frequent in CTS surgery in which a closed field technique is used. These same types of injuries also happen to occur sometimes in endoscopic surgery, but rarely in open field technique.

We will not include in this chapter the frequent injuries to the PCB of the median nerve and the rare occurrence of injury to a sensitive branch of the radial nerve, with the consequential formation of neuromas correlated to the cutaneous scar. These complications have been previously discussed (see p. 275).

Total or Partial Injuries of the Median or Ulnar Nerve and Their Branches

Data in the Literature for the Median Nerve and Its Branches

Semple and Cargill [94] reported 3 cases of sectioning of digital sensory nerves at the palm. Hybbinette and Mannerfelt [53] described 1 case in which there was a median nerve muscle branch injury. Das and Brown [31], reported 1 out of 6 reoperated cases, of scar compression of the median nerve muscle branch and another case of sectioning of the digital palmar sensitive branch for the cleft between the middle and ring finger. Conolly [29] described 2 cases of total sectioning of the median nerve and 1 case of sectioning of the median nerve muscle branch. Wadstroem and Nigst [106] reported 2 out of 40 reoperated cases of median nerve muscle branch injury. Lilly and Magnell [70] reported on 2 reoperated cases, in which they found both cases to have undergone an injury to the median nerve muscle branch. Luchetti et al. [74] reported on 1 case out of 15 reoperated patients, where there was a complete sectioning of the median nerve and 1 case where there was a partial sectioning of the median nerve and a complete sectioning of the muscle branch of the same nerve. Kern et al. [60], out of 16 reoperations, observed 1 case of median nerve muscle branch injury. Strasberg et al. [96], out of 50 reoperations, reported 2 cases where there was a complete injury to the median nerve, 1 to the muscle branch of the median nerve, and 3 cases of injury to the common digital nerve of the third web space. Condamine et al. [28] found that in 18 reoperations, there were 2 cases of complete sectioning of the median nerve. Chapman et al. [22] described 1 case in which there was a complete sectioning of the median nerve in a CTS surgery where a small incision was made and a carpal tunnel tome instrument was used.

Boekstyns and Sorensen [16], in a bibliographic research article on 54 CTS surgery studies that were published in the 1990s, reported that out of 1,203 total cases that were operated on with the open field technique, there was 1 reported case of a median nerve palmar branch injury.

The same authors reported that out of 9,516 total cases operated on with endoscopic surgery, there were 3 reported cases of a total injury and 4 of a partial injury to the median nerve, 1 reported case of a median nerve muscle branch injury, and 1 reported case of a median nerve palmar branch injury.

Data in the Literature for the Ulnar Nerve and Its Branches

Favero and Gropper [42] reported on 1 reoperated case where they found a sectioning of the muscle branch of the ulnar nerve and of the ulnar digital nerve to the little finger.

Terrono et al. [99] reported on 3 reoperations in which 2 cases presented with a complete sectioning of the ulnar nerve's muscle branch and in the third case, a partial injury to the same branch.

Boeckstyns and Sorensen [16], in a bibliographic research article on 54 CTS surgery studies that were published in the 1990s, reported that out of 1,203 total cases that were operated on with open field technique, there was only 1 reported case of an ulnar nerve muscle branch injury. The same authors, reported that out of 9,516 total cases operated on with endoscopic surgery, there was only 1 reported case of a total ulnar nerve injury and 1 reported case of an ulnar nerve muscle branch injury.

Data Taken from an American Questionnaire Concerning Injuries of the Median and Ulnar Nerve and Their Branches

The author has found the data that has been published by Palmer and Toivonen [86] to be very interesting. This questionnaire was sent to 1,253 members of the American Society for Surgery of the Hand, asking them to indicate the complications that they had observed in their years of surgical experience regarding CTS, whether or not they used traditional or endoscopic techniques from 1990 to 1995.

The questionnaire omitted two very important specifications. There was no way to determine if the surgery without endoscopic instruments was performed in an open or closed surgical field. In addition, the number of complications that were reported did not correlate to the number of surgeries performed. However, the responses that were derived from this questionnaire are extremely interesting and surprising.

Six hundred and sixteen surgeons who performed CTS surgery without the use of endoscopic instrumentation responded.

Iatrogenic injuries in CTS surgery without endoscopy were reported as follows:

Median nerve: 23 complete injuries, 102 partial and 22 muscle branch injuries
Ulnar nerve: 11 complete injuries, 15 partial and 3 muscle branch injuries
Digital palmar sensitive branches of the median or ulnar nerve: 54 injuries

This data is extremely important because it demonstrates that iatrogenic complications for CTS surgery, whether performed in an open field, but most of all in a closed surgical field, without the use of endoscopic instruments, occur much more frequently than that which is published in the literature.

If one takes into consideration the anatomical anomalies of the median nerve muscle branch that are often present, above all, those which are transligamentous [64, 68, 89], then some of these nerve injuries can be justified. Although, the number of injuries reported in the questionnaire is quite surprising for complete or partial injury to either the median or ulnar nerve and their digital palmar sensitive branches.

Seven hundred and eight surgeons, who used endoscopic techniques, responded to the same questionnaire [86].

Iatrogenic injuries in CTS endoscopic surgery were reported as follows:

Median nerve: 17 complete injuries, 28 partial, 5 muscle branch injuries, and 50 nonspecified
Ulnar nerve: 8 complete injuries, 8 partial, 5 muscle branch, and 66 nonspecified injuries
Digital palmar sensitive branches of the median or ulnar nerve: 77 injuries

Considering the medical-legal implications that are associated with iatrogenic injuries during CTS surgery, the surgeon must pay the utmost attention in preventing any type of injury from occurring.

From these reported experiences, one must absolutely take into account the possible dangers of performing this type of surgery using mini-incisions, in a closed field, or with the use of endoscopic instruments. A very careful evaluation of surgical indications is necessary, even when this surgery is being performed by well-experienced surgeons.

When performing an open field CTS surgery, it is important to respect that sectioning of the TCL is made on the ulnar side of the tunnel, in order to avoid an injury to the median nerve muscle branch (especially in the presence of anatomical anomalies), but at the same time, not too ulnarly, in order to avoid penetration into Guyon's canal instead of the carpal canal. According to Tunesi et al. [103], intraoperative findings of muscle fibers inside the TCL can indicate anomalies of the median nerve muscle branch pathway.

Vascular Complications

The severity of a hematoma, caused by a vascular injury, can be evaluated and a decision must be made concerning reoperation. When there is the presence of a severe iatrogenic vascular injury, surgical reintervention must be performed urgently, when possible, even during the surgery itself.

Hematomas from Nonsevere Vascular Injuries

A frequent cause of hematomas is correlated to the lack of small subcutaneous vessels cauterization. Such complication can easily arise when the incision is limited to the palm and the distal antebrachial fascia is sectioned subcutaneously [8].

Another cause of excessive bleeding can be from a radical tenosynovectomy, where a poor or incorrect hemostasis occurred [51, 61].

From a preventative point of view, Hunt and Osterman [51] underline the importance of following an accurate hemostasis after the removal of the brachial tourniquet.

When using a palmar incision, subcutaneous sectioning of the distal antebrachial fascia should be preceded by an atraumatic separating of the subcutaneous plane from the fascia [10].

Urbaniak [105] has underlined the importance of using a drainage system. However, the use of drains in CTS surgery is not frequently performed.

The American Society for Surgery of the Hand sent out a questionnaire to its members concerning the use of drains in CTS surgery. The results were published by Duncan et al. [36] and 414 surgeons (88.6%) responded they do not use any type of drainage system in CTS surgery.

Severe Vascular Injuries

The literature has reported that severe iatrogenic vascular injuries that occur during CTS surgery are quite rare.

Conolly [29] reported 2 cases of superficial palmar arch injuries. Mac Donald et al. [76] observed another 2 similar cases.

As we have seen for iatrogenic nerve injuries (see p. 278), even for iatrogenic vascular injuries, the responses to the questionnaires that have been published by Palmer and Toivonen [86] demonstrated that these complications in CTS surgery are not as rare in their occurrence as that which has been published in the medical literature.

From the responses of 618 members of the American Society for Surgery of the Hand, the following results have been collected concerning iatrogenic vascular injuries as a result of CTS traditional surgery (open or closed field), without the use of endoscopic instruments, from 1990 to 1995:

Superficial palmar arch: 21 injuries
Ulnar artery: 11 injuries
Radial artery: 2 injuries

In comparison, below are the results of 708 surgeons that have responded to the same questionnaire published by Palmer and Toivonen [86], regarding iatrogenic vascular injuries following CTS endoscopic surgery, also from 1990 to 1995:

Superficial palmar arch: 86 injuries
Ulnar artery: 34 injuries
Radial artery: 1 injury

The importance of taking into account the risks taken when performing endoscopic or closed field CTS surgery must be carefully considered after reviewing these statistics.

Superficial palmar arch injuries are highly correlated to the absence of a proper visual operating field, as well as the fear of performing an incomplete TCL distal sectioning.

In open field surgeries, it is of the utmost importance that maximum attention is paid to all the surrounding anatomical structures in order to avoid iatrogenic injuries from occurring.

When severe iatrogenic vascular injuries occur, an immediate and adequate surgical treatment must be followed.

Tendon Complications

Various tendon pathologies will be discussed in this paragraph. Scar adhesions between the flexor tendons without median nerve involvement, subcutaneous anterior subluxation of the flexor tendons, non-pre-existing trigger finger, ulnar subluxation of the flexor tendons outside of the carpal canal, and iatrogenic injury of the flexor tendons are all included.

Adhesions Between Flexor Tendons

In a previous paragraph, perinervous fibrotic scar proliferation was discussed (see p. 273), indicating that it had a strong attributing factor to causing scarring between the median nerve and the flexor tendons. The formation of adhesions between flexor tendons can also occur without median nerve involvement. In these cases, patients usually do not report neurological symptoms, but only a decrease in flexor tendon gliding that is associated with an eventual onset of decreased hand grip strength [76]. Generally, clinical symptoms do not require reoperation.

Such pathologies can be objectively diagnosed by CAT scan [109]. According to various authors [61, 76, 105], these type of adhesions frequently appear after a radical tenosynovectomy, where appropriate hemostasis has not been followed intraoperatively and/or in cases where early postoperative hand therapy for the fingers has been left out.

In order to avoid this complication, correct intraoperative hemostasis must be performed in conjunction with drain insertion. Postoperatively, these cases must be carefully followed-up with early finger rehabilitation while the wrist is immobilized at 15° of extension for 14 days.

Subcutaneous Anterior Subluxation of the Flexor Tendons

As has been previously mentioned, the normal postoperative course for CTS surgery includes a correct scar healing of the sectioned TCL. This allows for an increase in carpal canal volume, thus eliminating previous symptoms from median nerve compression, while, at the same time, maintaining correct functioning of the pulley system at the carpal canal level, guaranteeing that the nine flexor tendons and the median nerve are correctly housed in their canal.

Postoperative CAT scan follow-up exams [20, 108] have demonstrated that the reconstructed TCL is wider and more convex. There is an observable increase of the anterior-posterior canal diameter with a modest anterior repositioning of the flexor tendons and median nerve, which remain inside the tunnel.

Richman et al. [91] reported on 6-week follow-up postoperative MRI exams in 15 operated wrists and found an average increase in the anterior-posterior carpal canal diameter of 3.5 mm.

In normal healing conditions, subcutaneous anterior subluxation of the flexor tendons does not occur. Unfortunately, this subluxation may occur, in rare cases, where there has been a poor or lack of TCL scar formation and the finger flexor tendons tend to sublux anterior to the ligamentous plane and come in contact with the subcutaneous plane.

In perithenar incisions and TCL sectioning on the radial side, median nerve adhesions can be associated with cutaneous scar (see p. 276).

The clinical exam, in this case, demonstrates a cord-like effect (bowstringing) when activating the flexor tendons in active wrist and finger flexion.

This complication rarely occurs but can be found when a portion of the TCL has been removed and the wrist has been left in a flexed position postoperatively.

MacDonald et al. [76], summarized the results of 186 CTS operated wrists, and reported that in 34 various complications observed, there were two cases of flexor tendon anterior subluxation with tendon bowstringing. This complication is considered to be quite rare [51, 85, 105] and is generally nonsymptomatic. Usually it provokes a definitive reduction of hand grip strength (see p. 282).

In order to prevent this type of complication from occurring, the TCL must be sectioned on its ulnar side, without removing any portion of it and postoperatively the wrist should be at 15° of extension for 14 days, with the fingers completely free. This allows for proper TCL scar healing, thus preserving the correct functioning of the pulley system and maintaining the nine tendons and median nerve in their canal.

Non-pre-existing Trigger Finger

Mackinnon [77] has observed that after CTS surgery a possible trigger finger pathology, that had not been present prior to surgery, can occur. The author feels that this complication is correlated to an overloading of the finger flexor tendons at the metacarpophalanx pulley system level since there is a decreased pulley effect more proximally at the nonperfectly healed TCL.

In order to avoid this complication from occurring, it is reasonable to maintain the wrist at 15° of extension and leave the fingers free to move for 14 days. This posture guarantees proper healing of the TCL, thus maintaining the effect of the pulley system.

Ulnar Subluxation of Flexor Tendons Outside the Carpal Tunnel

Rarely do finger flexor tendons ulnarly sublux outside the carpal canal postoperatively (superficialis 5° and/or 4°), jumping over the hook of the hamate.

Tubiana [102] observed this complication in 2 cases where there was a subluxation of the fifth digit's flexor superficialis. Hunt and Osterman [51] reported a few cases of subluxation of the flexor superficialis tendons of the fourth and fifth digits.

This complication is symptomatic and develops into a chronic trigger finger. This pathology is caused by excessive ulnar sectioning of the TCL at the hook of the hamate insertion and the lack of postoperative wrist immobilization in moderate extension.

In order to avoid this complication from occurring, one should section the TCL on its ulnar side at about 3 mm from the bony insertion of the hook of the hamate and postoperatively maintain the wrist at 15° of extension for 14 days, thus facilitating correct TCL scar healing.

Injuries of the Flexor Tendons

Flexor tendon injuries during CTS surgery, whether or not it has been performed in an open or closed field, have been documented in the medical literature.

Terrono et al. [99] found during a reoperation that the fifth flexor superficialis tendon had been injured and was associated with a partial injury to the muscle branch of the ulnar nerve. Palmer and Toivonen [86] collected responses from their questionnaire and concluded that flexor tendon injuries in CTS surgery are not as exceptional in occurrence as that which has been published in the medical literature.

In fact, 616 surgeons, from the American Society for Surgery of the Hand that performed CTS operations without the use of endoscopic instruments during 1990–1995, reported:

19 tendon injuries of which 13 were complete and 6 partial

They did not specify the surgical approach or which tendons were involved in the iatrogenic injuries.

In comparison, 708 surgeons, from the American Society for Surgery of the Hand, that performed the CTS surgery using endoscopic equipment in the same period (1990–1995), reported:

69 tendon injuries of which 7 were complete and 62 partial

In order to avoid this complication from occurring, a careful evaluation of closed field and also of endoscopic surgery must be considered, due to the higher risk of iatrogenic injury.

In open field surgery it is sufficient if the surgeon is extremely attentive.

Reduction of Hand Grip Strength

In the first weeks after CTS surgery, one's hand grip strength decreases but can be gradually recuperated in the following months. Numerous studies have been conducted in order to determine why this phenomenon occurs.

Lluch [71] performed, after 2 and 8 years, a follow-up study of 220 CTS operated hands and observed that there was an average decrease in hand grip strength of 16%, with modest wrist extension, and of 24% with the wrist placed at 20° of flexion.

Gellman et al. [47] reported on 21 CTS cases and they found that after 6 weeks there was an average hand grip strength decrease of 27% and a successive average increase of 16% to that preoperatively after 6 months.

Katz et al. [59], in a prospective study of 35 patients that were operated on for CTS, found an average decrease of grip strength of 51.4% after 6 weeks, with an average recovery superior to 60.4% with respect to that taken preoperatively after 2 years.

Citron and Bendall [23], in a randomized prospective study of 47 CTS operated cases, found that 2 weeks after operation the average grip strength reduction was 34%, with complete recovery after 9 months.

Azzarà et al. [2] reported on 49 open field CTS surgery patients and found that after 1 month from surgery there was an average decrease of grip strength of 37% with a successive recovery superior to 36% with respect to preoperative strength values after 12 months.

Various authors have proposed a TCL lengthening-reconstruction in order to obtain a more rapid postoperative hand grip strength recovery.

Kapandji [57] planned a zig-zag incision on the TCL, obtaining two quadrangular shaped flaps that are sutured at their apex. This author observed that in 46 cases that were operated on using this technique, more rapid grip strength was recovered.

Jakab et al. [55] proposed a TCL reconstruction creating a distal radially-based flap and a proximal ulnarly-based flap. The apices of these flaps are approximated, lengthening the ligament 6–10 mm. In a group of 104 cases operated on using this technique, Jakab et al. [55] found in a follow-up control, at a distance of 2 and 7 years, that there was complete grip strength recovery with respect to the preoperative strength.

Karlsson et al. [58] proposed another surgical technique of TCL lengthening. The ligament is incised in a zig-zag fashion, making two triangular flaps on each side of the incision. The tips of the flaps are sutured together obtaining the release. These authors performed a retrospective study on 50 of their patients who were operated on only sectioning the TCL and 24 who underwent a TCL lengthening-reconstruction and they did not find any difference between these two groups concerning grip strength recovery.

Netscher et al. [83] proposed a TCL lengthening-reconstruction creating a proximally based transposition flap from the radial edge of the sectioned ligament. Successively the transposition flap is sutured to the ulnar edge of the TCL. In one of the randomized prospective studies, the authors made a comparison between a group of 17 patients who only underwent TCL sectioning and another group who underwent TCL reconstruction.

They observed that after 3 weeks there was an equal decrease in grip strength between the two groups, but after 6 weeks they found a more rapid strength recovery in the "TCL reconstruction" group. The authors also observed that after 12 weeks the "TCL sectioning" group had reached their average preoperative grip strength level and the "TCL reconstruction" group had surpassed it.

Azzarà et al. [2] followed a randomized prospective study on 49 cases that underwent a simple sectioning of the TCL and a second group of 48 cases who were operated on for TCL reconstruction according to Jakab et al.'s [55] technique. In a 1-month follow-up control, Azzarà et al. [2] found a decrease in grip strength by 37% in the first group and 46% in the second. By 3 months post operation, there was an average increase of grip strength by 14% and 15% respectively in the two groups and by 12 months, an increase in strength by 36% to the values taken preoperatively in both groups.

Particular interest has been voiced among hand surgeons concerning grip strength recovery comparing open field versus endoscopic surgical procedures for CTS.

A more rapid grip strength recovery has been reported in endoscopic surgery by some authors [1, 35, 39], but not confirmed by other authors.

Brown et al. [18] reported on a group of 85 open field surgical patients and a second group of 84 endoscopically treated patients (two-portal technique). In follow-up controls that were performed at 21, 42 and 84 days after surgery, the authors did not find significant differences in grip strength recovery between the two groups.

In a retrospective study done in 1992 by Bande et al. [4], 58 patients that were operated on using an open field technique and 44 patients using an endoscopic procedure (one portal technique) did not demonstrate statistical differences after 6 and 18 months with regard to their capacity to return to work, which was between 4 to 6 weeks postoperatively. MacDermid et al. [75] conducted a randomized study on CTS surgeries of which 91 were performed endoscopically and 32 open field. They found that the endoscopically treated group had better results 1 and 6 weeks after operation, while after 12 weeks the results were equal for both groups.

In conclusion, it seems to be quite evident that after CTS surgery, the reduced hand grip strength represents a transitory complication and it is correlated to a temporary loss of the TCL pulley system's function.

Only in rare cases of subcutaneous anterior subluxation of the flexor tendons with bowstringing, can one observe a definitive decrease in grip strength (see p. 280).

The temporary decrease in postoperative grip strength can also be due to thenar and hypothenar pain (see p. 276) or the formation of mini-neuromas in a painful palmar scar (see p. 275). As we have seen, in these pathologies, painful symptoms usually resolve themselves within a few months.

The preventative goal is to have rapid and correct TCL healing, so the temporary loss of grip strength is short-lived. The author feel that reconstruction of the TCL is not necessary and it is sufficient enough to maintain the wrist at 15° of extension for 14 days, while allowing for the immediate mobilization of the fingers.

Infection

Postoperative infection, (whether it be superficial and limited to only the skin and subcutaneous tissue or deep inside the canal) after CTS surgery has infrequently been reported in the medical literature.

Phalen [87] reported only 1 case (0.48%) out of 212 operated on, that was afflicted with a superficial infection. Other authors report more significant statistics.

Gainer and Nugent [45] found 26 cases (6%) of superficial infection out of 430 cases operated on for TCS, O'Malley et al. [84]: 1 case (5%) out of 20 reoperations, Clayburg et al. [24]: 2 cases (3.3%) out of 60 surgeries, Kluge et al. [63]: 5% of superficial infections out of 89 cases operated on.

Klein et al. [62] reported on 149 CTS surgeries performed in a closed field with a 1-cm incision, in which they found 3 superficial infections (2%).

Deep infections are also rarely documented.

Eason et al. [37] reported on 2 cases of deep infection, out of 47, which had suboptimal results, requiring hospitalization.

Hanssen et al. [49] reported, in a retrospective study, that out of 3,620 CTS surgeries from 1976 to 1985, they found 17 cases of deep infection (0.47%) that were diagnosed at an average of 13 postoperative days (minimum 2 days, maximum 35 days). In only one of the 17 cases antibiotics prophylaxis was performed. In 13 of the 17 cases tenosynovectomy, intracanal corticosteroid injection and/or drain insertion were performed. In 15 of these 17 cases staphylococcus aureus was the bacterial agent and in the only case where antibiotic prophylaxis was administered, the bacterial agent was pseudomonas aeruginosa.

A case of deep tunnel infection following CTS surgery is documented in Fig. 37.2.

In summary, by analyzing the data reported, we can see that superficial infections are not infrequent but deep ones rarely occur.

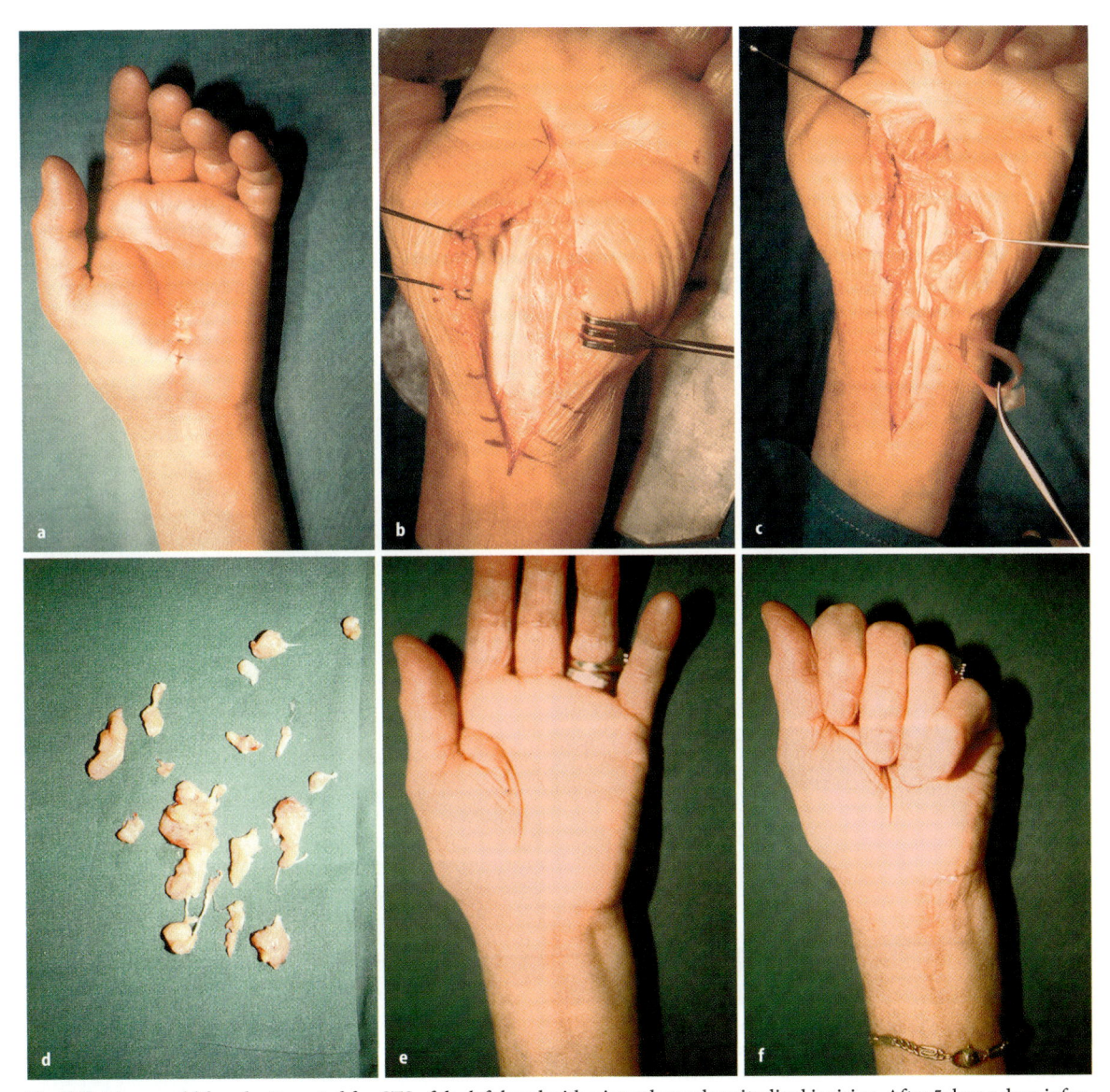

Fig. 37.2. 78-year-old female. Operated for CTS of the left hand with a interthenar longitudinal incision. After 5 days a deep infection developed. **a** Clinical aspect of the infected hand. **b** Immediate reoperation with palmar incision extending to the forearm. One can observe acute hypertrophic tenosynovitis. The median nerve appears integral. **c** A tenosynovectomy and median nerve external neurolysis are performed. **d** The synovial tissue is removed. **e, f** Healing of the infection with good hand function recovery 1 month after the time of surgery (This case has been generously lent to me by Dr. Riccardo Luchetti)

From both my experience and also from the medical literature, infective risk factors arise from hematomas, marginal cutaneous necrosis, and local intraoperative corticosteroid infiltrations.

In a questionnaire published by Duncan et al. [36], 64 out of 467 American surgeons habitually use intraoperative corticosteroid infiltrations as part of their treatment regime for their patients.

One of the most important elements for preventing CTS postoperative infections is essentially by avoiding the formation of hematomas (see p. 279).

Correct and atraumatic surgical techniques, well-equipped and sterile operating rooms, and avoiding the use of intraoperative corticosteroid infiltrations allow for an effective prevention of CTS surgical infections.

Antibiotic prophylaxis is not routinely used for this type of surgery [5].

Reflex Sympathetic Dystrophy (Algodystrophy)

Reflex sympathetic dystrophy or algodystrophy is essentially characterized by edema, by a loss of functional hand strength (primarily from pain and then from articular stiffness), by vasomotor instability, and lastly by trophic disturbances [34].

Various authors have reported on the occurrence of reflex sympathetic dystrophy as a CTS postoperative complication.

Phalen [87] cited 1 case of algodystrophy out of 219 surgeries operated on (0.5%).

Hybbinette and Mannerfelt [53] reported 3 out of 506 cases (0.6%.), Mac Donald et al. [76] 4 out of 186 cases (2.15%), Fissette and Onkelinx [44] 1 out of 45 cases (2.2%), Lichtman et al. [69] 5 out of 100 cases (5%), Clayburgh et al. [24] 3 out of 60 (5%), O'Malley et al. [84] 1 out of 20 cases (5%), and Azzarà et al. [2] 1 out of 100 cases (1%).

Duncan et al. [36] published some very interesting data taken from a questionnaire in which 467 member of the American Society for Surgery of the Hand responded. Three hundred and four surgeons (65.2%) responded that they consider reflex sympathetic dystrophy as a possible complication in CTS surgery, in a percentage that varies from 1% to 5% of cases operated on.

Blair [14] upholds that reflex sympathetic dystrophy represents a postoperative complication in at least 5% of CTS surgeries performed.

An algodystrophy case, secondary to CTS surgery, is documented in Fig. 37.3.

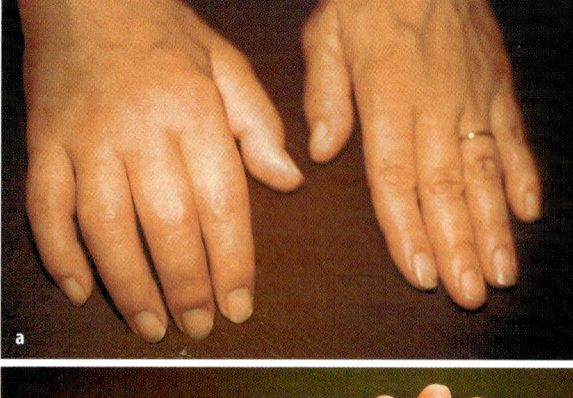

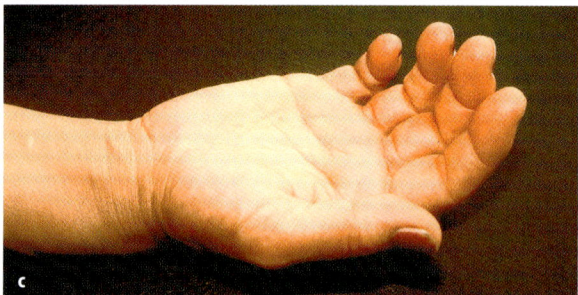

Fig. 37.3. (This case has been generously lent to me by Dr. Riccardo Luchetti). 53-year-old female. Operated for CTS on the right hand, reflex sympathetic dystrophy appeared after 20 days from the time of surgery. **a** The edema of the right hand is quite evident. **b** Significant hand function limitations, the patient was unable to make a complete fist. **c, d** Good functional results after 2 months. The reflex sympathetic dystrophy was treated immediately using pain blocking medication and guanethidine

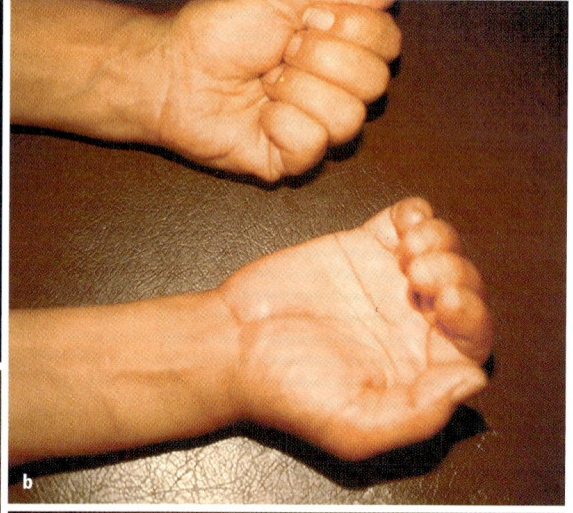

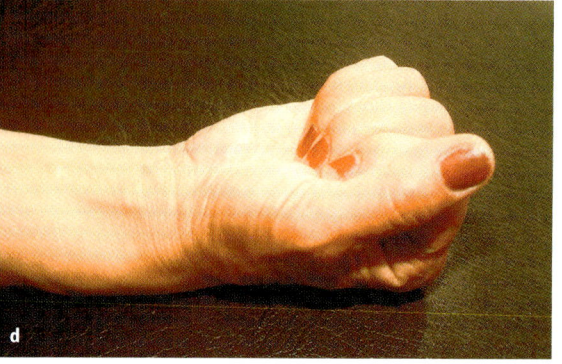

An important risk factor with regard to reflex sympathetic dystrophy is represented by an individual predisposition correlated to a psychological labile constitution [27] or to an unstable neuro-vegetative state of health [69]. This predisposition is also more frequently correlated to women.

Prolonged acute pain is another risk factor that is correlated with the onset of algodystrophy. This complication is often caused by hematomas and/or tight compressive bandages that have been worn for a prolonged period of time.

Duncan et al. [36] made a report on the responses derived from a questionnaire completed by members of the American Society for Surgery of the Hand, where 414 (88.6%) confirmed that they never used a drainage system in CTS surgery and 365 surgeons (78.1%) declared that they systematically apply a compressive bandage to the patient postoperatively. In particular, 119 surgeons apply this compressive bandage for 4–7 days, 45 surgeons for 8–10 days, and 76 surgeons for over 10 days.

In order to prevent algodystrophy from occurring, it has been suggested by Codega [27] that predisposed patients are treated pharmacologically with tranquilizers.

The author suggests that it is of fundamental importance that the surgeon prevents hematomas from occurring by using a correct hemostasis during surgery and the insertion of a drainage system postoperatively for 24 h.

In addition, the author feels that compressive bandages are dangerous to use and is in complete agreement with Urbaniak [105] that they should be abandoned.

Causalgia

Causalgia is a rare painful syndrome that is characterized by the onset of spontaneous pain which is constant, nonsubsiding, sharp, and often severely interferes with the personal life of the patient. It is generally correlated to a partial nerve injury [11].

This severe complication rarely occurs in the postoperative course of CTS surgery.

The main risk factors occur after an internal neurolysis, when the median nerve forms adhesions to the radial wall of the tunnel or to the reparative TCL scar.

The worst symptoms occur when an internal neurolysis has been performed, and the nerve subluxes anterior to the subcutaneous plane and forms adhesions directly with the cutaneous scar (see p. 276). In this case severe pain is elicited, even only when the superficial scar is slightly touched. Generally, a true causalgia occurs after two or three reoperations and is aggravated by the precarious condition of the nerve and perinervous scar adhesions.

In the author's experience, he remembers at least two severe cases of causalgia. Both cases had been operated on two times and the median nerve was bare of its epineurium along a portion of its tract. In one of the cases, the nerve was anteriorly subluxed and adherent to the cutaneous perithenar cutaneous scar; in the other case, the nerve was adherent to the radial wall of the tunnel and to the flexor pollicis longus tendon.

Luchetti et al. [74] reported one case of causalgia after CTS surgery. The patient had already been operated with a median nerve internal neurolysis and presented perinervous adhesions to the TCL reparative scar. The patient underwent two successive interposition surgeries, one surgery with a muscle flap and the other with a fascial ulnar island flap, neither of which improved the causalgia.

One of the characteristics of the causalgia, above all in its advanced phase, is that it is irreversible, even in front of the most sophisticated surgical and microsurgical techniques.

Various authors have underlined that an internal neurolysis of the median nerve, in the course of CTS surgery, is an important risk factor leading to causalgia [53, 88, 105].

Curtis and Eversmann [30] point out the utility in CTS surgery of performing an internal neurolysis, but the latest clinical research that has been conducted by medical experts in this subject [15, 46, 73], indicates that internal neurolysis useless and dangerous.

Another pathological situation that, although rarely occurring, can provoke a causalgia is an iatrogenic injury to the PCB of the median nerve or to a sensitive branch of the radial nerve (see p. 275). If a painful neuroma develops and is not adequately treated in a timely manner, or if it is reoperated on without success, it can set off a vicious causalgia.

In order to prevent causalgia from occurring, one must absolutely avoid any type of iatrogenic injury, abstain from performing internal neurolysis of the median nerve, and make sure the TCL has a chance to heal correctly, by positioning the wrist at 15° of wrist extension for 14 days, with the fingers free to move.

It is absolutely necessary that, in the postoperative period, nerve origin pain is treated in a timely and adequate manner and not left to resolve itself spontaneously, otherwise there is a higher risk of the patient ending up with a causalgic syndrome.

Conclusions

From all that has been reported and statistically documented in this chapter, it appears that possible complications occurring from CTS surgery are numerous and of variable severity and duration.

The author upholds that it is very important that the surgeon, when deciding what surgical technique to employ, thoroughly evaluates which complications arise more frequently with the associated technique. The surgeon must be aware if these possible complications are temporary and will resolve themselves in a few weeks or months, or are irreversible.

The author has summarized the complications associated with specific surgical CTS techniques by grouping them into complications with the tendency to resolve themselves and those which tend to be irreversible.

Complications That Spontaneously Resolve Within 6 Months, Frequently Associated With Open Field Surgical Technique

Mini-neuromas from the sectioning of palmar cutaneous terminal endings of the median nerve and/or ulnar nerve

The severity and duration of this complication is minor if the incision is performed along the fourth digital palmar ray axis.

Thenar and hypothenar pain (pillar pain)
Reduction of hand grip strength

These complications are the consequence of TCL sectioning. The resolution of these disturbances is proportional to a correct TCL scar healing.

Complications That Are Not Spontaneously Reversible, Frequently Associated With Open Field Surgical Technique

Perinervous fibrotic scar proliferation
Cutaneous scar pathology
Neuroma from the sectioning of the palmar cutaneous branch of the median nerve or of a sensitive branch of the radial nerve
Cutaneous scar adhesions to the median nerve
Adhesions between flexor tendons
Subcutaneous anterior subluxation of the flexor tendons
Ulnar subluxation of flexor tendons outside the carpal tunnel

These various complications are evitable when a correct and attentive surgical technique is used under a wide visual surgical field and followed by a correct postoperative treatment, which allows for the TCL to heal correctly and at the same time leaves the fingers free to move.

Complications That Are Not Spontaneously Reversible and Are More Frequently Occurring in the Closed Field and Endoscopic Surgical Technique

Incomplete or complete lack of median nerve decompression

Total or partial injuries of the median or ulnar nerve and their branches
Severe vascular injuries
Injuries of the flexor tendons

Such complications are not always avoidable even when the procedure is performed by a surgeon who has expertise in this technique.

Hypertrophic tenosynovitis of the flexor tendons

The closed field surgical technique and the endoscopic surgery are not indicated when the patient has a pre-existing condition of synovial hypertrophy. This condition can be confirmed both clinically and instrumentally.

Complications That Are Not Spontaneously Reversible and Are Not Correlated to the Surgical Approach

Piso-triquetral pain
Non-pre-existing trigger finger

These complications are rare in occurrence and can be avoided if a correct TCL scar healing process takes place. However, they can be resolved with a successive modest surgical intervention.

Complications That Are Not Specific to CTS Surgery and Are Not Correlated to the Surgical Approach

Hematomas from nonsevere vascular injuries
Infection
Reflex sympathetic dystrophy (algodystrophy)

These complications can generally be avoided if a correct surgical technique is performed and an adequate postoperative functional rehabilitation program is followed.

Severe Complication, Rare, Nonspecific, and Not Correlated to the Surgical Approach

Causalgia

This complication usually occurs from a prolonged and intense painful syndrome caused often by a partial nerve injury. It can be avoided by not provoking a nerve injury, abstaining from performing an internal neurolysis of the median nerve and treating painful nerve symptoms in an adequate and timely fashion, both surgically and with modern pain therapy methods.

At the end of this complex chapter, the author states that he prefers to treat CTS with an open field surgical approach.

The personal technique that he improved on the course of his experience, includes the following steps:

1. Palmar cutaneous incision of 4- to 5-cm length along the fourth digital ray axis
2. Complete sectioning of the TCL on its ulnar side about 3 mm from the hook of the hamate insertion
3. Atraumatic separation of the antebrachial fascia from the subcutaneous tissue moving proximally for 2–3 cm to the distal flexor crease of the wrist
4. Subcutaneous sectioning of the distal part of the antebrachial fascia, ulnar to the median nerve, always under visual control, for 2–3 cm
5. Careful external neurolysis of the median nerve
6. Nonradical tenosynovectomy, when synovial hypertrophy of the flexor tendons is present
7. Accurate hemostasis, when removing the brachial tourniquet
8. Atraumatic suturing of the skin
9. Drain insertion
10. Gauze and cotton sterile medication and application of a noncompressive bandage with placement of a plaster volar valve which immobilizes the wrist at 15° of extension and leaves the fingers completely free to move
11. Twenty-four hours postoperatively: medication, drain removal, noncompressive bandage and application of plaster volar valve or dorsal thermoplastic splint at 15° of extension, starting with functional rehabilitation of the fingers
12. Fourteen days postoperatively: removal of the plaster valve or the thermoplastic splint, medication, removal of sutures, beginning of wrist functional re-education and continuing of hand rehabilitation under the guidance of a hand therapist

By following this specific protocol for many years in the surgical treatment of CTS, the author observed optimal results at long-distance follow-ups.

Specifically, he has found the disappearance of irreversible complications and a noticeable reduction in the severity and duration of spontaneously reversible complications.

The author would like to underline that when using a closed field or endoscopic technique, the risk of provoking severe and irreversible complications is always present.

CTS surgery complications are generally infrequent but unfortunately, in some circumstances, unavoidable complications do arise even when the surgeon is an expert.

Personally, the author does not feel that one should use surgical techniques which can increase the possibility of severe and irreversible complications from occurring.

In closing, the author would like to advise young surgeons never to consider CTS treatment to be a banal surgery.

References

1. Agee JM, Mc Carroll HR, Tortosa RD et al. (1992) Endoscopic release of the carpal tunnel: A randomized prospective multicenter study. J Hand Surg 17A: 987–999
2. Azzarà A, Altissimi M, Mancini GB, Romeo F (1997) Variazioni di forza dopo semplice sezione e dopo allungamento e ricostruzione del legamento trasverso del carpo nella sindrome del tunnel carpale. Riv Chir Mano 34: 343–344
3. Bagatur AE (2002) Analysis of the causes of failure in carpal tunnel syndrome surgery and the results of reoperation. Acta Orthop Traumatol Turc 36:346–353
4. Bande S, De Smet L, Fabry G (1994) The results of carpal tunnel release: open versus endoscopic technique. J Hand Surg 19B: 14–17
5. Bedeschi P (1983) Limiti della profilassi antibiotica nella chirurgia ortopedica e traumatologica. In: Galli PA and Montanari GD (eds) Prevenzione antimicrobica in chirurgia. Piccin, Padova, pp 201–208
6. Bedeschi P (1986) Un nuovo segno clinico nella diagnosi della sindrome del tunnel carpale: la rilevazione palpatoria dell' aumento della tensione locale. Atti 12° Congresso Soc It Ric Chir, 20–22 novembre 1986, Modena. Monduzzi, Bologna, pp 113–116
7. Bedeschi P (1997) La resezione della prima filiera del carpo. In: Monografie SICM (ed) Lo Scafoide. Mattioli, Fidenza, pp 225–233
8. Bedeschi P (2001) Le complicanze e gli insuccessi nella Chirurgia della Sindrome del tunnel carpale. Riv Chir Mano 38: 197–204
9. Bedeschi P (2002a) Complicanze postoperatorie correlate alla sezione e/o alla cicatrizzazione del legamento traverso del carpo nella chirurgia della sindrome del tunnel carpale e loro prevenzione. Ortop Traumatol 44: 30–34
10. Bedeschi P (2002b) Complicanze del trattamento chirurgico a cielo aperto o a cielo chiuso senza ausilio endoscopico. In: Luchetti R (ed) Sindrome del tunnel carpale. Verduci, Roma, pp 217–236
11. Bedeschi P, Mingione A, Luchetti R, De Santis G (1981) Il dolore negli esiti del trattamento chirurgico delle lesioni dei nervi periferici. Riv Chir Mano 18: 409–416
12. Berzero GF, Genovese E, Bertolotti M et al. (1994) La RMN nella definizione delle compressioni estrinseche e delle lesioni intrinseche del nervo mediano al polso e al terzo distale di avambraccio. Riv Chir Mano 31: 163–166
13. Biyani A, Downes EM (1993) An open twin incision technique of carpal tunnel decompression with reduced incidence of scar tenderness. J Hand Surg 18B: 331–334
14. Blair SJ (1988) Avoiding complications of surgery for nerve compression syndromes Orthop Clin North America 19: 125–130
15. Blair WF, Goetz DD, Ross MA et al. (1996) Carpal tunnel release with and without epineurotomy: a comparative prospective trial. J Hand Surg 21A: 655–661
16. Boeckstyns MEH, Sorensen AL (1999) Does endoscopic carpal tunnel release have a higher rate of complications than open carpal tunnel release? J Hand Surg 24B: 9–15
17. Braun RM, Rechnic M, Fowler E (2002) Complications related to carpal tunnel release. Hand Clinics 18: 347–357
18. Brown RA, Gelberman RH, Seiler JG et al. (1993) Carpal tunnel release. J Bone Joint Surg 75A: 1265–1275
19. Carroll RE, Green DP (1972) The significance of the palmar cutaneous nerve at the wrist. Clin Orthop 83: 24–28
20. Chaise F, Roger B, Laval-Jeantet M, Alhomme Ph (1986) Exploration tomodensitométrique des modifications anatomiques du poignet entraînées par la section du ligament annulaire antérieur. Rev Chir Orthop 72: 297–302

21. Chang B, Dellon AL (1993) Surgical management of recurrent carpal tunnel syndrome. J Hand Surg 18B: 467–470
22. Chapman CB, Ristic S, Rosenwasser MP (2001) Complete median nerve transection as a complication of carpal tunnel release with a carpal tunnel tome. Am J Orthop 30: 652–653
23. Citron ND, Bendall SP (1997) Local symptoms after open carpal tunnel release. A randomized prospective trial of two incisions. J Hand Surg 22B: 317–321
24. Clayburgh RH, Beckenbaugh RD, Dobyns JH (1987) Carpal tunnel release in patients with diffuse peripheral neuropathy. J Hand Surg 12A: 380–383
25. Cobb TK, Amadio PC (1996) Reoperation for carpal tunnel syndrome. Hand Clinics 12/2: 313–323
26. Cobb TK, Dalley BK, Posteraro RH, Lewis RC (1993) Anatomy of the flexor retinaculum. J Hand Surg 18A: 91–99
27. Codega G (1987) La patologia del polso. Piccin, Padova
28. Condamine JL, Marcucci L, Rosas MH et al. (1998) Repetitive release of the median nerve at the carpal tunnel. Analysis of a series of 18 cases. Rev Chir Orthop 84: 323–329
29. Conolly WB (1978) Pitfalls in carpal tunnel decompression. Aust NZ J Surg 48: 421–425
30. Curtis RM, Eversmann WW (1973) Internal neurolysis as an adjunct to the treatment of the carpal tunnel syndrome. J Bone Joint Surg 55A: 733–740
31. Das SK, Brown HG (1976) In search of complications in carpal tunnel decompression. The Hand 8: 243–249
32. Da Silva MF, Moore DC, Weiss AC et al. (1996) Anatomy of the palmar cutaneous branch of the median nerve: clinical significance. J Hand Surg 21A: 639–643
33. De Smet L (1993) Recurrent carpal tunnel syndrome. Clinical testing indicating incomplete section of the flexor retinaculum. J Hand Surg 18B: 189
34. Dirheimer Y (1993) Algodystrophie du membre supérieur post-traumatique et post-chirurgicale. In: SFCM (ed) Cahier d' enseignement de la SFCM (5), Expansion Scientifique Francaise, Paris, pp 21–39
35. Dumontier C, Sokolow C, Leclercq C, Chauvin P (1995) Early results of conventional versus two-portal endoscopic carpal tunnel release. A prospective study. J Hand Surg 20B: 658–662
36. Duncan KH, Lewis RC, Foreman KA, Nordyke MD (1987) Treatment of carpal tunnel syndrome by members of the American Society for Surgery of the Hand. Results of a questionnaire. J Hand Surg 12A: 384–391
37. Eason SY, Belsole RJ, Greene TL (1985) Carpal tunnel release: analysis of suboptimal results. J Hand Surg 10B: 365–369
38. Engber WD, Gmeiner JG (1980) Palmar cutaneous branch of the ulnar nerve. J Hand Surg 5: 26–29
39. Erdmann MWH (1994) Endoscopic carpal tunnel decompression. J Hand Surg 19B: 5–13
40. Eversmann WW (1988) Entrapment and compression neuropathies. In: Green DP (ed) Operative Hand Surgery, 2nd ed, Churchill Livingstone, New York pp 1423–1478.
41. Fairplay T, Urso G (2002) Trattamento postoperatorio dopo decompressione a cielo aperto o endoscopica. In: Luchetti R (ed) Sindrome del tunnel carpale. Verduci, Roma, pp 205–213
42. Favero KJ, Gropper PT (1987) Ulnar nerve laceration. A complication of carpal tunnel decompression: case report and review of the literature. J Hand Surg 12B: 239–241
43. Ferrari GP, Gilbert A (1991) The superficial anastomosis on the palm of the hand between the ulnar and median nerves. J Hand Surg 16B: 511–514
44. Fissette J, Onkelinx A (1979) Treatment of carpal tunnel syndrome. Comparative study with and without epineurolysis. Hand 11: 206–210
45. Gainer JV, Nugent GR (1977) Carpal tunnel syndrome: report of 430 operations. South Med J 70: 325–328
46. Gelberman RH, Pfeffer GB, Galbraith RT et al. (1987) Results of treatment of severe carpal tunnel syndrome without internal neurolysis of the median nerve. J Bone Joint Surg 69A: 896–903
47. Gellman H, Kan D, Gee V et al. (1989) Analysis of pinch and grip strength after carpal tunnel release. J Hand Surg 14A: 863–864
48. Gilliatt RW, Wilson TG (1953) A pneumatic-tourniquet test in carpal tunnel syndrome. Lancet i: 595–597
49. Hanssen AD, Amadio PC, De Silva SP, Ilstrup DM (1989) Deep postoperative wound infection after carpal tunnel release. J Hand Surg 14A: 869–873
50. Hobbs RA, Magnussen PA, Tonkin MA (1990) Palmar cutaneous branch of the median nerve. J Hand Surg 15A: 38–43
51. Hunt TR, Osterman AL (1994) Complications of the treatment of carpal tunnel syndrome. Hand Clin 10: 63–71
52. Hunter JM (1991) Recurrent carpal tunnel syndrome, epineural fibrous fixation, and traction neuropathy. Hand Clin 7: 491–504
53. Hybbinette CH, Mannerfelt L (1975) The carpal tunnel syndrome. A retrospective study of 400 operated patients. Acta Orthop Scand 46: 610–620
54. Inglis AE (1980) Two unusual operative complications in the carpal tunnel syndrome. A report of two cases. J Bone Joint Surg 62A: 1208–1209
55. Jakab E, Ganos D, Cook FW (1991) Trasverse carpal ligament recostruction in surgery for carpal tunnel syndrome: a new technique. J Hand Surg 16A: 202–206
56. Jones SMG, Stuart PR, Stothard J (1997) Open carpal tunnel release. Does a vascularized hypothenar fat pad reduce wound tenderness ? J Hand Surg 22B: 758–760
57. Kapandji AI (1990) La plastie d' agrandissement du ligament annulaire antérieur du carpe dans le traitement du syndrome du canal carpien. Ann Chir Main 9: 305–314
58. Karlsson MK, Lindau T, Hagberg L (1997) Ligament lengthening compared with simple division of the transverse carpal ligament in the open treatment of carpal tunnel syndrome. Scand J Reconstr Hand Surg 31: 65–69
59. Katz JN, Fossel KK, Simmons BP et al. (1995) Symptoms, functional status, and neuromuscolar impairment following carpal tunnel release. J Hand Surg 20A: 549–555
60. Kern BC, Brock M, Rudolph KH, Logemann H (1993) The recurrent carpal tunnel syndrome. Zentralbl Neurochir 54:80–83
61. Kessler FB (1986) Complications of the management of carpal tunnel syndrome. Hand Clinics 2: 401–406
62. Klein RD, Kotsis SV, Chung KC (2003) Open carpal tunnel release using a 1-centimeter incision: technique and outcomes for 104 patients. Plast Reconstr Surg 111:1616–1622.
63. Kluge W, Simpson RG, Nicol AC (1996) Late complications after open carpal tunnel decompression. J Hand Surg 21B: 205–207
64. Kozin SH (1998) The anatomy of the recurrent branch of the median nerve. J Hand Surg 23A: 852–858
65. Kuhlmann N, Tubiana R, Lisfranc R (1978) Apport de l' anatomie dans la compréhension des syndromes de compression du canal carpien et des séquelles des interventions décompressives. Rev Chir Orthop 64: 59–70
66. Kulick MI, Gordillo G, Javidi T et al. (1986) Long-term analysis of patients having surgical treatment for carpal tunnel syndrome. J Hand Surg 11A: 59–66
67. Langloh ND, Linscheid RL (1972) Recurrent and unrelieved carpal tunnel syndrome. Clin Orthop 83:41–47
68. Lanz U (1977) Anatomical variations of the median nerve in the carpal tunnel. J Hand Surg 2: 44–53

69. Lichtman DM, Florio RL, Mack GR (1979) Carpal tunnel release under local anesthesia: evaluation of the outpatient procedure. J Hand Surg 4: 544–546
70. Lilly CJ, Magnell TD (1985) Severance of the thenar branch of the median nerve as a complication of carpal tunnel release. J Hand Surg 10A: 399–402
71. Lluch A (1987) El sindrome del tunel carpiano. Mitre, Barcelona, pp 139–140
72. Louis DS, Greene TL, Noellert RC (1985) Complications of carpal tunnel surgery. J Neurosurg. 62: 352–356
73. Lowry WE, Follender AB (1988) Interfascicular neurolysis in the severe carpal tunnel syndrome: a prospective, randomized, double-blind, controlled study. Clin Orthop 227: 251–254
74. Luchetti R, Soragni O, Pederzini L et al. (1993) Trattamento delle complicanze della sindrome del tunnel carpale. Riv Chir Mano 30: 155–161
75. MacDermid JC, Richards RS, Roth JH et al. (2003) Endoscopic versus open carpal tunnel release: a randomized trial. J Hand Surg 28A:475–480
76. Mac Donald RI, Lichtman DM, Hanlon JJ, Wilson JN (1978) Complications of surgical release for carpal tunnel syndrome. J Hand Surg 3: 70–76
77. Mackinnon SE (1991) Secondary carpal tunnel surgery. Neurosurg Clinics North America 2: 75–91
78. Martin CH, Seiler III JG, Lesesne JS (1996) The cutaneous innervation of the palm: an anatomic study of the ulnar and median nerves. J Hand Surg 21A: 634–638
79. Matloub HS, Yan J-G, Mink Van Der Molen AB et al. (1998) The detailed anatomy of the palmar cutaneous nerves and its clinical implications. J Hand Surg 23B: 373–379
80. Murphy RX, Chernofsky MA, Osborne MA, Wolson AH (1993) Magnetic resonance imaging in the evaluation of persistent carpal tunnel syndrome. J Hand Surg 18A: 113–120
81. Naff N, Dellon AL, Mackinnon SE (1993) The anatomical course of the palmar cutaneous branch of the median nerve, including a description of its own unique tunnel. J Hand Surg 18B: 316–317
82. Nakamichi K, Tachibana S (1993) The use of ultrasonography in detection of synovitis in carpal tunnel syndrome. J Hand Surg 18B: 176–179
83. Netscher D, Steadman AK, Thornby J, Cohen V (1998) Temporal changes in grip and pinch strength after open carpal tunnel release and the effect of ligament reconstruction. J Hand Surg 23A: 48–54
84. O'Malley MJ, Evanoff M, Terrono AL, Millender LH (1992) Factors that determine reexploration treatment of carpal tunnel syndrome. J Hand Surg 17A: 638–641
85. Omer GE (1992) Median nerve compression at the wrist. Hand Clin 8: 317–324
86. Palmer AK, Toivonen DA (1999) Complications of endoscopic and open carpal tunnel release. J Hand Surg 24A: 561–565
87. Phalen GS (1966) The carpal tunnel syndrome. Seventeen years' experience in diagnosis and treatment of six hundred fifty-four hands. J Bone Joint Surg 48A: 211–228
88. Phalen GS (1972) The carpal tunnel syndrome. Clinical evaluation of 598 hands. Clin Orthop 83: 29–40
89. Poisel S (1974) Ursprung und Verlauf des R. muscularis des Nervus digitalis palmaris communis (N. medianus). Chir Praxis 18: 471–474
90. Povlsen B, Tegnell I (1996) Incidence and natural history of touch allodynia after open carpal tunnel release. Scand J Plast Reconstr Surg 30: 221–225
91. Richman JA, Gelberman RH, Rydevik BL et al. (1989) Carpal tunnel syndrome: morphologic changes after release of the transverse carpal ligament. J Hand Surg 14A: 852–857
92. Rigoni G (1990) Presentation of 25 cases of the pisotriquetral syndrome occurring in 600 cases of carpal tunnel release. Proceedings of the annual congress of the Swiss Society for Surgery of the Hand, Lausanne, 23rd-24th march 1990. Ann Hand Surg 9: 389
93. Rose EH, Norris MS, Kowalski TA et al. (1991) Palmaris brevis turnover flap as an adjunct to internal neurolysis of the chronically scarred median nerve in recurrent carpal tunnel syndrome. J Hand Surg 16A: 191–201
94. Semple JC, Cargill AO (1969) Carpal tunnel syndrome. Results of surgical decompression. Lancet i: 918–919
95. Seradge H, Seradge E (1989) Piso-triquetral pain syndrome after carpal tunnel release. J Hand Surg 14A: 858–862
96. Strasberg SR, Novak CB, Mackinnon SE, Murray JF (1994) Subjective and employment outcome following secondary carpal tunnel surgery. Ann Plast Surg 32: 485–489
97. Strickland JW, Idler RS, Lourie GM, Plancher KD (1996) The hypothenar fat pad flap for management of recalcitrant carpal tunnel syndrome. J Hand Surg 21A: 840–848
98. Taleisnik J (1973) The palmar cutaneous branch of the median nerve and the approach to the carpal tunnel. J Bone Joint Surg 55A: 1212–1217.
99. Terrono AL, Belsky MR, Feldon PG, Nalebuff EA (1993) Injury to the deep motor branch of the ulnar nerve during carpal tunnel release. J Hand Surg 18A: 1038–1040
100. Tinel J (1915) Le signe du "fourmillement" dans les lésions des nerfs périphériques. Presse Med 47: 388–389
101. Tomaino MM, Plakseychuk A (1998) Identification and preservation of palmar cutaneous nerves during open carpal tunnel release. J Hand Surg 23B: 607–608
102. Tubiana R (1990) Carpal tunnel syndrome: some views on its management. Ann Hand Surg 9: 325–330
103. Tunesi D, Di Giuseppe P, Ajmar R, Fassi PL (1997) Implicazioni chirurgiche delle anomalie della branca tenare del nervo mediano nella sindrome del tunnel carpale. Riv Chir Mano 34: 13–17
104. Upton ARM, McComas AJ (1973) The double crush in nerve entrapment syndromes. Lancet i: 359–361
105. Urbaniak JR (1991) Complications of treatment of carpal tunnel syndrome. In: Gelberman R (ed) Operative nerve repair and reconstruction. Lippincott, Philadelphia, vol 2, pp 967–979.
106. Wadstroem J, Nigst H (1986) Reoperation for carpal tunnel syndrome. A retrospective analysis of forty cases. Ann Chir Main 5: 54–58
107. Watchmaker GP, Weber D, Mckinnon SE (1996) Avoidance of transection of the palmar cutaneous branch of the median nerve in carpal tunnel release. J Hand Surg 21A: 644–650
108. Zanlungo M, Martelli A, Uggetti C, Consoli C (1988) Interesse della tomografia computerizzata (TC) nelle recidive al trattamento chirurgico della sindrome del canale del carpo. Arch Ortop Reum 101: 327–332
109. Zanlungo M, Locatelli G, Consoli C, Frati A (1998) Le recidive al trattamento chirurgico della sindrome del carpo. Atti Giornate Magentine di Aggiornamento in Chirurgia della Mano, Magenta 27–28 marzo 1998. Boehringer Mannheim, Milano, pp 130–137

38 Complications Following Endoscopic Treatment

G. Pajardi, G. Pivato, L. Pegoli, D. Pisani

Introduction

The introduction of a new diagnostic or therapeutic method, particularly a surgical one, creates a great deal of both perplexity and enthusiasm, at least until the protocol is finished and the use of the technique achieves a strict application of the protocol itself.

This is exactly what happened with the endoscopic release of the carpal annular ligament (generally for the whole hand surgery, especially for the wrist, it has been universally accepted).

It's difficult to understand the reason for this situation; in fact, the arthroscopic method for the treatment of wrist ligament lesions seems to date back before the history of other joint surgeries such as on the knee or the shoulder. The concern regarding the presence of the nerve makes it much more difficult to accept this technological innovation in the pathology we are talking about.

We can not forget that the wide diffusion of carpal tunnel syndrome (CTS) surgical treatment, not only in the hand surgery field but also in plastic surgery and orthopedics, caused a return to clinical malpractice and carelessness.

Surgeries have been performed by nonspecialists in an effort to prove that technical experience was not necessary when performing endoscopic procedures. It resulted, instead, in irremedial damage to the patients.

This is the primary statement underlying the following chapter, where we will have to use scientific rigor to distinguish between real complications and technical or indication mistakes [2, 11, 18].

This is not an easy job considering the volume of literature concerning this matter. In fact, the huge diffusion of the pathology and the current wide distribution of many endoscopic instruments showed that there are many pathological situations not solved by endoscopy itself [4]; this resulted in inadequate data collection and obviously made proper evaluation of the problem difficult. A more updated evaluation of complications, which can not be ignored in this work, was described by Prof. Bedeschi with his usual lucidity and synthesis.

The introduction of the endoscopic technique moved toward the closed technique, due to the necessity of obtaining the transversalis carpal ligament dissection in the less aggressive approach towards soft tissues [1, 2, 18, 24, 27].

The different endoscopic techniques enabled direct visualization of the ligament, resulting in a smaller incidence of iatrogenic lesions than that with the closed techniques. This statement makes the literature analysis confused.

Later on we will try to report schematically the data collected during training and congressional meetings.

Complications of the Endoscopic Treatment

Some of clinical situations defined as "complication" cannot be considered as follows.

The symptom persistence due to an incomplete decompression of the median nerve can be considered an inadequacy of the technique rather than strictly a complication of the surgical treatment. In fact, if the ligament is not released the symptoms will persist or, more commonly, even get worse [8, 20].

Accordingly, we should consider as "complications" only those events theoretically or statistically linked to the pathology or to the surgical technique. To help the reader we will apply Bedeschi's classification, which analyzes all the causes of failure or partial success of the surgery, in order to guide daily clinical evaluation. In line with this classification we do not consider mistaes due to a wrong diagnosis. These, in fact, will always exist, but they are included in the diagnostic field, which is widely and effectively treated in this text.

Analysis of Complications Using Bedeschi's Classification

Persistence of Symptoms

We should consider here only those cases in which we suppose that the absence of clinical improvement is really due to technical defects. As analyzed in the previous chapters concerning clinical and instrumental diagnosis, the lesion of the nerve can be so advanced that it would not allow an improvement in the clinical setting [12, 25]. These are the cases where surgery has a real palliative purpose, and its only aim is to avoid a definitive paralysis, being irreversible damage at this step.

Incomplete or Nonexistent Decompression of the Median Nerve

An incomplete decompression of the nerve is the most frequent consequence of a missing or partial opening of the carpal annular ligament. In this second case the symptomatology tends to get even worse, because all of the compression forces converge on only one point of the nerve According to the literature, such an situation has "a major incidence with the closed techniques" compared to the mini-invasive technique [4, 19]. In fact, the lack of direct visualization of the whole ligament due to an incorrect or "timorous" use of the optical fibers results in a tendency to cut only the proximal part of the ligament, and considering it as a complete surgical operation. This is the most common situation that occurs during the learning curve of the endoscopic procedure, surely more compelling than the two-portal techniques and less than the single-port technique as described by Agee [1, 2, 16, 17].

Incomplete Section of the Carpal Annular Ligament

This is the most common complication in the endoscopic dissection of the ligament, due to the difficult visualization of the distal edge of the ligament by an inexperienced operator. The fear of causing a vascular or nervous lesion, the presence of adipose membrane distally to ligament usually not well identified, and the inflammation of the peritendinous tissues are considered to be among the most common reasons.

In fact, a perfect execution of the procedure avoids this complication: as a consequence, when some traversal fibers persist in the distal part of the ligament, the already-opened proximal part assumes a V-shape, while the final result of the operation must have a U-shape.

Whenever a V-shaped conformation at the end of the surgical procedure is seen, an incomplete distal opening of the ligament should be suspected [15]. Nevertheless, the section of the remaining fibers can not be easy, especially in more severe stages because of the herniated nerve in the operational field. For this reason some maneuvers with the endoscopy are required to move the nerve just for the time needed for the dissection of the ligament, without causing any kind of trauma, and particularly without being tempted to use the instrument in an incorrect manner, as though it were a classic endoscopy. For this reason it is advisable, during the learning curve, in case of failure or malfunction during the operation, to proceed with the traditional opening of the carpal annular ligament (conversion of the technique).

Whenever there is a persistence of the symptoms after the operation, without any kind of clinical evolution and with a positive Tinel test as described by Luchetti, it is advisable to proceed with a surgical review, which must be done with a traditional and complete lancing.

Incomplete Distal Section of the Antebrachial Fillet

This really rare case happens when opening of the transverse carpal ligament (TCL) occurs following Agee's technique, modified by Foucher [15]. As a matter of fact, preserving the interthenar muscular fascia allows a quick recovery of strength, but does not allow the nerve to emerge too close to the surface and makes the section of the antebrachial fascia not useful as described by Peiner.

For this reason, and due to the fact that no complications of any kind are described in the literature, those surgeons who have been using this technique in the last 5 years have abandoned the subcutaneous section of the antebrachial fascia.

Missing Section of the LTC

This event should not be considered as a complication, because it is more likely to be a mistake in the procedure itself: paradoxically it is a complication which requires resolution by the same operation that generated it.

Nevertheless, it must be included in the complications for this treatment. This consequence, in fact, excludes the chance to proceed with the endoscopic technique, making necessary the open one, and furthermore prevents the patient from taking advantage of a therapeutic opportunity.

This consequence is due only to the inability of surgeons and can occur with any method, open or closed.

Recurrence of Symptoms

Gilbert recently stated that when a recurrence of symptoms occurs this simply masks a technical incapacity. Whichever approach in opening of the TCL is used, in every operation cicatricial fibrous perinervous proliferation should be checked by an expert operator. Bedeschi describes, in all second stage procedures, flexor tendons hypertrophic tenosynovitis.

A surgical technique, protecting nervous and tendinous structures, together with a postoperative rehabilitation protocol without articular immobilization and with a progressive strengthening of the involved structures, permits a good nerve and tendon sliding. In this way the newly formed scar tissue will not be an obstacle to the operated structures.

Only if another major disease is present (such as patients with rheumatoid arthritis or in patients under dialysis) hypertrophy could cause a new compression on the nerve. This latter event is, however, clinically described and documented, thus not being often considered as a "complication."

In all cases, endoscopic technique highly reduces such situations compared to open procedures [10, 27]. Furthermore, perspective studies revealed an incidence of 11% for the open procedure and 4% for endoscopic ones. Even not considering statistical data and surgeon experience, it is clear that all endoscopic procedures are superior with respect to managing the anatomy.

The New Symptoms Appearance

According to Bedeschi's classification analysis, this subsection appears to be the most important concerning complications. In fact, we admit it may be concerning the "real" ones. Indeed, we disagree with the analysis that complications could be defined as an incorrect diagnosis or an incorrect technical execution. On the other hand, we consider as complications the appearance of new symptoms in comparison to the clinical preoperative situation and not as "necessary" for pathology resolution. The clinical setting could be the most important source of complications.

It's easy to understand that the appearance of a single scar cannot be considered a complication, because every surgical approach results in a scar, whatever the size. A decrease in strength could not be defined as a complication, because such clinical reduction is caused by the pathology itself; in any case, lack of strength is itself an unavoidable price to be paid for disease resolution. Some controversies arise from this last sentence: perspective studies showed endoscopic technique as having faster and better strength recovery compared to open techniques [9, 21, 24, 27].

It may seem a philosophical matter, but it is important that definitions and contents are very well understood for scientific rigor, with regard to a new operation, or just for inevitable legal implications.

Cutaneous Scar Pathology

The less aggressive cutaneous approach is the main advantage for using the endoscopic technique.

Absence of a palmar cutaneous scar determines the quality of the postoperative period: in the early days after surgery, thanks to the absence of sutures and medications, and later to the absence of complications like hypertrophic scar, pain, or edema [9].

Aesthetic reasons and good potential for treatment make distal wrist fold the ideal site of surgical approach.

Regarding this subject, we must consider the slight attention paid by the majority of authors to dermal treatment.

It is a common idea of plastic hand surgeons that scarring must be treated in every case without distinctions about the site, extension, and accidental damage caused by surgical instruments. If scarring is not properly treated, it will always cause pain, dysesthesia, and discomfort that could make the postoperative results aleatory. Massage is the only known effective treatment, specifically "pressotherapy," where salve and ointment treatment is just a way to increase the execution sliding. If the scar is not treated, both at the level of the palm or wrist, major consequences can arise. Once again, according to our philosophy, we must remember that the correct performance of an adequate postoperative protocol produces the best results.

Painful Symptomatology of Nervous Origin Related to Cutaneous Scar

For the same reasons mentioned above, with the use of endoscopy this kind of complication seems to be decreased and related only to a low learning curve.

We must emphasize that in comparison with the procedure originally described by Agee, nowadays the cutaneous incision is shorter than 1 cm at the ulnar side from the palmaris gracilis, so the possibility of finding and damaging cutaneous palmar branches is merely theoretic [2, 5].

Painful Symptomatology Not Related to Cutaneous Scar

Thenar and Hypothenar Pain

This is probably the most interesting section concerning symptoms related to the endoscopic treatment of CTS.

In our opinion [5–7, 22, 24], this kind of operation shows an incidence of the so-called pillar pain that is higher than the one reported in literature with the open procedure. Obtaining exact quantification of this incidence is actually very difficult, since it is correct to rely only on those patients who are particularly reliable. Moreover, the pillar pain definition is itself far from being unequivocal, as is evidenced by major discrepancies in the literature (see Chap. 37, "Carpal Tunnel Syndrome Surgical Complications"). Moreover, pillar pain is not mentioned as being among postoperative complications by some authors, demonstrating that it has not been investigated for lack of quality in the investigation. Therefore, this will make the whole case-report evaluation completely unreliable.

As regards pillar pain etiology, in our opinion the most qualified hypothesis is postoperative edema. In fact, the theory that it could derive from temporary unsteadiness of thenar and hypothenar muscles attachments is definitively contradicted by our systematic preservation of muscular attachments while sectioning the carpal transverse ligament, according to Agee's technique modified by Foucher [13–15]. For this reason, postoperative protocols based on immobilization, even for short periods, are not any more scientifically correct. On the other hand, it is clear that edema within carpal tunnel occurring with endoscopy is greater than that occurring after open procedures. This is the reason why pillar pain is systematically present in the postoperative period, sometimes stronger, sometime weaker. Despite what we wrote at the beginning of this section, we think [22] that this kind of pain can be found in more than 80% of patients, even if limited only to the first days of the postoperative period. In all cases, it undergoes a high reduction within the second month, disappearing within the sixth month. On this subject, as demonstrated by our prospective studies, this period can be greatly shortened by a suitable rehabilitative protocol based on immediate mobilization, lymph drainage, and muscular improvements, all under the direct guide of a specialized therapist.

Piso-Triquetral Pain

While the literature is replete with papers dealing with pillar pain, not much is written about piso-triquetral pain. Actually, as already emphasized in this chapter and in the literature, in our opinion, for those cases of CTS treated by open technique, this symptomatology could be present before surgical treatment, but not documented by a careless presurgical examination. In fact, while there are serious and accurate prospective studies about cases of CTS treated endoscopically, on the other hand, there are only retrospective studies regarding cases treated with open procedure. Furthermore, we have to consider that most operated cases show a severe painful symptomatology; in this way the patient is able to be sufficiently reliable or detailed in describing his own symptomatology before the operation.

We do not believe that this complication could justify a systematic radiological examination in order to diagnose an eventual pre-existent piso-triquetral arthritis. Similarly, we do not believe that an echographic examination should be indicated, apart from monolateral juvenile cases. The low incidence of this complication does not justify a higher medical expense and this kind of instrumental examination does not add anything to the surgical treatment.

Onset of New Symptoms Related to Other Nervous Complications

In Professor Bedeschi's chapter (Chap. 37, "Carpal Tunnel Syndrome Surgical Complications") there is a careful analysis of the most updated literature concerning the median and ulnar nerves lesions. From its beginning, it has been thought that the endoscopic technique has increases these lesions, and this hypothesis seemed to be confirmed by the preliminary data. Such data is difficult to obtain from the eastern part of the world, where they do not use to distinguish among the different endoscopic techniques.

Actually, as shown by Palmer and Gilbert [23], after 10 years we can say that there are more iatrogenic lesion reports due to open than to endoscopic technique (Figs. 38.1–38.3). However, endoscopic supporters cannot report such statistics authoritatively, because it will take at least 10 years to have a sufficient number of cases to be able to compare the two techniques.

In our opinion those closed techniques not endoscopically assisted must not be allowed; in fact, a partial or total lesion of the median nerve, seen directly

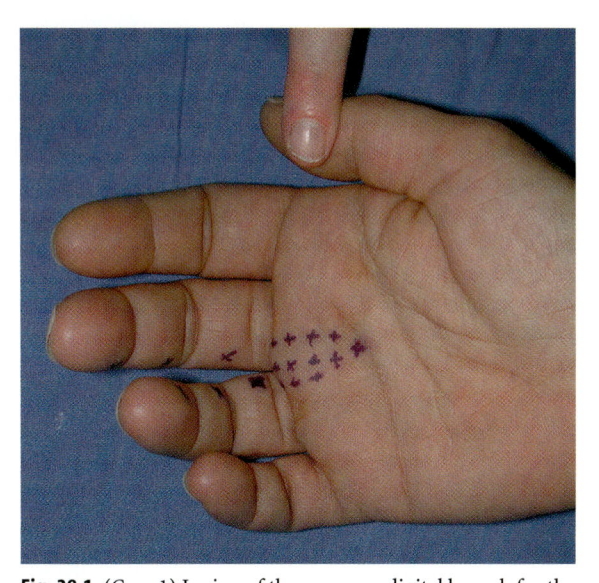

Fig. 38.1. (Case 1) Lesion of the common digital branch for the third interdigital space: area of hypo-anesthesia

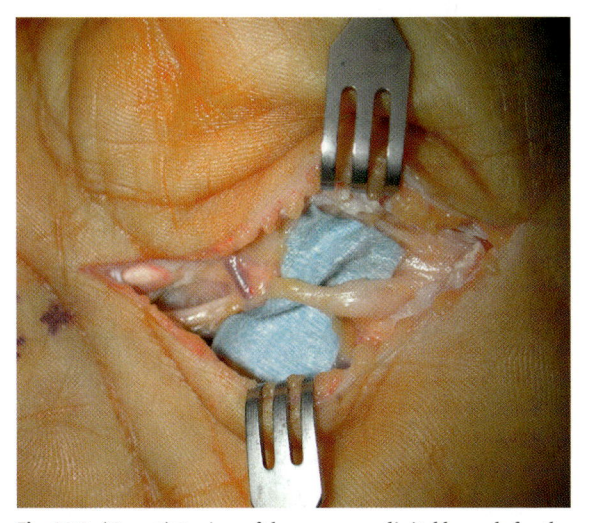

Fig. 38.2. (Case 1) Lesion of the common digital branch for the third interdigital space: identification of neuroma in the point of section

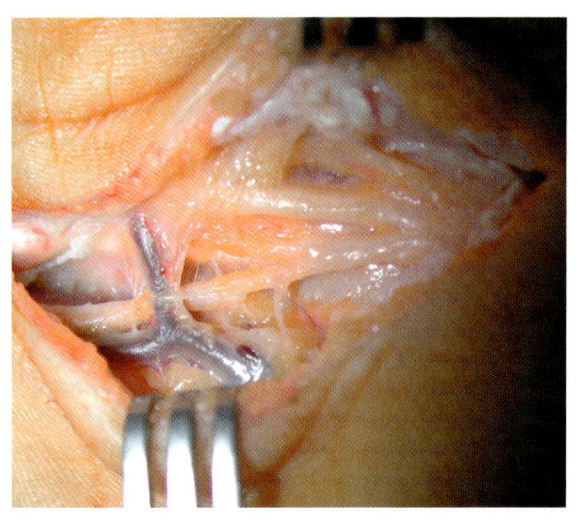

Fig. 38.3. (Case 1) Lesion of the common digital branch for the third interdigital space: neurolysis and microsurgical repair

with an open technique or with a camera in endoscopy, cannot be considered a lack of surgical skill nor a mistake due to erroneous technical education.

As already said above and in previous chapters, we must never forget that in choosing a surgical procedure any permanent nervous lesions are completely unacceptable in a merely painful or moderately invalidating syndrome.

New Onset Compression of the Ulnar Nerve in the Guyon Canal

When an endoscopic procedure is performed, compression of the ulnar nerve in the Guyon canal is as frequent an event as pillar pain, even if it generally resolves itself within the first month. Varying patient reliability prevents distinguishing between compression of the ulnar nerve in the Guyon canal and pillar pain. Not even clinical examination by the surgeon or instrumental examination by the neurophysiologist will succeed in evaluating bilaterally the ulnar nerve at different levels.

Remission of symptoms related to the median nerve, and certainly more severe symptoms, may reveal a pre-existent ulnar compression not previously mentioned by the patient and not adequately evaluated.

This kind of complication, similar to pillar pain, probably involves a compressive mechanism by edema within the tunnel, particularly with endoscopy.

Nevertheless, in our opinion, the systematic opening of the Guyon canal, described by several authors, cannot be justified by the incidence of this complication, because this could represent the basis for a hypothetic "precautionary surgery."

Vascular Complications

Hematoma Resulting from Minor Vascular Lesions

A surgical procedure performed with optical magnifying instruments, as always should be the case in hand surgery, and direct vision of the surgical field both open and endoscopic, do not involve major vascular structure lesions. We have not been releasing the tourniquet, except after the final dressing, for more than 10 years, and have never performed hemostasis nor employed a drain, regardless of the surgical technique. An accurate prospective study of our cases, realized in order to gather the data necessary to study endoscopic release and involving more than 5,000 cases operated on with open or endoscopic technique, did not show any hematoma that could be considered a complication.

Major Vascular Lesions

What we wrote about nervous lesions above can also be applied to major vascular lesions. Ulnar artery lesions must be attributed to an incorrect introduction of the tool in the Guyon canal, instead of the carpal tunnel, or to a incorrect use of the tool in the tunnel, with too distal or ulnar section of the ligament itself. At this level it is easier to produce a superficial palmar arch lesion, which usually resolves itself in a few days. In any case, even if vascular lesions are usually without complications, compared with nervous ones, we cannot accept this surgical risk, being that the latter is strongly related to an improper technique of the surgeon.

Tendinous Complications

As written in the section regarding complications related to cutaneous scar, there are very few objective considerations about tendinous lesions. In fact, we cannot include adhesion problems; these are not found using either endoscopy or open procedure, since we have been avoiding the systematic synovectomy of flexor tendons for 12 years. Furthermore, anterior dislocation of flexor tendons was found using the endoscopic procedure.

It is worth mentioning the continuation of trigger finger in the postoperative period. We have not been convinced, from a statistic point of view, by explanations reported in literature and based on the biomechanical analysis of tendon movement, in particular by the theory which states that the A1 pulley, without the carpal ulnar ligament, may undergo on overload. It is more reasonable to think that the co-pathology could be pre-existent, although lacking in clinical signs, or not researched by the surgeon, as we wrote about compression of the ulnar nerve in the Guyon canal. Otherwise, we can suppose that the inflammatory disease, idiopathic or not, which is at the base of CTS, could in turn cause a trigger finger soon after the surgical operation.

In conclusion, the same can be said for tendinous lesions reported in literature as for iatrogenic nervous and vascular lesions.

Decrease of Hand Prehension Strength

Among complications due to endoscopic treatment of CTS, decrease of hand prehension strength is totally absent, since the main indication for the use of this procedure is keeping and increasing hand strength [9, 21]. Various published prospective studies, including ours recruiting 710 patients, demonstrate that there is not any strength loss during the postoperative period and that within 6 months after the operation is a recovery of 50% of the strength according to preoperative values. This is in agreement with results established during the Groupe d'Etude de la Main (GEM) Congress in 1999 [24].

This is actually the parameter we must evaluate, since the severity of the pathology primarily influences postoperative results, when we use a surgical procedure which does not itself decrease hand strength. On this subject, even if data are not homogenous enough, we must emphasize with scientific objectivity that a deep difference regarding timing and quality of recovery does exist, depending on if postoperative rehabilitation protocol is applied or not. (Fig. 38.4)

Infections

The analysis of our personal experience shows that the occurrence of infection is not significant among complications following the treatment of CTS, regardless of the technique performed. However, any infectious complications that do occur should be mainly ascribed to an incorrect performance of the surgical act, which is often executed in an unsuitable place and with unsuitable instruments. This is evidenced by a lack of cases in the literature of major infections due to the endoscopic procedure, which is only performed in a properly equipped and aseptic setting.

Algodystrophy

An estimation of the incidence of algodystrophic complications is probably impossible due to the disparity in the acquisition of data. In fact, while the French consider as a beginning algodystrophy any edema or pain persisting even very little over the accepted maximum, on the other hand, we too often discover this complication in its advanced stage, after it has been wrongly diagnosed as postoperative edema or beginning infection or edema from stasis with associated infection, and so on.

Furthermore, both definition of this syndrome and, even more, its etiology seem not to be univocal.

If we accept that algodystrophy is usually related neither to intensity nor to characteristics of the surgical trauma, it could seem to be pretentious if we prove different incidences, changing on the basis of surgical procedure performed.

However, we can suppose that the more delicate the surgery, especially when involving nervous structures, the smaller the occurrence of algodystrophy, and that a delicate and precise surgery involving lack of immobilization and only a 8–10 days dressing contributes furthermore to reduce this occurrence [13]. After these considerations, we can accept that the great decrease of cases of algodystrophy is one of the main indications for the endoscopic technique, as shown in the literature. However, we think that the incidence of this complication can be decreased by proper and essential surgery, that is, not only by endoscopic or other techniques. In fact, algodystrophy is a complication usually following rough or unsuitable surgery.

Causalgia

As perfectly described in the literature by Bedeschi and afterwards confirmed by Luchetti, causalgia is an unrestrainable painful syndrome that does not allow the patient to have a normal life and relationships. It seems to be often related to one or more surgical operations on peripheral nervous structures. Therefore, causalgia can be hardly ascribed in a specific way to CTS, but it has to be recognized as a warning from a potentially incorrect surgical act.

Conclusions

In our opinion [5–7, 21, 22, 24], an analysis of the preceding sections enables the creation of some guidelines, which we consider reliable, in that they were developed with great scientific rigor and derived from

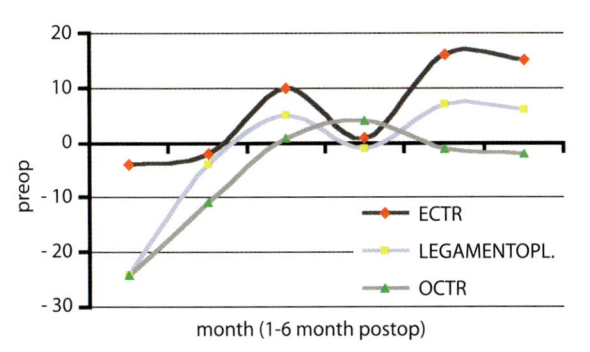

Fig. 38.4. Grip strength evaluation of our study: modification of strength after CTS treatment. After 6 months strength is near to normal only in ECTR

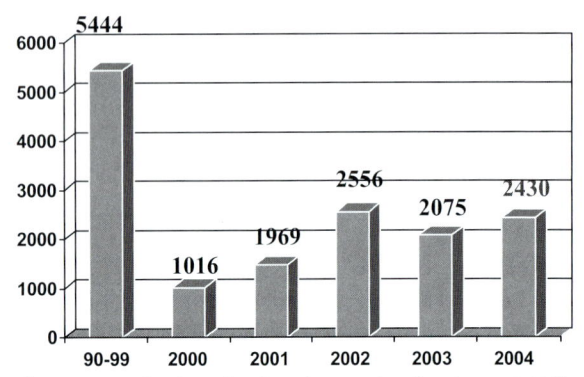

Fig. 38.5. Distribution of patients by year (total patients 15,490)

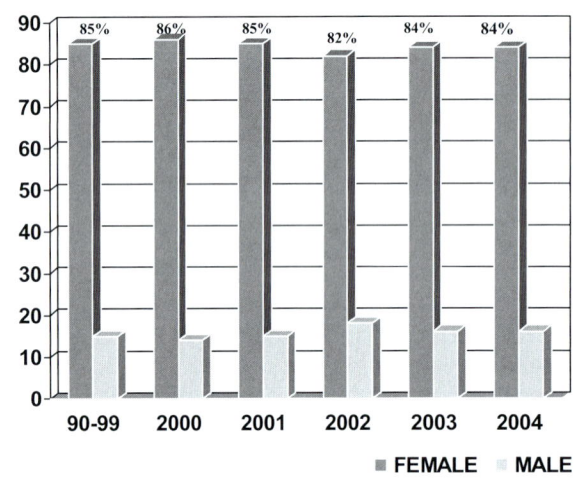

Fig. 38.6. Distribution of sex by year

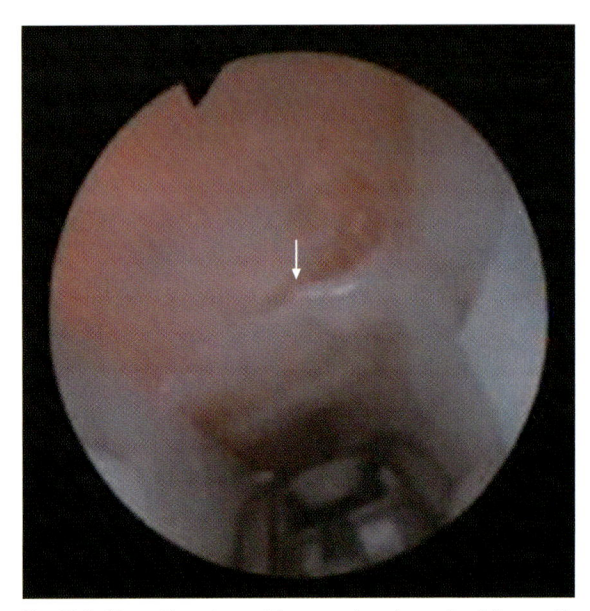

Fig. 38.7. (Case 2) patient with anomalous branch of the median nerve identified during endoscopic approach: a conversion into an open technique was performed. The *arrow* shows the anomalous branch of the median nerve

15,490 operated cases from April 1990 to December 2004. There were 13,062 women (84%) and 2,428 males (16%), for 9,101 right hands and 6,389 left. We have performed 12,702 (82% of cases) endoscopic carpal tunnel releases (ECTR; Table 38.1, Figs. 38.5, 38.6); in this series only 59 patients (0.46%, which is not a statistically significant rate), underwent a conversion to open surgery (Fig. 38.7). We had recurrences in 46 patients (0.3%); of these only 12 cases (0.1%) after ECTR. We observed major complications only in 6 cases (0.04%) (Tables 38.2–38.4; Figs. 38.1, 38.2).

The learning curve shows that the trial period to learn the operating technique is very short. In our data, we can demonstrate that the period in which we had a decrease in the total number of ECTR (73%), was the period in which we had new members of our team on trial. In only 1 year we returned up to 80%, which is the standard in our Department. (Fig. 38.8). Furthermore, this procedure can be performed also when the CTS is

Table 38.1. General distribution of our data

	Female R	L	Male R	L	Total	
CTS	6302	4534	1223	938	12997	84%
CTS+TG	923	449	88	86	1546	10%
CTS+CMCJ	202	157	10	11	380	2.4%
CTS+DQ	198	120	7	7	332	2.1%
CTS+.....	110	67	38	20	235	1.5%
Partial	7735 (59%)	5327 (41%)	1366 (56%)	1062 (44%)		
Total	13062		2428		15490	100%

Table 38.2. Causes of conversion ECTR → OCTR

Changes of technique	59
Difficult view for synovial bands	32
Muscular interpositions	20
Lipomas	4
Difficult insertion of the blade	3

Table 38.3. Causes of recurrences after ECTR

Recurrences	12
Incomplete dissection of LTC	6
Incomplete dissection of LTC + hypertrophy of endoscopic scar	2
Hypertrophy of endoscopic scar	3
Nerve adhesion	1

Table 38.4. Causes of major complication during ECTR

Major complications	6
Painful neuromas of palmar cutaneous branch of median nerve + partial section of the motor branch for the opponent muscle	1
Complete lesion of the common digital branch for the third interdigital space	3
Painful neuromas of palmar cutaneous branch of median nerve muscle	2

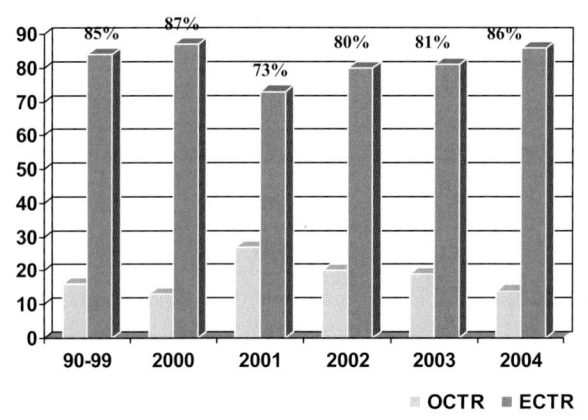

Fig. 38.8. Distribution of percentage of ECTR/OCTR by year

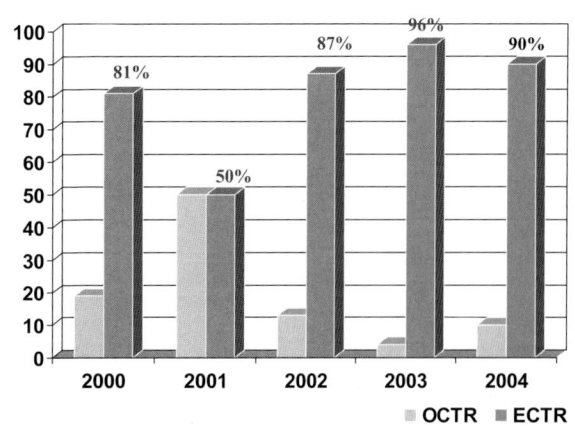

Fig. 38.9. Distribution of ECTR for STC associated with carpometacarpal joint

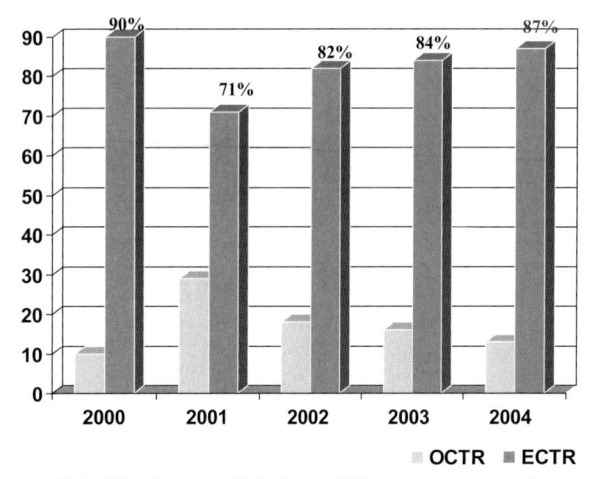

Fig. 38.10 Distribution of ECTR for STC associated with trigger finger

associated with other pathologies of the hand, obtaining good results and less discomfort for the patients (Figs. 38.9, 38.10) [16–18, 22, 24, 26, 27].

1. It is known by anyone confident with this pathology that it is necessary to make the surgical procedure as least invasive as possible [5]. In fact, CTS is essentially associated with a painful symptomatology and therefore the persistence of pain must be considered as a real failure.
2. The treatment of CTS does not allow any nondefinitive solution or iatrogenic lesion, which are both unacceptable and easily avoided in a clinical situation, as is widely shown in the literature.
3. The introduction of endoscopy makes unsuitable any closed procedure not endoscopically assisted, since it enables the surgeon to choose between a direct (open) or an indirect (closed) view of the nerve. In any case, with endoscopy no surgery is appropriate if performed without any view of the nerve.
4. There are no prospective studies in the literature that enable a reliable evaluation of the clinical results related to the open procedure. However, there is enough experience regarding the open procedure within areas of specialty that this gap can be filled. Conversely, prospective studies about the endoscopic technique seem to be rigorous and analytical.
5. Based on all of the above, we think we can objectively state that the eternal dilemma between supporters and opponents of endoscopy must cease and that endoscopy itself must be considered nothing but a surgical procedure which must be perfectly performed by every hand surgeon, just like microsurgery or osteosynthesis. The clinical indication established by the surgeon, based on his experience [3, 15, 16, 21], will allow him/her to choose between open or closed techniques, without any prejudice towards one or the other, which prejudice is totally unacceptable in the modern scientific world.

References

1. Agee JM, McCarroll HR (1994) North ER Endoscopic carpal tunnel release using the single proximal incision technique. Hands Clinics 10:647–659
2. Agee JM, McCarroll HR, Tortosa RD et al. (1992) Endoscopic release of the carpal tunnel: a randomized prospective multicenter study. J Hand Surg 17A:987–995
3. Atroshi I, Axelsson G, Gummesson C, Johnsson R (2000) Carpal tunnel syndrome with severe sensory deficit: endoscopic release in 18 cases Acta Otrthop Scand 71(5).484–7
4. Boeckstyns MEH, Soresen AI (1999) Does endoscopic carpal tunnel release have a higher rate of complication than open carpal tunnel release? J Hand Surg (Br) 24B:1: 9–15
5. Campiglio GL, Pajardi G (1998) Carpal tunnel release with short incision. Plast Reconstr Surg 101: 1151
6. Campiglio GL, Pajardi G, Rafanelli G (1996) Sezione endoscopica del legamento anulare del carpo Minerva Ortop Traumat 47,XX
7. Campiglio GL, Ravanelli G, Colombelli J et al. (1998) Il trattamento endoscopico della sindrome del canale carpale con il sistema £M Agee; revisone critica di 4 anni di esperien-

za(611 casi su 2800 operati) Atti 47° Congresso Nazionale S.I.C.P.R.E. Palermo Sept 23–26, 425–430
8. Cartotto MD, Mc Cabe S, Mackinnon Se (1992) Two devasting complication of carpal tunnel surgery Ann Plast Surg 28:472–4
9. Chen HT, Chen HC, Wei FC (1999) Endoscopic carpal tunnel release Chang Keng I Hsueh Tsa Chih 22(3):386–391
10. Citron ND, Bendall SP (1997) Local symptoms after open carpal tunnel release J Hand Surg 22B:317–321 Bene per trattamento cicatrice
11. Concannon MJ, Brownfield ML, Puckett CL (2000) The incidence of recurrence after endoscopic carpal tunnel release. Plast Reconstr Surg 105(5):1662–5
12. DeStefano F, Nordstrom DL, Vierkant RA (1997) Long-Term Symptom outcomes of carpal tunnel syndrome and its treatment J Hand Surg 22A:200–210
13. Erhard L, Foucher G (1990) Quoi de neuf au sujet du syndrome du canal carpien? Ann Chir Plast Esthet 43:6: 600–605
14. Erhard L, Ozalp T, Citron N, Foucher G (1999) Carpal tunnel release by Agee endoscopic technique Results at 4 year follow-up J Hand Surg (Br) 24(5):583–5
15. Foucher G, Pajardi G, Campiglio GL (1994) Agee endoscopic treatment of CTS: a series of 280 cases. Riv Chir Riab Mano Arto Sup 31(2):151–156
16. G. Eder (2003) Endoscopic carpal tunnel release without iatrogenic complication-a report about 1000 procedures. Handchir Mikrokir Plast Chir 35(1): 57–62
17. G. Eder (2003) Reply to the invited commentary of R.G.H. Baumeister to the article of G. Eder: Endoscopic carpal tunnel release without iatrogenic complication-a report about 1000 procedures. Handchir Mikrokir Plast Chir 35(6):403
18. Jimenez DF, Gibbs SR, Clapper AT (1998) Endoscopic treatment of CTS: a critical review J Neurosurg 88(5):817–826
19. Macdermid JC, Richards RS, Roth JH et al. (2003) Endoscopic versus open carpal tunnel release: a randomized trial J hand Surg 28(3):475–80
20. Mackinnon SE (1991) Secondary carpal tunnel surgery. Neurosurgery Clinics of North America 2:75–91
21. Pajardi G, Campiglio GL, Rafanelli G et al. (1998) Il trattamento della sindrome del canale carpale per via endoscopica: la nostra esperienza dopo 5 anni. Acta Orthopaedica Italica volXXI:52–56
22. Pajardi G, Rafanelli G, Pivato G, Colombelli J (1998) Sezione endoscopica del legamento anulare del carpo: esperienza personale di 4 anni Atti XXVI Congresso S.I.M.F.E.R. Brescia Jun 15–17, 207–209
23. Palmer AK, Toivonen DA (1999) Complication of endoscopic and open carpal tunnel release J Hand Surg 24A: 561–565
24. Pivato G, Colombelli J, Rafanelli G et al. (1999) Endoscopic treatment of canal carpaltunnel sindrome: A critical review of cases (710 in 5 years) and our indications J Hand Surg suppl. 1, p. X
25. Rosen B, Lundborg G, Abrahamsson SO et al. (1997) I Sensory function after median nerve decompression in carpal tunnel syndrome J Hand Surg 22B:5:602–605
26. Timothy A, Straub MD: Endoscopic carpal tunnel release: a prospective analysis of factors associated with uninsatisfactory results
27. Trumble TE, Diao E, Abrams RA, Gilbert-Anderson MM (2002) Single-portal endoscopic carpal tunnel release compared with open release J Bone Joint Surg 84A(7):1107–1115

Role of Neurosensory Testing in Differential Diagnosis of Failed Carpal Tunnel Syndrome

J. H. Coert, A. L. Dellon

Conflict of interest statement: A. Lee Dellon has a proprietary interest in the Pressure-Specified Sensory Device

Introduction

Carpal tunnel syndrome is the most frequently encountered nerve compression. The diagnosis is based on a combination of subjective (history) and objective (physical examination and sensory testing) criteria. Interestingly, a positive history and electro-diagnostic study (EDS) often suffices to schedule surgery. In mild carpal tunnel syndrome it has been shown that 30% of symptomatic patients may have a normal EDS [1]. In acute and chronic nerve compressions, simple tests of cutaneous pressure and vibratory threshold have been proven to be less reliable [2, 3]. For example, Semmes-Weinstein (SW) nylon monofilaments only test one-point static touch threshold. Therefore, with the SW-monofilaments, mild nerve compressions will not be detected. Another disadvantage of the SW monofilaments is that the tip of the filaments is not uniform in size. A recent carpal tunnel meta-analysis showed a large heterogeneity in outcome measures and inadequate reporting of results due to the widespread use of so many different measurement methods [4].

Neurosensory testing (NST) with a device that can measure both the distance required for two-point discrimination and the pressure of the application of the two "points" or prongs is needed to overcome these limitations and to warrant reproducibility to allow for comparison between different authors [5–7]. Diagnosing recurrent or failed carpal tunnel syndrome will be facilitated by NST. It is the purpose of this chapter to describe our experience using neurosensory testing with the Pressure-Specified Sensory Device (PSSD) to document the presence of a recurrent carpal tunnel syndrome.

Patient Examples of Neurosensory Testing

A mild degree of compression of median nerve at the wrist can be diagnosed (Figs. 39.1, 39.2). The test results demonstrate that an early nerve compression translates into an elevated application pressure (36.4 g/mm^2) to discriminate a 3-mm static two-point measurement at the tip of the involved index finger compared to the uninvolved side (1 g/mm^2). For a severe carpal tunnel syndrome the application pressure is higher (67.0 g/mm^2) (Figs. 39.3, 39.4). These PSSD results for different degrees of median nerve compression at the wrist demonstrate the feasibility to confirm the diagnosis [7, 8].

However, for a recurrent or failed carpal tunnel syndrome one must rule out a radial sensory nerve entrapment, a proximal median nerve compression, and a neuroma of the palmar cutaneous branch of the median nerve. Each of these three problems is related to nerves that may cause the same complaints as recurrent carpal tunnel syndrome. The PSSD is helpful in diagnosing a pronator syndrome [9]. Besides elevated application pressures of the index finger (42.7 at the 3 mm s-2PD), the thenar eminence shows elevated pressures (70.1 g/mm^2 at 9 mm s-2PD) (Figs. 39.5–39.8). Of course, a failed carpal tunnel syndrome can occur together with a pronator syndrome (index finger 66.8 g/mm^2 at 8 mm s-2PD; thenar eminence 60.6 at 9 mm s-2PD) (Figs. 39.7, 39.8). Radial sensory nerve entrapment can be differentiated from carpal tunnel syndrome showing normal values for the thenar eminence and the index pulp, but abnormal values for the dorsal radial skin (Figs. 39.9, 39.10).

Discussion

The ability of traditional electro-diagnostic studies to evaluate recurrent carpal tunnel syndrome remains open to question. One reason is that following decompression of a peripheral nerve, it rarely will have remyelination to the normal degree, so there is often abnormal distal latency or conduction velocity even when the patient is asymptomatic. Electrodiagnostic testing is utilized extensively in the literature for nonrecurrent compressions, where it does provide a diagnosis with a high specificity; however, its sensitivity may be as low as 66% [1]. Neurosensory testing with the PSSD offers advantages over traditional electro-diagnostic studies, in that it will measure a given piece of skin without regard to which nerve innervates it, and therefore correlate with the patient's symptoms.

Fig. 39.1. Mild CTS

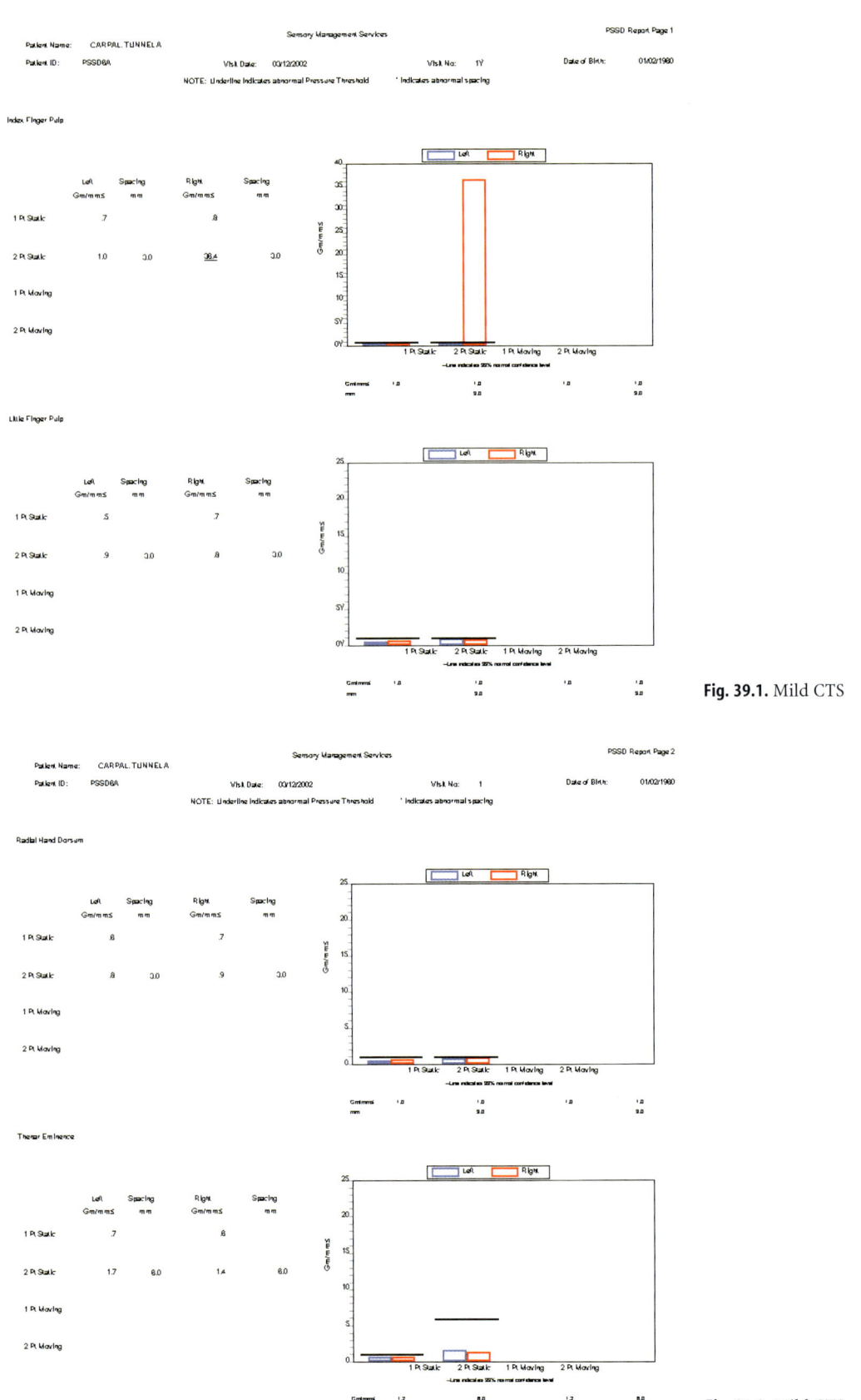

Fig. 39.2. Mild CTS

39 Role of Neurosensory Testing in Differential Diagnosis of Failed Carpal Tunnel Syndrome

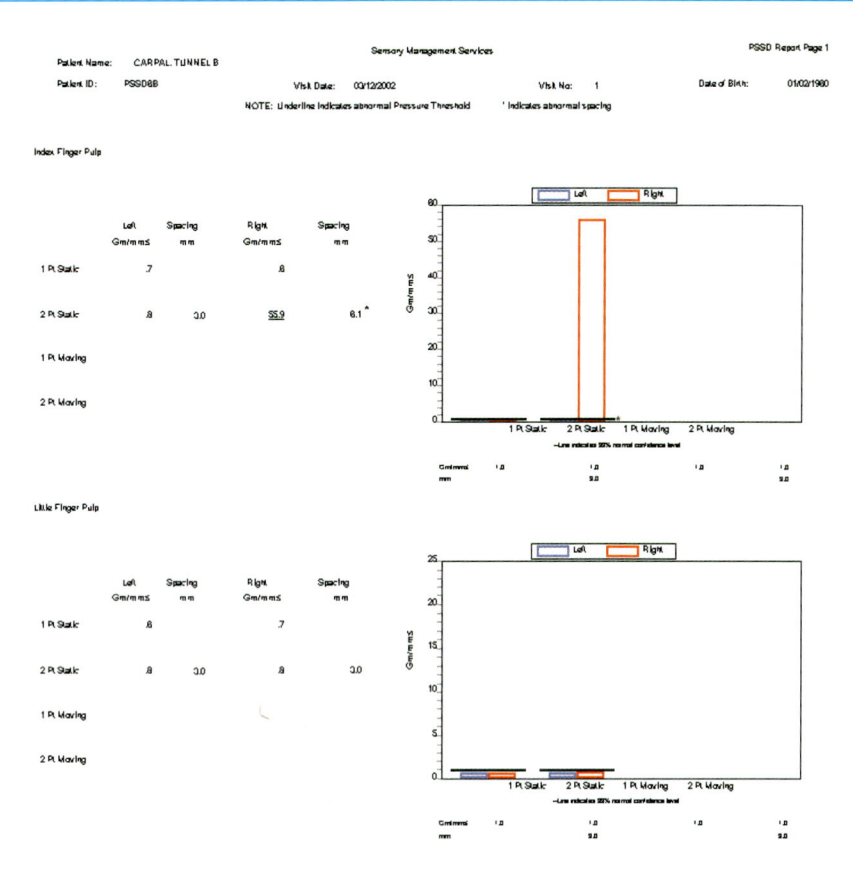

Fig. 39.3. Severe CTS

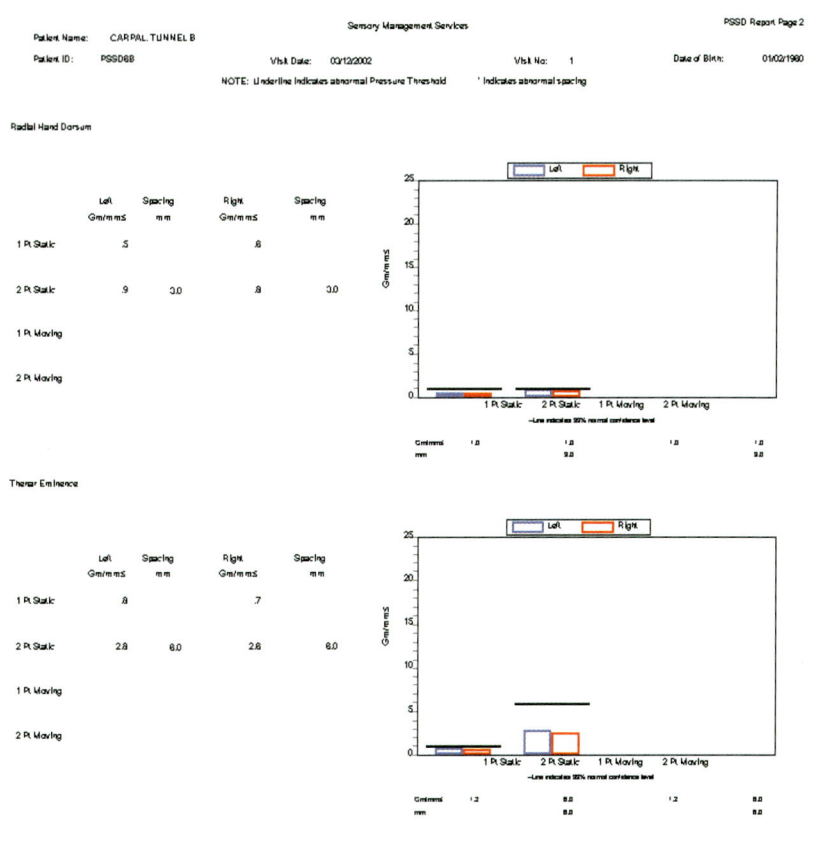

Fig. 39.4. Severe CTS

Fig. 39.5. Pronator

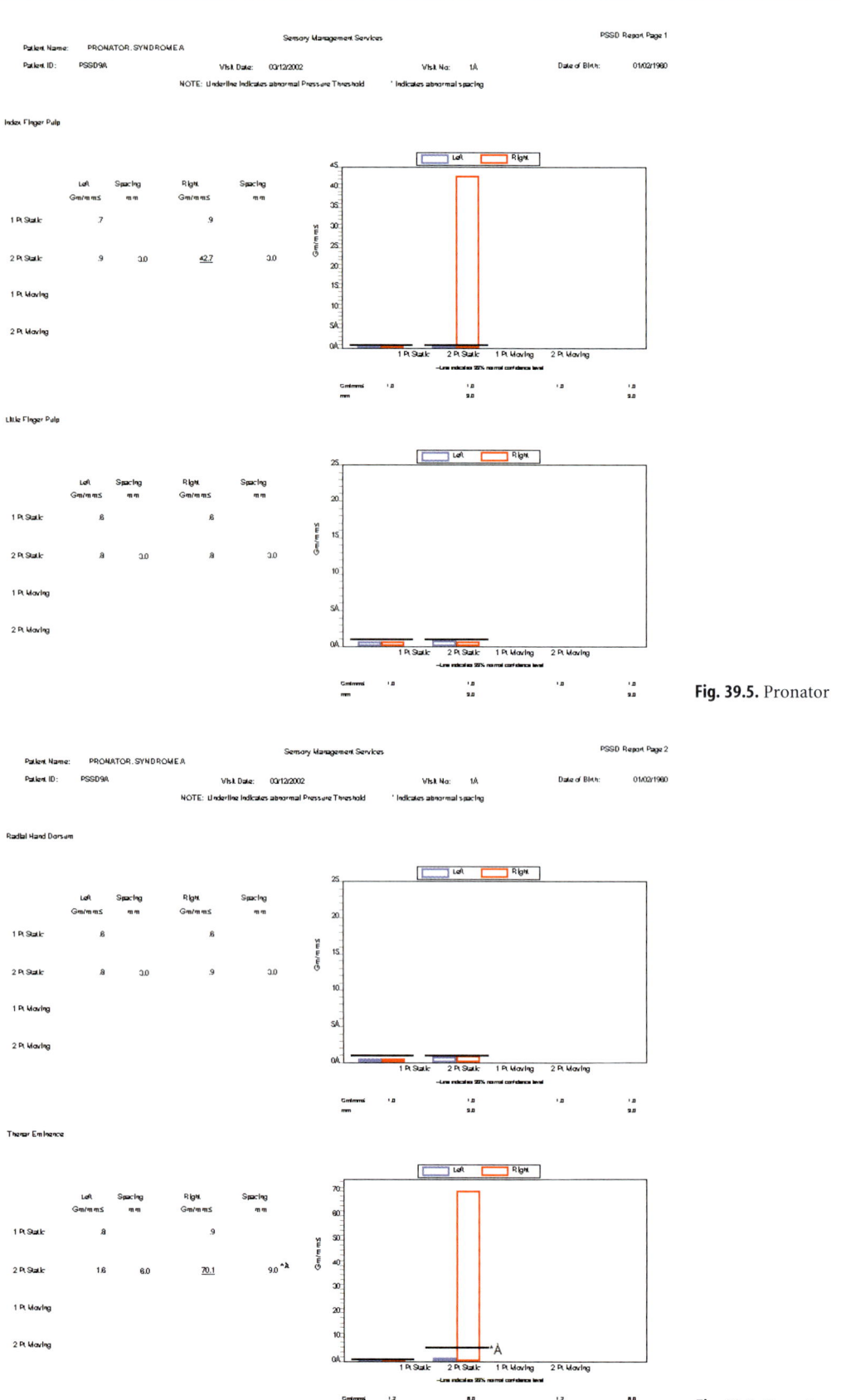

Fig. 39.6. Pronator

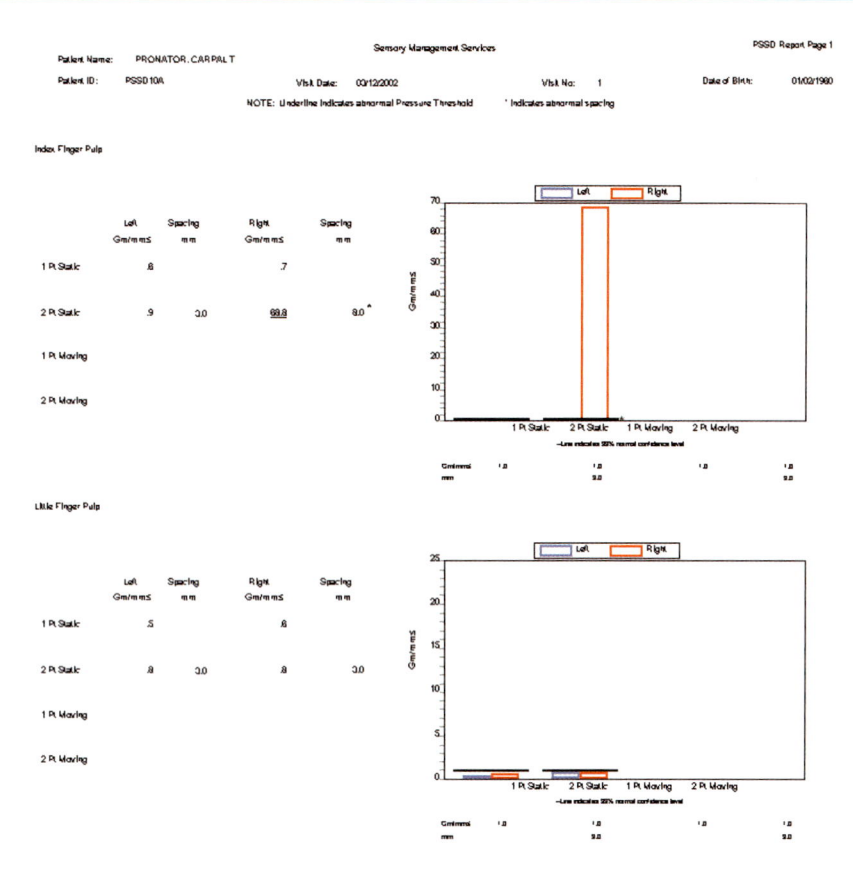

Fig. 39.7. Pronator and CTS

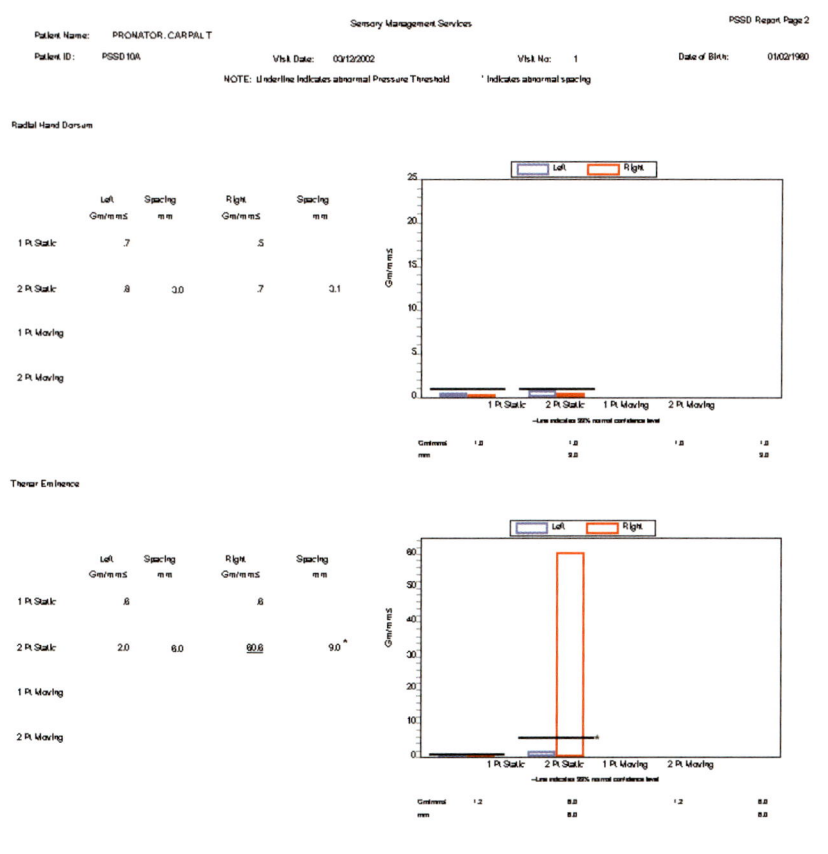

Fig. 39.8. Pronator and CTS

304 **V Complications**

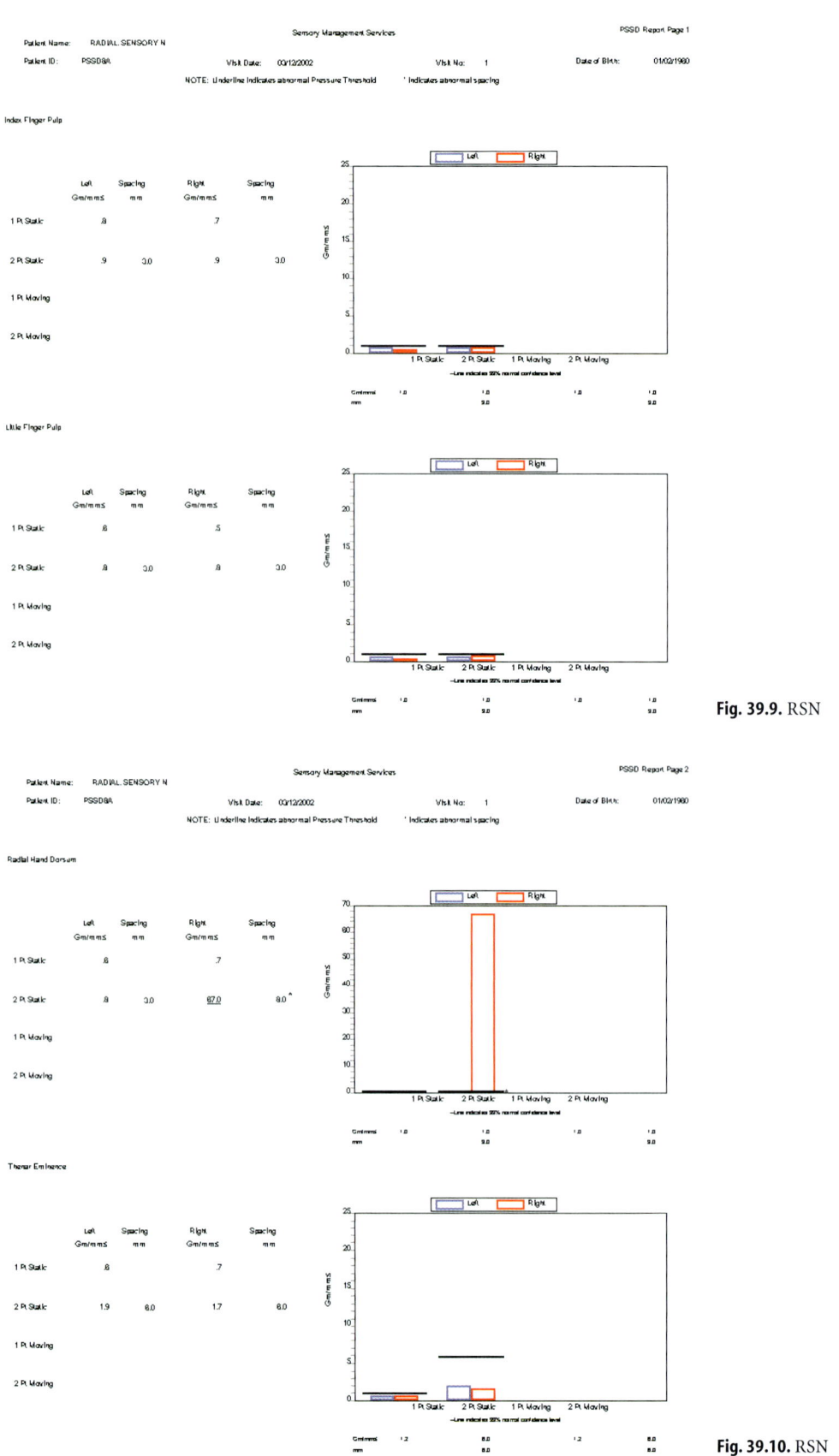

Fig. 39.9. RSN

Fig. 39.10. RSN

39 Role of Neurosensory Testing in Differential Diagnosis of Failed Carpal Tunnel Syndrome

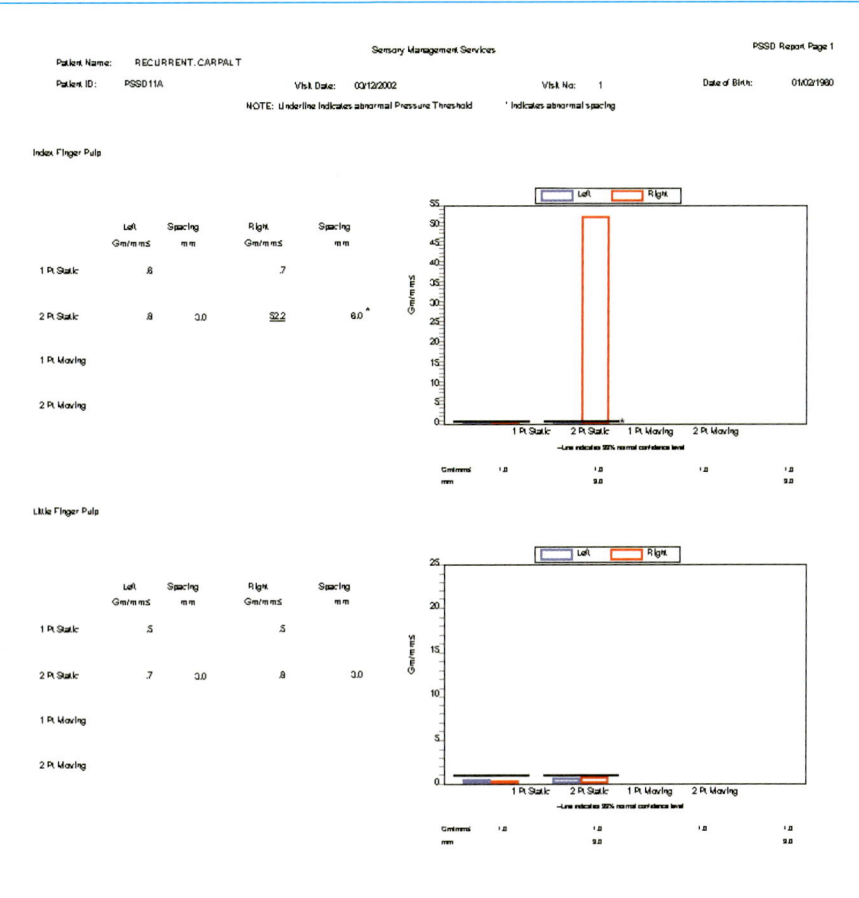

Fig. 39.11. Recurrent CTS

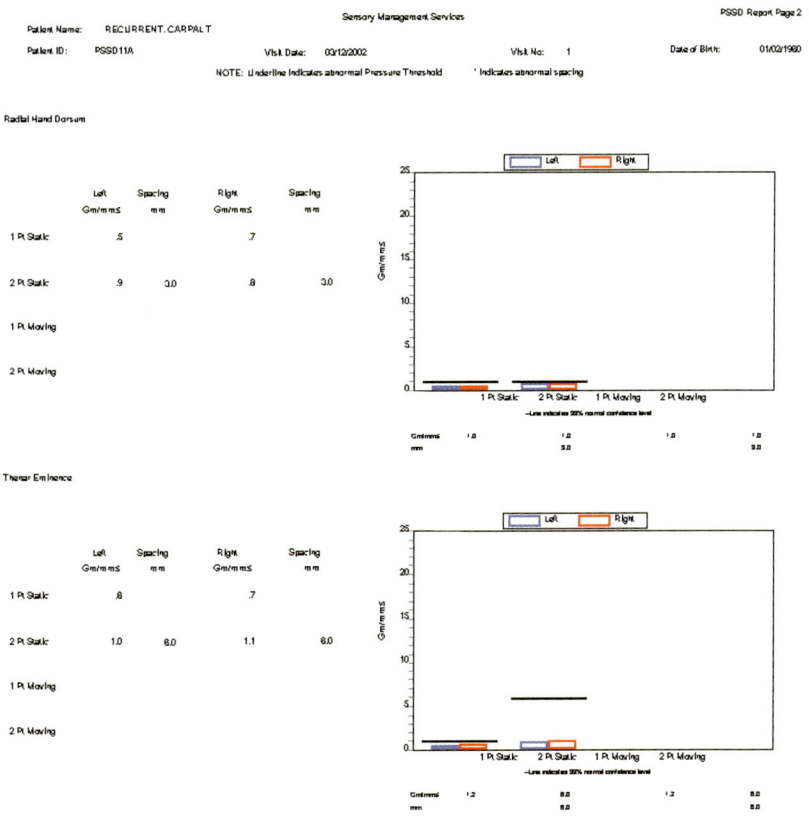

Fig. 39.12. Recurrent CTS

A recurrent carpal tunnel syndrome will show abnormal values for just the index pulp and normal values for thenar eminence and radial sensory nerve (Figs. 39.11, 39.12).

The PSSD will identify the earliest stages of nerve compression and neuropathy at a time when traditional electro-diagnostic testing will not be able to detect a change in peripheral nerve function, and therefore the PSSD will correlate better with patient symptom [9, 10]. The PSSD is a painless and a noninvasive test. Patients tolerate repeated tests easily. Frequently, patients refuse electro-diagnostic tests due to discomfort. In the postoperative follow-up, 11 from our group of 28 patients refused to undergo these tests [11]. Therefore, it can be used to follow serially progression or improvement of the condition with a high degree of patient acceptance.

In recurrent or failed carpal tunnel syndrome a radial sensory nerve entrapment, a proximal median nerve compression, and a neuroma of the palmar cutaneous branch of the median nerve should be considered. Often in worker's compensation cases a failed carpal tunnel syndrome and a pronator syndrome can coexist [13]. Electro-diagnostic testing usually cannot identify proximal median nerve compressions. The palmar cutaneous branch of the median nerve arises 5–7 cm proximal to the carpal tunnel, so that abnormal sensibility of the thenar eminence can be measured and used to identify pronator syndrome The PSSD has shown to be very helpful in these cases [9]. A neuroma of palmar cutaneous branch of the median nerve would cause pain in the scar of the carpal tunnel release mimicking a failed or recurrent carpal tunnel syndrome. Sensation in the thenar eminence will be abnormal and should be differentiated from pronator syndrome [9]. In this situation, a neuroma of the terminal branch of anterior interosseous nerve could be a source of wrist pain [14].

Summary

Neurosensory testing with the Pressure-Specified Sensory Device is a valuable tool in diagnosing failed or recurrent carpal tunnel syndrome. It offers the possibility to differentiate this diagnosis from radial sensory nerve entrapment and proximal median nerve compression. This is often difficult to obtain by traditional electrodiagnostic testing.

References

1. Jablecki CK, Andary MT, So YT et al. (1993) Literature review of the usefulness of nerve conduction studies and electromyography for the evaluation of patients with carpal tunnel syndrome. AAEM Quality Assurance Committee. Muscle Nerve 16:1392–414
2. Szabo RM, Gelberman RH, Dimick MP (1984) Sensibility testing in patients with carpal tunnel syndrome. J Bone Joint Surg [Am] 66:60–64
3. Gelberman RH, Szabo RM, Williamson RV, Dimick MP (1983) Sensibility testing in peripheral-nerve compression syndromes. An experimental study in humans. J Bone Joint Surg [Am] 65:632–638
4. Gerritsen AMA, De Vet HCM, Scholten RJPM et al. (2002) Enabling meta-analysis in systematic reviews on carpal tunnel surgery. J Hand Surg 27A: 828–832
5. Dellon AL (1999) Management of peripheral nerve problems in the upper and lower extremities using quantitative sensory testing. Hand Clinics 15:697–715
6. Dellon AL (2001) Clinical grading of peripheral nerve problems. Neurosurg Clinics N. Amer 12: 229–240
7. Seiler D, Barrett SL, Dellon AL (2003) Interpretation Guide to Neurosensory and Motor Testing, Sensory Management Services, Baltimore, Maryland
8. Dellon AL, Keller KM (1997) Computer-assisted quantitative sensory testing in carpal and cubital tunnel syndromes. Ann Plast Surg 38:493–502
9. Rosenberg D, Conolley J, Dellon AL (2001) Thenar eminence quantitative sensory testing in the diagnosis of proximal median nerve compression. J Hand Ther 14:258–65
10. Tassler PL, Dellon AL (1995) Correlation of measurements of pressure perception using the pressure-specified sensory device with electrodiagnostic testing. J Occupat Med 37; 862–866
11. Weber R, Weber RA, Schuchmann JA, Ortiz J (2000) A prospective blinded evaluation of nerve conduction velocity versus pressure-specified sensory testing in carpal tunnel syndrome. Ann Plast Surg 45:252–7
12. Wong KH, Coert JH, Robinson PH, Meek MF. A comparison of diagnostic tools to score recovery of function after median nerve lesions. Submitted J Hand Ther
13. Coert JH, Meek MF, Gibeault D, Dellon AL (2004) Documentation of posttraumatic nerve compression in patients with normal electrodiagnostic studies. J Trauma 56: 339–44
14. Dellon AL, Mackinnon SE, Daneshvar A (1984) Terminal branch of anterior interosseous nerve as source of wrist pain. J Hand Surg 9B:316–22

Secondary Carpal Tunnel Surgery

T.H.H. Tung, S.E. Mackinnon

Carpal tunnel syndrome was first described by Sir James Paget [1] in 1854. The first carpal tunnel release is credited in most historical reviews to Learmonth in 1929 for a patient with posttraumatic nerve compression [2]. However, a review of the Mayo Clinic records by Amadio [3] indicates that the first surgical release of the transverse carpal ligament for median nerve compression was done by Drs. Herbert Galloway and Andrew Mackinnon in Winnipeg, Manitoba, Canada in 1924, also for a patient with a posttraumatic neuropathy. The following is a description from those records: "On February 21, 1924, Drs. Galloway and Mackinnon explored the median nerve downward for an inch & upward for two inches from the wrist crease. The patient continued to have pain and was seen at Mayo by Dr. A.W. Adson, who diagnosed median neuritis. On August 27, 1925, Dr. Galloway reoperated and found that the palmar cutaneous nerve was excised. The patient had some improvement but continued to have some difficulty." It would appear that the earliest case of carpal tunnel surgery began with a significant and unfortunately still common complication of injury to the palmar cutaneous branch of the median nerve. The recognition and popularization of spontaneous carpal tunnel syndrome as a diagnostic entity has only been as recent as the late 1940s and 1950, and this occurred largely through the writings of George Phalen [2]. In 1951, he initially described his technique using a transverse incision at the distal wrist crease, with proximal and distal extension as needed [4]. Not until the 1970s through the work of Taleisnik [5] and others did the longitudinal incision along the line of the ring finger become the recommended approach.

Carpal tunnel syndrome remains the most understood and the commonest of peripheral compression neuropathies and as it continues to be diagnosed with increasing frequency, it remains the most common hand operation performed [6]. The open method remains the standard surgical approach for patients who have failed to improve satisfactorily with conservative measures. More recently, two alternative approaches have been reported: the endoscopic carpal tunnel release and limited incision techniques [7]. The latter came about in response to concerns about the safety of the endoscopic approach. Both of these approaches may be performed through one or two smaller incisions. The reported advantages, especially of the endoscopic approach, have included a faster return of preoperative strength, less midpalm and scar tenderness, and more rapid return to work in non-workers' compensation patients [2]. However, the higher incidence and severity of the reported complications with the endoscopic technique and the subsequent need for secondary surgery has continued to generate much controversy.

The simple release of the transverse carpal ligament consistently relieves symptoms in most patients. A small but significant group of patients, however, will have similar symptoms following surgery or will experience new symptoms in the postoperative period. Problems following the surgical treatment of carpal tunnel syndrome that may lead to secondary surgery can be classified into three general areas (Table 40.1). Symptoms may be persistent after surgery with little or no improvement. Alternatively, there may be significant improvement or relief of symptoms but only temporarily with eventual recurrence of the same problem. Finally, new symptoms may arise following surgery which are distinct from the initial complaints.

Table 40.1. Indications for secondary carpal tunnel surgery

Complaints	Etiology
Persistent symptoms	Inadequate release of flexor retinaculum or antebrachial fascia Proximal median nerve compression (forearm, neck) Wrong diagnosis
Recurrent symptoms	Pathological scar formation around median nerve Reformation of flexor retinaculum Proximal median nerve compression
New symptoms	Iatrogenic injury

From [52] with permission

Complications Following Carpal Tunnel Surgery

Persistent Symptoms

The persistence of preoperative complaints is the most common complication of carpal tunnel release with an incidence of 7%–20% (Table 40.2) [8–17]. This may occur for three primary reasons. Most commonly, the transverse carpal ligament (flexor retinaculum) is incompletely released with the problem usually in the most distal portion of the ligament (Fig. 40.1) [18–20]. This may be due to inadequate exposure or visualization as in the endoscopic approach or with limited inci-

Table 40.2. Results of treatment of carpal tunnel syndrome by decompression

Study	No patients followed	Staging	Decompression alone	Symptomatic relief complete	Atrophy corrected	Weakness corrected	Sensory "loss" corrected	2PD corrected	Recurrence (n)
Paine, 1963	133	N/A	100%	99%	0%	25%*	50%*	ND	1
Patrick, 1965	32	N/A	100%	100%	N/A	N/A	N/A	N/A	2
Phalen, 1966	212	Minimal-moderate, 44%	100%	N/A	–	N/A	78%	ND	2
		Severe, 56%	100%	N/A	68%	83%	78%	ND	
Cruez et al., 1966	313	N/A	95%	46%	ND	N/A	81%	ND	0
Reitz, Önne, 1967	65	Minimal-moderate, 40%	100%	100%	–			–	
		Severe, 60%	50%	92%	75%			ND	
Semple, Cargill, 1969	150	N/A	100%	75%		N/A	N/A	N/A	ND
Posch, Marcotte, 1976	681	N/A	100%	91%		N/A	N/A	N/A	ND
Eversmann, Retsick, 1978	51	Moderate, 86%	100%			†			
Graham, 1983	214	Minimal-moderate, 44%	100%	75%	N/A	N/A	N/A	ND	
Gelberman et al., 1987	33	Severe, 100%	100%	62%	65%	90%		85%	31%
Kulick et al., 1986	100	Minimal-moderate, 80%	100%	85%‡		70%	N/A	ND	6
		Severe, 20%	100%‡	35%	5%		N/A	ND	

Abbreviations: N/A, data not available; ND, examination not done; 2PD, two-point discrimination
* Estimated
† Ninety-one percent of these patients had improvement in motor conduction latencies, the only parameter tested
‡ Epineurotomy added
From [40] with permission

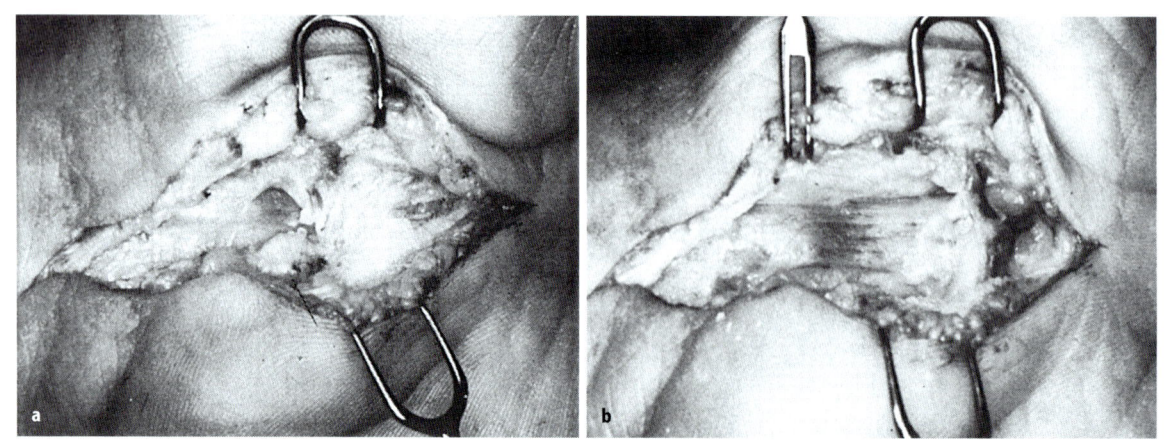

Fig. 40.1. a This patient underwent a left carpal tunnel release via a proximal transverse incision which was complicated by persistence of preoperative symptoms. This photograph of the left carpal tunnel shows the distal portion of the transverse carpal ligament which was not previously released. **b** Significant compression of the underlying median nerve is demonstrated after release of the distal portion of the carpal ligament (from [40] with permission)

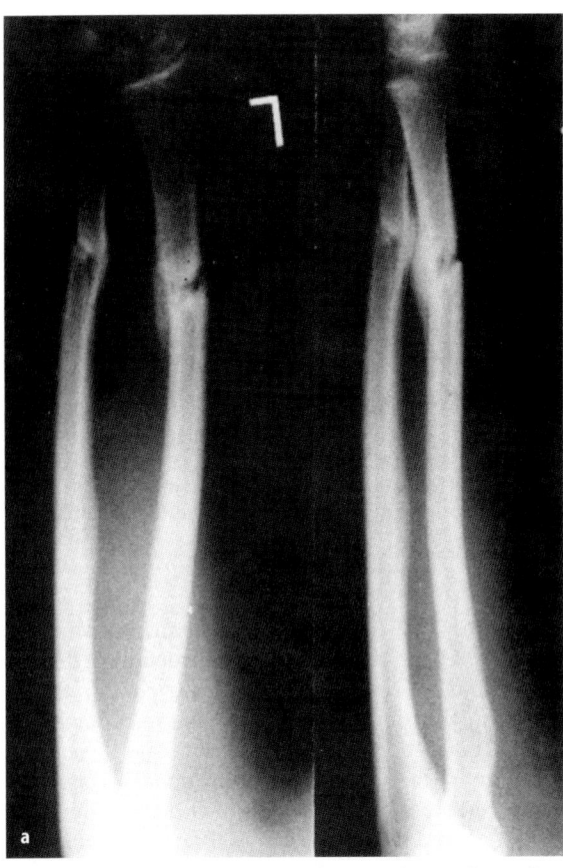

Fig. 40.2. a This patient experienced sensory loss in the median nerve distribution subsequent to radius and ulnar fractures. A previous carpal tunnel release was performed but with no improvement. **b** During re-exploration, the thickened antebrachial fascia is also seen to compress the median nerve. The surgical instrument is being inserted in the palm distal to the scarred forearm fascia, which will be released proximally up to the level of the fracture site (from [40] with permission)

sion techniques. Continued compression on the median nerve may also occur more proximally by inadequate release of the most distal portion of the antebrachial fascia. Patients who develop carpal tunnel symptoms following trauma to the wrist and hand may be particularly prone to proximal compression as the fascia may be scarred and thickened (Fig. 40.2).

Secondly, preoperative symptoms may persist because of compression of the median nerve further proximally in the forearm or the neck. There is a well-established association between carpal tunnel syndrome and cervical disc disease [21]. These regions must be thoroughly examined preoperatively to rule out additional areas of compression that may be contributing to the patients' complaints. Patients with work-related symptoms in particular may have multiple areas of nerve entrapment and are often improved following carpal tunnel surgery. A number of workers' compensation patients, however, continue to have problems after surgical management and may respond best to a different job that does not involve the use of vibration tools or repetitive activities.

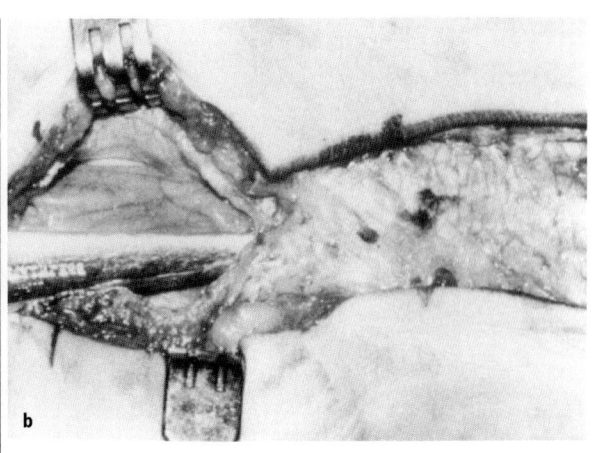

Of course, patients whose symptoms are initially misdiagnosed as carpal tunnel syndrome will respond poorly to carpal tunnel surgery. These patients often have more vague, diffuse, and atypical carpal tunnel complaints.

Recurrent Symptoms

Many patients may do well initially after surgery only to have the same preoperative symptoms recur, often after a few months. Postoperative scarring may be significant in many of these patients. The scar tissue may involve the median nerve directly by formation around and entrapping the nerve. Contributory factors may include poor hemostasis and hematoma formation, prolonged postoperative immobilization, or inadequate range-of-motion exercises and therapy. Excess scar tissue may also indirectly affect the nerve by leading to reformation of the transverse carpal ligament (Fig. 40.3).

Alternatively, preoperative symptoms may recur because of compression of the median nerve at a more proximal level as in the pronator syndrome. According to the theory of the multiple-crush syndrome, release of a distal site of compression, such as the carpal tunnel, may unmask a more proximal site of compression, such as at the proximal forearm, which preoperatively may not have been diagnosed as a clinically significant area of entrapment.

New Symptoms

A third group of patients with postoperative problems experience symptoms different from their original complaints. These can be broadly classified into the general areas of neurological, vascular, tendon, and wrist complaints (Table 40.3).

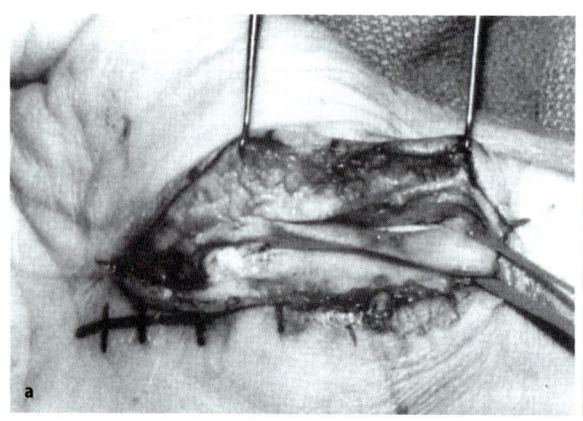

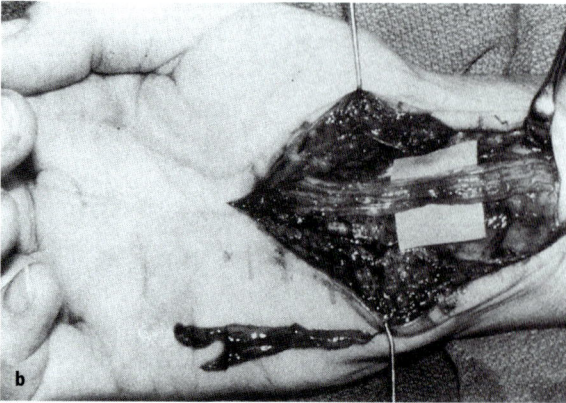

Fig. 40.3. a Secondary carpal tunnel surgery was performed on this diabetic patient after median nerve function was lost following primary release. The flexor retinaculum was found to have reformed from scar tissue and the median nerve, adherent to its underside, was compressed. **b** The gross appearance of the nerve improved with neurolysis. The resected epineurium is seen on the hypothenar eminence. The patient ultimately experienced return of median nerve function but required a full 10 months with recovery at a rate of 1 inch per month (from [40] with permission)

Table 40.3. Complications following carpal tunnel release

Neurologic complications
Injury to median nerve
Palmar cutaneous branch (compression, neuroma)
Recurrent motor branch
Median nerve

Injury to ulnar nerve
Ulnar palmar cutaneous neuroma
Main ulnar nerve
Communicating ramus between median and ulnar nerves
Reflex sympathetic dystrophy

Vascular injury
Ulnar artery
Superficial palmar arch
Palmar hematoma

Wrist pain
Carpal arch alteration
Pillar pain
Piso-triquetral syndrome

Tendon problems
Trigger finger
Bowstringing of flexor tendons
Flexor tendon adhesions

Wound complications
Infection, wound dehiscence
Hypertrophic or painful scar

From [52] with permission

Neurologic Complications

New neurologic problems usually involve one of the branches of the median nerve and less commonly the median nerve itself. Injury to the palmar cutaneous branch or one of its branches is most frequently the problem. A more radially placed incision is more likely to cross the distribution of the palmar cutaneous branch with subsequent injury and neuroma formation (Fig. 40.4). A tender hypertrophic scar is likely to be the result of injury to small cutaneous branches [22–25]. A primary entrapment neuropathy of the palmar cutaneous branch has been reported [26], as well as secondary compression following carpal tunnel release. Transection of the transverse carpal ligament may not release pressure on the palmar cutaneous branch because it may have its own distinct tunnel to the hand, and postoperative swelling and edema may lead to compression of this tunnel (Fig. 40.5). Other branches that may be injured include the recurrent motor branch [22, 23, 27] and common digital nerves (Fig. 40.6) [21–23]. Direct injury to the median nerve itself can occur and unfortunately, even complete transection of the nerve during carpal tunnel surgery has been reported [28]. The portion of the median nerve to the third webspace is frequently injured, especially with the endoscopic release. Patients complain of burning, pain, and numbness in the long and ring fingers. Additionally, a rare but clinically significant problem that has been described as a sequela of carpal tunnel release is "bowstringing" or "anterior dislocation" of the median nerve [29].

▷
Fig. 40.6. a Prior carpal tunnel release was performed using the incision outlined and complicated by pain at the wrist consistent with a neuroma of the palmar cutaneous branch, loss of thenar muscle function, loss of thumb sensation and altered sensation in the index finger. **b** The median nerve was explored and the following findings were noted: injury of the sensory branches to the thumb and index finger (distal visibility background), injured recurrent motor branch, and neuroma of the palmar cutaneous branch (proximal background, at *upper right*). The palmar cutaneous branch will be transposed proximally into the forearm musculature, the sensory branch to the index finger neurolysed, and the sensory and motor branches to the thumb will be reconstructed with nerve grafts (from [52] with permission)

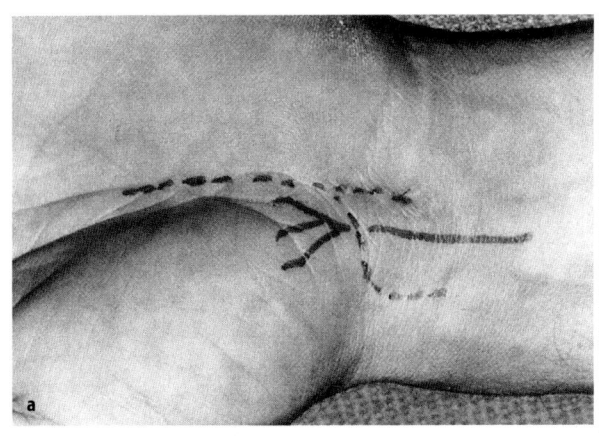

Fig. 40.4. a The scar from previous carpal tunnel surgery may be indicative of the type of release and also possible nerve injury. The incisions previously used in this patient are outlined. One portion of the scar intersects the path of the palmar cutaneous branch of the median nerve at the wrist and exploration revealed an injury to this nerve. **b** In another patient, transection of the palmar cutaneous branch had occurred. **c** A closeup view demonstrates neuroma formation of the proximal palmar cutaneous branch between the tendons of the palmaris longus and the flexor carpi radialis (from [52] with permission)

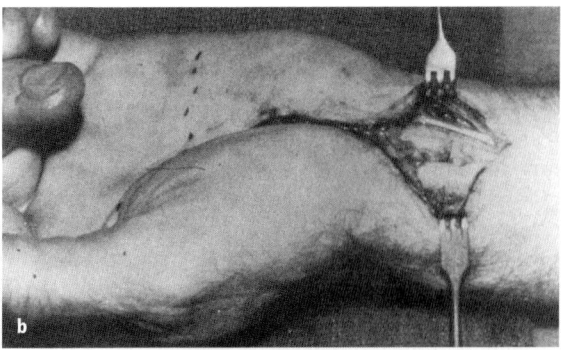

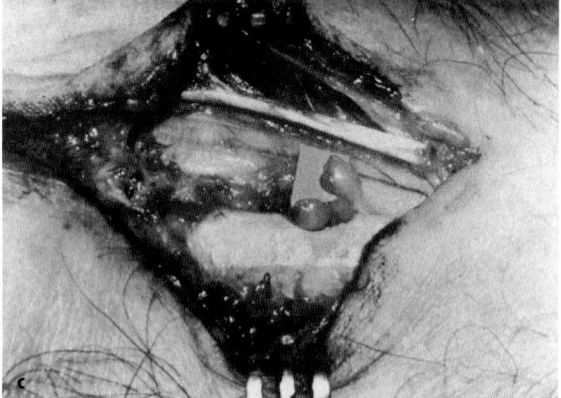

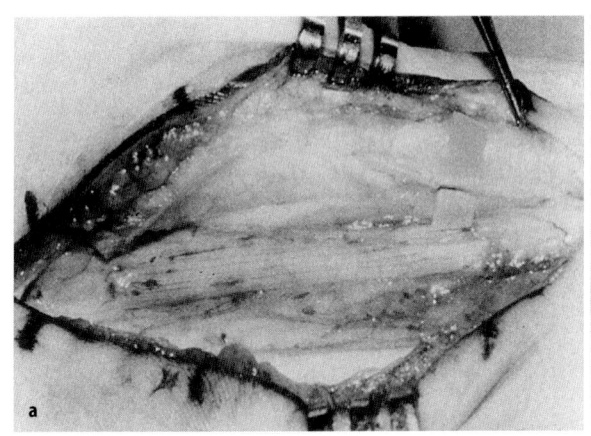

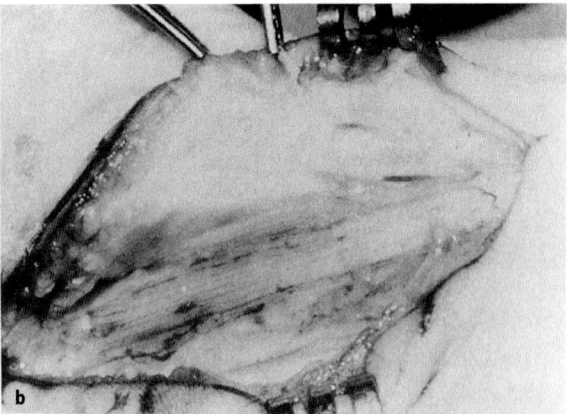

Fig. 40.5. a After carpal tunnel release, this patient developed symptoms consistent with a neuroma of the palmar cutaneous branch of the median nerve. The palmar cutaneous branch, seen with the visibility background, was not damaged but compressed in its own tunnel. **b** The patient's symptoms resolved after release of this separate tunnel (from [40] with permission)

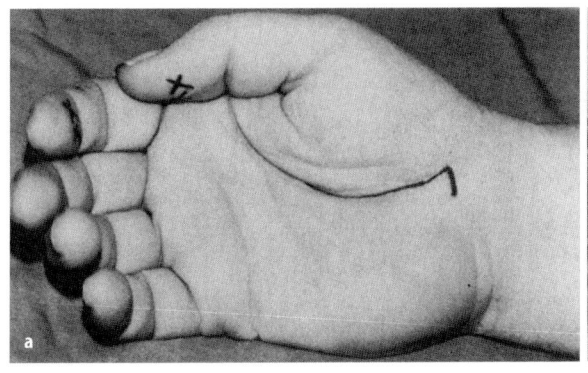

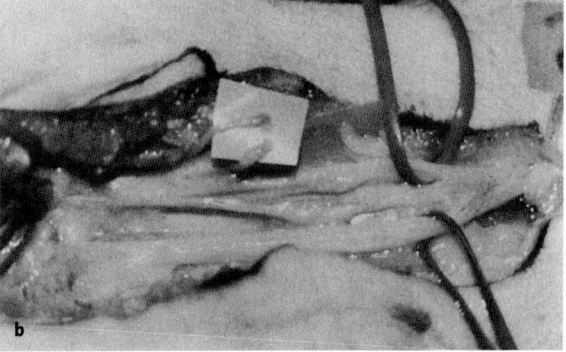

Other neurologic complications may include injury to the ulnar nerve, especially its palmar cutaneous branch and a communicating branch between the median and ulnar nerves [30], the radial sensory nerve with neuroma formation [24], and multiple nerve dysfunction [31]. Injury to the ulnar nerve is more common with the endoscopic release. Reflex sympathetic dystrophy (RSD) is rare but may follow carpal tunnel surgery [22, 25, 32], or alternatively, may be caused or exacerbated by carpal tunnel syndrome. In the latter case, surgical treatment with carpal tunnel release may actually improve rather than worsen the RSD. Of course, caution should be exercised in these patients and a satisfactory response to surgical management will be facilitated by a thorough preoperative psychological evaluation and pre-, intra- and postoperative sympathetic blockade.

Vascular Injury

Injury to the superficial palmar arch may be insignificant if recognized or may lead to accumulation of a hematoma in the palm [22, 25]. If not managed in a timely manner, this has been reported to progress to massive necrosis of the palmar skin and require a free flap for coverage [28].

Wrist Pain

Various entities have been reported following carpal tunnel release and include carpal arch alterations [33, 34], pillar pain, and pisotriquetral [35] syndrome. In an attempt to minimize these effects, some advocate reconstruction of the transverse carpal ligament either by resuturing one side of the carpal ligament (usually radial) to the opposite side of the palmar aponeurosis

Table 40.4. Incidence of new complaints following carpal tunnel release

Study	Total no. of cases	No. of cases affected	IN-COMP DIV	PCM	Thenar	Digital	Fibrosis	Injury	Bowstring	Ulnar Ramus	Radial Nerve	Multiple Nerves	RSD	Hem	Inf	Scar	Bow	Adhsns	PTP
Crow, 1960	40	2	2																
Goodman, Gilliatt, 1961	20	2	2																
Paine, 1963	119	1																	
Goodwill, 1965	55	6	6																
Patrick, 1965	32	1	1																
Phalen, 1966	212	4	3										1						
Langloh, Linscheid, 1972	2053	34	21				22											14	
Das, Brown, 1976	120	10	2	4	1	1								2					
MacDonald, 1978	186	34	12	11								4	2		2	2	1		
Conolly, 1978		35	9	4	1		2	2					1	2		1		2	
Inglis, 1980		2						2											
May, 1981		1								1									
Eason et al., 1985		47	4	3				2						2				3	
Lilly, Magnell, 1985	249	2			2														
Louis et al., 1985		26		14				3			2					3			
Kessler, 1986 (review)																			
Crandall, Weeks, 1988		1											1						
Seradge, Seradge, 1989	500	5																	5
Hanssen, 1989	3620	12												17					

Abbreviations: *Incomp div* incomplete division of carpal ligament; *Hem* palmar hematoma; *Adhsns* adhesions; *Bow* bowstringing; *Inf* infection; *Scar* hypertrophic painful scar; *PTP* piso-triquetral pain (from [52] with permission)

(ulnar) by a step lengthening type of transection, or by the use of transposition flaps from the carpal ligament. Such reconstruction, however, has been associated with reformation of the carpal tunnel and the subsequent recurrence of symptoms.

Tendon Problems

There seems to be a higher frequency of trigger finger after carpal tunnel surgery. A possible explanation is that the transverse carpal ligament may also normally function as a tendon pulley. When this is released, greater forces are then transmitted to the first annular ligament, which is now the most proximal pulley and may contribute to triggering at this site. Anterior dislocation or bowstringing of the flexor tendons [25] has already been mentioned, and flexor tendon adhesions can also be a problem [19]. Table 40.4 summarizes the complications reported in the literature after carpal tunnel surgery. Table 40.5 shows the results of a recent survey of the members of the American Society for Surgery of the Hand undertaken by Palmer and Toivonen regarding the complications of the endoscopic as well as the open approach [36].

Clinical Evaluation of the Patient with Failed Carpal Tunnel Release

An accurate assessment of the status of the median nerve after primary carpal tunnel surgery can usually be made from a thorough history and careful sensory examination. If the initial complaints were not resolved after the first surgery, the persistent symptoms are probably due to incomplete release either at the carpal tunnel or at the distal antebrachial fascia, or a more proximal compression. If the initial complaints were relieved after surgery but then recur after a period of time, the etiology is likely to be either pathologic scar formation around the median nerve or scarring with subsequent reformation of the transverse carpal ligament. More rarely, there may be a point of compression in the proximal forearm [21] which previously was not clinically significant until after the carpal tunnel was released. If the presenting symptoms are new and different than the initial complaints, such as pain or motor weakness, an iatrogenic nerve injury should be considered.

Physical Diagnosis

Pressure provocative tests are helpful to determine the area of compression of a peripheral nerve, since an entrapped nerve will be more sensitive to mechanical pressure [37, 38]. Digital pressure just proximal to the level of entrapment, such as the carpal tunnel or the pronator teres, will cause paresthesias in the territory of the median nerve if there is ongoing compression at that site. Other maneuvers that may produce paresthesias in the median nerve distribution from a compression in the proximal forearm include maximum passive supination of the forearm, resisted pronation, and resisted contraction of the flexor digitorum superficialis (FDS).

If an iatrogenic injury to the median nerve is being considered, then each region of the nerve should be evaluated separately. Potential problems can often be anticipated by the location of the scar from the first carpal tunnel release. An injury to the palmar cutaneous branch of the median nerve, which runs between the FCR tendon and the palmaris longus tendon, can often be suspected if the initial incision was placed inappropriately radially crossing the territory of the nerve. The recommended approach ideally is well ulnar to the distribution of the palmar cutaneous branch. We advocate the use of the interthenar depression, which is the deepest point between the thenar and hypothenar eminences, as a reliable and constant landmark. The thenar crease anatomy is too variable and the ring finger axis will also vary depending on whether the digit is flexed or extended. The palmar cutaneous branch is located approximately 5 mm radial to the interthenar depression on average [39] and our approach is approximately 5 mm ulnar to the interthenar depression. Symptoms consistent with an injury to the palmar cutaneous branch will usually include abnormal sensation in the territory of the nerve and a Tinel sign at the level of the injury. Sometimes there may be entrapment of the palmar cutaneous nerve itself in its own separate tunnel and the presentation will be similar to a neuroma [40]. The presentation of an injured recurrent motor branch is usually straightforward and will consist of weakness or atrophy of the abductor pollicis brevis muscle. A partial injury to the median nerve itself will present with abnormal sensation in the territory of the injured fascicles. The most superficial or anteriorly located fascicles

Table 40.5. Complications of endoscopic and open carpal tunnel release

Complication	ECTR	OCTR
Median nerve lacerations	100	147
Palmar cutaneous branch lacerations	17	117
Ulnar nerve lacerations	88	29
Digital nerve lacerations	77	54
Tendon lacerations	69	19
Superficial arch lacerations	86	21
Ulnar artery lacerations	34	11
Total complications	**455**	**283**
Total respondents	**708**	**616**

Data from Palmer AK, Toivonen DA: Complications of endoscopic and open carpal tunnel release. Presented at the 50th Annual Meeting of the American Society for Surgery of the Hand. San Francisco, September 16, 1995 of the median nerve are the most vulnerable to injury and these usually supply the third web space. A Tinel sign radiating to the territory of the injured nerve will help to identify the level of the injury. We have found a simple clinical test which is useful in determining what nerve(s) is injured. It is important that all of the nerves involved are identified and appropriately managed to ensure the best possible result. A Tinel-like response can be elicited 2–4 inches *proximal* to the actual area of injury. Frequently, palpation *at* the level of injury is so painful that the patient has difficulty accurately describing the distribution of the pain [41]. For example, gentle tapping between the FCR and palmaris longus starting proximal to the level of the scar will illicit a response into the distribution of the palmar cutaneous branch if it is involved. A careful physical examination should also include sensibility testing of the autonomous zone of each digital nerve to further determine which nerves are involved. Our sensory examination consists of testing for innervation density (moving and static two-point discrimination) and threshold tests (vibration and pressure monofilaments) [40].

Painful sequelae of carpal tunnel surgery require careful pre- and postoperative management. Patients should become familiar with the techniques of desensitization on a nonpainful area prior to secondary surgery so that desensitization can be started early following surgery. If the pain is significant, a pain evaluation scale will help determine the extent of nonorganic, functional, or psychological components contributing to the problem [42]. Patients should have a complete understanding of the nature of their injury and potential risks and benefits of having secondary surgery.

Surgical Techniques in Secondary Carpal Tunnel Surgery

Internal Neurolysis

We advocate internal neurolysis in practically all patients undergoing secondary carpal tunnel release. With the use of microsurgical instrumentation, the external and internal epineurium is opened until a normal fascicular appearance with visible perineurial markings (bands of Fontana) is seen. Injured fascicles may be identified in this manner. The extent of internal neurolysis required for each case will vary with the amount of scarring and fibrosis within each nerve (Fig. 40.7). Opening the perineurium is avoided because it is an anatomical site of the blood-nerve barrier. The benefit of internal neurolysis during *primary* carpal tunnel surgery has been examined in a prospective randomized study [6]. No benefit could be shown over simply transecting the transverse carpal ligament in the setting of primary carpal tunnel surgery. The role of internal neurolysis in secondary carpal tunnel release has yet to be evaluated but it is a technique we use in all secondary carpal tunnel cases.

Median Nerve Compression in the Forearm

If the physical exam supports a diagnosis of median nerve compression in the proximal forearm, then exploration at this level and decompression should be considered. The entrapment usually involves the pronator teres and less commonly the FDS muscle [43]. The superficial and deep heads of the pronator teres muscle often form a tendinous arch around the median nerve (Fig. 40.8). Slightly more distally, the FDS muscle may have a fibrous leading edge that also compresses the nerve.

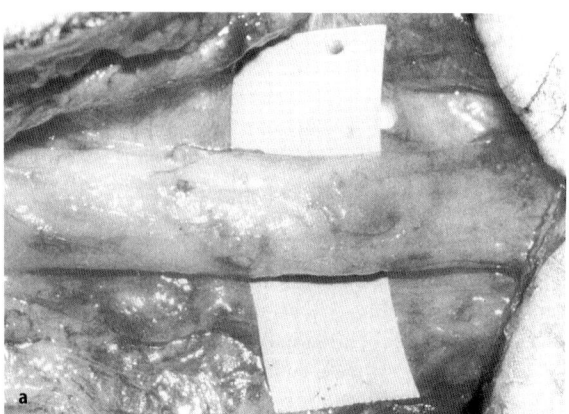

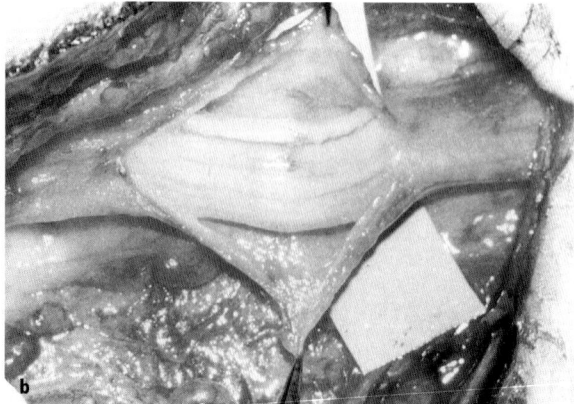

Fig. 40.7. a Secondary surgery often reveals a significantly scarred and thickened nerve. In secondary carpal tunnel surgery, the median nerve is usually adherent to the radial undersurface of the transverse carpal ligament. **b** Opening and excision of the thickened epineurium is performed standard microneurosurgical internal neurolysis technique (from [52] with permission)

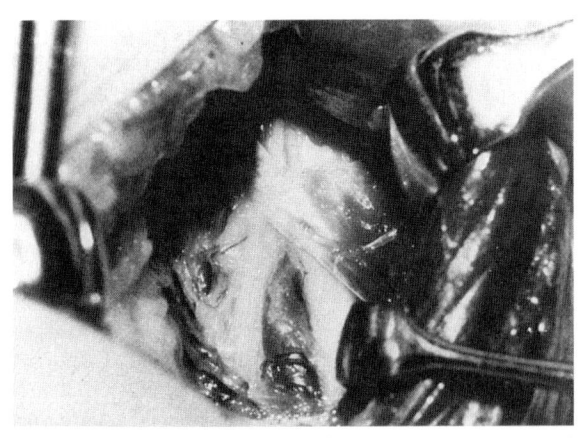

Fig. 40.8. Compression of the median nerve in the proximal forearm can occur from a fibrous arch formed by the superficial and deep heads of the pronator teres (from [52] with permission)

Neuroma of the Palmar Cutaneous Branch of the Median Nerve

The surgical management of painful nerve injuries is based on experimental studies using primates which showed that a neuroma is both spontaneously active and mechanically sensitive [44]. By excising the neuroma and inserting the nerve stump in an area that will minimize its exposure to mechanical stimulation, the nerve will be much less likely to be clinically problematic. The regenerative potential and behavior of an injured nerve has been shown by other experimental work to be influenced by its environment and tissue bed [45]. While proximity to denervated skin will encourage sprouting and attempts at regeneration by trophic influences, innervated muscle, on the other hand, will inhibit such nerve activity.

The surgical management of an injured palmar cutaneous nerve therefore includes the identification and excision of the neuroma, and dissection of this branch proximally from the main trunk of the median nerve by microsurgical internal neurolysis. This permits a long enough segment of the nerve to be transposed further proximally between the deep and superficial layers of the flexor muscles. This provides an environment for the nerve stump in an innervated muscle bed as far away as possible from the overlying skin and scar. We also coagulate the end of the nerve using microbipolar cautery prior to transposing the nerve. Much less commonly, the palmar cutaneous branch may simply be compressed in its own distinct tunnel, in which case the release of this tunnel will be all that is required. However, if it is at all unclear whether the nerve has been actually injured or not, then an injury should be assumed and the nerve transposed proximally as in the case of a neuroma.

Nerve Grafting

Management of an injury to the main portion of the median nerve itself will usually require an interposition nerve graft (Fig. 40.9). Again, microsurgical technique is used to evaluate the extent of damage and to identify the injured portion. A thorough preoperative evaluation should have given a good idea of the components of the nerve that are uninjured, those that are only partially injured, and those that are not functioning at all. The median nerve is then managed as a sixth degree injury, dissecting and replacing only the affected portion of the nerve (Fig. 40.10). Our first choice of donor nerve in these cases is usually the anterior branch of the medial antebrachial cutaneous nerve. The landmark for finding the medial antebrachial cutaneous nerve is the adjacent basilic vein located along the medial border of the biceps muscle. The anterior branch supplies sensation to the ulnar volar aspect of the forearm and the posterior branch which supplies the elbow is left intact. The ulnar medial location of the scar on the forearm is a less visible and more cosmetically acceptable location and the area of sensory loss diminishes with time. In cases where a short nerve graft is needed, the lateral antebrachial cutaneous nerve may be used instead. It lies adjacent to the cephalic vein along the medial border of the brachioradialis muscle in the proximal forearm, and the donor scar therefore is more visible. The use of the sural nerve for grafting should be reserved for cases in which long grafts or multiple cable grafting will be needed. The resulting scar and sensory deficit are more unsatisfactory, and the formation of a problematic neuroma in the lower leg where the distal end is in proximity to the Achilles' tendon or the overlying scar is likely if just a short segment of sural nerve is harvested. Recently we have used the terminal branch of the anterior interosseous nerve as a donor nerve graft. We harvest this nerve just proximal to the pronator quadratus muscle. Because it is an expendable motor nerve there is no sensory loss.

The same general principles of nerve grafting apply to secondary carpal tunnel surgery as well. Sufficient length of nerve graft should be harvested to avoid any tension at the repair sites and also to permit a full range of motion at the wrist. Postoperatively, the wrist is immobilized and the metacarpal phalangeal joints blocked for 2 weeks. Active motion should be continued at the distal and proximal interphalangeal joints as well as finger flexion to permit gliding of the flexor tendons and minimize scarring to the nerve and graft.

Tissue Interposition Flaps

For patients with significant pain and hyperalgesia at the proximal palm and wrist, a flap of innervated mus-

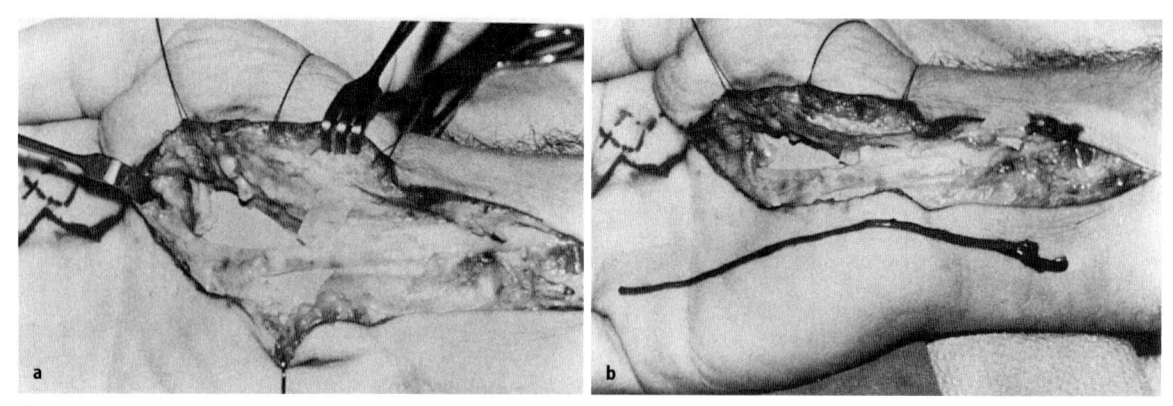

Fig. 40.9. a A prior release of the carpal tunnel was done in this patient through a transverse incision. Release of the distal carpal ligament without appropriate exposure was complicated by transection of both the motor and sensory branches of the median nerve to the thumb. **b** Reconstruction of these branches will be performed using the anterior branch of the medial antebrachial cutaneous nerve, seen lying on the hypothenar eminence, as an interposition nerve graft (from [52] with permission)

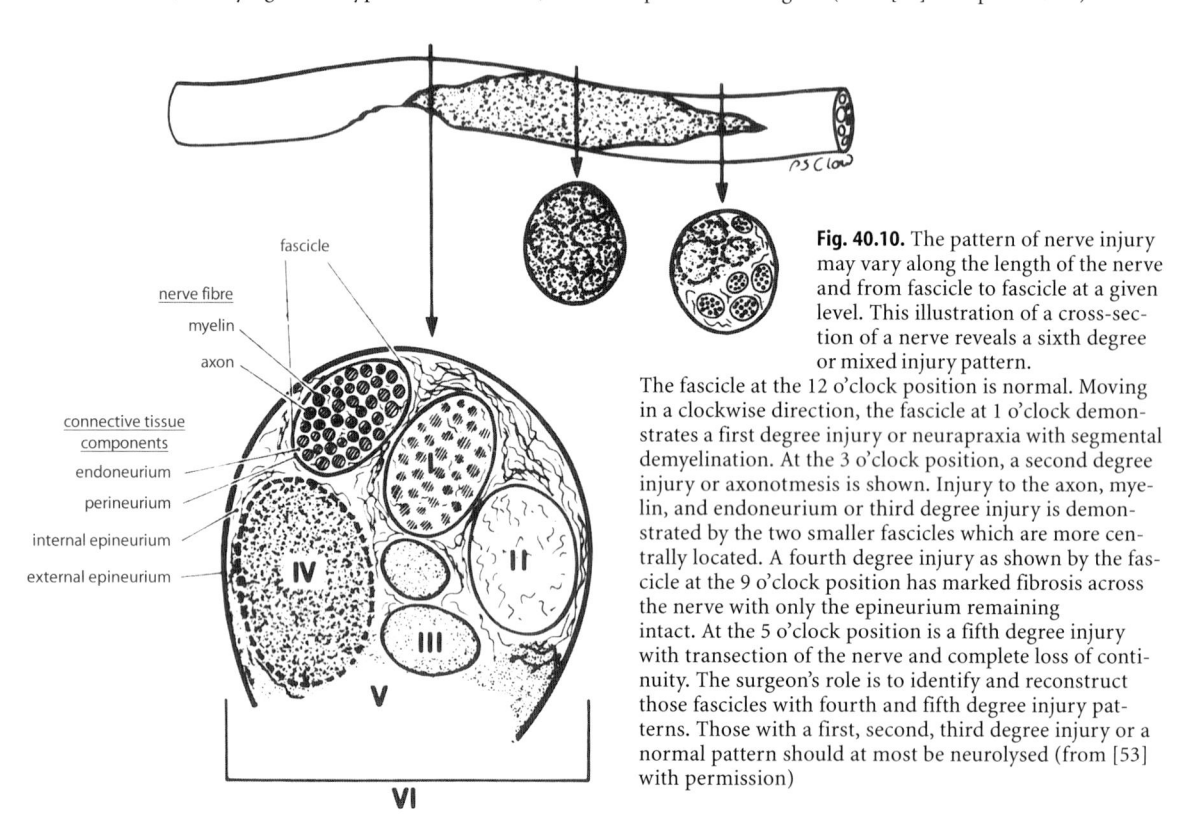

Fig. 40.10. The pattern of nerve injury may vary along the length of the nerve and from fascicle to fascicle at a given level. This illustration of a cross-section of a nerve reveals a sixth degree or mixed injury pattern.

The fascicle at the 12 o'clock position is normal. Moving in a clockwise direction, the fascicle at 1 o'clock demonstrates a first degree injury or neurapraxia with segmental demyelination. At the 3 o'clock position, a second degree injury or axonotmesis is shown. Injury to the axon, myelin, and endoneurium or third degree injury is demonstrated by the two smaller fascicles which are more centrally located. A fourth degree injury as shown by the fascicle at the 9 o'clock position has marked fibrosis across the nerve with only the epineurium remaining intact. At the 5 o'clock position is a fifth degree injury with transection of the nerve and complete loss of continuity. The surgeon's role is to identify and reconstruct those fascicles with fourth and fifth degree injury patterns. Those with a first, second, third degree injury or a normal pattern should at most be neurolysed (from [53] with permission)

cle or soft tissue can be raised and inset over the median nerve to provide padding and interposition tissue beneath the sensitive skin. The hypothenar fat pad flap is an easy dissection through the same incision and with good results in some cases [46]. However, it provides only a small amount of tissue. Several donor muscle flaps have been described including the abductor digiti minimi (ADM), the pronator quadratus, the palmaris brevis, and the first or second radial lumbrical muscles. The ADM is easily dissected and is our coverage flap of choice (Fig. 40.11). The pronator quadratus requires a more tedious mobilization but can provide better coverage more proximally in the distal forearm [40]. It has a very limited reach distally and we rarely use it. The palmaris brevis is rather thin and somewhat variable in its size and thickness. The use of the first or second radial lumbrical muscles has also recently been reported without any obvious motor deficit or weakness [47]. We have not used these muscles.

More aggressive approaches have also been described mostly as salvage procedures for particularly recalcitrant cases. A reverse radial artery fascial flap

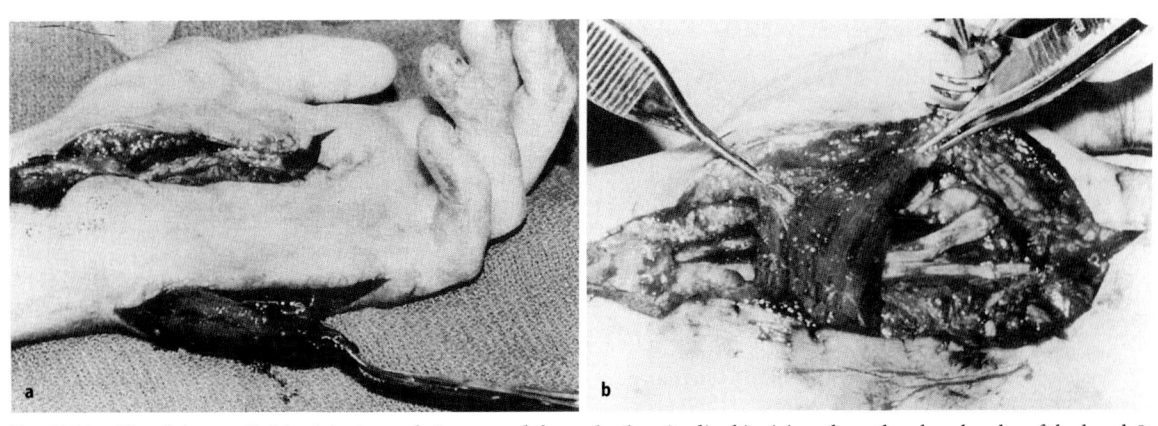

Fig. 40.11. a The abductor digiti minimi muscle is exposed through a longitudinal incision along the ulnar border of the hand. It is mobilized with a pedicle based on the proximal neurovascular bundle. **b** The muscle can then be transferred across the carpal tunnel to provide coverage for the median nerve (from [52] with permission)

has been used to envelop the median nerve and restore a suitable gliding bed with reportedly good results [48]. Free tissue transfers have included a thoracodorsal fascial flap from the latissimus dorsi muscle [49], and the omentum. The use of these flaps attests to the potential severity of the complications from carpal tunnel surgery and the dilemma which the patient and the surgeon may experience. In our experience, coverage of painful median nerve injury or nerve graft with a free muscle flap will not necessarily relieve pain. In these recalcitrant cases, if a psychological evaluation is acceptable and anesthesia nerve block of the median nerve relieves symptoms, then a peripheral nerve stimulator inserted on the median nerve is recommended.

Conclusion

Carpal tunnel release successfully resolves symptoms for most patients but a small group continues to have problems. The majority of these patients will have persistent or recurrent symptoms similar to the initial complaints, and secondary surgery to complete the decompression or decompression in the proximal forearm will relieve their symptoms.

A final group of patients however will present with new and different symptoms following their carpal tunnel release. In many of these cases the etiology will be an iatrogenic nerve injury. A contributing factor to this problem as well as incomplete carpal ligament release will often be a surgical approach, such as the endoscopic [50, 51] and limited incision techniques [7], that provides suboptimal exposure and visualization of the important structures. These cases are much more difficult and complex, and will require careful preoperative sensory and psychological pain assessment as well as meticulous intraoperative microsurgical technique to accurately determine the extent of injury. The techniques and principles of internal neurolysis, neuroma-in-continuity assessment, neuroma management, nerve grafting, and muscle flap or tissue interposition grafting can reliably improve most of these patients [52]. In the severe pain patient, a nerve stimulator should be considered.

Carpal tunnel surgery is considered by many to be a simple and easy procedure. However, significant complications can occur and an increasing awareness of their frequency and potentially disabling nature should continue to encourage greater respect for the procedure.

References

1. Paget J (1854) Lectures on Surgical Pathology, ed 2. Philadelphia, Lindsay and Blakiston, pp 42
2. Deune EG, Mackinnon SE (1996) Endoscopic carpal tunnel release: The voice of polite dissent. Clin Plast Surg 23(3): 487–504
3. Amadio PC (1992) The Mayo Clinic and carpal tunnel syndrome. May Clin Proc 67(1):42–48
4. Phalen GS (1951) Spontaneous compression of the median nerve at the wrist. JAMA 145:1128
5. Taleisnik J (1973) The palmar cutaneous branch of the median nerve and the approach to the carpal tunnel: An anatomical study. J Bone Joint Surg [Am] 55:1212–17
6. Mackinnon SE, McCabe S, Murray JR, et al. (1991) Internal neurolysis fails to improve the results of primary carpal tunnel decompression. J Hand Surg [Am] 16(2):211–8
7. Mirza MA, King ET (1996) Newer techniques of carpal tunnel release. Orthop Clin North Am 27(2):355–71
8. Creuz JA, Thomas JE, Lambert EH, et al. (1966) Long-term results of operation for carpal tunnel syndrome. Mayo Clinic Proc 41:232–241
9. Eversmann WW Jr, Retsick JA (1978) Intraoperative changes in motor nerve conduction latency in carpal tunnel syndrome. J Hand Surg 3:77–81
10. Gelberman RH, Pfefier GB, Galbraith RT, et al. (1987) Results of treatment of severe carpal tunnel syndrome without internal neurolysis of the median nerve. J Bone Joint Surg [Am] 69:896–903

11. Graham RA (1983) Carpal tunnel syndrome: A statistical analysis of 214 cases. Orthopedics 6:1283–7
12. Kulick MI, Gordillo G, Javidi T, et al. (1986) Long-term analysis of patients having surgical treatment for carpal tunnel syndrome. J Hand Surg [Am] 11:59–66
13. Paine KWE (1963) The carpal tunne syndrome. Can J Surg 6:446–9
14. Posch JL, Marcotte DR (1976) Carpal tunnel syndrome: An analysis of 1201 cases. Orthop Rev 5:25–35
15. Reitz KA, Onne L (1967) Analysis of sixty-five operated cases of carpal tunnel syndrome. Acta Chir Scand 133:443–7
16. Rhodes CE, Mowery CA, Gelberman RH (1985) Results of internal neurolysis of the median nerve for severe carpal tunnel syndrome. J Bone Joint Surg [Am] 67:253–6
17. Semple JC, Cargill AO (1969) Carpal tunnel syndrome: Results of surgical decompression. Lancet 1:918–9
18. Hudson AR, Kline D, Mackinnon SE (1987) Entrapment neuropathies. In Horowitz NH, Rizzoli HV (eds): Postoperative Complications of Extracranial Neurological Surgery. Baltimore, Williams & Wilkins, pp 260–82
19. Langloh ND, Linscheid RL (1972) Recurrent and unrelieved carpal tunnel syndrome. Clin Orthop 83:41–7
20. Patrick J (1965) Carpal-tunnel syndrome. BMJ 1:1377
21. Eason SY, Belsole RJ, Greene TL (1985) Carpal tunnel release: Analysis of suboptimal results. J Hand Surg [Br] 10:365–69
22. Conolly WB (1978) Pitfalls in carpal tunnel decompression. Aust N Z J Surg 48:421–5
23. Das SK, Brown HG (1986) In seach of complications in carpal tunnel decompression. Hand Clin 2:243–49
24. Louis DS, Greene TL, Noellert RC (1985) Complications of carpal tunnel surgery. J Neurosurg 62:352–6
25. MacDonald RI, Lichtman DM, Hanlon JJ, et al. (1978) Complications of surgical release of carpal tunnel syndrome. J Hand Surg 3:70–6
26. Buckmiller JF, Rickard TA (1987) Isolated comparison neuropathy of the palmar cutaneous branch of the median nerve. J Hand Surg [Am] 12:97–99
27. Lilly CJ, Magnell TD (1985) Severance of the thenar branch of the mdian nerve as a complication of carpal tunnel release. J Hand Surg [Am] 10(3):399–402
28. Cartotto R, McCabe S, Mackinnon SE (1992) Two devastating complications of carpal tunnel surgery. Ann Plas Surg 28(5):472–4
29. Inglis AE (1980) Two unusual operative complications in the carpal tunnel syndrome: A report of tow cases. J Bone Joint Surg [Am] 62:1208–9
30. May JW Jr (1981) Division of the sensory remus communicans between the ulnar and median nerves, a complication following carpal tunnel release: A case report. J Bone Joint Surg [Am] 63:836–8
31. Crandall RE, Weeks PM (1988) Multiple nerve dysfunction after carpal tunnel release. J Hand Surg [Am] 13:584–9
32. Phalen GS (1966) The carpal tunnel syndrome: Seventeen years experience in diagnosis and treatment of 654 hands. J Bone Joint Surg [Am] 48:211–28,
33. Bloem JJ, Pradarajardja CL, Vuursteen PJ (1986) The post carpal tunnel syndrome, causes and Prevention. Neth J Surg 38:52–55
34. Gartsman GM, Kovach JC, Crouch CC, et al. (1986) Carpal tunnel alteration after carpal tunnel release. J Hand Surg [Am] 11: 372–4
35. Seradge H, Seradge E (1989) Piso-triquetral pain syndrome after carpal tunnel release. J Hand Surg [Am] 14(5):858–73
36. Palmar AK, Toivonen DA (1995) Complications of endoscopic and open carpal tunnel release. Presented at the 50th Annual Meeting of the American Society for Surgery of the Hand, September 16
37. Novak CB, Mackinnon SE, Brownlee R, Kelly L (1992) Provocative sensory testing in carpal tunnel syndrome. J Hand Surg [Br] 17(2):204–8
38. Williams T, Mackinnon SE, McCabe S, et al. (1992) Verification of the pressure provocative test in carpal tunnel syndrome. J Hand Surg [Am] 29(1):8–11
39. Watchmaker GP, Weber D, Mackinnon SE (1996) Avoidance of transection of the palmar cutaneous branch of the median nerve in carpal tunnel release. J Hand Surg [Am] 21(4): 644–50
40. Mackinnon SE, Dellon AL (1988) Surgery of the Peripheral Nerve. New York, Thieme Medical Publishers, pp 164
41. Mackinnon SE (1998) Neuromas. Foot Ankle Clin 3(3):385–404
42. Novak CB, Mackinnon SE (1999) Evaluation of the patient with thoracic outlet syndrome. Chest Surg Clin North Am, in press
43. Dellon AL, Mackinnon SE (1987) Evaluation of musculotendinous variations about the median nerve in forearm. J Hand Surg [Br] 12:359–65
44. Meyer RA, Raja SN, Campbell JN et al. (1985) Neural activity originating from a neuroma in the baboon. Brain Res 325:255–60
45. Mackinnon SE, Dellon AL, Hudson AR et al. (1985) Alteration of neuroma formation by manipulation of neural environment. Plast Reconstr Surg 76:345
46. Strickland JW, Idler RS, Lourie GM, Plancher KD (1996) The hypothenar fat pad flap for management of recalcitrant carpal tunnel syndrome. J Hand Surg [Am] 21(5): 840–8
47. Koncilia H, Kuzbari R, Worseg A et al. (1998) The lumbrical muscle flap: Anatomic study and clinical application. J Hand Surg [Am] 23(1):111–9
48. Tham SKY, Ireland DC, Riccio M, Morrison WA (1996) Reverse radial artery fascial flap: A treatment for the chronically scarred median nerve in recurrent carpal tunnel syndrome. J Hand Surg [Am] 21(5):849–54
49. Wintsch K, Helaly P. (1986) Free flap of gliding tissue. J Reconstr Microsurg 2:143–51
50. Chow JC (1989) Endoscopic release of the carpal ligament: A new technique for carpal tunnel syndrome. Arthoscopy 5(1):19–24
51. Okutsu I, Ninomiya S, Takatori et al. (1989) Endoscopic management of carpal tunnel syndrome. Arthroscopy 5(1):11–18
52. Mackinnon SE (1991) Secondary carpal tunnel surgery. Neurosurg Clin North Am 2(1):75–91
53. Mackinnon SE (1989) Surgical management of the peripheral nerve gap. Clin Plast Surg 16:589

Hypothenar Fat-Pad Flap

R. Giunta, U. Frank, U. Lanz

Introduction

The treatment of scarring of the median nerve in the carpal tunnel following open carpal tunnel release, trauma, or infection presents the hand surgeon with a difficult problem, since adhesions between the nerve and scar tissue in the tunnel impair its longitudinal mobility. Measured in specimens, this amounts to between 7 and 14 mm in a longitudinal direction [1, 2] and some dorso-palmar and radio-ulnar excursion also [3, 4]. In some cases the median nerve is even prolapsed and scared between the two ligamentous stumps of the flexor retinaculum after open carpal tunnel release.

However, loss of this mobility can give rise to a wide spectrum of symptoms from slight dysesthesia to complete loss of function of the hand because of severe algodystrophy. Careful neurolysis is often insufficient to prevent new scar formation. In severe cases it is therefore necessary where possible to build up a "cushion" between the nerve, the rest of the retinaculum, and the skin, which can serve both as a sliding surface for mechanical protection and as a barrier for sprouting nerve fibers.

Historical Background

Various operative procedures based on these principles of treatment have been described [5]. The treatment ranges from local pedicled flaps of muscle or fascia [6–9] over synovial flaps [15] to free microvascular reanastomosed flaps [10]. Some of these operations are technically very demanding, they employ muscles of insufficient size, or have an unacceptable donor site defect. In the present article we summarize our experience [11, 11a] with the local vascular pedicled hypothenar fat-pad flap [12], to our knowledge first introduced by Cramer in 1985 [13], in support of this useful alternative.

Technique

Following the direction of the existing scar, the skin is incised in the direction of the ring finger from the proximal palmar flexion crease to that of the wrist joint. An oblique extension is carried in the direction of the ulnar end of the forearm, producing a triangular flap with its apex pointing in an ulnar direction. Under loupe magnification, neurolysis of the median nerve, starting from an unscarred region and running toward the scar (i.e., from proximal to distal), is now possible (Fig. 41.1). After the nerve, together with its thenar branch, has been completely freed from the scar tissue of the carpal tunnel, the hypothenar fat-pad flap is harvested. Dissection is then continued through the subcutaneous fatty tissue immediately below the skin, and carried in an ulnar direction as far as the fascia of the abductor digiti minimi (Fig. 41.2). From here the flap, including the palmaris brevis muscle, is dissected in a radial direction as far as Guyon's canal. While mobilizing the fatty tissue, the palmar branch of the ulnar nerve and the palmar digital nerves, which are often buried in the fat, must be carefully preserved. The ulnar nerve and artery lie within the Guyon's canal, and here it is important to preserve the fine end branches of the ulnar artery which ensure the blood supply of the flap. When completed, the flap measures about 4 × 3 cm. On the radial side it is pedicled by the branches of the ulnar artery, where it is hinged like the page of a book, and can be used to cover the scarred region of the median nerve (Fig. 41.3). What was formerly the ulnar side of the flap is now stitched with absorbable sutures to the radial wall of the carpal canal and fixed immediately below within the carpal tunnel. In this way the median nerve is protected from further palmar displacement and cushioned by a sufficiently thick fatty layer against the hollow of the palm (Fig. 41.3). The nerve is now in a position to slide freely backward and forward.

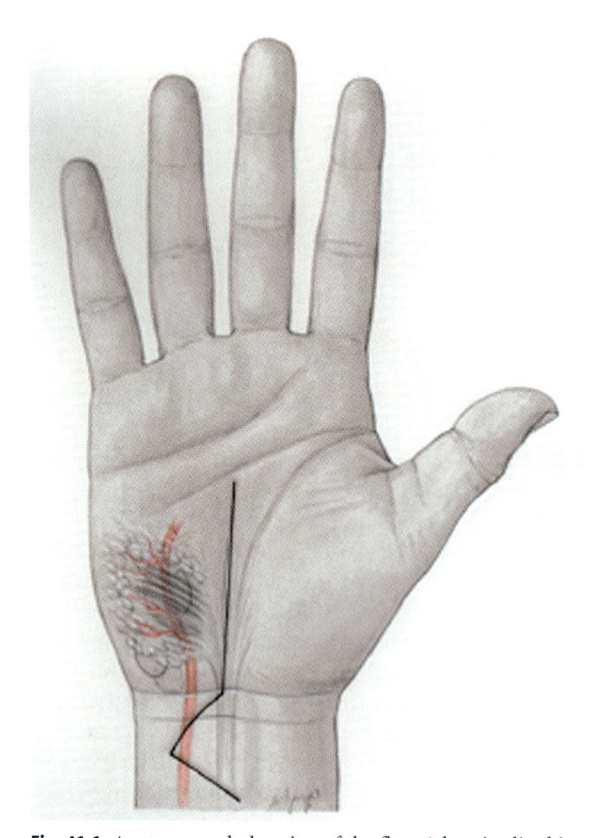

Fig. 41.1. Anatomy and planning of the flap. A longitudinal incision from the proximal palmar flexion crease to that of the wrist joint. Approach to the forearm through a radially pedicled triangular flap. The ulnar artery and its end branches to the palmaris brevis and hypothenar fatty tissue can be seen near Guyon's canal (from [11] with permission)

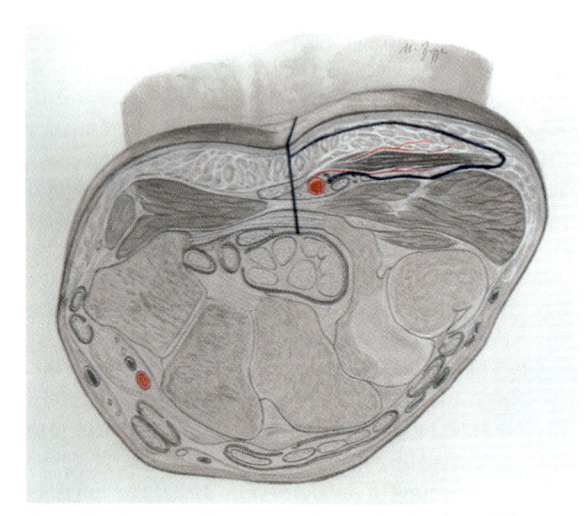

Fig. 41.2. Anatomy in cross section and planning of the flap. The palmaris brevis and hypothenar fatty tissue are raised as a flap. Dissection is continued as far as the fascia of the abductor digiti minimi or Guyon's canal (from [11] with permission)

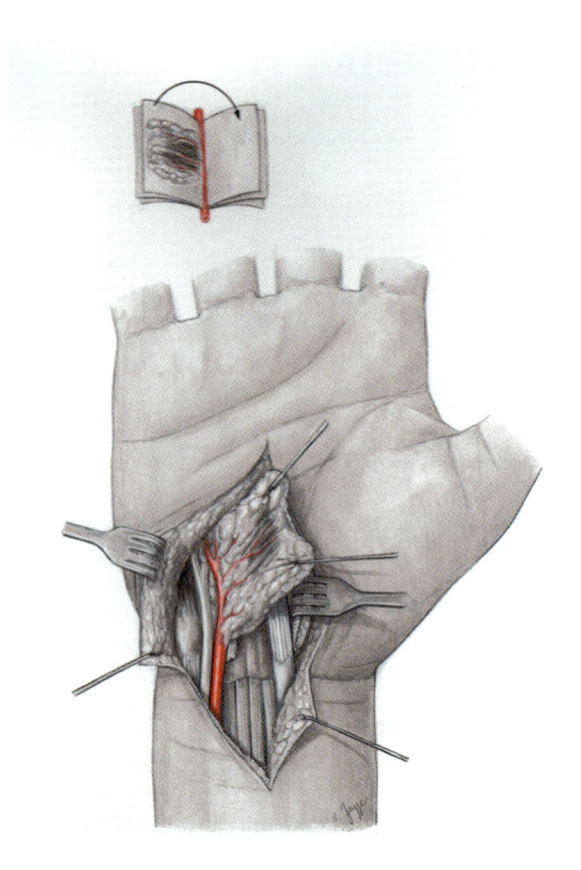

Fig. 41.3. Transposition of the flap. The hypothenar fat-pad flap is turned across like the page of a book and used to cover the median nerve (from [11] with permission)

Rehabilitation

Postoperatively, a palmar splint is applied for 1 week, with the wrist joint in the neutral position. Starting on the first postoperative day, physiotherapy to the wrist joint is necessary in order to maintain the free sliding movement of the newly embedded nerve.

Indications/Contraindications

In general, the first step in dealing with chronic wrist pain after open carpal tunnel release is to repeat the neurolysis and attempt to leave the nerve covered by any remaining loose tissue. If this is impossible, or has already been unsuccessfully attempted, a flap is the simplest way to restore mobility and cushion the nerve. The advantages and disadvantages of the available techniques must be carefully weighed against one another. Basically, the choice lies between a muscular and a fat-pad flap. We are against the use of synovial tissue from the flexor tendons to cover the nerve [15] because

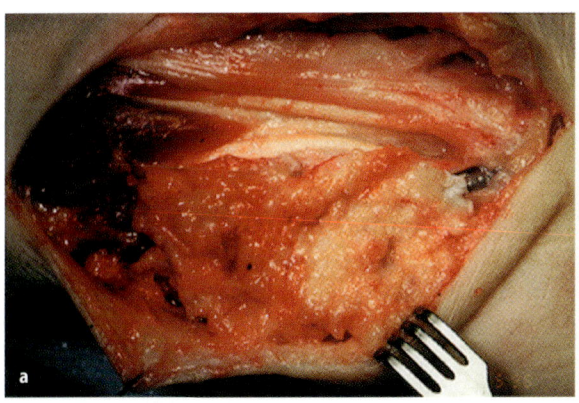

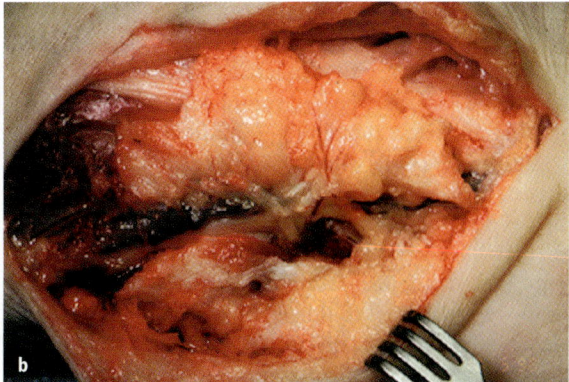

Fig. 41.4. Clinical case. **a** The hypothenar fat-pad flap has been harvested by the ulnar side. **b** The hypothenar fat-pad flap is rotated to cover the median nerve

of its known tendency to fibrose and form scar tissue. Muscle flaps [6–9, 17] have the advantage of bringing a good blood supply to a damaged median nerve and thus helping it to regenerate. If the muscles are fairly large – as with a flap from the abductor digiti minimi [9] or the pronator quadratus [7] – there is good cushioning against mechanical pressure from the hollow of the palm. The disadvantage, compared with the method described here, is the donor site defect which causes loss of muscle function, and the greater expenditure of tissue. Flaps involving smaller muscles (the lumbricals [6], or palmaris brevis [16]) are mostly suitable for smaller defects. In contrast to the muscle flaps, the fat-pad flaps are, because of the reduced likelihood of scar formation, particularly suitable for restoring a sliding sheath [10]. The hypothenar fat-pad flap presented here combines the advantage of a highly vascularized sliding tissue with that of requiring less tissue with an acceptable donor site defect. Our results have shown that in two thirds of the cases a significant reduction of the all-important pain syndrome is possible, and with this a considerable improvement in trophism, the ability to grip, and sensory input from the hand can be achieved. Complete freedom from pain cannot be obtained. This is expressed by the persistence of the Hoffmann-Tinel sign in the majority of cases, which indicates a continuing if somewhat reduced irritation of the median nerve. On the basis of these results we consider the hypothenar fat-pad flap to be suitable simply as a salvage procedure only in the presence of severe scarring of the median nerve at the wrist joint. It shows reproducible results which confirm those reported in the literature [16–19]. However, there is certainly no indication for a prophylactic hypothenar fat-pad flap as an additional part of open carpal tunnel release [21].

Results

Within 2 years we treated 11 patients (9 women and 2 men) with marked scar formation in the carpal tunnel which was seriously interfering with the motor and sensory function of the median nerve. The results were published in *Annales de la Chirurgie de la Main* [11]:

In 8 cases the right hand was affected, in 3 the left. The mean age at the time of operation was 50 years (28–82 years).

In the large majority of cases ($n=8$) the carpal tunnel had been previously released by open decompression. In 2 cases a chronic pain syndrome had appeared following infection of the flexor tendon sheath, and in a further case there had been a severe primary crush injury of the hand. In each case a repeated operation with renewed neurolysis of the median nerve had already been undertaken without success.

All patients suffered from a limitation of coarse and fine motor activity due to a severe chronic pain syndrome, and the function of the hand was impaired. This was accompanied by severe autonomic dysfunction, with increased sweating of the skin, sensitivity to cold, and a reduced skin temperature in comparison with the contralateral limb. It was possible to follow up 9 of the patients for periods of from 3 to 24 months after the operation.

Skin and Trophism

In 7 of the cases examined the preoperative thenar atrophy was already disappearing. In 5 of the 9 patients the scar was fully mature and free from irritation. Two other patients showed slight or marked hypertrophic scar formation. As a parameter revealing satisfactory trophism in the hand, normal secretion of sweat was present in 8 cases. In one case it was still reduced. The skin temperature showed no marked bilateral difference in 7 cases ("reduced" in 2 cases). The blood supply of the skin was assessed as "good" in 5 cases, "moderate" in 2 cases, and "poor" in 2 cases.

Pain and Sensibility

The marked sensitivity to touch in the region of the carpal tunnel roof disappeared completely in two thirds of the patients, the remaining 3 patients continued to complain of pain, which was nevertheless reduced. Static two-point discrimination was elicited from the tips of the thumb, index, and middle fingers. Improvement was recorded in 5 cases, 3 showed no change, and one showed a deterioration. Dysesthesia over the roof of the carpal tunnel could be elicited from all but 2 patients, while in the remaining 7 the Hoffmann-Tinel sign was still positive, but subjectively less marked than before the operation. The Phalen provocation test was negative in two thirds of the cases. In 6 patients no paresthesias were produced by full extension of the wrist joint [12].

Hand Function and Grip

Fist closure was completely present postoperatively in 6 cases and finger extension in 7. In 7 of the patients pinch grip and key grip with the index finger were possible. The remaining patients showed impairment of these functions.

Power grip, measured with the Jamar dynamometer, was significantly improved in 8 cases, and in 5 of these there had been an improvement of between 80% and 90% of the value on the contralateral side (50%–80% $n=1$, 30%–50% $n=3$).

Subjective Assessment of the Operative Result

Eight of the 9 patients would again have chosen to have the operation were the preoperative conditions to be repeated. Two assessed the result of the operation as "very good" and 3 as "good." A further 3 considered it to be "satisfactory" and one "poor."

Complications

In 3 cases the donor site defect caused problems to the patients: In 2 patients paresthesia, hypesthesia, or cold intolerance was reported for the hypothenar. A livid discoloration of the donor site was found in one patient.

Tips and Tricks

If chronic irritation of the median nerve due to scarring appears at the wrist joint, it is most often after open carpal tunnel release. In general this is referred to as a "recurrence" of the carpal tunnel syndrome [14–19]. In our opinion such a description is not correct, since it implies that the pain is still due to external compression of the nerve. In fact, however, operative exploration reveals that the trouble is caused by scarring of the nerve within the carpal tunnel, or outside and involving the flexor retinaculum. The reason for this is usually that the original incision for opening the carpal tunnel roof was placed too far radially. This leads to a division of the flexor retinaculum immediately palmar to the median nerve. After pressure in the tunnel has been released, the nerve can then become displaced toward the surface, and this leads to cicatrization with the connective tissue of the roof and, finally, to possible loss of freedom of longitudinal movement. Investigations on specimens [1–2] and MRT examination of living subjects [3, 4, 20] have revealed a physiological excursion of the median nerve in all planes and have thus emphasized the importance of free sliding. If the sheath of the nerve is scarred, movements of the wrist joint result in unconscious traction on the nerve and this produces pain [12].

We conclude from our results [11] that the appearance of such (frequently iatrogenic) conditions of chronic pain can and should be avoided. To avoid this attention must be paid to the supposedly simple opening of the roof of the carpal tunnel by cutting the retinaculum on the ulnar side of the median nerve. If the nerve shows a tendency to prolapse forwards even during the operation, we believe that a cast in extension of the wrist should be applied for 2 weeks.

References

1. Wilgis EFS, Murphy R (1984) The significance of longitudinal excursion in peripheral nerves. Hand Clin, 2, 761–766
2. Szabo RM, Bay BK, Sharkey NA, Gaut C (1994) Median nerve displacement through the carpal canal. J Hand Surg, 19A, 901–906
3. Nakamichi K, Tachibana S (1992) Transverse sliding of the median nerve beneath the flexor retinaculum. J Hand Surg, 17B, 213–216
4. Skie M, Zeiss J, Ebraheim NA, Jackson WT (1990) Carpal tunnel changes and median nerve compression during wrist flexion and extension seen by magnetic resonance imaging. J Hand Surg, 15A, 934–939
5. Wilhelm K, Putz R, Hierner R, Giunta R (1997) Lappenplastiken in der Handchirurgie – Anatomische Grundlagen, Operationstechniken und Differentialtherapie. Munich Vienna Baltimore, Urban & Schwarzenberg Verlag
6. Wilgis EFS (1984) Local muscle flaps in the hand anatomy as related to reconstructive surgery. Bull Hosp Jt Dis, 44, 552–557
7. Dellon AL, Mackinnon SE (1984) The pronator quadratus muscle flap. J Hand Surg, 9A, 423–427
8. Ulmer J, Buck-Gramcko D (1988) Der neurovaskulär gestielte Abductor digiti minimi-Muskellappen zur Abdeckung des N. medianus oder seiner Äste. Handchir, 20, 338–341
9. Milward TM, Scott WG, Kleinert HE (1977) The abductor digiti minimi muscle flap. Hand, 9, 82–85
10. Wintsch K, Helaly P (1986) Free flap of gliding tissue. J Reconstr Microsurg, 3, 143–151

11. Giunta R, Frank U, Lanz U (1998) The hypothenar fat-pad flap for reconstructive repair after scarring of the median nerve at the wrist joint. Ann Chir Main 17:107–112
11a. Stutz N, Gohritz A, van Schoonhoven J, Lanz U (2006) Revision surgery after carpal tunnelrelease – analysis of the pathology in 200 cases during a 2 year period. J Hand Surg (Br) 31:68–71
12. Hunter JM (1991) Recurrent carpal tunnel syndrome, epineural fibrous fixation, and traction neuropathy. Hand Clin, 7, 491–504
13. Cramer LM (1985) Local Fat Coverage for the Median Nerve. In: Lankford LL (ed.): Correspondence Newsletter for Hand Surgery, 35
14. Mathoulin CH, Bahm J (1996) Treatment of recalcitrant carpal tunnel syndrome with the hypothenar fat flap. J Hand Surg, 21B (Suppl), 12
15. Wulle CH (1996) The synovial flap as treatment of the recurrent carpal tunnel syndrome. Hand Clin, 12, 379–388
16. Rose EH, Norris MS, Kowalski TA et al. (1991) Palmaris brevis turnover flap as an adjunct to internal neurolysis of the chronically scarred median nerve in recurrent carpal tunnel syndrome. J Hand Surg, 16A, 191–201
17. Plancher KD, Idler RS, Lourie GM, Strickland JW (1996) Recalcitrant carpal tunnel syndrome. Hand Clin, 12, 337–349
18. Rose EH (1996) The use of the palmaris brevis flap in recurrent carpal tunnel syndrome. Hand Clin, 12, 389–395
19. Strickland JW, Idler RS, Lourie GM, Plancher KD (1996) The hypothenar fat pad flap for management of recalcitrant carpal tunnel syndrome. J Hand Surg, 21A, 840–848
20. Rath TH, Millesi H (1990) Das Gleitgewebe des N. medianus im Karpalkanal. Handchir Mikrochir Plast Chir, 22, 203–205
21. Jones SMG, Stuart PR, Stothard J (1997) Open carpal tunnel release – Does a vascularized hypothenar fat pad reduce wound tenderness? J Hand Surg, 22B, 758–760

42 Management of Recurrence of Carpal Tunnel Syndrome by Using the Abductor Digiti Minimi Muscle Flap to Cover the Median Nerve

J. H. Coert, A. L. Dellon

Introduction

Recurrent carpal tunnel syndrome is a clinical problem that continues to be a challenge in the hand surgery practice. It is a different entity with less favorable successes in diagnosis and treatment compared to primary carpal tunnel syndrome. Results after surgery depend on the strategy chosen to address the problem. A second, more ulnar incision has been propagated [1, 2]. Intraoperative findings consist of extensive fibrosis with nerve adhesions with flexor tendons or the roof of the tunnel. This implies that pathophysiology may be the lack of nerve gliding as well as compression of the nerve. Besides neurolysis it might be worthwhile bringing vascularized tissue to the bed of the median nerve [3].

To create a barrier against adhesions we have several options, that be summoned as a so-called reconstructive ladder: local tissue, distant and pedicled tissue (e.g., posterior interosseous artery flap, reversed radial forearm flap) and free vascularized tissue.

Examples of treatment of recurrent carpal tunnel syndrome with local tissue are the so-called palmaris brevis turnover flap [4], the pedicled hypothenar fat flap [5–8], the synovial flap [9], and the abductor digiti minimi flap [10]. Besides autologous tissue allogenic, absorbable barriers have been used to reduce to recurrence rate [11].

A recent study compared the coverage of the median with free and pedicled flaps. They concluded that local vascularized tissue, preferably ulnar-based fat flap, may be worthwhile [12]. This chapter presents our experience with the abductor digiti minimi muscle flap as alternative pedicled, local flap.

Surgical Approach and Example Cases

The incision is planned ulnar to previous standard incision (usually between the third and fourth metacarpal) (Fig. 42.1). In this fashion the scarred area will be avoided. Next an external neurolysis is performed using adequate magnification (Fig. 42.2). The abductor digiti minimi (ADM) muscle is harvested through lazy-S incision over the hypothenar (Fig. 42.3). The muscle is

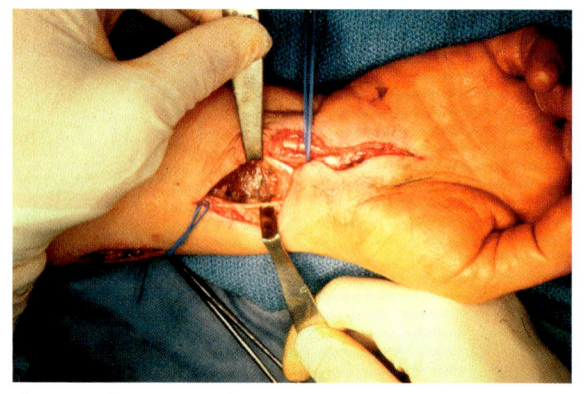

Fig. 42.1. The incision ulnar to old incision

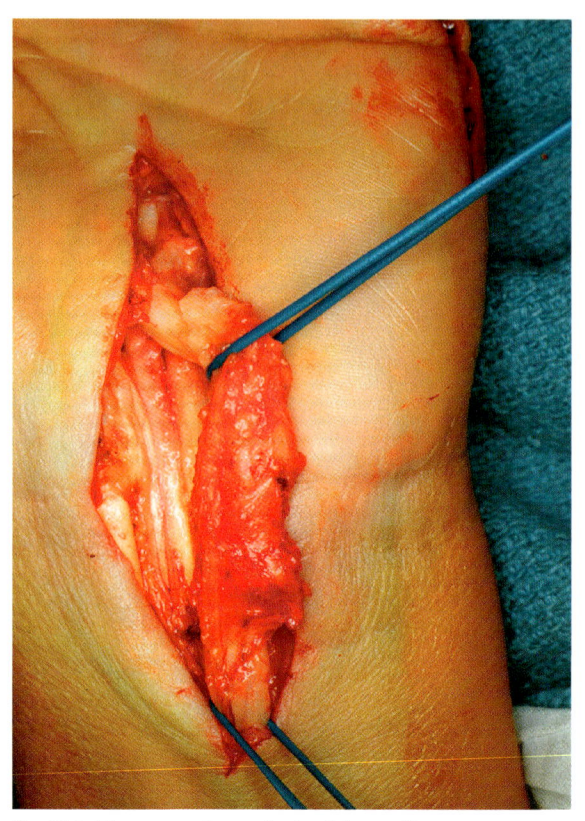

Fig. 42.2. The external neurolysis of the median nerve

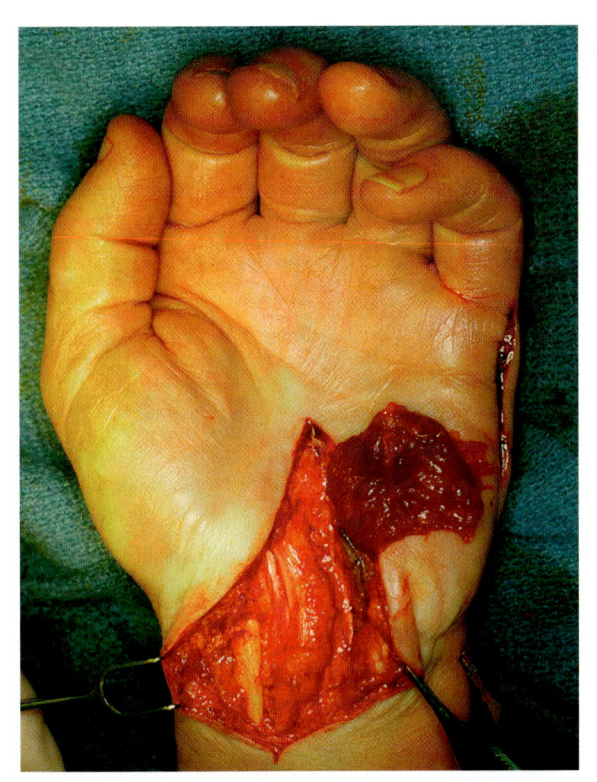

Fig. 42.3. The tunneling of the ADM flap

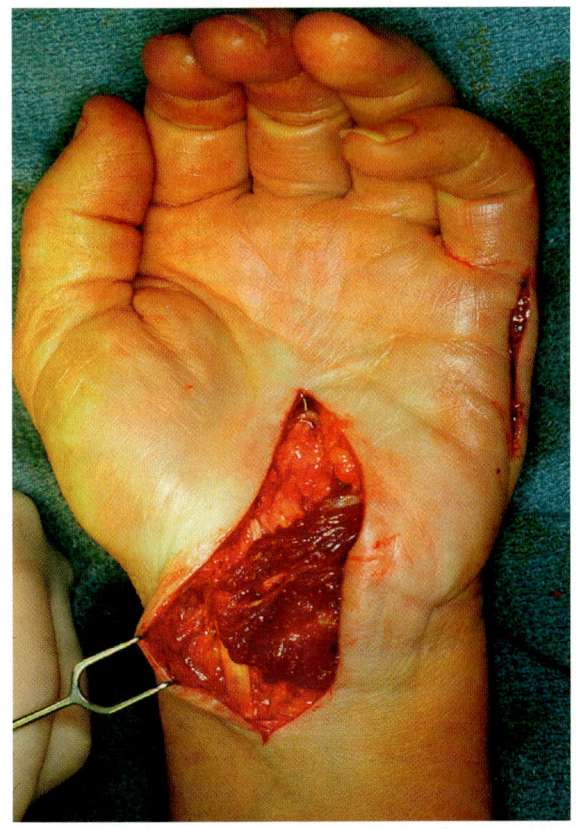

Fig. 42.4. The adequate reach of the flap, the mobilization of radial and ulnar skin, and the fixation to the flexor carpi radialis

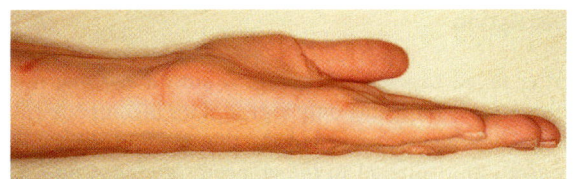

Fig. 42.5. The acceptable scar on the hypothenar

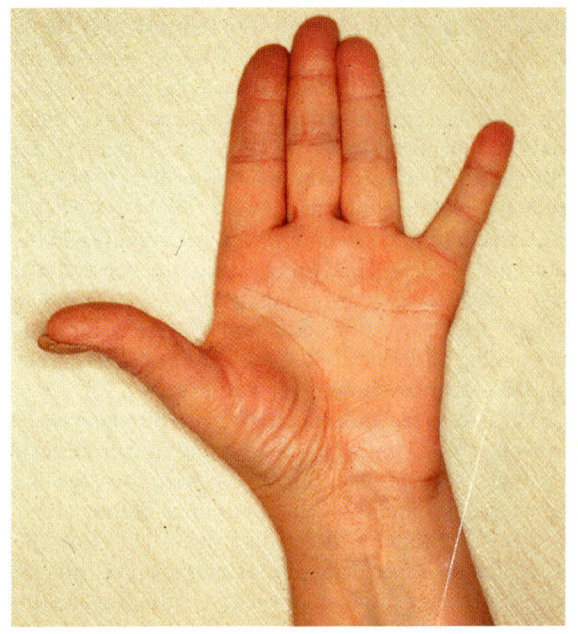

Fig. 42.6. The intact abduction of the little finger after harvesting the flap

elevated from distal to proximal. To allow adequate mobilization and to prevent tethering, the insertion on the pisiform bone is taken down. To accommodate the flap and to prevent compression, the radial and ulnar skin are undermined. The ADM flap will reach proximal to the wrist crease. It is sutured to the flexor carpi radialis (Fig. 42.4).

In our series, all of the 12 patients were incapacitated by persistent or recurrent pain in the palmar aspect of the hand and wrist. By employing an ADM muscle flap, successful relief of pain was aided. It should be emphasized that the first step in treating recurrent carpal tunnel syndrome should be a thorough microsurgical neurolysis (including internal neurolysis) with simple skin closure. Early range of motion should commence for the fingers on the first and the wrist at the eighth postoperative day. The muscle flap is only utilized as a so-called salvage procedure.

Eleven of the 12 patients (92%) achieved good to excellent results in terms of relief of pain, plus either return to their previous job or vocational rehabilitation. Donor-site morbidity was minimal with an acceptable scar on the hypothenar and with intact abduction of the little finger (Figs. 42.5, 42.6).

Discussion

After failed carpal tunnel surgery simply redoing the decompression seems only logical if an incomplete release has been performed. If the median nerve is scarred and adhered to the adjacent tendons and the transverse carpal ligament, creating a barrier between the nerve and its surrounding structures after neurolysis is indicated. Interposing well vascularized tissue should reduce scarring around the nerve, decrease direct pressure on the nerve, and will facilitate gliding when the wrist moves. Local muscle flaps (e.g., palmaris brevis turnover flap [4], abductor digiti minimi flap [10]) will fulfill these requirements. Local fat flaps (e.g., pedicled hypothenar fat flap [5–8]) are not as well vascularized and may give more scarring resulting in diminished excursion and protection of the nerve. Local fascial flaps (e.g., synovial flap [9]) have the advantage of good vascularization and a smooth surface facilitating gliding of the nerve, but they are thin and do not provide adequate padding for the nerve.

The abductor digiti minimi flap has also been used to treat wound dehiscence after carpal tunnel surgery, coverage of defects after tumor resection, coverage of a damaged median nerves and neuromas of the palmar cutaneous branch of the median nerve [13–18]. The ADM flap is superior to the palmaris brevis muscle flap, because of the easy dissection, sufficient muscle volume, and excellent vascularization.

References

1. Dellon AL, Chang BW (1992) An alternative incision for approaching recurrent median nerve compression: at the wrist. Plast Reconstr Surg 89(3):576–8
2. B, Dellon AL (1993) Surgical management of recurrent carpal tunnel syndrome. J Hand Surg [Br] 18(4):467–70
3. Duclos L, Sokolow C (1998) Management of true recurrent carpal tunnel syndrome: is it worthwhile to bring vascularized tissue? Chir Main. 17(2):113–7; discussion 118
4. Rose EH, Norris MS, Kowalski TA et al. (1991) Palmaris brevis turnover flap as an adjunct to internal neurolysis of the chronically scarred median nerve in recurrent carpal tunnel syndrome. J Hand Surg [Am]. 16(2):191–201
5. Mathoulin C, Bahm J, Roukoz S (2000) Pedicled hypothenar fat flap for median nerve coverage in recalcitrant carpal tunnel syndrome. Hand Surg 5(1):33–40
6. De Smet L, Vandeputte G (2002) Pedicled fat flap coverage of the median nerve after failed carpal tunnel decompression. J Hand Surg [Br] 27(4):350–3
7. Frank U, Giunta R, Krimmer H, Lanz U (1999) Relocation of the median nerve after scarring along the carpal tunnel with hypothenar fatty tissue flap-plasty. Handchir Mikrochir Plast Chir 31(5):317–22
8. Strickland JW, Idler RS, Lourie GM, Plancher KD (1996) The hypothenar fat pad flap for management of recalcitrant carpal tunnel syndrome. J Hand Surg [Am] 21(5): 840–8
9. Wulle C (1996) The synovial flap as treatment of the recurrent carpal tunnel syndrome. Hand Clin 12(2): 379–88
10. Spokevicius S, Kleinert HE (1996) The abductor digiti minimi flap: its use in revision carpal tunnel surgery. Hand Clin 12(2):351–5.
11. Loick J, Joosten U, Lucke R (1997) Implantation of oxidized, regenerated cellulose for prevention of recurrence in surgical therapy of carpal tunnel syndrome. Handchir Mikrochir Plast Chir 29(4):209–13
12. Dahlin LB, Lekholm C, Kardum P, Holmberg J (2002) Coverage of the median nerve with free and pedicled flaps for the treatment of recurrent severe carpal tunnel syndrome. Scand J Plast Reconstr Surg Hand Surg 36(3):172–6
13. Milward TM, Stott WG, Kleinert HE (1977) The abductor digiti minimi muscle flap. Hand 9(1):82–5
14. Reisman NR, Dellon AL (1983) The abductor digiti minimi muscle flap: a salvage technique for palmar wrist pain. Plast Reconstr Surg 72, 6: 859–65
15. Ulmer J, Buck-Gramcko D (1988) The neurovascular pedicled abductor digiti minimi muscle flap for covering the median nerve or its branches. Handchir Mikrochir Plast Chir 20(6):338–41
16. Leslie BM, Ruby LK (1988) Coverage of a carpal tunnel wound dehiscence with the abductor digiti minimi muscle flap. J Hand Surg [Am] 13(1):36–9
17. Evans GR, Dellon AL (1994) Implantation of the palmar cutaneous branch of the median nerve into the pronator quadratus for treatment of painful neuroma. J Hand Surg [Am] 19(2):203–6
18. Bloom RJ, Kane AJ, Maxwell R (1997) The abductor digiti minimi flap: a case report and review. Aust N Z J Surg 67(8):582–3

Protection of the Median Nerve with the Pronator Quadratus and Palmaris Brevis Muscle Flaps

B. Battiston, P. Tos, R. Adani

Introduction

Patients who have a residual lesion of the median nerve at the level of the wrist despite a surgical decompression, or even due to the surgery itself, pose a difficult problem, i.e., freeing the nerve anew while also improving its local vascularization.

Therefore, the surgeon is prompted to take advantage of local flaps, that are able not only to offer a mechanical protection against the formation of new scar tissue, but also to provide further vascular support.

Literature reports the use of various local flaps to this aim, of which the pronator quadratus muscle flap [2] and the palmaris brevis [9] seem to be able to offer very good results. Indeed, as both flaps may be transferred along with their own innervation, they are able to inhibit the formation of new neuromas as described by some authors [3], in as much as the nerve is surrounded by innervated muscle.

However, if the nerve has not been treated in the correct manner, including the use of such procedures as freeing it from the scar, carrying out an accurate neurolysis and resecting the neuroma and grafting if required, then the transposition of these muscles will not suffice to resolve a condition of hyperalgesia.

The pronator quadratus muscle flap may be used to cover lesions up to the wrist flexion fold or a more proximal lesion [4], while the palmaris brevis may be used more distally.

Pronator Quadratus Muscle Flap

Basic Anatomy

The pronator quadratus muscle is a transverse muscle that forms part of the deep anterior compartment of the forearm and is taut between the radius and the ulna, in the distal quarter.

This muscle is always thicker on the radius side and usually inserts into the radius and ulna at the same level. The vascularity of this muscle derives mainly from the anterior interosseous artery that reaches the proximal border of the muscle about 5 cm from the radiocarpal joint, even if it does also receive support from some of the arterial radial and ulnar branches which are, in fact, periosteal muscle branches. At insertion into the muscle, the anterior interosseous artery is about 2 mm [5] and is accompanied by two venae comitantes that guarantee the flow out from the muscle itself (Fig. 43.1a). This muscle is innervated by a branch of

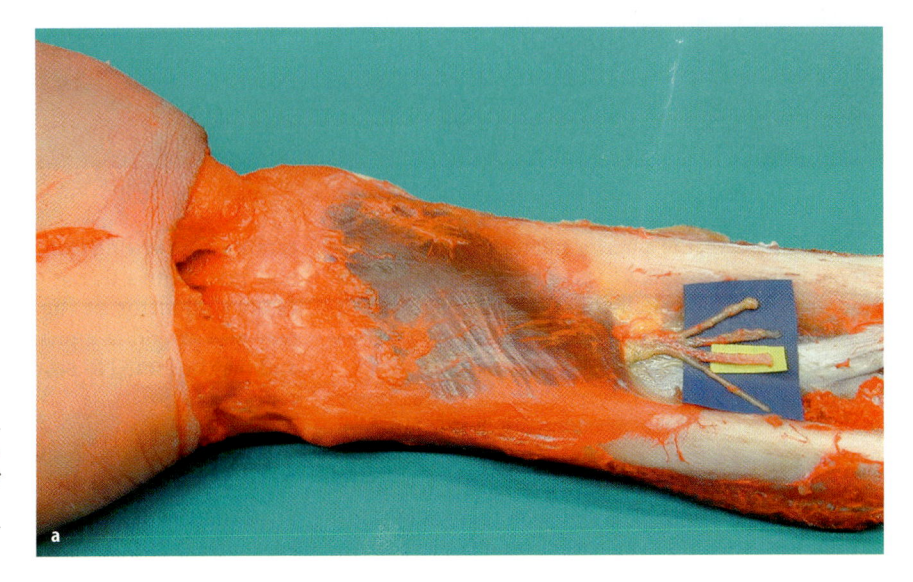

Fig. 43.1. a The pronator quadratus muscle is supported by a neuro-vascular pedicle composed by the anterior interosseous artery, two venae comitantes and the anterior interosseous nerve

328 V Complications

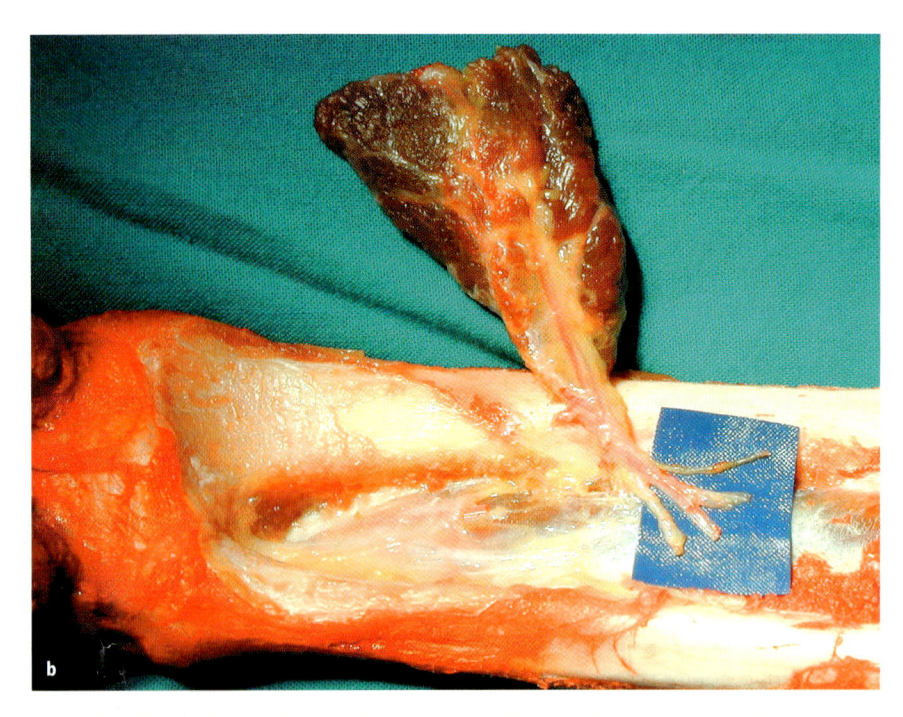

Fig. 43.1. b The pronator quadratus is raised as an island flap on its neurovascular bundle

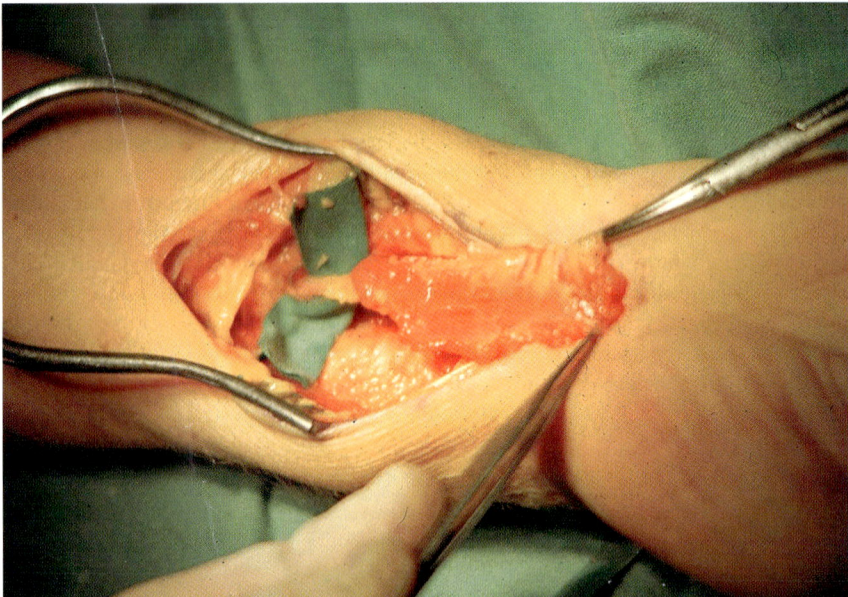

Fig. 43.2. The pedicle may be freed very proximally so as to permit the muscle to be moved up to a distance of 2 cm

the median nerve, the anterior interosseous nerve. The pronator quadratus muscle may be elevated as an island flap, about 7–8 cm long [2], pivoted on its neurovascular pedicle (anterior interosseous nerve and vessels) (Fig. 43.1b).

In very rare instances, even when the radius is normal, the absence of the pronator quadratus has been noted [6]. It is occasionally laminated into two or more layers consisting of fasciculi running in different directions. It may be continued down on the carpus or metacarpus, in some cases as an ulnar carpal fasciculus. Aberrant fibers arising from the distal edge of the muscle may insert into a thenar muscle mass and act as an accessory adductor of the thumb. Pronator quadratus may also extend in a proximal direction on the radius and may be joined to pronator teres or to a flexor carpi radialis brevis.

Surgical Technique

The pronator quadratus muscle and its pedicle can be approached through an anterior longitudinal incision in the distal third of the forearm. This incision may be carried out along any pre-existing scar and goes from the distal wrist flexion fold, in a proximal direction for about 12 cams. The muscle can then be accessed between the flexor carpi radialis tendon laterally and the palmaris gracilis medially. In this way access can be obtained by localizing the interval between the flexor digitorum profundus and flexor carpi ulnaris. Dissection starts from the distal border, taking care to tie all the vascular branches going to the deep palmar arch. The muscle can then be easily lifted on the ulnar side thereby exposing the neuro-vascular pedicle. The same procedure is carried out, with a little more difficulty, at its insertion border on the radius. Its pedicle is then freed as proximally as possible so as to permit the muscle to be moved up to a distance of 2 cm (Fig. 43.2). Small incisions are made along the proximal radius margin so as to slant the muscle slightly distal in order to access the wrist area more easily.

Advantages

The dissection of this flap is extremely simple, with an easily accessible valid vascularized pedicle at one's disposal. The pronator quadratus is then "transformed" into an island flap that may be rotated amply. The use of this flap does not compromise the pronation and/or function of the forearm in any way.

Disadvantages

The pronator quadratus muscle flap allows only for a coverage of areas involving the median nerve close to the wrist flexor fold and not a more distal application.

Palmaris Brevis Muscular Flap

Basic Anatomy

The palmaris brevis is a thin trapezoidal muscle which lies superficially subcutaneous on the ulnar side of the palm of the hand. It inserts into the flexor retinaculum and the margin of the central palmar aponeurosis and ends in the dermis on the ulnar side of the hand, superficially to the ulnar nerve and artery, thus forming part of the roof of Guyon's canal. Although this muscle is of little significance, it is absent in only 2% of the population [6] and is responsible for tensing the palm of the hand, deepening the groove of the palm, and, therefore, enhancing grip. Two fascicles can be observed in this muscle, each one with its own individual nerve/vascular support [9]. The two supporting arterial branches usually originate from the deep volar branch of the ulnar artery close to the bifurcation that starts at the deep palmar arch. The innervation takes place thanks to a branch that comes directly from the ulnar nerve and one that comes from the IV intermetacarpal sensitive nerve. Indeed, strange as it may seem, the motor control is governed by a branch that is considered, in general, to be purely a sensitive branch.

Surgical Technique

The incision is made parallel to the thenar eminence flexion fold and becomes transverse proximally when reaching the wrist flexion fold. When lifting the skin flap, care must be taken to remain just below the dermis in order to avoid damage to the cutaneous branches of the median nerve in the palm. After turning the skin flap onto the ulnar side of the wrist, the muscle is evident. The dissection is then started from this side dividing its insertions from the hypothenar dermis (Fig. 43.3a–d). At this point care must be taken not to damage the neurovascular ulnar bundle underneath. The muscle is, therefore, further isolated with a proximal/distal transversal incision, maintaining only the radial connections at the palmar aponeurosis, so as to be able to turn over the flap. This is made possible by separating the dorsal bundle from the underlying hypothenar muscles. Once the dissection has been completed, the muscle can be turned over and sutured to the remaining radials of the transverse carpal ligament.

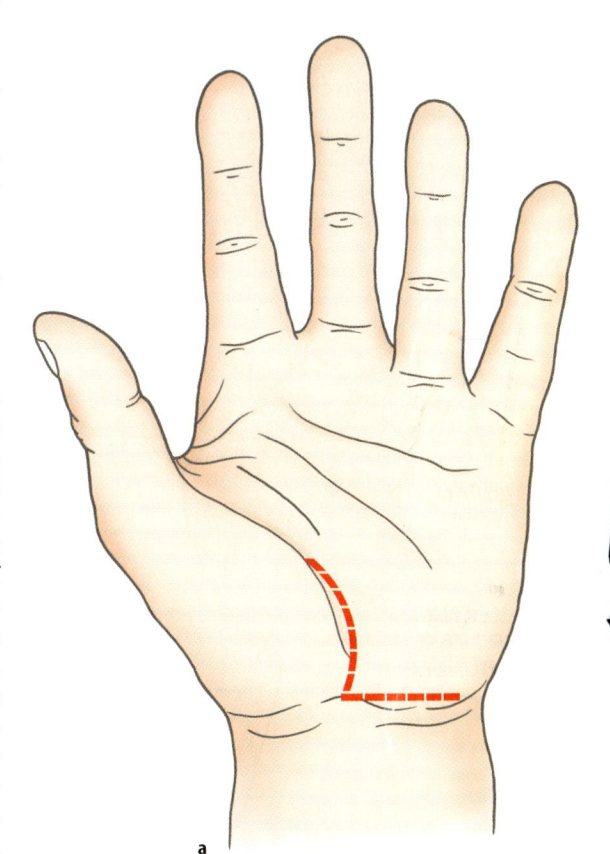

Fig. 43.3. Design of the skin incision (**a**)

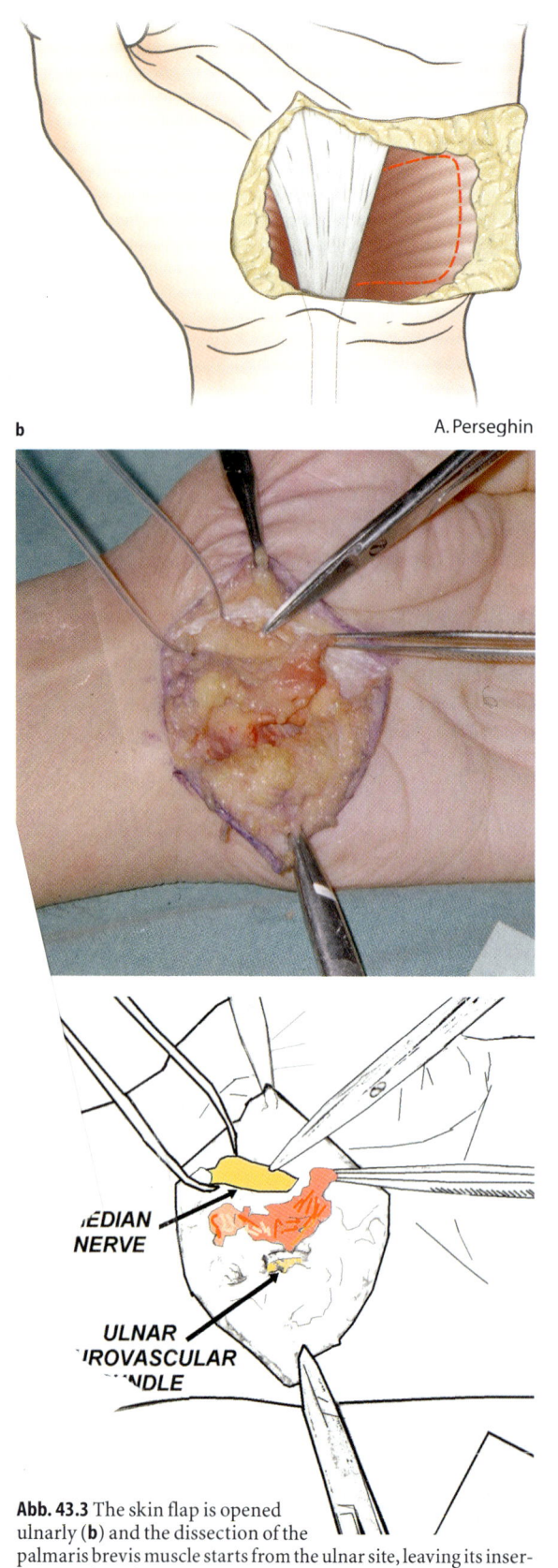

Fig. 43.4. The muscle flap is turned over as a book page to cover the median nerve (**a**). Scheme and vascular axis (**b**)

In this way the median nerve, that has been freed from its "old scar tissue," can be covered (Fig. 43.4a, b).

Advantages

One of the main advantages of the use of this technique is the extreme proximity of the muscle to the area where the surgical approach is to be made, thus making it possible to turn the flap over without extensive dissection or the need for a more complex surgery involving the use of free flaps, etc. When harvesting this flap no motor deficit is created. Although without its roof, the ulnar neuro-vascular bundle is well protected by the thick layer of the subcutaneous tissue that remains.

Abb. 43.3 The skin flap is opened ulnarly (**b**) and the dissection of the palmaris brevis muscle starts from the ulnar site, leaving its insertions to the palmaris aponeurosis intact at the radial site (**c, d**)

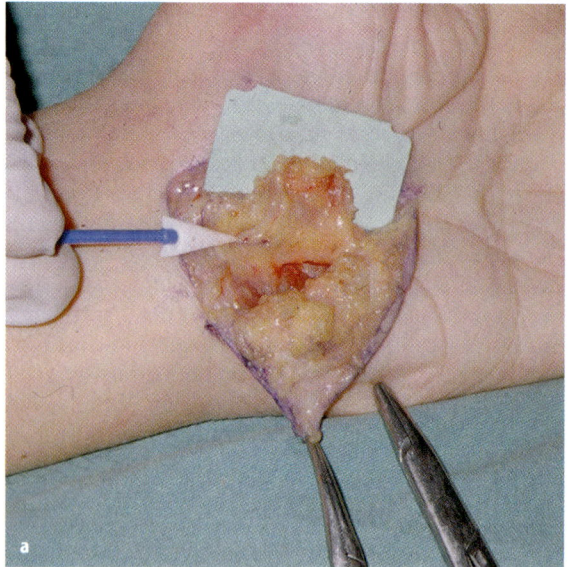

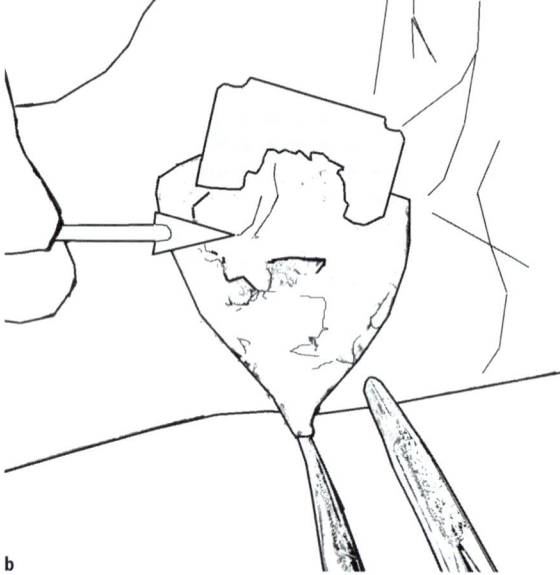

Disadvantages

As the palmaris brevis muscle is thin, it requires a delicate resectioning technique so as to conserve it without damage. Moreover, although its small dimensions do allow it to be placed between the median nerve and the scar tissue, it is not able to protect large lesions of the nerve itself.

Discussion

The literature reports studies by various authors [7] which have clearly demonstrated that the presence of a large postsurgical scar may interfere not only mechanically with the peripheral nerve trunks, thus causing compression, but may also have a biological effect resulting in an alteration of the intraneural microcirculation. Although a good neurolysis is able to resolve the mechanical compression, it cannot completely restore problems of local circulation. Therefore, when revision surgery is carried out on the median nerve at the wrist utilizing a protective flap, it should be of use not only from a mechanical point of view, but also should be able to improve local vascularization.

The use of muscular flaps rich in vascularization can be of great help when this is an objective, as reported by many authors [7, 9]. Indeed, it has been demonstrated experimentally that no neuromas develop when an injured nerve is surrounded by innervated muscles [8]. A so-called cellular cap is formed at the muscle-nerve interface and less connective tissue grows inside the nerve itself. This would explain the extensive successful use of muscular flaps described in literature, when they are placed between the injured nerve and the overlying scar tissue [10].

As to the pronator quadratus flap, we used it in the last 5 years in 9 patients [1] with a partial or total injury of the median nerve leading to a painful incontinuity neuroma. All patients except 1 had pain relief and in 4 patients there was also improvement of sensory function (Fig. 43.5a–d).

Our experience has led us to the conclusion that, although there is a choice of local flaps available to this aim, the use of pronator quadratus muscle flap offers the best results when dealing with this kind of operative scar and its "complications" in the wrist flexor fold region. When dealing with a more distal scar, the palmaris brevis muscular flap is a valid solution. It is easy to harvest and leaves no residual functional damage,

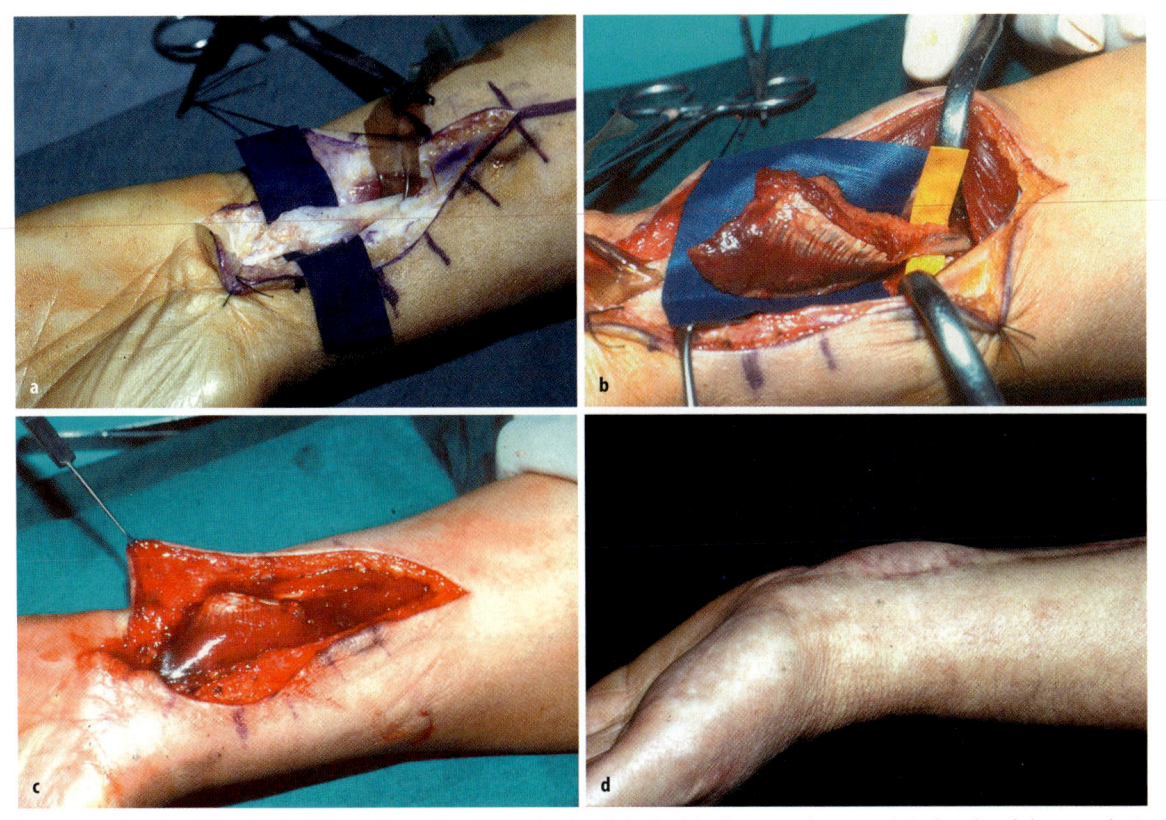

Fig. 43.5. a Painful median nerve incontinuity neuroma at the distal third of the forearm: the nerve is isolated and the neurolysis started. **b** The pronator quadratus muscle flap is raised. **c** The neurolysed median nerve is protected with the muscle flap. **d** Final clinical result with complete pain disappearance and complete regained mobility

while the use of the equally adequate abductor digiti minimi flap results in a reduced abduction of the small finger and loss of some gripping of the hand.

References

1. Adani R, Tarallo L, Battiston B, Marcoccio I (2002) Management of neuromas in continuity of the median nerve with the pronator quadratus muscle flap. Annals of Plast Surg 48:35–40
2. Dellon AL, MacKinnon SE (1984) The pronator quadratus muscle flap. J Hand Surg [Am], 3: 423–427
3. Dellon AL, MacKinnon SE, Pestronk A (1984) Implantation of sensory nerve into muscle: preliminary clinical and experimental observations on neuroma formation. Annals of Plast Surg, 12: 30–40
4. Evans GRD, Dellon AL (1994) Implantation of the palmar cutaneous branch of the median nerve into the pronator quadratus for tretment of painful neuroma. J Hand Surg 19A: 203–206
5. Fontaine C, Millot F, Blancke D, Mestdagh H (1992) Anatomic basis of pronator quadratus flap. Surg Radiol Anat, 14: 295–299
6. Le Double AF (1897) Traitè des variations du systeme musculaire de l'homme. Paris, Reinwald, 170–171
7. MacKinnon SE, Dellon AL (1988) Surgery of the peripheral nerve. Stuttgart-NewYork, George Thieme Verlag
8. MacKinnon SE, Dellon AL, Hudson AR, Hunter DA (1985) Alteration of neuroma formation by manipulation of its microenvironment. Plast Reconstr Surg, 76, 345–352
9. Rose EH, et al. (1991) Palmaris brevis turnover flap as an adjunct to internal neurolysis of the chronically scarred median nerve in recurrent carpal tunnel syndrome. J Hand Surg [Am], 16: 191–200
10. Wilgis EFS (1984) Local muscle flaps in the hand. Anatomy as related to reconstructive surgery. Bull Hosp J Dis Orthop Inst, 44, 552–557

Vein Wrapping of the Median Nerve

D.G. Sotereanos, N.A. Darlis

Introduction

Carpal tunnel syndrome is the most common entrapment neuropathy of the upper extremity with an incidence of 99 per 100,000 [1]. Surgical decompression by releasing the flexor retinaculum is the established treatment for this syndrome. Although surgical decompression is generally considered effective, recurrence of symptoms is not uncommon. Rates of treatment failures or recurrence have been reported to be as high as 32% [2–9]. There are several reasons for persisting or recurrent pain following surgical decompression; incomplete release, injury to the nerve trunk or its branches resulting in neuromas, reflex sympathetic dystrophy, and scarring of an intact nerve. Incomplete release can be addressed with repeated decompression; neuromas are rare and are usually treated with neurolysis, resection, and possibly grafting, and for reflex sympathetic dystrophy treatment must be individualized. Scarring of the nerve is by far the most difficult condition to treat since attempts at repeated decompression and internal neurolysis further enhance scar tissue formation and recurrence is inevitable [10].

Pain resulting from postoperative epineural scarring is caused by mechanical constriction, nerve ischemia, and impairment of nerve gliding on the adjacent tissues. Intraneural scarring also develops and aggravates symptoms. The term "traction neuropathy" was coined to describe the resultant chronic neuropathy [4]. Although this term is clinically relevant (pain is usually exacerbated with motion of the adjacent joints), it describes only one of the mechanisms (lack of gliding) that lead to pain.

The treatment of "traction neuropathy" would ideally be to transfer the affected nerve segment to a new well-vascularized bed but the median nerve is restricted at the carpal tunnel in a confined space between tendons and the carpal bones. In this setting most investigators agree that soft tissue coverage is necessary to prevent this phenomenon and several options have been suggested [11–15] and are discussed in detail in other chapters. The hypothenar fat pad flap can produce good results and is uncomplicated in most cases [11]. Pedicle or free flaps, including the groin flap, lateral arm flap, and posterior interosseous flap, provide excellent protection of the nerve, but the technique is complex and the result is not always satisfying [11, 12]. Small local flaps, such as the abductor digiti minimi, the palmaris brevis, and the pronator quadratus, also have been used [13, 14]. The dissection of these flaps, however, is not always easy; nerve coverage is sometimes inadequate, and skin closure problems may occur. A more conservative approach using implanted nerve stimulators or anesthetic reservoirs [16, 17] has failed to consistently produce good results and was associated with complications.

Another approach to this problem is to wrap the affected nerve segment with a substance that would act as a barrier to scar formation. Several materials have been used for inhibition of adhesion formation including gelatin, fascia, polyglactin, and silicone sheets or tubes. Most of these were tried in the nerve repair setting to prevent adhesion formation but their efficacy in preventing adhesion recurrence is controversial.

The first clinical report of vein wrapping of a scarred peripheral nerve is attributed to Masear [18]. Subsequent reports in the early 1990s [12–19] discussed the clinical applications of both autograft and glutaraldehyde-preserved allograft vein wrapping and the experimental confirmation of these clinical observations followed.

Basic Science

The effect of wrapping scarred nerves with autogenous vein graft was studied by our group in the late 1990s [22, 23] in an experimental chronic nerve compression model. The sciatic nerve of rats was first constricted with a silicone tube and nerve deficits were confirmed at 8 months. Animals were then randomly allocated in a vein wrapping or a control group. Functionally (using the sciatic function index, SFI), the sciatic nerves in the vein-wrapped group showed greater improvement than those in the non-vein-wrapped group. In electrophysiologic testing the latency was significantly shorter in the vein-wrapped group. Histologic evaluation showed marked nerve degeneration and scar tissue formation around the nerves in the non-vein-wrapped group but not in the vein-wrapped group. These studies showed that vein wrapping in a chronic nerve compression model could improve the functional recovery of the nerve and prevent scar in-growth.

Clinical observations from re-exploration of vein grafted nerves further support this conclusion. Masear and Colgin [21] found no significant scarring external to allograft umbilical vein and thus believed that the barrier to scar is external to the vein graft. In a re-exploration of an autogenous vein grafted ulnar nerve [24], we found very few adhesions between the adventitia of the vein and surrounding tissues and no adhesions between the intimal surface of the vein and the ulnar nerve. In a histopathologic analysis Campbell et al. [25] showed that autogenous saphenous vein wrapping of the tibial nerve in the setting of recalcitrant tarsal tunnel syndrome effectively protected the nerve from intrinsic and extrinsic scar formation because there was no fibrous reaction noted within or around the wrapped nerve microscopically. In a biopsy taken from a vein-wrapped median nerve [26], we found neovascularization of the vein graft and structural transformation of the vein endothelium which was noted to be hyperproliferative and elevated into multiple papillary projections. Thus the vein was considered live tissue rather than an interposition.

Although good clinical results have been reported with the use of allograft vein wrapping [19, 21], Ruch et al. [27] in an animal study using rats compared the effect of femoral vein autograft with a glutaraldehyde-preserved allograft and found a significant increase in inflammatory cells and scar tissue associated with the allograft. It seems that the difference between autograft and allograft vein wrapping is that an autologous vein graft creates fewer adhesions between the vein and the nerve compared with a vein allograft. If allograft vein adheres to the nerve, the gliding between the nerve and vein might be impaired, which may possibly have a negative effect on recovery.

In summary, although the exact mechanism of both extrinsic and intrinsic scar prevention with this technique are still unclear, recent basic research has shown that prevention of epineurial adhesions, preservation or restoration of intrinsic epineurial vascularity, and formation of a gliding surface between the nerve and the surrounding tissues contribute to the good clinical results. It is hypothesized that locally produced bioactive molecules could play a significant role in the structural changes observed [26].

Preoperative Assessment

Patients usually present with recurrent symptoms after an adequate primary decompression. The history of initial temporary relief after the primary decompression or a subsequent neurolysis is highly indicative of scar formation. Their complaints are usually that of pain worsening with activities and paresthesias. Severe pain (5 or above in a visual analogue scale) is their chief complaint. Numbness is also an important patient concern.

A positive percussion test over the carpal tunnel is the rule and in our experience most of the patients have abnormal static two-point discrimination. Muscular atrophies are not very common and when present they are indicative of more severe intrinsic scarring of the nerve. Electrodiagnostic testing often shows decreased electrical amplitude and sensory conduction after stimulation of the median nerve; muscle denervation is seen less often. It should be noted that median nerve scarring can be present even with normal two-point discrimination and electrodiagnostic findings, but in that setting worker's compensation and litigation issues should be carefully taken into consideration. Cases involved in litigation must be carefully evaluated.

An initial period of nonoperative treatment to reduce pain (especially in patients without a measurable sensory or motor deficit) is advisable. This can include splinting, injections, desensitization, scar massage, and/or nerve stimulation. Narcotic analgesics are avoided since these patients can easily become dependent.

The primary indication for vein wrapping is significant epineurial scarring and although it can be suspected preoperatively, it is verified intraoperatively. We usually reserve vein wrapping for the multiply operated patients and the ones with unrelenting symptoms following carpal tunnel release. Patients who present for their first reoperation and have moderate pain can be effectively treated with other soft tissue coverage procedures and the hypothenar fat flap is our choice in such instances.

Operative Technique

General anesthesia is used for this procedure because of the need to have two operating fields (in the upper extremity and in the lower extremity). The incision used for the primary procedure or the revisions is usually used and it is slightly extended both proximally and distally. The median nerve should be identified in healthy tissues both proximally and distally and then dissected towards the scarred section. Dissection is painstaking and is performed under loop magnification. Internal neurolysis under the operating microscope is performed as necessary. Indications for internal neurolysis included severe compression and thinning of the nerve, lack of epineurial vascularity, and muscle wasting.

The ipsilateral or contralateral lower extremity is used for harvesting of the greater saphenous vein. The required length of the vein is approximately four times the scarred length of the nerve. The length taken is usually 25–30 cm. The position of the great saphenous vein can be usually palpated and is marked on the skin prior to tourniquet inflation. An incision is made 1 cm anterior to the medial malleolus and the greater saphenous vein is identified. Care is taken not to injure branches of the saphenous nerve. The vein is ligated distally and a small longitudinal phlebotomy is made. A vein stripper is introduced through the phlebotomy and is advanced proximally to the predetermined length. A second 1-cm incision is made over the stripper proximally; the vein is ligated and cut and the graft is retrieved by pulling the stripper (Fig. 44.1). Alternatively, the vein can be harvested through a continuous incision or interrupted incisions and dissection without the use of a vein stripper.

After the saphenous vein is harvested, it is incised and opened longitudinally (Fig. 44.2). The adventitia side of the vein graft is marked with a marking pen longitudinally as it is important that the intimal side of the graft comes in contact with the scarred nerve. One of the ends of the vein graft is tacked distal to the scarred portion of the nerve on a tissue that is not mobile, with the intima against the nerve, using a 7-0 or 8-0 nylon stitch. The wrapping proceeds circumferentially as described by Masear et al. [18] from distal to proximal, while care is taken not to make the wrap too snug and thus constrict the nerve (Fig. 44.2). After each complete circle on the nerve, the vein is stabilized with a loose 7-0 or 8-0 nylon stitch to the adjacent ring of vein (Figs. 44.2, 44.3). If enough vein graft length has been obtained, each loop of the vein graft around the nerve can partially overlap the previous loop. Ensuring that the intima side is apposed to the nerve after each loop is important. The other end of the vein graft is tacked proximal to the scarred segment of the nerve on unscarred tissue (Fig. 44.4). The coverage of the scarred nerve segment must be complete and must extend slightly to an unscarred segment to prevent recurrent compression.

Fig. 44.1. Harvesting of the greater saphenous vein in the lower extremity using two incisions and a vein stripper

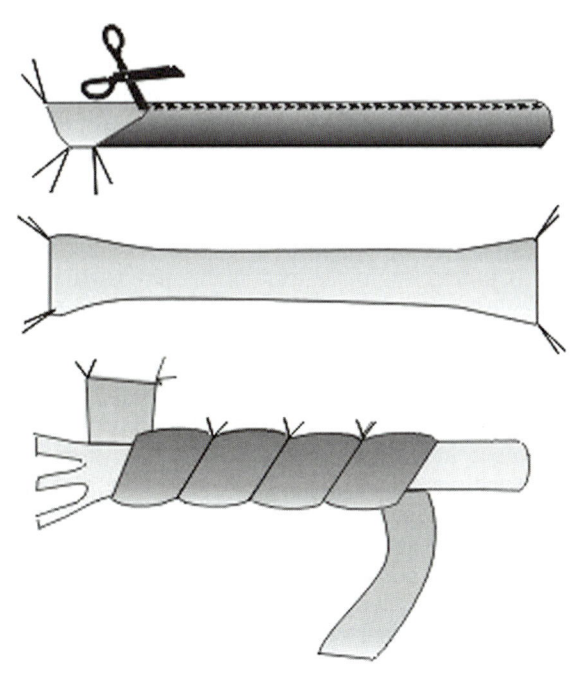

Fig. 44.2. The technique used for vein wrapping of the median nerve. The saphenous vein is split longitudinally, and is opened to form a rectangle. The saphenous vein is then wrapped around the scarred portion of the nerve in a spiral pattern with its intima on the surface of the nerve

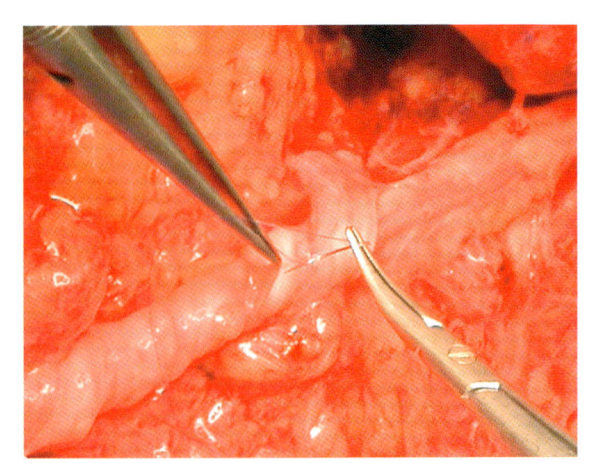

Fig. 44.3. Each ring of the wrapped vein is secured to the adjacent rings with a 7-0 nylon stitch. Care is taken to ensure that the intima of the vein is apposed to the scarred nerve epineurium with each turn

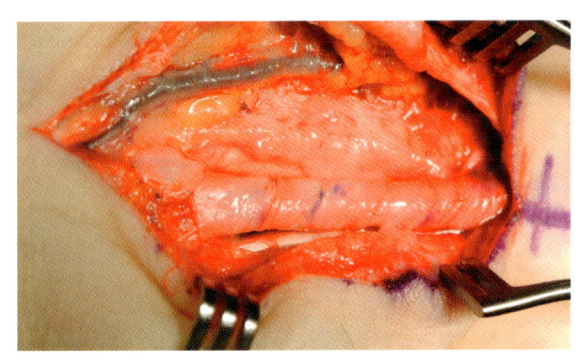

Fig. 44.4. The entire scarred portion of the median nerve is covered with the saphenous vein

For the median nerve, the wrist is immobilized after surgery for 1 week in slight extension. Active and passive motion exercises are started immediately after the splint is removed.

Results

The results of autogenous vein wrapping to treat recurrent compressive neuropathy using the aforementioned technique have been rewarding [28, 29]. Fifteen patients with recurrent carpal tunnel syndrome were reviewed after a mean follow-up of 43 months. The mean number of previous procedures was 3, with a minimum of 2 and a maximum of 5 for each patient. Previous procedures included simple nerve decompression, tenosynovectomy, internal neurolysis, hypothenar fat pad flap, and local flaps. All patients experienced pain relief (in a visual analogue scale all patients rated their pain at the last follow-up between 2 and 6 compared to preoperative pain which was rated between 6 and 9). Sensation was improved by more than 2 mm of two-point discrimination in 80% of the patients, although some continued to experience mild median nerve distribution numbness. In 8 patients that had nerve conduction studies performed, improvement was noted in all, although none returned to completely normal. Grip strength improved in 80% of the patients. No complications due to saphenous vein harvesting were noted other than mild discomfort and swelling at the incision site that resolved by approximately 4 months. Fourteen out of 15 patients were satisfied with the procedure.

In summary, autologous vein wrapping is an excellent option for the multiply operated patient with chronic median nerve compression secondary to cicatrix formation. It is a simple technique that causes minimal complications in the donor area. In addition, the donor vein is readily available and harvesting is easy. It consistently provides pain relief. Sensation is also improved, although return to normal is infrequent. Both experimental and clinical results support its use for recurrent compressive neuropathy of the median nerve at the wrist.

References

1. von Schroeder HP, Botte MJ (1996) Carpal tunnel syndrome. Hand Clin 12:643–655
2. Cobb TK, Amadio PC, Leatherwood DF et al. (1996) Outcome of reoperation for carpal tunnel syndrome. J Hand Surg 21A:347–356
3. Gelberman RH, Pfeffer GB, Galbraith RT et al. (1987) Results of treatment of severe carpal-tunnel syndrome without internal neurolysis of the median nerve. J Bone Joint Surg 69A:896–903
4. Hunter JM (1991) Recurrent carpal tunnel syndrome, epineural fibrous fixation, and traction neuropathy. Hand Clin 7:491–504
5. Yu G-Z, Firrell JC, Tsai T-M (1992) Pre-operative factors and treatment outcome following carpal tunnel release. J Hand Surg 17B:646–650
6. Haupt WF, Wintzer G, Schop A, Löttgen J et al. (1993) Long-term results of carpal tunnel decompression: assessment of 60 cases. J Hand Surg18B:471–474
7. Mackinnon SE (1991) Secondary carpal tunnel surgery. Neurosurg Clin North Am 2:75–91
8. Gelberman RH, Eaton R, Urbaniak JR (1993) Peripheral nerve compression. J Bone Joint Surg 75A:1854–1878
9. Kessler FB (1986) Complications of the management of carpal tunnel syndrome. Hand Clin 2:401–406
10. Rhoades CE, Mowery CA, Gelberman RH (1985) Results of internal neurolysis of the median nerve for severe carpal-tunnel syndrome. J Bone Joint Surg 67A:253–256
11. Urbaniak JR (1991) Complications of treatment of carpal tunnel syndrome. In: Gelberman RH (ed) Operative nerve repair and reconstruction, JB Lippincott, Philadelphia, pp 967–979
12. Gould JS (1991) Treatment of the painful injured nerve incontinuity. In: Gelberman RH (ed) Operative nerve repair and reconstruction, JB Lippincott, Philadelphia, pp 1541–1549
13. Botte MJ, von Schroeder HP, Abrams RA, Gellman H (1996) Recurrent carpal tunnel syndrome. Hand Clin 12: 731–743

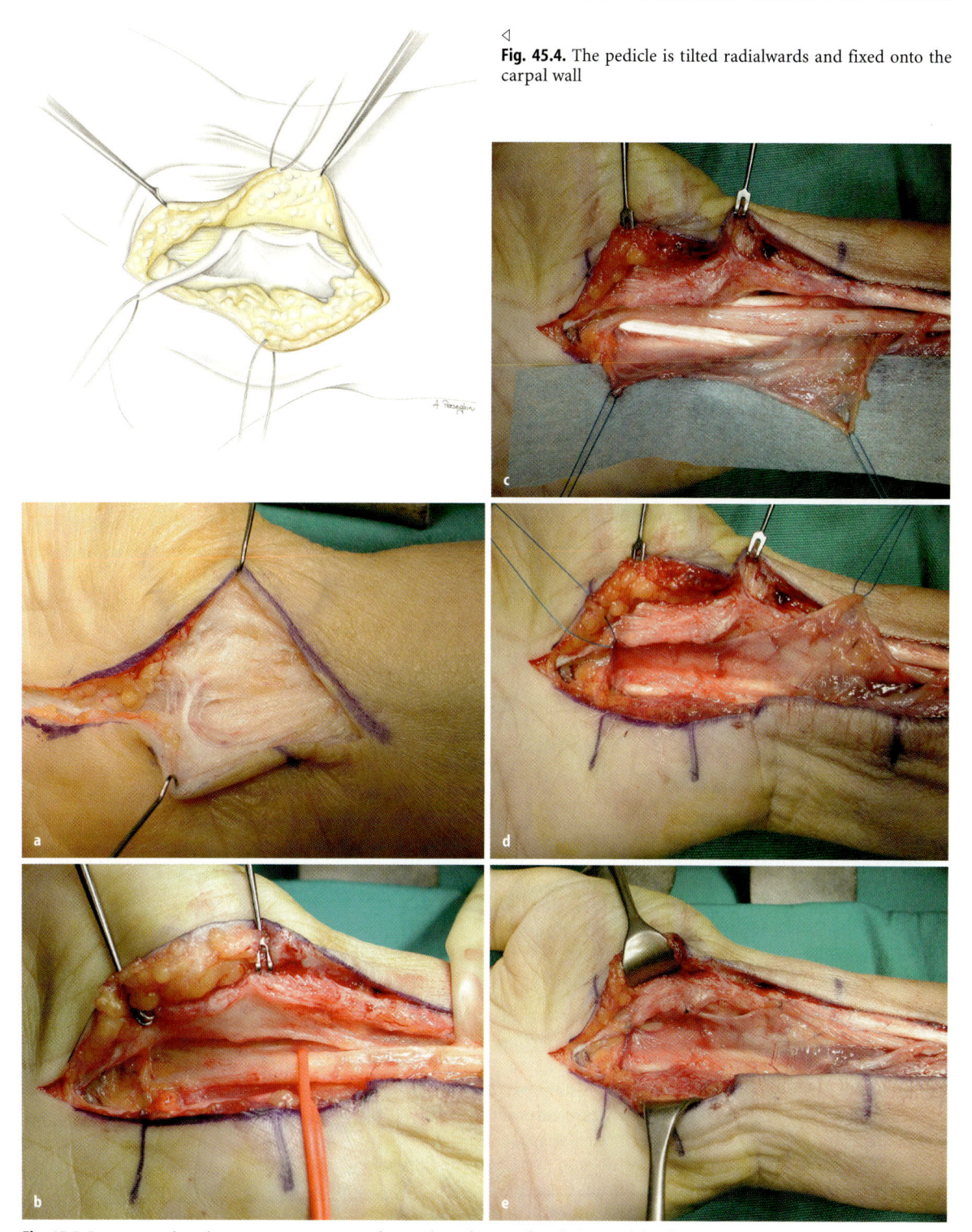

Fig. 45.4. The pedicle is tilted radialwards and fixed onto the carpal wall

Fig. 45.5. Intraoperative pictures: recurrent carpal tunnel syndrome after division of the flexor retinaculum and palmar plate removal for distal radius fracture. **a** Before neurolysis. **b** After Neurolysis. **c** Synovial flap dissection. **d** Flap tension and wideness testing. **e** Flap fixation

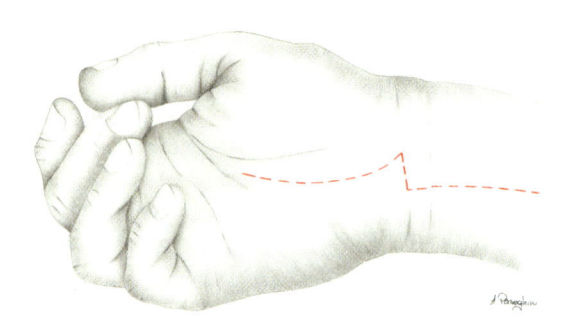

Fig. 45.1. Surgical approach

flexion wrist crease by forming an ulnarly directed "L" and extends for a further 4 cm proximally from here. The ulnar incision allows us to avoid lesions of the palmar cutaneous branch of the median nerve and of those small branches of it, which Taleisnik [8] describes going ulnarwards.

Neurolysis (Figs. 45.2, 45.5a, b)

After opening of the *antebrachial fascia* we look for the median nerve by working on its ulnar border. We identify the *palmar cutaneous branch* and perform, if necessary, a neurolysis of it. If we find a neuroma, instead of a neurolysis, we prefer to do a neurectomy [9]. The *opening of the roof of the carpal tunnel* is so performed strictly on the *ulnar* border of the median nerve. This has mainly two reasons:

- *Avoiding lesions of the motor branch,* which can differ very much in its course [10]. The lysis of the motor branch is necessary whenever it seems to be compressed: the blunt tips of the preparation scissors should be easily moved between the entrance point of the motor branch into the thenar and its muscular fibers.
- The *flexor retinaculum is thinner* on this side [11].

Depending on the progression of the "fibrosis" of the median nerve, we perform an *epineurotomy,* a *resection of the palmar hemicircumference of the epineurium* or an *"epineurial neurolysis"* [12]. These procedures are part of the *external neurolysis*. In the extremely rare cases in which the fibrosis extends into the interfascicular space, we perform an *internal neurolysis*: we do not dissect each axonal fascicle, but we remove the fibrous tissue between fascicle groups, as recommended by Millesi [13].

The median nerve, which has been freed of the fibrotic tissue, needs now protection. The tissue we need for this purpose should have the following main properties. It *should not*:

- Cause compression
- Obstruct the lumen of the carpal tunnel

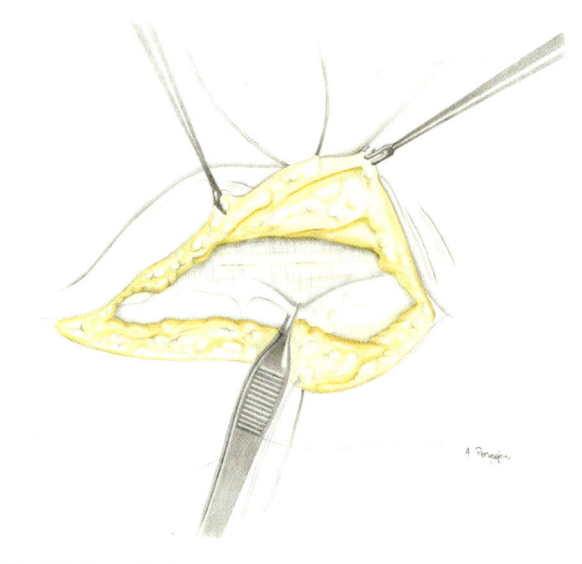

Fig. 45.2. Neurolysis

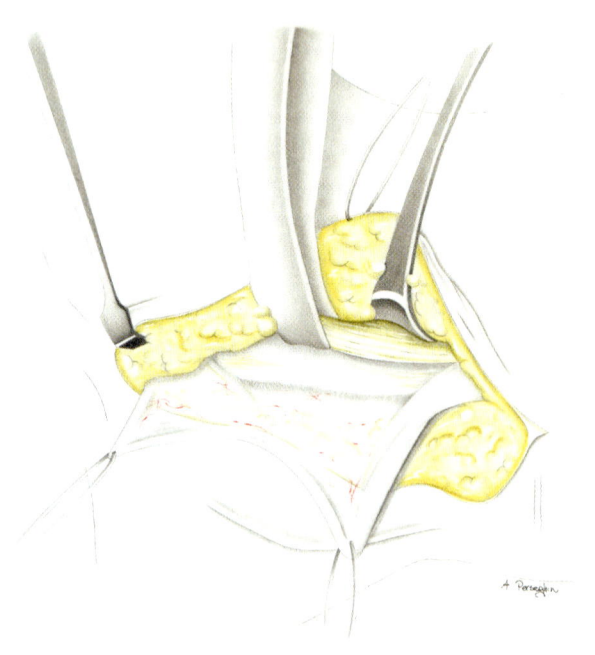

Fig. 45.3. The synovial flap is pedicled ulnarwards and is as wide as possible

Forming and Fixing the Synovial Flap (Figs. 45.3 – 45.5c–e)

The flap, which is taken from the flexor tendon sheaths, should be as wide as possible in the distal-proximal direction. We fix it with two or three single stitches radially (for example with absorbable 6-0 monofil thread), using the radial margin of the carpal canal as a fixation point. Two technical details have now to be observed:

1. The synovial flap must be *as wide as possible*, in order to obtain a good nerve covering and to avoid strictures that could cause a secondary compression.

45 Synovial Flap Plasty as a Treatment of Recurrent Carpal Tunnel Syndrome

D. Espen

Introduction

In 1980, Christhild Wulle, Hand Surgeon of the Hand and Plastic Surgery Department of the Kliniken Dr. Erler in Nürnberg, described for the first time the synovial flap plasty ("Synovialislappenplastik") and compared this technique with many others. Her paper was striking for its clear indications and very simple principle of the technique. We have been using Christhild Wulle's synovial flap technique since 1993 and are going to describe its indications and performance.

Definition of "Recurrence"

Depending on the *pathogenesis* [1–2] we can describe three types of recurrence:

1. Incomplete division of the flexor retinaculum: The complaints did not subside or did so only partially after surgery, or even worsened. We call this "carpal tunnel *persistence*."
2. The flexor retinaculum was divided completely; the patient showed gradual improvement and, in some cases, the complaints even subsided fully. The symptoms may recur because of a new cause, e.g., a fracture of the distal radius, hypertrophic synovitis of the flexor tendon sheaths, or recurrent swelling of the hand.
3. After complete release of the flexor retinaculum, extensive local fibrosis caused scar fixation of the median nerve – a true recurrence. Complaints and symptoms subsided partly or completely, but recurred shortly after surgery and may become progressive in the following months.

We are not talking about a recurrence, when:

1. The median nerve or one of its branches has been injured during the first surgery. This would cause local sensibility or motion (opposition) disturbance. In some cases a neuroma formation can occur.
2. Scar pain or pain in the region of the thenar and hypothenar base is present.
3. A second median nerve compression is present, e.g., underneath the pronator teres muscle or the lacertus fibrosus or the scalenus muscle.
4. Pain is caused by other concomitant diseases such as arthrosis of the carpometacarpal joint of the thumb or the intercarpal joints, radiocarpal arthrosis, arthrosis of the digital joints, and synovitis of the flexor tendon sheaths in the carpal or distal regions.

Method

1. The *principle* of our surgical technique is the covering of the damaged median nerve by means of a vascularized synovial flap which is taken from the flexor tendons and has an ulnar pedicle. Tubiana [3], Bonnard and coworkers [4], and Millesi and coworkers [5] describe nerve covering after neurolysis by muscular flaps which are either pedicled (m. abductor digiti minimi, m. pronator quadratus) or free (free fascial grafting from the subscapular area). Our flap is turned over the median nerve in order to avoid its further fibrosing and scar formation with the tissue.
2. The *indication* for this technique is the recurrence of carpal tunnel syndrome with fibrosis of the median nerve. The *contraindications* are given by the condition of the synovial membrane: in the case of a rheumatoid disease or when a synovectomy has been previously performed, our technique can not be performed.
3. The intraoperative *complications* that can occur depend on some technique details, such as the fixation of the flap on the radial rim of the flexor retinaculum. It is mandatory to check intraoperatively how the synovial tissue works during finger motion.

Surgical Technique [6–7]

Approach (Fig. 45.1)

We work in general or plexus anesthesia and ischemia. The skin incision passes parallel to the thenar crease, 2–3 mm ulnarly from it. Proximally it crosses the distal

14. Rose EH, Norris MS, Kowalski TA et al. (1991) Palmaris brevis turnover flap as an adjunct to internal neurolysis of the chronically scarred median nerve in recurrent carpal tunnel syndrome. J Hand Surg 16A: 191–201
15. Jones NF (1996) Treatment of chronic pain by "wrapping" intact nerves with pedicle and free flaps. Hand Clin 12: 765–772
16. Nashold BS, Goldner JL, Mullen JB, Bright DS (1982) Long-term pain control by direct peripheral-nerve stimulation. J Bone Joint Surg 64A:1–10
17. Monsivais JJ, Monsivais DB (1996) Managing chronic neuropathic pain with implanted anesthetic reservoirs. Hand Clin 12:781–786
18. Masear VR, Tullos JR, St Mary E, Mayer RD (1990) Venous wrapping of nerve to prevent scarring. J Hand Surg 15A: 817–818
19. Koman LA, Neal B, Santichen J (1995) Management of the postoperative painful median nerve at the wrist. Orthop Trans 18:765
20. Sotereanos DG, Giannakopoulos PN, Mitsionis GI et al. (1995) Vein-graft wrapping for the treatment of recurrent compression of the median nerve. Microsurgery 16:752–756
21. Masear VR, Colgin S (1996) The treatment of epineural scarring with allograft vein wrapping. Hand Clin 12: 773–779
22. Xu J, Sotereanos DG, Moller AR (1998) Nerve wrapping with vein grafts in a rat model: a safe technique for the treatment of recurrent chronic compressive neuropathy. J Reconstr Microsurg 14:323–330
23. Xu J, Varitimidis SE, Fisher KJ et al. (2000) The effect of wrapping scarred nerves with autogenous vein graft to treat recurrent chronic nerve compression. J Hand Surg 25A:93–103
24. Vardakas DG, Varitimidis SE, Sotereanos DG (2001) Findings of exploration of a vein-wrapped ulnar nerve: Report of a case J Hand Surg 26A:60–63
25. Campbell JT, Schon LC, Burkhardt LD (1998) Histopathologic findings in autogenous saphenous vein graft wrapping for recurrent tarsal tunnel syndrome: a case report. Foot Ankle Int 19:766–769
26. Chou KH, Papadimitriou NG, Sarris I, Sotereanos DG (2003) Neovascularization and other histopathologic findings in an autogenous saphenous vein wrap used for recalcitrant carpal tunnel syndrome: A case report. J Hand Surg 28A:262–266
27. Ruch DS, Spinner RM, Koman LA (1996) The histologic effect of barrier vein wrapping of peripheral nerves. J Reconstr Microsurg 12:291–295
28. Varitimidis SE, Vardakas DG, Goebel F, Sotereanos DG (2001) Treatment of recurrent compressive neuropathy of peripheral nerves in the upper extremity with an autologous vein insulator. J Hand Surg 26A:296–302
29. Varitimidis SE, Riano F, Vardacas DG, Sotereanos DG (2000) Recurrent compressive neuropathy of the median nerve at the wrist: Treatment with autogenous saphenous vein wrapping. J Hand Surg 25B:271–275

2. *No tension should result* while you are going to fix the flap. Mobilizing fingers intraoperatively during and after flap fixation is therefore mandatory.

This important step allows us to verify the flap tension: once we have reached the shape of the flap, we fix it to the radial carpal tunnel wall as described. Now we verify dynamically, by flexing and extending every single long finger and the thumb, how these structures glide within the synovial flap. We do not complete the flap fixation unless this test removes all doubt. We repeat this procedure after tourniquet opening.

Postoperative Management

A dorsal below-the-elbow splint at 20° of wrist extension is positioned for about 1 week. Immediate finger movement and fist closing is recommended. After removing the splint, the patient is allowed to do activities of daily living and should avoid heavy work for 1 month. An electromyography is performed after 3 months.

Evaluation

The original protocol by Christhild Wulle [1-2] takes sensibility, strength, function, and electrodiagnostic parameters into account (Table 45.1). It also considers the subjective judgment of the patient. In our patient revision [6] we added the DASH score (Germann et al.) [14], the Padua EMG evaluating system [15], and the modified Mayo Wrist Score [16].

Table 45.1. Evaluation protocol according to Christhild Wulle [1-2].

Assessment	Evaluation parameters
Excellent	Normal sensitivity Normal function and strength EMG improvement
Good	Residual paresthesia Improved sensitivity Normal function and strength EMG improvement
Satisfactory	Paresthesia Improved sensitivity Absent hypoesthesia's Slight m. opponens weakness, diminished strength EMG improvement
Poor	Persisting paresthesia Hypesthesia Thenar atrophy Thenar atrophy Disturbed prehensile function, diminished strength EMG unchanged

Different Treatment Options for Recurrence

In the literature many different methods of covering the damaged median nerve are described: from the transposition of the abductor digiti minimi (Milward and co-workers [17, 18]), to the "palmaris brevis-turn-over-flap" [19], to the m. pronator quadratus-transposition [20], until the muscular lumbrical flap [21], the subcutaneous hypothenar fat flap [22, 23], the interposition of a radial forearm flap [24], the free flap of gliding tissue [25], until the free fat flap [26] or the Vein Wrapping [27].

Discussion

The mentioned techniques present with two main problems: the increase of volume of the carpal canal on one side and a possible decrease of strength on the other side. The subcutaneous hypothenar fat flap or the palmaris brevis turnover flap have less influence on the carpal canal volume, they rather are a disturbing factor of the scar healing of the flexor retinaculum. This could cause strength impairment or instability. The synovial flap plasty not only brings vascularized, but also little bulky tissue as a coverage of the median nerve. Consequently there are no problems concerning the increase of volume in the carpal canal. On the other hand, the healing process of the flexor retinaculum has no obstacle.

If the indication is correct, the prognosis is good. A bad prognosis must be given in the case of the primary recurrent fibroplastic hyperplasia [28].

Acknowledgements. Miss Alessia Perseghin performed the anatomical drawings, which are very useful for better understanding some principles of technique. Mr. Konrad Faltner helped create the DVD of the surgical technique. I would like to thank them.

References

1. Wulle Ch (1980) Die Synovialislappenplastik beim Rezidiv eines Medianus-Kompressions-Syndroms. Zeitschrift für Plastische Chirurgie 4:266-271
2. Wulle Ch (1996) The Synovial Flap as Treatment of the Recurrent Carpal Tunnel Syndrome. HandClin Vol 12, 379-388
3. Tubiana R (1990) Carpal tunnel syndrome: some views on its management. Ann Hand Surg 9, n05, 325-330
4. Bonnard C, Egloff DV, Simonetta C, Narakas A (1991) Le syndrome du tunnel carpien. Helv.chir.Acta 58, 419-423
5. Millesi H, Zöck G, Rath Th (1990) The gliding apparatus of peripheral nerve and its clinical significance. Ann Hand Surg 9, 87-97
6. Espen D (2003) Indication, Technique and Results of Revision Sugery after Carpal Tunnel Sindrome with Video.

Talk at the Annual Spring Meeting of the Austrian Society for Surgery of the Hand, Amstetten-Austria, March 8
7. Espen D (2002) Nerve Cover with Synovial Flap, Chapter in "Sindrome del Tunnel Carpale," Editor Riccardo Luchetti, Verduci, Rome
8. Taleisnik J (1973) The Palmar Cutaneous Branch of Median Nerve and the Approach to the Carpal Tunnel. J Bone Jt Surg 55-A, 1212 – 1217
9. Mannerfelt L, Oetker R (1986) Die chirurgische Bedeutung des ramus palmaris n.mediani. In: Nigst (Hrsg.): Nervenkompressionssyndrom an der oberen Extremität. Bibliothek für Handchirurgie, Hippokrates Verlag, Stuttgart
10. Schmidt H-M, Lanz U (1992) Chirurgische Anatomie der Hand. Hippokrates Verlag
11. Denman EE (1981) The Anatomy of the Incision for the Carpal Tunnel Decompression. Hand 13 17 – 28
12. Nigst H (1981) Nervenkompressionssyndrome an den oberen Gliedmassen. In: Nigst, H., Buck-Gramcko, D., Millesi, H.(Hrsg.): Handchirurgie. Georg Thieme, Stuttgart Kap. 17.9).
13. Millesi H (1988) personal comunication to Baranowski D, Klein W, Grünert J
14. Germann G, Wind G, Harth A (1999) The DASH Survey – A new instrument for the assessment of treatment results on the upper extremity. Handchir Mikrochir Plast Chir 31: 149 – 152
15. Padua L, Padua R, Lo Monaco M et al. (1999) Multiperspective assessment of carpal tunnel syndrome – A multicenter study. Neurology 53:1654
16. Krimmer H (2001) Post-traumatic carpal collapse – Occurrence and therapy concept; Contributions to the journal "Der Unfallchirurg," Berlin, Heidelberg, New York: Springer
17. Milward TM, Stott WG, Kleinert HE (1977) The Abductor Digiti Minimi Muscle Flap. Hand 9 82 – 85
18. Reismann NR, Dellon AL (1983) The abductor digiti minimi Muscle Flap: A Salvage Technique for Palmar Wrist Pain. J Plast Reconstr Surg 72 859 – 865
19. Rose EH, Norris MS, Kowalski TA et al. (1991) Palmaris brevis turnover Flap as an Adjunct to Internal Neurolysis of the Cronically Scarred Median Nerve in recurrent Carpal Tunnel Syndrome. J Hand Surg 16 A 191 – 201
20. Dellon AL, Mackinnon SE (1984) The Pronator quadratus Muscle Flap. J Hand Surg 9 A 423 – 427
21. Wilgis EFS (1984) Local Muscle Flaps in the Hand Anatomy as Related to Reconstructive Surgery. Bull Hosp Joint Dis 44 552 – 557
22. Cramer LML (1985) Local Fat Coverage for the Median Nerve. Correspondence Newsletter American Society for Surgery of the Hand No. 35
23. Frank U, Giunta R, Krimmer H, Lanz U (1999) Neueinbettung des N.medianus nach Vernarbung im Karpalkanal mit der Hypothenar-Fettgewebslappenplastik. Handchir Mikrochir Plast Chir 31 317 – 322
24. Poell JG, Büchler U (1985) Anwendung des radialen Vorderarmlappens bem Rezidiv-Karpaltunnelsyndrom. Lecture for the Annual Congress of the Swiss Society for Plastic Surgery
25. Wintsch K, Helaly P (1986) Free Flap of Gliding Tissue. J Reconstr Microsurg 2 143 – 151
26. McClinton MA (1996) The Use of Dermal-Fat Grafts. Hand Clin 12 357 – 364
27. Soteranos DG, Jiangming X (1997) Vein Wrapping for the Treatment of Recurrent Carpal Tunnel Syndrome. Techniques in Hand and Upper Extremity Surgery 1 (1): 35 – 40
28. Büchler U, Goth D, Haußmann P et al. (1983) Karpaltunnelsyndrom: Bericht über 56 Nachuntersuchungen. Handchir Mikrochir Plast Chir 15 Suppl, 3 – 12

Reverse Island Forearm Flaps for the Coverage of the Median Nerve in Recurrent Carpal Tunnel Syndrome

M. Riccio, A. Bertani, W.A. Morrison

Introduction

The use of fascial or fasciocutaneous flaps for treating recalcitrant carpal tunnel syndrome has repeatedly demonstrated itself to be a reliable surgical treatment method for resolving severe clinical problems, in terms of pain and functional deficits, that originate directly from a median nerve compression injury, at the carpal level.

Trauma to the median nerve and its surrounding soft tissue, with the eventual formation of scar tissue, and nerve entrapment, is a typically occurring carpal tunnel syndrome (CTS) complication after incorrect carpal tunnel release (CTR) and multiple surgical neurolysis.

These events have been well documented in the literature with an incidence that ranges from 0.3% to 20% of treated cases [24, 32, 41, 42, 57, 76]. CTS symptoms can be ongoing and persistent in nature or can reappear within a 1–1.5 year period from the time of initial surgery [34]. Typically, median nerve compression symptoms exacerbate progressively and develop into persistent neuralgia that is localized around the median nerve innervation zone. Cases that have a predisposition to residual symptoms are usually those where an initial surgical error has occurred during the median nerve decompression.

- One of the most common causes for reoperation is due to the incomplete sectioning of the transverse carpal ligament, especially in the palm's most distal portion [42].
- Incorrect reconstruction of the transverse carpal ligament can produce a compression syndrome [29].
- Imprecise skin incisions [29] that are made in direct correspondence to the median nerve with sectioned portions of the transverse carpal ligament can cause an entrapment or favor the formation of adhesions between the nerve and the radial half of the sectioned ligament.

In all these cases, excessive surgical nerve manipulation, when performing an aggressive neurolysis, is a strong contributing factor for causing residual symptoms and leading to the formation of adhesive scar tissue and nerve trunk devascularization in the carpal canal.

Residual intraoperative findings may include epineural fibrotic scarring with superficial adhesions of the transverse carpal ligament and the development of fibrotic scar tissue. Consequently, these findings cause extrinsic nerve compression and nerve trunk ischemia.

In severe cases, nerve entrapment occurs where the nerve is strangled by scar tissue. This tissue must be divided from the nerve and removed and replaced with a well-vascularized flap similar to the surrounding loose connective tissue sheath, which has been described by Lang as "conjunctiva nervorum" [33], and successively defined as "adventitia" [75] or "paraneural sheath" [31]. We define it "perineurium."

The "perineurium" represents a single anatomical structure and is the most important element of the gliding mechanism. It is wrapped around the peripheral nerve trunk and plays the double role of facilitating passive nerve gliding, as well as providing blood supply to the nerve. A major vascular network connects the epineural surfaces with the endoneural compartment [39].

The median nerve's gliding mechanism has about 3 cm of excursion thus allowing for passive nerve adaptation when the wrist is flexed or extended [50]. The difference between the median nerve's length when the wrist is flexed, as opposed to when the upper extremity is held in an extended position is about 20% [49]. The peripheral nerve must be able to adapt to these sudden wrist dynamic movement changes by employing its passive sliding mechanism, which is equal to about 15% of the excursion difference. Fiber lengthening compensates for these adaptations by 4.5% [47].

Therefore, the infiltration of scar tissue around and into the nerve's gliding mechanism limits its capacity to passively adapt to the limb's flexion and extension movements and presents itself in the form of dynamic limb movement pain. The severity of this pain is proportional to the amount of scar tissue that surrounds and invades the median nerve's endoneural architecture. Fibroblastic invasion in the perifascicular space causes mechanical dysfunction, edema, and chronic endoneural ischemia. The evolution of this pathology is characterized by progressive nerve fasciculi strangulation up until there is complete sensory nerve fiber amputation. This pathology has been defined by Lundborg as "Miniature Compartment Syndrome" [39], and it is clinically dominated by painful symptoms. Initially, the pain can be described as neuralgic due to sensitive fiber mechanical compression. Therefore, it is acute, sometimes sharp and spontaneous and can easily be elicited by tapping over the painful area, causing the pain to radiate outward from the percussion site. Successively, in about 15% of patients [38, 69], the pain becomes persistent and resistant to pharmacological treatment. This pain can become so severe that it interferes with the patient's activities of everyday living. In addition to these painful symptoms, other symptoms can appear, such as vasomotor disturbances, trophic and/or neurovegetative states, typical of Reflex Sympathetic Dystrophy (RSD), recently redefined as Sympathetic Maintained Pain Syndrome (SMPS) [43].

Numerous surgical methods based on nerve coverage and protection have been proposed in order to avoid the occurrence of these type of complications. Techniques that have been proposed create the interposition of a well-vascularized protective tissue barrier between the nerve and its surrounding area, therefore physically impeding scar tissue from penetrating the epineurium and fighting against the formation of new fibrotic adhesions and ischemic compression. Numerous citations can be found in the medical literature regarding these types of local flaps: Pronator Quadratus muscle flap, Abductor Digiti Minimi muscle flap, Lumbrical muscle flap, Palmaris Brevis flap, Hypothenar Fat Pad flap, Synovial flap, Becker-Gilbert Ulnar flap, and "Vela Quadra" flap [1, 13, 14, 27, 30, 35, 43, 52, 56, 58, 60, 62–64, 66, 68, 74, 78, 81] and many authors have suggested the use of free flaps: Subscapular gliding tissue flap, Great omentum flap, Scapular flap, Lateral arm flap, Superficial temporal fascial flap, Latissimus Dorsi flap, and Tensor Fascia Lata flap [3–6, 17, 21–23, 26, 28, 67, 79, 80]. For the most part, the local flaps that have been proposed have important application limits, one of which is an insufficient rotational arc, which is not able to reach the median nerve in its entire carpal segment length and wide enough to wrap around it for its entire circumference, not to mention the tendency for these tissue flaps to be bulky. Frequently, they are not compatible with the anatomical carpal tunnel space. These technical limits can also be associated with important functional complications, one of which is the loss of muscle flap motor function and a random vascularization. Therefore, they are not compatible with the goal of "revascularization" of nerve structures that have been affected by chronic ischemia. These structures would gain major benefit by being treated with axial vascularized flaps.

On the other hand, the use of "barrier material" which is made up of vein autografts and silicone membrane, has yet to demonstrate itself to be statistically sufficient and homogeneous. In particular, Masear enthusiastically proposed nerve segment insertion, after undergoing neurolysis, in the lumen of the saphenous vein [45] with a success rate of 79% of his treated cases. The success rate of this procedure has been partially reevaluated in a more recent survey [18] that has pointed out the right perspective of this technique. The temporary use of a silicone barrier, which is removed 3 weeks after its implantation, is done in an attempt to reproduce a perineural connective tissue sheath that permits passive nerve sliding. This procedure is somewhat analogous to what is done in a two-stage hand flexor tendons reconstruction procedure, but lacks repetitive surgical experience and its follow-up results are still quite limited [44, 74].

In comparison, due to a nonresolved clinical problem, Wintsch [79, 80], was the first to introduce the use of a flap made from specialized gliding tissue that was ideal for circumferential reconstruction of peritendinous and perineural tissue which had been obliterated by fibrotic tissue proliferation. He substituted the simple concept of covering and protecting the injured nerve with the tenacious project of reconstructing the peripheral nerve's entire gliding mechanism. The "subscapular fascial flap" has been defined as an ideal tissue

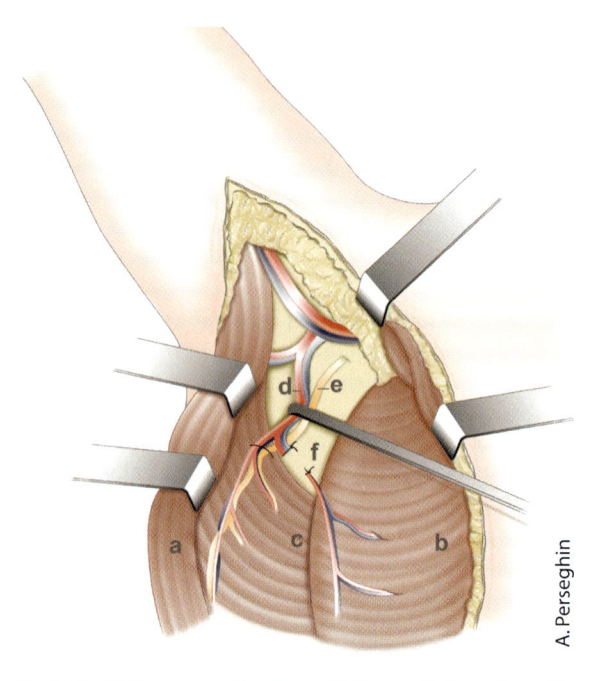

Fig. 46.1. Gliding connective tissue (*f*) it extends from the axilla into the space made by the latissimus dorsi and serratus posterior muscle. (*a*) latissimus dorsi muscle. (*b*) Serratus anterior muscle. (*c*) Serratus posterior muscle. (*d*) Thoracodorsal artery. (*e*) Thoracodorsal nerve. (*f*) Gliding connective tissue

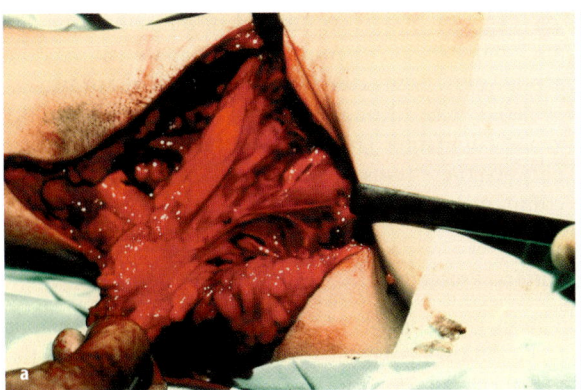

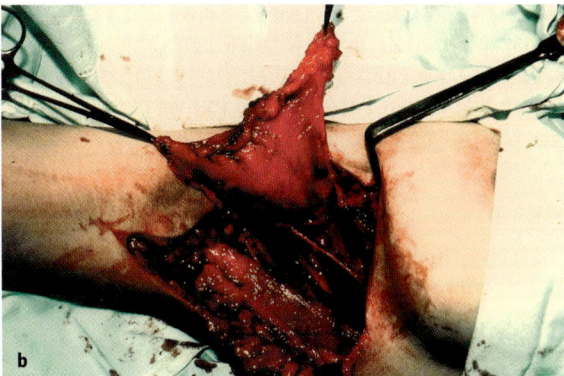

Fig. 46.2. a Dissection of the gliding connective tissue. **b** Harvesting of the subscapular gliding tissue flap (Wintsch procedure), vascularized by the thoracodorsal artery

that can be wrapped around the tendon and nerve trunks of the upper extremity after lysis or reparative surgery. This flap comes from an elastic connective tissue that is located between the intermuscular space that separates the latissimus dorsi from the serratus posterior muscle (Fig. 46.1). The subscapular fascial flap is vascularized by collateral branches of the thoracodorsal artery (Fig. 46.2a, b).

The main anatomical characteristics of this flap, according to Wintsch, is that it has the specific function of tissue gliding and is characterized by an elevated intertissue gliding coefficient, due to its ratio of elasticity to connective tissue thickness, whereas the coefficient expresses the flap's elastic connective tissue thinness thus reducing friction that is produced during the tissue's passive movements.

H. Millesi successfully used the same flap for reconstructing the gliding system of the wrist's median nerve and for protecting the brachial plexus after extensive neurolysis [46, 48].

With the same strategy in mind, various free flaps have been proposed in the medical literature, prevalently fascial in nature [3, 22, 23, 26, 28], in the conviction that loose epifascial areolar connective tissue possesses the characteristics for obtaining passive gliding as has been described by Wintsch. The Greater Omentum Flap [4–6, 67] must be added to the list of fascial flaps since, at a perineural level, it has the intrinsic characteristic of reducing friction during passive movements of the abdominal organs.

W. Millesi [51] subsequently reaffirmed the concept of the ubiquitous gliding tissue, pointing out that interpectoral connective tissue has the same characteristics and proposing its use in brachial plexus protection. This flap is known as a "subpectoral island flap" and is vascularized from the interpectoral thoraco-acromial artery.

The advantage of this method is the use of a nearby gliding connective tissue island flap, so that it can be raised and turned to cover the injured nerve, avoiding the risk of a free flap failure due to the thrombosis of the microvascular anastomoses.

By applying these same principles in the treatment of the recurrent CTS, we propose the use of the reverse island forearm flaps, which are made up of an epifascial surface derived from loose areolar connective tissue. These flaps can easily reach the median nerve and circumferentially wrap themselves around the length of the nerve in the carpal tunnel.

We feel that three fundamental objectives must be performed to accurately complete this flap procedure:

- Complete separation of the median nerve from its surrounding tissue for its entire circumferential length inside the carpal tunnel.
- Accurate surgical dissection of the flap by carefully respecting the epifascial areolar connective tissue's integrity so that passive gliding of the epineurium can be allowed.
- Provide a nutritional supply to the ischemic nervous tissue, by means of a rich intrinsic axial vascularization. Besides immediately increasing blood supply, this also allows for appropriate nerve structure revascularization by creating a neoangiogenesis mechanism.

Various reverse forearm, fascial, and fasciocutaneous flaps can be classified (Radial artery flap, Retrograde radial fascial flap, Ulnar artery flap, Posterior interosseous flap), in order of their capacity to satisfy these objectives. We uphold that the reverse island radial artery flap has the greatest reliability and practicality [72].

The Forearm Radial Artery Flap

The Reverse Island Forearm Radial Artery Flap is used the most in the treatment of hand pathologies that require tissue reintegration. We will classify the radial flaps on the basis of their composition as, fascial, adipofascial, and fasciocutaneous [7, 8, 15, 16, 19, 25, 53, 61, 65, 82]. In addition, we will distinguish the standard Reverse Island Forearm Radial Artery Flap, from the Retrograde Radial Forearm Flap in that the radial artery remains intact when the flap is raised [2, 77].

Anatomy

The harvesting of a radial flap, from the forearm, essentially requires the dissection of the radial portion of the antebrachial fascia. This portion represents not only the flap's main structure in all its variations, fascial and fasciocutaneous, but even the flap's vascular axes. The arterial supply to the skin is from the radial artery via small cutaneous branches passing along the fascial septum or mesentery which emerges from the cleft between the extensor muscles radially and flexor muscles ulnarwards, specifically between brachioradialis muscle and flexor carpi radialis [10] (Fig. 46.3).

The relevant arterial septal branches tend to be in three groups with three associated and anastomosing perfusion zones, respectively concentrated in the proximal third, medial third, and distal third of the radial artery tract. These vessels are quite sporadically located in the middle third, but are extremely concentrated at the forearm's proximal and distal portions [73]. The perforating septal branches directly nourish a system of fascia axial vessels. The epifascial plexus is made up of a very dense vessel network. It is prevalently localized to the superficial side of the fascia and intimately connected, by means of numerous vertical vessels, with the adipose tissue's vascular system. In this way, a three dimensional, rich and branching vascular network is established, from which it is possible to harvest fascial and fascio-adipose flaps that are reliable and well vascularized. The venous drainage is from the venae comitantes of the radial artery and the superficial veins which course through the flap in the subcutaneous plane. Specifically the venous drainage of the radial fascia is assured by a dense network of venae that run parallel to the arterial network, and are confluent with the septal veins. Each arterial perforator has one or two associated veins through which blood can pass into the venae comitantes [10, 73]. The multiple anastomoses between these veins permit reversal of flow in the venae comitantes without valvular obstruction [36].

Surgical Procedure

The surgery consists of harvesting the radial fascial or fasciocutaneous island reverse flap by sacrificing the radial artery in the forearm's proximal segment. A preoperative Allen test must be performed to confirm the patency of the ulnar artery and its capacity to supply blood to the hand [9]. The operation can be performed with general anesthesia or brachial plexus nerve block anesthesia. A pneumatic tourniquet is applied to the arm by the surgeon. The limb is exsanguinated and the pneumatic tourniquet inflated to 50 mm Hg above the patient's systolic pressure in order to maintain a bloodless operating field.

The incision should widely expose the median nerve while also providing a wide opening of the carpal tunnel beyond its normal anatomical limits. It is advisable to perform a longitudinal curvilinear incision that begins at the palm, located ulnarly, under the fourth digital ray axis, and crosses over the interthenar sulcus directed radially towards the wrist's flexor crease and moves in gentle diagonal direction toward the radial aspect of the forearm. The cutaneous incision should not invade the skin area that holds the flexor carpi radialis and the palmaris longus where the palmar cutaneous branch runs [71]. Therefore, when the incision reaches the palmaris longus, it is direct proximally, parallel to the long axis of the forearm. Dissection of the median nerve from the surrounding scar tissue is made, particularly undersurface of the radial half of the transverse carpal ligament, and ensuring adequate decompression, neurolysis including epineurotomy is performed. An interfascicular neurolysis should only be associated with this procedure when absolutely necessary, when a severe intraneural fibrosis is altering the fascicles' anatomy [47]. Therefore, if intraoperative findings demonstrate severe median nerve scar entrapment, the surgeon should proceed with harvesting a reverse island forearm radial artery flap.

To proceed with the reverse island fascial radial artery flap, a linear incision is made in a disto-proximal direction extending proximally to within a few centimeters of the elbow flexion crease. Two skin flaps are harvested from the antebrachial fascia, in both a radial and ulnar direction with a 2 cm width. The interval between the fat and the fascia must not be violated as it contains the epifascial vascular plexus network and an adipose tissue layer, which must be preserved

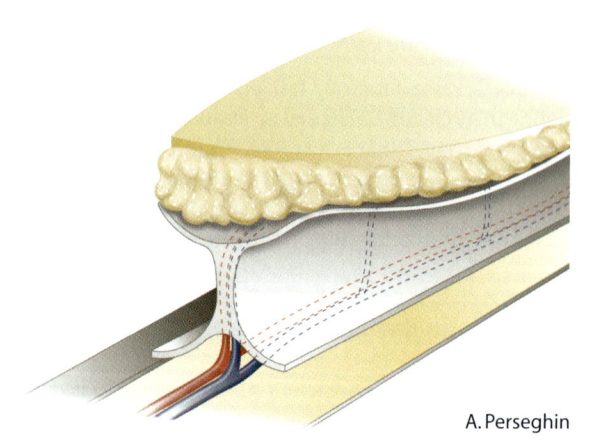

A. Perseghin

Fig. 46.3. Septal fasciocutaneous flap diagram: radial artery forearm flap

Fig. 46.4. a–c Exposure of the forearm fascia. **b** Radial artery forearm fascial flap raised with vascular pedicles intact proximally and distally. **c** Radial artery fascial flap elevated with distal radial artery and venae comitantes intact distally

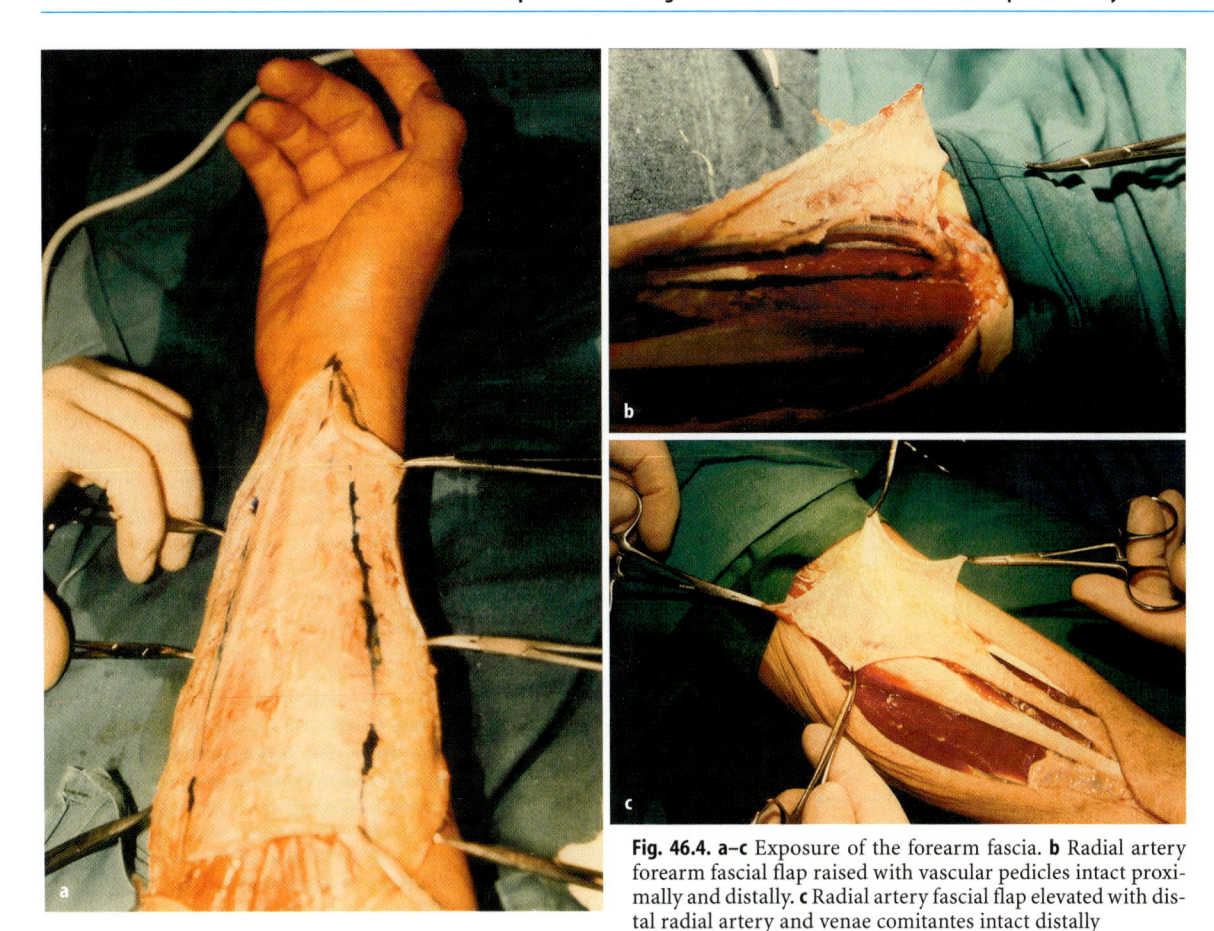

(Fig. 46.4a). The fascia is incised at its periphery and dissected at a plane immediately above the forearm muscle's epimysium and extends ulnarly, as well as radially towards the radial artery septum. The fascial flap is taken on the radial artery, 5 cm in length and 4 cm in width (Fig. 46.4b).

Once the flap has been raised, the radial artery and the venae comitantes are sectioned to the flap's proximal extremity (Fig. 46.4c). The fascial flap is turned down distally and buried under the flexor carpi radialis muscle in such a way that its gliding surfaces wrap around the median nerve in a dorso-volar direction, enveloping its entire circumferential length within the carpal tunnel [72] (Fig. 46.5). Its pivot point is about 4 cm proximal to the radial styloid.

The flap margins are sutured with 6/0 reabsorbable noncontinuous sutures and accurately making sure that the suture border slide towards the tunnel's ulnar side in order to exclude the possibility of adhesions forming between the three layers: epineurium, fascia, and skin.

The tourniquet is then removed and the vitality of the flap can be determined once accurate hemostasis has been established. The skin is closed with noncontinuous suturing. The donor site is closed first and an aspirating drain is fixed in place.

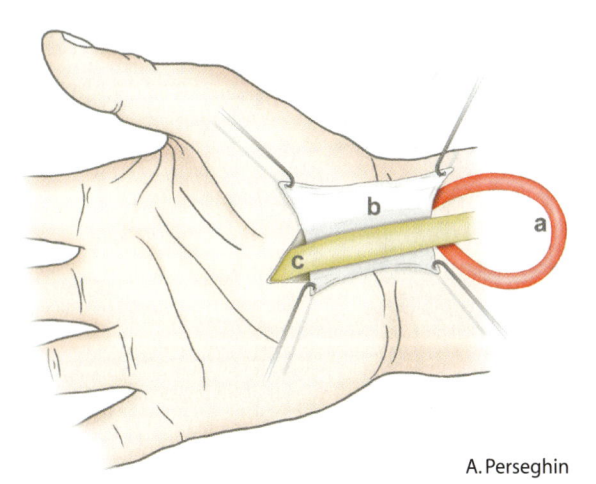

A. Perseghin

Fig. 46.5. The radial artery island fascial flap is rotated towards the carpal tunnel. The epifascial surface is circumferentially wrapped around the median nerve. *a* Radial artery. *b* Radial forearm fascial flap. *c* Scarred median nerve

Finally, the hand is wrapped in a medicated bandage, a plaster valve is applied to immobilize the anterior aspect of the wrist and maintain it in a rest position for about 2 weeks before initiating functional re-education.

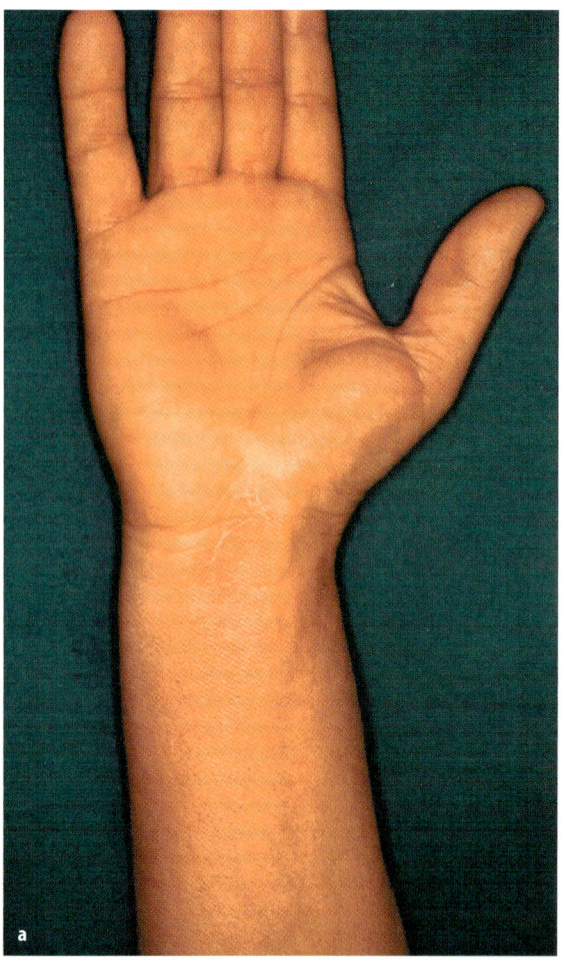

This surgical technique needs to be modified, in cases in which, due to incorrect CTR and multiple neurolysis, the preoperative clinical exam indicates that the thenar and hypothenar eminence have become close together due to a tenacious scar retraction. In such cases the surgeon needs to harvest a reverse island fasciocutaneous radial artery flap. This method is comparable to the previously described technique with the only difference being in the harvesting of an elliptical-shaped antebrachial island skin flap that measures about 5 cm by 3 cm. It is slightly longer than the carpal tunnel's cutaneous area, therefore, it can be positioned between the thenar and hypothenar eminence in order to avoid the recurrence of skin retraction in the palm and the compression of the median nerve. In addition, it can be used as a convenient indicator as to the flap's vitality [26] (Fig. 46.6). The skin flap's elliptical axis will be situated exactly on the long axis of the flap. During the dissection it is useful to raise a fascial flap extended in width some centimeters in a radial direction thus maintaining the cutaneous island slightly off center on the ulnar side of the fascial flap. In this way, the fascia can be evenly wrapped around the median nerve's entire circumference and ensuring that the suture margins fall on the tunnel's ulnar side, maintaining the skin island precisely in the interthenar zone. The same medicated bandage and plaster valve are applied and a functional reeducation postoperative program is initiated 2 weeks later.

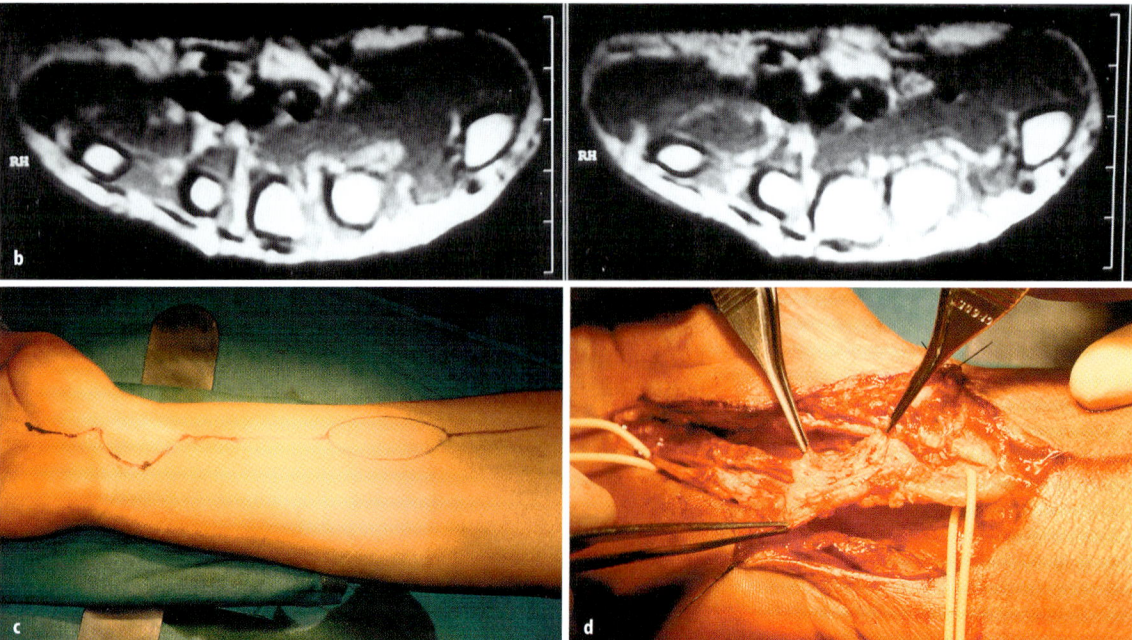

Fig. 46.6. a Residual scarring after three CTR operations. **b** A preoperative NMR image indicating median nerve scar adhesions. **c** Preoperative procedure planning. **d** After external neurolysis of the median nerve in the carpal tunnel the penetrating scar tissue inside the nerve with interruption and dislocation of the nerve fasciculi is evident

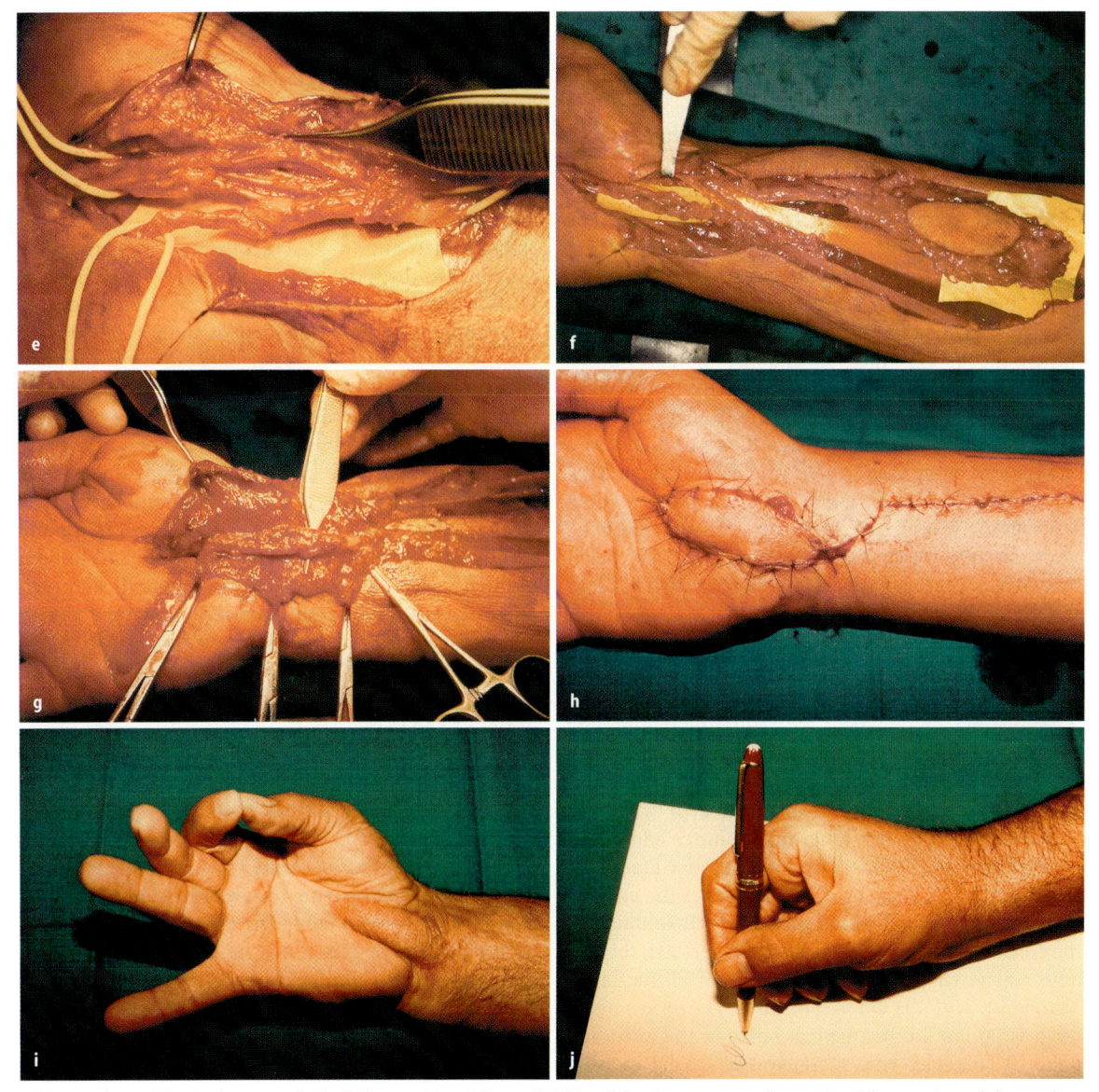

Abb. 46.6. e Interfascicular neurolysis. **f** Harvesting of the radial island fasciocutaneous flap. **g** Fascial wrapping of the median nerve. **h** Immediate postoperative result. **i, j** Long term follow-up functional results

The Retrograde Radial Forearm Flap

The retrograde radial forearm flap is a distally based adipofascial flap that can be distinguished from the most commonly described reverse radial artery forearm flap since it can be harvested without having to sacrifice the radial artery [2, 77].

Anatomy

Direct flap vascularization is established by numerous ascending branches that come from the distal third of the radial artery and go into the antebrachial fascia, enriched by perforating branches of muscle origin. The retrograde blood flow supplies additional circulation to the flap through collateral vessels that traces the blood flow's origin back to a thick epifascial and extrafascial vessel plexus that comes from the radial aspect of distal forearm and wrist. It develops in a disto-proximal direction along the antebrachial fascia and the epifacial adipose tissue which is also rich with vessels, thus an adipofascial flap is able to be harvested.

Surgical Procedure

This surgery can be performed under brachial plexus or general anesthesia. It is better to perform this surgery in a bloodless operating field by emptying the veins so that vein dissection is accurate. In order to achieve this, a pneumatic tourniquet can be applied to the arm and inflated to 50 mmHg above the patient's systolic pressure.

The surgery begins by exposing the median nerve, respecting the same standard techniques that have already been described for harvesting the reverse fascial radial artery flap. This incision is compatible with the progressive operative phases that will take place in the palm and along the longitudinal axis of the fourth ray towards the interthenar sulcus. The direction and location of the incision is followed out in order to limit ulterior scar adhesions by establishing a distance between the cutaneous axis incision and the median nerve's course. The incision extends proximally to the wrist flexors, deviating itself slightly radially at the intersection with the palmaris brevis. It then continues in a straight line along the forearm's medial portion until it reaches the flap's pivot point, (which is located about 4 cm from the radial styloid), up until the forearm's proximal third which is a few centimeters from the elbow crease. The two flaps are cut out respectively, ulnar and then radial, so that the antebrachial fascia is amply exposed and the epifascial surfaces are carefully preserved by maintaining a thin layer of adipose tissue. Since the dissected-out tissue is of minimal thickness it is compatible, on one hand, in facilitating flap gliding and on the other, for avoiding the presence of an excessive depression at the donor site. Therefore, a rectangular adipofascial flap can be harvested, of which its length is traced by two longitudinal ulnar and radial parallel incisions. It differs from the standard radial island fascial flap, since its diameters cover the entirely exposed antebrachial fascial surface and it contains all the epifascial vascular network, which perfuses the flap both collaterally and distally. The width of the flap is compatible with the amount of surface coverage needed to wrap around the median nerve at the wrist and palm. It coincides with a transversal fascial incision that is located at the end of the flap in proximity to the elbow crease. The thickness of the dissection plane must always include adipofascial tissue in the incision in order to preserve the adipofascial vessels' integrity. They collect in the virtual space situated between the adipose tissue and fascia and assure that the flap is vascularized in a three-dimensional manner, passing over the forearm flexor muscles' anterior surface.

As the flap is elevated, the radial artery is not transected; it is protected and remains intact below the flap. A few small perforating vessels coming off the radial artery to the fascia at the proximal and midforearm level may be transected safely during elevation of the flap. In this phase of surgical dissection, as that which occurs in the standard technique, it is necessary to pay particular attention to respect and preserve the portion of the radial nerve that emerges from the brachioradialis muscle's ulnar border and the forearm's lateral cutaneous branch. The nerve must be identified when performing a proximal third fascial radial border incision, so that it is protected during the fascia's transverse incision, as well as isolating it from the adipose tissue when cutting out the flap in a proximal distal direction. The retrograde radial flap's pivot point will be located slightly proximal to that of the standard one, since the flap remains viable because of the radial artery's distal perforating vessels and the distal collateral circulation, just proximal to the wrist, which proceeds in a retrograde fashion within the raised adipofascial flap. These vessels supply the adipofascial flap at about 5–8 cm from the wrist flexor crease. It is necessary to verify the presence and integrity of the distal vessels once the flap has been harvested, in order to verify if they are sufficient in number for providing proper perfusion to the flap.

The flap is elevated and turned distally towards the carpal tunnel, assuring 90°–180° of rotation, so that a gliding surface will be ample enough to wrap around the median nerve. The flap will be housed and sutured in the tunnel, analogous to that which has been previously described in the standard technique. The tourniquet is then removed and the vitality of the flap can be determined once accurate hemostasis has been established. The donor site is closed first and an aspirating drain is fixed in place.

The Forearm Ulnar Artery Flap

The ulnar artery flap, described by Lovie [37], is a fasciocutaneous flap overlying the proximal and central one third of the forearm along the course of the ulnar artery, which can be raised in a similar fashion to the radial artery flap. Guimberteau [20] has developed this flap to its maximum potential so that regarding the reliability it can be compared to a " Chinese flap" and may replace it in most circumstances. The ulnar artery flap has important advantages: the skin paddle is thinner than the radial equivalent, pliable, without adipose tissue, and virtually hairless. It is much more compatible with the thickness and skin type quality of the palm. Nevertheless, it should be stressed that the mesenteric attachment of the flap to the ulnar artery is much more tenuous than the radial artery flap and consists of one or two small branches.

The donor site is more acceptable because it offers better aesthetic results than the radial equivalent since it allows for an easier and less taut closure. The scar, which is positioned laterally, is less apparent and has a lower incidence of complications, such as hypertrophy and pain, whereas a skin graft easily roots itself to a well-padded muscular bed. The ulnar flap's rotation point is located more distally than that of the radial flap. It is located up by the palm and can totally compensate for its minor rotation arc which is under anatomical obligation due to the position of the septal perforators. The sacrifice of the ulnar artery does not cause ulnar nerve devascularization and does not cause symptomatic functional disturbances.

Notwithstanding such advantages, many authors are reluctant to use this type of retrograde flap on the basis that there is a presumed dominance of the ulnar artery, with respect to the radial artery, in the blood supply of the hand.

Anatomy

Ulnar Artery Flap vascularization comes from ascending branches of the ulnar artery that vary from one to three in number and are usually in the middle and proximal third of the forearm. They are situated in the fascial septum between the flexor carpi ulnaris and the flexor digitorum superficialis of the fourth and fifth fingers. These perforators usually directly supply the fascia but sometimes can follow an indirect ascending course perforating the surface of the flexor carpi ulnaris. Cases have been documented where there has been a complete lack of ascending branches from the ulnar artery to the overlying fascia [72]. The ulnar island flap's venous drainage is through the deep venae comitantes which, like the radial flap, has a retrograde flow, and is made up of a complex vessel network found around the ulnar artery. It is through this network that hematic flow is able to avoid valve obstructions due to its continual change in direction, assuring the venous return to the flap.

Surgical Procedure

The surgery consists of harvesting the reverse fascial or fasciocutaneous ulnar flap by sacrificing the ulnar artery in the forearm's proximal segment. A preoperative Allen test must be performed to confirm the patency of the radial artery and its capacity to supply blood to the hand [9]. The operation can be performed with general anesthesia or brachial plexus nerve block anesthesia. A pneumatic tourniquet is applied to the arm by the surgeon. The limb is exsanguinated and the pneumatic tourniquet inflated to 50 mm Hg above the patient's systolic pressure in order to maintain a bloodless operating field.

The operative method is similar to that which has already been described for harvesting the radial artery flap. The first phase includes wide exposure and dissection of the median nerve from the surrounding scar tissue at the palm and wrist. The longitudinal incision begins at the palm, along the fourth digital ray axis, and moves toward the palmaris longus tendon. When the incision reaches the palmaris longus, it is direct proximally, parallel to the long axis of the forearm. The longitudinal axis of the flap is centered over the course of the ulnar artery in the cleft between flexor carpi ulnaris ulnarwards and on the radial side by the palmaris longus. The course of this longitudinal axial line is from the pisiform bone inferiorly to the medial epicondyle superiorly. The skin and subcutaneous tissue are incised linearly along this axis until it reaches the proximal third of the forearm in proximity to the elbow crease, and the antebrachial fascia is exposed on the forearm's ulnar side.

The fascial flap, eventually with an elliptical shaped skin island, is raised from the forearm's middle and proximal third junction where the septal perforators are usually found.

The radial side of the fascial flap is first incised and the radial half of the flap should be lifted up along the subfascial plane, passing into the intermuscular cleft between flexor carpi ulnaris on the ulnar side and palmaris longus and flexor superficialis on the radial side. Once the location of the ascending branches of the ulnar artery is confirmed, the ulnar side of the flap is elevated and dissected from the subfascial plane up until the intermuscular septum, where it passes over the ulnar nerve. The dissection continues under the mesenteric attachment of the flap, developing down to the ulnar vessels proper. Sometimes the ascending branches do not directly reach the antebrachial fascia. They cross over and penetrate the most superficial portion of the flexor carpi ulnaris, making it more difficult to dissect out the vessels, often making it necessary include the superficial margin of the muscle within the flap. At this point, a transversal incision is made on the fascia, attaching and sectioning the ulnar artery to the flap's proximal extremity, after having verified that the vessel has been sectioned distal to the bifurcation of the common interosseous artery. Proceeding, the flap is lifted in a distal direction by dissecting it out until it reaches the wrist's ulnar artery, which must be separated by the adjacent ulnar nerve, taking care to limit it as much as possible from being devascularized.

Once the flap is rotated, it is used for reconstructing the median nerve's gliding system and for interthenar skin island coverage. This part of the surgical procedure is analogous to that which has been described for the radial flap (Fig. 46.7).

The rotation arc of the ulnar artery flap is shorter than the radial artery flap. It is determined by the location of the bifurcation of the common interosseous artery. In order to completely cover the median nerve at the carpal tunnel level, the flap's pivot point can be distally displaced, by extending the ulnar artery's dissection up until the palm.

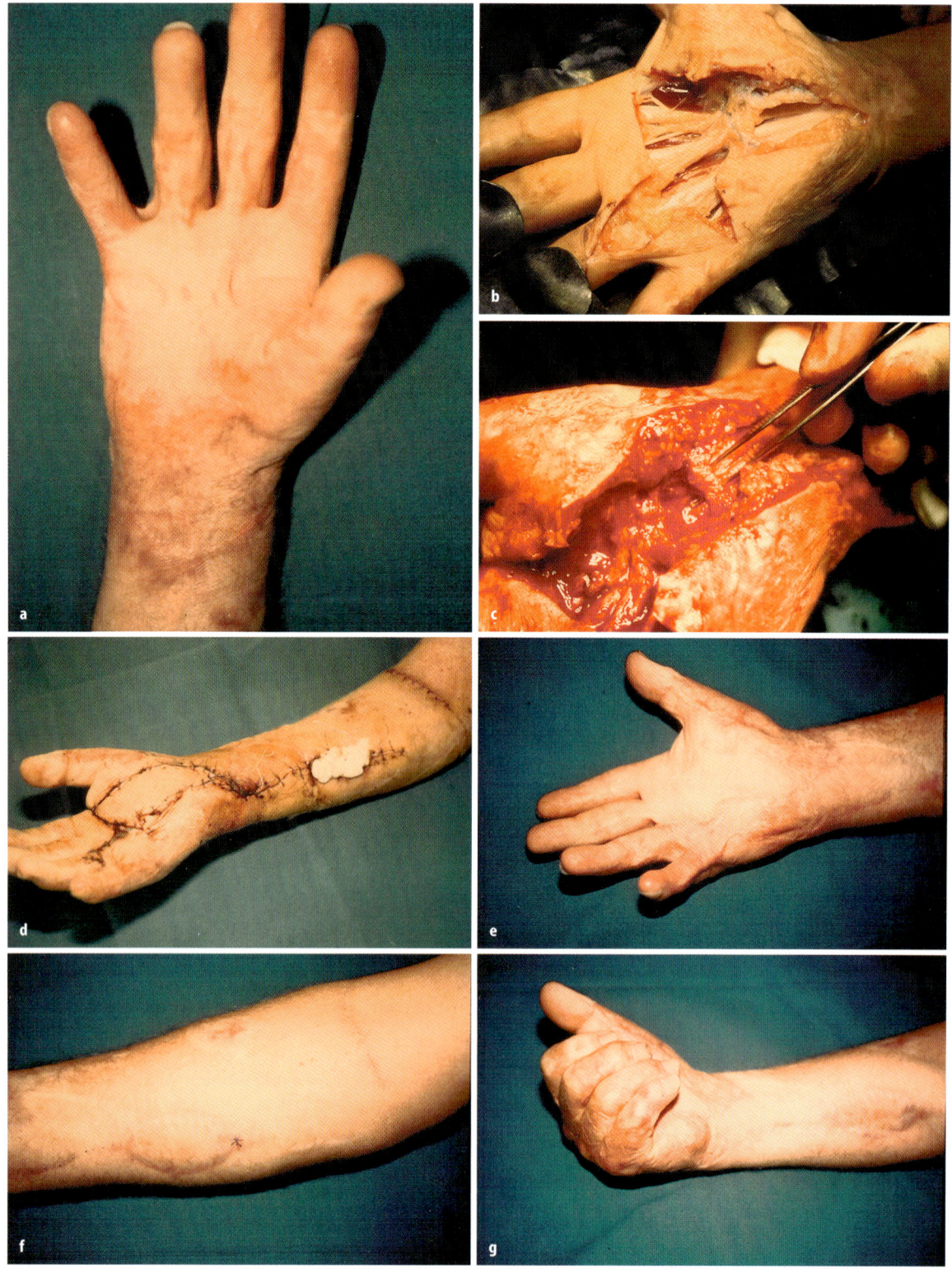

Fig. 46.7. a CTS after thermal burn to the palm and wrist (preoperative). **b** Cross incision of the palm with median nerve exposure at the carpal tunnel level. Release of transverse carpal ligament adhesions to the median nerve. **c** Raising of the hypothenar fat pad flap, rotated to protect the median nerve at the wrist. **d** The distally based forearm ulnar artery flap has been rotated onto the palm: the fascia covers the median nerve, the skin island has reconstructed the palm. Postoperative result. **e** Long-term follow-up result at the palm. **f** Long-term follow-up result at the donor site. **g** Long-term follow-up functional result

The Posterior Interosseous Flap

This flap has been described by Zancolli and Angrigiani [83, 84] and furthermore, specifically elaborated on by numerous authors [11, 12, 59] regarding its vascular anatomy and its multiple applications. This flap has been accepted with enthusiasm for its use in traumatic hand treatments, since it holds the same applicative advantages as that of the other island flaps harvested from the forearm's anterior side, but it also differs in that it has the enormous advantage of not sacrificing a major artery to the hand.

Anatomy

The distally based island posterior interosseous flap is supplied by multiple small septocutaneous ascending branches which originate from the posterior interosseous artery. It arises from the common interosseous artery in the proximal third of the forearm and continues dorsally, passing between the chorda obliqua and the interosseous membrane in the forearm's posterior portion at the junction between the two distal thirds and the proximal third. Its course goes in a proximal-distal direction towards the wrist from the lateral epicondyle humeri to the ulnar head, and collects in the septum between the extensor carpi ulnaris and the extensor digiti minimi muscles. The posterior interosseous artery, in proximity to the wrist, runs laterally to the ulnar head and is adherent to the periosteum. It then terminates itself by branching into the carpal dorsal arch after having formed an anastomosis under the extensor tendons with the anterior interosseous artery, whose presence is fundamental for the elevation of the posterior interosseous island reverse flap. The posterior interosseous artery, along its course in the muscle septum, originates collateral branches that supply the abductor longus, the extensor pollicis longus, and extensor proprius indicis. It also gives off numerous fasciocutaneous septal perforators which emerge through the muscular septum in the posterior interosseous segment included between the ulnar head and the recurrent interosseous artery that penetrate the supinator muscle. Three distinct patterns of these septocutaneous vessels have been identified [11]:

- Pattern I: is characterized by two perforator branch groups; one is distal and the other proximal, adjacent to the origin of the recurrent artery, each one is made up by three or four ascending vessels.
- Pattern II: multiple small branches arising at 1–2 cm intervals along the total length of the posterior interosseous artery. This is the most common vascular pattern.
- Pattern III: is characterized by sporadic and distant distal perforators arising from the posterior interosseous artery with a large proximal perforator that is adjacent to the recurrent interosseous artery, which often shares the same origin. This perforator has a larger diameter than the remaining septocutaneous vessels and supplies the fascia via small several branches. This is a more infrequently found anatomical situation.

In all the vascular patterns, the largest septocutaneous perforator is found distal to the supinator, arising from the proximal segment of the artery. Analogous to what occurs for radial artery and ulnar artery flaps, all the septocutaneous vessels anastomoses in the superficial layer of the dorsal deep fascia, creating a rich vessel network with numerous longitudinal anastomoses. A rich venule plexus is located at the septal veins that drain into the two main venae comitantes of the vascular pedicle.

The fascial plexus supplies a large area of skin on the posterior aspect of the forearm. The reverse posterior interosseous island flap is supplied via the dorsal carpal arch and via the anastomosis between the posterior interosseous and the anterior interosseous arteries.

Surgical Procedure

A distally based fascial or fasciocutaneous island flap can be raised based on the posterior interosseous artery and will easily reach the dorsum of the hand, the first web space of the thumb, the metacarpophalangeal joints, and the carpal region up until the palm.

The flap is centered on a line between the lateral epicondyle of the humerus and the distal radial ulnar joint with the forearm in full pronation. The flap base is located 4–6 cm inferior to the lateral epicondyle and a point approximately 9 cm distal to the lateral epicondyle marks the center of the skin island.

At the inferior edge of the skin island margin a vertical incision extending to the level of the distal radial ulnar joint is required for elevation of the vascular pedicle to its pivot point. At the wrist, the extensor carpi ulnaris and the extensor digiti minimi muscles are identified and separated in order to isolate the posterior interosseous artery and the associated venae comitantes in its most distal tract, on the dorsal surface of the interosseous membrane. Care is required to show the distal anastomosis with the anterior interosseous artery. The incision is extended proximally through the flap radial margin and deep fascia to the superficial dorsal forearm extensor musculature. The flap is dissected out until it includes the fascia that covers the finger extensor communis. The fascia is sutured to the skin so that the flap does not come apart. By proceeding in this manner it is possible to adapt the flap dissection based on the location of the underlying perforators, by modifying the raising of the flap in a distal and proximal direction to extend the dissection so that at least one or

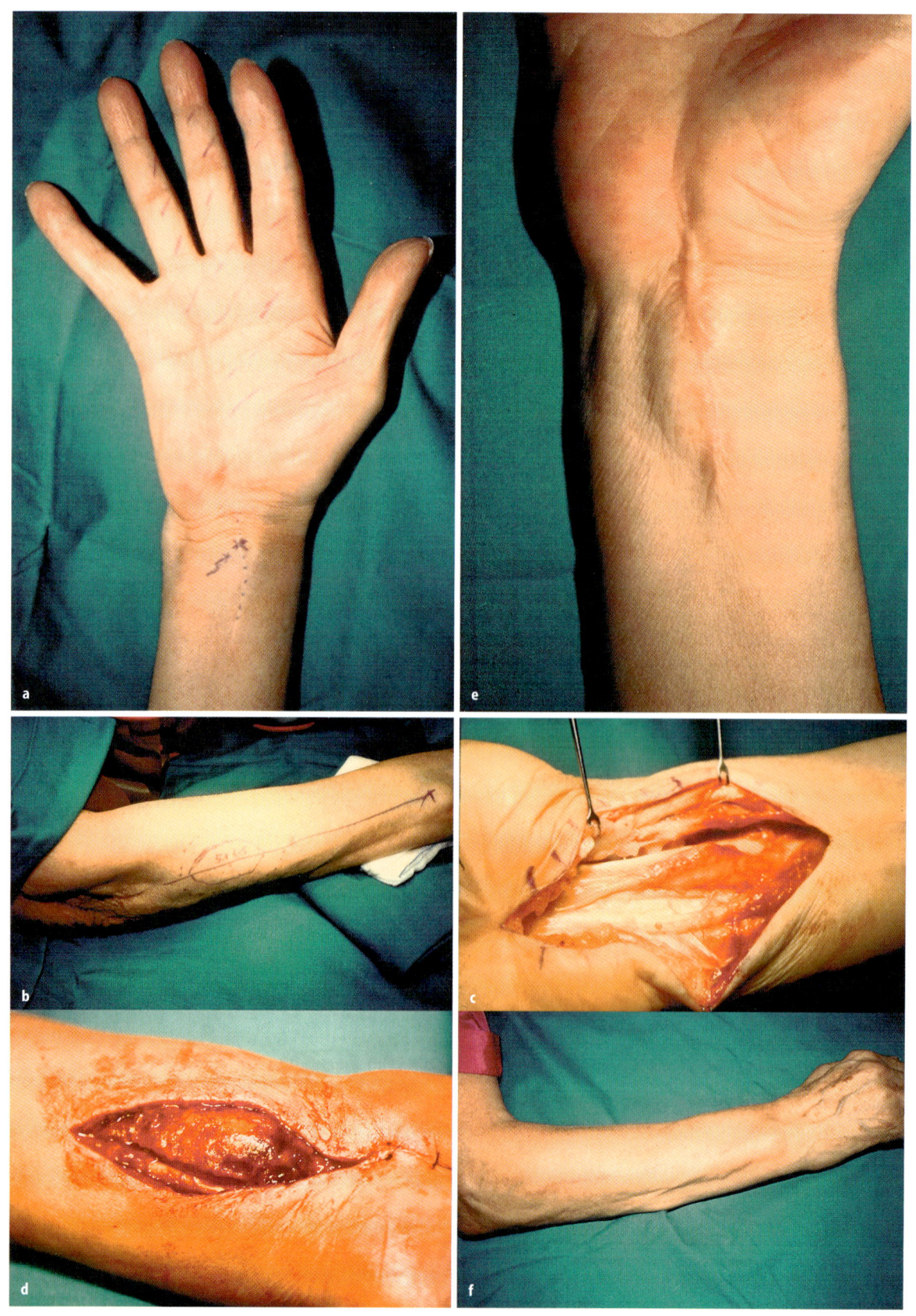

Fig. 46.8.

two large perforators are included in the flap. Once the position of the perforators has been identified, the skin island is incised on the ulnar side through deep fascia to the underlying extensor carpi ulnaris and extensor digiti minimi muscle bellies, until the muscle septum is completely exposed. At the distal flap edge located in the proximal forearm these muscle bellies are separated to visualize the underlying supinator muscle. Immediately distal and deep to the supinator muscle the posterior interosseous artery and associated venae comitantes are identified, tied, and sectioned, immediately after the origin of the large proximal perforator so it is included within the flap. The adjacent posterior interosseous nerve is identified too, and preserved. If the motor branch to the extensor carpi ulnaris from the deep radial nerve crosses superficial to the posterior interosseous artery, it is necessary to tie and divide the vascular pedicle distal to this motor branch. If an exclusively fascial flap has been dissected out, the cutaneous incision should be made along the flap axis exposing the fascia, by adequately elevating the two radial and ulnar cutaneous flaps, then the transfascial incision and the pedicle dissection follow the previously described techniques.

The flap dissection is completed in a proximal-distal direction elevating the septum extending between the extensor carpi ulnaris and extensor digiti minimi muscle and the overlying deep fascia to include the posterior interosseous artery and its septal ascending branches into the flap. At the forearm's distal third, the pedicle is usually wrapped in a osteo-fibrous sheath which is adherent to the ulna's periosteum. Care is required to complete the dissection, preserving the vascular pedicle, and to avoid the interruption of the T-shaped distal anastomosis with the anterior interosseous artery. It is an important anatomical landmark of the flap's pivot point because of the important role in perfusing the vascular pedicle of the flap. The flap is ready for transposition to the carpal region, or through a subcutaneous tunnel which has an adequate width and accurate hemostasis, or in an open surgical field by incising the skin at the ulnar bridge in a dorso-volar and also a proximo-distal direction (Fig. 46.8).

The exposure of the median nerve at the carpal tunnel and its entire circumference wrapping is done using a standard technique. However, this technique must always take into account the dimensional limitations of the posterior flap with respect to the radial artery or ulnar artery flap, since it has an inferior amount of fascia surface that is available for median nerve wrapping and an inferior distal extension for the length of the nerve.

Clinical Case Reports

Between October, 1989 and December, 2001, 18 patients were operated on by the authors. They were 11 women and 7 men, aged 38–76 years (mean 56 years). All the patients complained of severely painful symptoms in the median nerve area after multiple and/or aggressive operations of CTR.

Thirteen patients had two previous CTRs, 4 patients had three prior releases; 1 patient had only one CTR with a wide exposure of the median nerve and an aggressive neurolysis including epineurotomy and interfascicular neurolysis.

All patients complained of symptoms that impeded them from performing their usual activities of daily living. Only three of these patients reported that they had been symptom free for a few months after their first operation (Recurrent CTS); the other ones complained of a continuing morbidity (Persistent CTS). After the second CTR, often associated with external neurolysis of the median nerve, each patient achieved transient relief of symptoms never lasting more than 6 months from the time of surgery. Only 1 out of 4 patients reported having undergone symptom remission after the third operation.

The patients referred to their painful symptoms as wrist paresthesia at the thumb, index, and middle fingers. The patients described their pain as spontaneous and intractable or as throbbing and sharp, following light tactile skin stimulation around the median nerve zone.

The patients frequently described their hyperalgesic pain in terms of "electric shocks" or "intense burning."

One of the patients attempted suicide due to his intolerance of such strong symptoms.

Thenar eminence atrophy was present in 11 of the patients and 14 patients presented with a positive Tinel and Phalen sign. Only 1 of the 18 patients treated had vague clinical signs.

Regarding the treatment, a preoperative Allen test is always performed to assess the patency of the ulnar and radial arteries. An open CTR is then carried out, performing an accurate dissection of the median nerve from the surrounding scar tissue, particularly at the undersurface of the radial half of the transverse carpal ligament, ensuring an adequate decompression and external neurolysis of the median nerve. All patients showed severe scarring and wasting of the median nerve. An inadequate proximal release was found in 6

◁
Fig. 46.8. a Recurrent CTS. The *arrow* indicates the site of a positive Tinel sign and suspicion of a neuroma. The *broken line* indicates the area of palmar paresthesia. **b** Preoperative design for distally based island posterior interosseous fasciocutaneous flap harvesting: the fascia will be used to reconstruct the gliding system of the median nerve. **c** Median nerve exposure at the wrist; a neuroma incontinuity is present. **d** Five days after surgery the ischemic skin island is removed and it is possible to verify good perfusion of the fascial wrap that has been placed around the median nerve. **e** Postoperative results at the surgical site. **f** Postoperative results at the donor site.

patients, a neuroma of the palmar cutaneous branch of the median nerve in 2 and a large neuroma of the median nerve involving the digital nerves to the index and long finger was found in 3 patients. In all these cases a decision to proceed with an antebrachial reverse island flap to reconstruct the median nerve's altered gliding mechanism was made after decompression and external neurolysis of the nerve.

The fascial flap raised from the anterior surface of the forearm (radial artery and ulnar artery flap) or from its posterior aspect (posterior interosseous flap), is turned down distally towards the carpal tunnel. The median nerve is enveloped by the fascia with the gliding surface of the flap interfacing the nerve. Usually, we use the reverse radial artery flap because the full length of the nerve throughout the carpal tunnel, including its extension proximally and distally, is wrapped circumferentially by the fascia, which is approximated with 6/0 reabsorbable suture. Specifically, we used the fascial radial artery flap in 10 patients, preferring to use the fasciocutaneous radial artery flap in 6 cases on which the preoperative clinical exam showed a tenacious scar retraction at the interthenar area. The skin island positioned between the thenar and hypothenar eminence permits avoiding the recurrence of skin retraction in the palm. We limited the use of the ulnar artery flap and of the posterior interosseous flap to the treatment of specific problems. For example, in one case characterized by a neuroma of the palmar cutaneous branch of the median nerve without scar entrapment of the nerve, the posterior interosseous flap permitted the circumferential wrapping of the proximal segment of the median nerve after neurolysis and neuroma excision, while the 18th case had a particularly different clinical story and reconstruction of the palm was indicated in order to correct a functional deficit that was caused by a previous burn scar in conjunction with median nerve compression. In this case, the reverse ulnar artery fascio-cutaneous island flap was used.

Results

The patients periodically underwent clinical examination, according to a protocol based on the comparison of pre- and postoperative data about pain, numbness, Tinel sign, Phalen sign, scar tenderness, and Weber and Dellon tests.

Sensibility changes were documented by comparing two-point discrimination scores and the patient's paresthesia description pre- and postoperatively. The patients were asked to respond to a VAS test that was aimed at quantifying the severity of their painful symptoms both preoperatively and postoperatively by means of a subjective, graded test in which "0" represented no pain (asymptomatic) to "10" (intolerable pain). The patients were also asked to describe their capacity to perform activities of daily living and more specifically, those required in their work. Furthermore, the place of initial injury was documented, specifically if it had occurred at their workplace and if worker's compensation was being received by the patient. The authors acquired this information by means of the Quick-DASH ("Disability of the Arm, Shoulder and Hand") questionnaire [55].

The average follow-up time was 4 years with a range between 12 and 61 months. Four groups were classified at the end of the follow-up:

- *Excellent results* (4 pts): complete relief of symptoms and a normal postoperative two-point discrimination. The patient returned to their prior work level.
- *Good results* (12 pts): symptomatic patient with long periods of well-being followed by a period of pain, but not severe enough to impede the full use of their hand. These patients suffered mild intermittent pain, numbness, or scar tenderness.
- *Fair results* (2 pts): pain and persistent paresthesia but of a reduced intensity with respect to their preoperative symptoms.
- *Poor results* (0 pts): unmodified or aggravated symptoms from the surgery.

All the treated patients were able to return to unrestricted use of their hand with tactile sensibility improvement.

Four patients obtained excellent results, reporting both complete disappearance of their symptoms and full return to work, in addition to full recovery of their finger tip discrimination capacity. Good results were obtained in 12 of the 18 patients that were treated. These results statistically underline that return of hand function is probable but it is preceded by a period of spontaneous intermittent painful finger paresthesia and wrist scar tenderness that was easily evoked by even the lightest touch.

In 2 patients fair results were obtained and were characterized by slight symptom intensity reduction to which they learned to adapt. Nevertheless, these patients developed an evident psychological intolerance and a chronic pathological state where they reported no periods of well-being. Specifically, one of these patients complained prior to the initial surgery of a very severe pain that was causing him to go into a state of deep depression and led him to an attempted suicide.

Two of the 12 patients, who reported good surgical outcomes, were pursuing medical-legal insurance and civil compensation.

Discussion

Recalcitrant CTS is frequently reported in the literature with an incidence that ranges from 0.3% to 20% of treated cases [24, 32, 41, 42, 57, 76].

Particularly, persistent CTS is characterized by unrelieved or transient relief of symptoms and is most often due to incomplete section of the transverse carpal ligament. The patient tends to complain of postoperative finger paresthesia and hypoesthesia, and sharp pain. These symptoms are highly associated with positive electromyography results for median nerve compression. In these cases, a revision carpal tunnel surgery with a correct CTS release enables recovery.

Recurrent CTS, characterized by return of symptoms more than 3 months after surgery, is usually associated with fibrous proliferation within the carpal tunnel and scar adhesion of the median nerve to the radial half of the transverse carpal ligament.

In such cases the surgical treatment requires a wide exposure of the median nerve, the dissection of the nerve from the surrounding scar tissue, particularly at the undersurface of the radial half of the transverse carpal ligament, and the transposition of a flap over the injured median nerve to protect it from the formation of new scar adhesions and certainly to prevent reinnervation of the overlying scarred and denervated skin. This will markedly reduce the possibility of redevelopment of hyperalgesia in the skin. Usually, we use the hypothenar fat pad flap to cover the median nerve distal to the proximal wrist crease, while the pronator quadratus flap or the palmaris brevis flap can be used to cover the nerve more proximal to this level.

Sometimes the intraoperative findings demonstrate a severe circumferential median nerve scar entrapment. After multiple neurolysis, median nerve compression and the nerve scar entrapment are associated with the formation of fibrotic endoneural scarring that causes severe structural suffering: torsion and amputation of the fascicles and amputation of the vessels. These repetitive and chronic lesions determine an increase in endoneural fluid pressure [39, 54, 70] ("miniature compartment syndrome" [39, 40]) and leads to a severe ischemic nerve injury, which is associated with a severe and pharmaco-resistant pain syndrome.

The pain becomes intractable, sharp, and increased in its intensity with movements of the hand and wrist. Successively, the pain becomes continuous, intolerable, and completely interferes with the patient performing their daily life. At this point, usually all pharmacological treatments fail to reduce the pain. Often, reflex sympathetic dystrophy symptoms begin to appear in this phase and the patient reports both immobility and complete lack of functional hand strength.

In such cases the simple concept of covering and protecting the injured nerve from the surrounding scar tissue to prevent new adhesions after a superficial neurolysis is not enough to recover the severe pain syndrome. The scarred median nerve requires "interfascicular neurolysis," with microneurosurgical techniques, in order to completely detach the median nerve from its surrounding scar tissue and reconstruct the nerve's entire gliding mechanism by means of a gliding tissue flap able to easily reach the median nerve and circumferentially wrap itself around the entire length of the nerve in the carpal tunnel.

We suggest the use of the reverse radial artery fascial flap.

Once the median nerve has been freed from its scar tissue, the surgeon proceeds to reconstruct the nerve's gliding mechanism by wrapping the reverse radial artery fascial flap around the nerve. This not only separates the median nerve from the surrounding scar tissue, but also allows for the nerve to move pain-free within the canal and to revascularize itself by neoangiogenesis.

In our opinion, the reverse radial artery flap has several advantages over the other island and pedicled forearm flaps [72]:

1. A long arc of rotation
2. A significant size
3. A reliable blood supply

It makes it possible to raise a well-vascularized, wide fascial flap adequate to cover both the length and circumference of the involved median nerve along the entire carpal tunnel, shaping the gliding bed for the median nerve.

The disadvantages of this flap are the long scar and the radial artery sacrifice.

A preoperative Allen test was performed in all our patients to confirm adequate ulnar arterial supply to the hand after radial artery sacrifice [9]. None of our patients complained of postsurgical morbidity (cold intolerance, claudication pain).

Patient Selection for Surgery

Our results in the reconstruction of the gliding mechanism of the median nerve in recurrent CTS are certainly encouraging in this small, selected group of patients, with good results in most of them (12 pts), excellent results in 4 patients, and few fair results.

Nevertheless, this technique is much more complex than the simple CTR and can be the source of some postoperative discomfort in the patients, different from that expected. With the aim to inform preoperatively the patients on the surgical procedure, it is important to clinically distinguish between a persistent CTS resulting from an incorrect surgical procedure and a recurrent CTS, as well as from cases in which scarring has completely obliterated the nerves capacity to glide. The surgeon should recognize preoperatively the ideal candidate of this treatment.

In our opinion the patient's type of pain is the fundamental symptom that helps the surgeon to make the differential diagnosis and to distinguish between different pathological situations. Only after a thorough evaluation has been performed and the differential diagnosis has been made can the correct reconstructive surgery be scheduled. When analyzing the characteristics of each patient's pain, it must be associated with an objective evaluation that includes other clinical parameters and diagnostic instruments (EMG, NMR). This will allow the surgeon to clarify the pathological situation which correspond to the most appropriate surgical candidate of our therapeutic approach.

Unfortunately, in this phase, psychological disturbances begin to appear and render the differential diagnosis between organic pain and psychogenic pain almost impossible to decipher.

It is particularly difficult, during the differential diagnosis, to distinguish when the patient is affected by organic pain associated with a strong psychogenic-emotional component that easily can amplify their symptoms and pain perception. In these patients reoperation is strongly contraindicated. Every surgical treatment that is aimed at resolving a severely painful syndrome which has been generated by a median nerve injury, must be preceded by an analytic patient evaluation, in order to quantify the functional pain component. It must be precisely distinguished, prior to surgery, which patient is suffering from organic pain associated with severe pathological alterations of the nerve structures and which is suffering prevalently from functional pain, in which case the surgery is destined to fail. It is also important to distinguish which cases are characterized by a psychogenic amplification of pain, which is often quite controversial especially when workers' compensation or litigation is involved.

Before any surgical procedure for severe pain of the hand in the patients with recurrent CTS, we use a screening test helpful in separating the "organic" from the "functional" pain patient and capable of rating a surgical candidate on the basis of three broad parameters [43].

A Numerical Scale reflects the answers the patient give to a "pain questionnaire." A score of more than 14 points suggests that the patient is prevalently affected by functional pain and therefore surgical treatment is contraindicated.

The body diagram pain drawing determines if the pain described by the patient follows any known anatomic pattern. The patient is asked to draw on a body diagram his pain distribution; if the patient refers to pain in an anatomical distribution that is not compatible with the nerve injury, the test is considered positive for a considerable functional overlay.

The pain descriptors indicate the number of adjectives the patient uses to describe the pain. The test is considered positive for a considerable functional overlay if the patient chooses more than three adjectives from the pain description list to describe his pain.

The synthesis of such conclusions is reported in a Venn diagram that has three interconnecting circumferences. Each one of them expresses one parameter.

By interpreting the graph, it is evident that the patient whose scores place him outside of all the circles is the ideal surgical candidate.

If the patient's scores result in a situation where all scores are positive, surgery is absolutely contraindicated.

Finally, the patient who scores positive on one or two of the three portions of the test is in need of a psychiatric consultation.

Conclusions

As idiopathic CTS has become one of the most common peripheral neuropathies in the upper extremity, the incidence of the open carpal tunnel release increases. Simultaneously, the incidence of failure of this surgical procedure increases with incorrect surgical manipulation of the median nerve.

Unnecessary manipulation of the median nerve, neurolysis, and epineurotomy during the initial CTR should be avoided as these add little to the outcome but may increase the risk of recurrent CTS, as do incorrect skin incision and a carpal transverse ligament sectioning [72].

When a severe fibrous proliferation within the carpal tunnel produces median nerve entrapment and/or endoneural fibrotic scarring that alters the fascicles' anatomy and destroy its gliding mechanism, the surgical procedure requires neurolysis, including epineurotomy and "interfascicular neurolysis" if necessary, in order to completely detach the median nerve from its surrounding scar tissue. It is important to underline that interfascicular neurolysis is reserved for cases which have been carefully selected and where intraoperative findings indicate a tenacious interfascicular fibrosis, because it is an aggressive technique that will result in the development of residual endoneural scar and nerve ischemia [47]. The operation continues, raising the reverse radial artery fascial flap turned towards the carpal tunnel to wrap circumferentially the median nerve along the entire length of the canal. This technique makes it possible to restore the gliding bed of the median nerve, which acts as a barrier between the nerve and the surrounding scarred structures, particularly the transverse carpal ligament, thereby improving the blood supply of the ischemic neural tissue.

The improvement of the pain syndrome indicates the recovery of the gliding ability of the median nerve.

References

1. Becker C, Gilbert A (1988) The ulnar flap. In: Tubiana R (ed), The Hand. Saunders Philadelphia, Vol 3, pp 149–151
2. Braun RM, Rechnic M, Neill Cage DJ et al. (1995) The retrograde radial fascial forearm flap: surgical rational, technique, and clinical application. J Hand Surg 20A: 915–922
3. Brent B, Upton J, Acland RD et al. (1985) Experience with the temporoparietal fascial free flap. Plast Reconstr Surg 76:177–188
4. Brunelli G (1980) Neurolysis and free microvascular omentum transfer in the treatment of prostactinic palsies of the branchial plexus. Int Surg 65:515
5. Brunelli G, Brunelli F (1985) Surgical treatment of actinic brachial plexus lesion: free microvascular transfer of the greater omentum. J Reconstr Surg 1:197
6. Brunelli G, Battiston B, Brunelli F (1988) Free greater omentum transfer in ionizing radiation lesions of the brachial plexus. In: Brunelli G (ed) Texbook of Microsurgery. Masson Milano pp 825–831
7. Chang SM (1990) The distally based radial forearm fascial flap. Plast Reconstr Surg 85: 150–1
8. Cherup LL, Zachary LS, Gottlieb LJ et al. (1990) The radial forearm skin graft-fascial flap. Plast Reconstr Surg 85: 898–902
9. Coleman SS, Anson BJ (1961) Arterial patterns in the hand based upon a study of 650 specimens. Surg Gynecol Obstet 113: 409
10. Cormack GC, Lamberty BGH (1984) A classification of fascio-cutaneous flaps according to their patterns of vascularisation. Br J Plast Surg 37:80–7
11. Costa H, Soutar DS (1988) The disatlly based island posterior interosseous flap. Br J Plast Surg 41: 221–7
12. Costa H, Smith R, McGrouther DA (1988) Thumb reconstruction by posterior interosseous osteocutaneous flap. Br J Plast Surg 41:228–233
13. Cramer LM (1985) local fat coverage for the median nerve. In: Lakford LL (ed) American Society for Surgery of the Hand Correspondence Newsletter, p 35
14. Dellon AL, Mackinnon SE (1984) The pronator quadratus muscle flap. J Hand Surg (Am) 9:423–7
15. Fatah MF, Davies DM (1984) The radial forearm island flap in upper limb reconstruction. J Hand Surg 9B: 234
16. Fouher G, Van Genechten F, Merle N et al. (1984) A compound radial forearm flap in hand surgery: an original modification of the Chinese forearm flap. Br J Plast Surg 37: 139
17. Gilbert A, Teot L (1982) The free scapular flap. Plast Reconstr Surg 69:601–4
18. Gould JS (1991) Treatment of the painful injured nerve in continuity. In: Gelberman RH (ed) Operative Nerve Repair and Reconstruction. JB Lippincott, Philadelphia, New York, pp 1541–50
19. Groenevelt F, Schoorl R (1985) The reversed forearm flap using scarred skin in hand reconstruction of the flexor apparatus in the forearm. Br J Plast Surg 38:398–402
20. Guimberteau JC, Goin JL, Panconi B et al. (1988) The reverse ulnar artery forearm island flap in hand surgery: 54 cases. Plast Reconstr Surg 81:925–932
21. Hill H, Nahai F, Vasconez C (1978) The tensor fascia lata myocutaneous free flap. Plast Reconstr Surg 61:517–22
22. Holmberg J, Ekerot L (1993) Post-traumatic neuralgia in the upper extermity treated with extraneural scar excision and flap cover. J Hand Surg 18B:111–114
23. Holmberg J, Ekerot L, Salgeback S (1986) Flap coverage for post-traumatic nerve pain in the arm. Scand J Plast Reconstr Surg 20:285–288
24. Hybbinette CH, Mannerfelt L (1975) The carpal tunnel syndrome: a retrospective study of 400 operated patients. Acta Orthop Scand 46:610–20
25. Jin WT, Guan WX, Shi TM et al. (1992) Reversed island forearm fascial flap in hand surgery. Ann Plast Surg 15: 340–7
26. Jones NF, Shaw WW, Katz RG (1997) Circumferential wrapping of a flap around a scarred peripheral nerve for salvage of end-stage traction neuritis. J Hand Surg 22A: 527–35
27. Jones SMG, Stuart PR, Stothard J (1997) Open carpal tunnel relase. Does a vascularized hypothenar fat pad reduce wound tenderness? J Hand Surg 22B:758–760
28. Katsaros J, Schusterman M, Beppu M et al. (1984) The lateral upper arm flap: anatomy and clinical application. Ann Plast Surg 12: 489–570
29. Kessler FB (1976) Complications of the management of carpal tunnel syndrome. Hand Clin 2:401–6
30. Koncilia H, Kuzbari R, Worseg A et al. (1998) The lumbrical muscle flap: Anatomic study and clinical application. J Hand Surg 23A:111–119
31. Krstic R (1978) Die Gewebe des Menschen und der Säugetiere. Springer-Verlag, Berlin
32. Kulick MI, Gordillo G, Javidi T et al. (1976) Long term analysis of patients having surgical treatment for carpal tunnel syndrome. J Hand Surg 11A:59–66
33. Lang J (1962) Über das Bindegewebe und die Gefäße der Nerven. Anat Uud Embryol 123:61
34. Langloh ND, Linscheid RL (1972) Recurrent unrelieved carpal tunnel syndrome. Clin Orthop 83:41–7
35. Leslie BM, Ruby LK (1988) Coverage of a carpal tunnel wound dehiscence with the abductor digiti minimi muscle flap. J Hand Surg 13A: 36–39
36. Lin SD, Lai CS, Chiu CC (1984) Venous drainage in the reverse forearm flap. Plast Reconstr Surg 74: 508
37. Lovie MG, Juncan GM, Glasson JW (1984) Ulnar artery forearm free flap. Br J Plast Surg 37: 486
38. Loeser JD (1983) Definition, etiology, and neurological assessment of pain originating in the nervous system following deafferantation. In: Bonica JJ, Lindblom U, Iggo A (eds) Advances in pain research and therapy. Raven Press, New York, Vol 5, pp701–11
39. Lundborg G (1979) The intrinsic vascularization of human peripheral nerves: structural and functional aspects. J Hand Surg 4(1):34–41
40. Lundborg G, Myers R, Powell H (1983) Nerve compression injury and increased endoneurial fluid pressure: a "miniature compartment syndrome." J Neurol Neurosurg Psychiatry 46:1119–24
41. MacDonald RI, Lichtman DM, Hanlon JJ et al. (1978) Complications of surgical release for carpal tunnel syndrome. J Hand Surg 3:70–6
42. MacKinnon SE (1991) Secondary carpal tunnel surgery. Neurosurg Clin N Am 2:75–91
43. MacKinnon SE, Dellon AL (1988) Painful sequelae of peripheral nerve injury. In: MacKinnon SE, Dellon AL (eds) Surgery of peripheral nerve. Meriscola, New York, pp 455–519
44. MacKinnon SE, Dellon AL, Hudson AR et al. (1985) Alteration of neuroma formation by manipulation of neural environment. Plast Reconstr Surg 76:345–85
45. Masear VR, Tulloss JR, St Mary E et al. (1989) Venous wrapping of nerves to prevent scarring. In: Proceedings of the American Society of Surgeons of the Hand, 44th annual meeting. Seattle, WA
46. Millesi H (1986) Invited discussion in Wintsch K and Helany P: free flap of gliding tissue. J Reconstr Microsurg 2:143–50

47. Millesi H (1990) Progress in peripheral nerve reconstruction. World J Surg 14: 733–747
48. Millesi H, Rath T (1985) Pain syndromes after nerve repair. Treatment by transplantation of gliding tissue. Paper presented at the 8th symposium of the International Society of Reconstructive Microsurgery, Paris
49. Millesi H, Beer R, Reishner R et al. (1986) Stress and strain in peripheral nerves. Paper presented at the 3rd Congr Int Federation of Societies for Surg of the Hand, 3–8 nonembre 1986 Tokyo
50. Millesi H, Zoch G, Rath T (1990) The gliding apparatus of peripheral nerve and its clinical significance. Ann Hand Surg: 9(2):87–97
51. Millesi W, Schobel G, Bochdansky T (1994) Subpectoral gliding tissue flap. Plast Reconstr Surg 93: 842–51
52. Milward TM, Scott WG, Kleinert HJE (1977) The abductor digiti minimi muscle flap. Hand 9:82–85
53. Muhlbauer W, Herndl E, Stock W (1982) The forearm flap. Plast Reconstr Surg 70: 336
54. Ochoa J, Fowlel TJ, Gilliatt RW (1972) Anatomical changes in peripheral nerves compressed by a pneumatic tourniquet. J Anat 113:433–55
55. Padua R, Padua L, Ceccarelli E et al. (2003) Italian version of the disability of the arm, shoulder and hand (DASH) questionnaire. Cross-cultural adaptation and validation. J Hand Surgery 28B(2):179–186
56. Pagliei A, Taccardo G, Tulli A et al. (1997) "Vela quadra" flap: a new fascioadipose flap in hand surgery. J Hand Surg. 22-B (Suppl):34
57. Phalen GS (1970) Reflections on 21 years' experience with the carpal tunnel syndrome. JAMA 212:1365–7
58. Plancher KD, Idler RS, Lourie GM et al. (1996) Recalcitrant carpal tunnel. The hypothenar fat pad flap. Hand Clin 12:337–349
59. Ponteado CV, Masquelet AC, Chevrel JP (1986) The anatomic basis of the fasciocutaneous flap of the posterior interosseous artery. Surg Radiol Anat 8:209
60. Reisman NR, Dellon AL (1983) The abductor digiti minimi muscle flap: a salvage technique for palmar wrist pain. Plast. Reconstr. Surg. 72:859–863
61. Reyes FA, Burkhalter WE (1988) The fascial radial flap. J Hand Surg 13A: 432–5
62. Rose EH (1996) The use of the palmaris brevis flap in recurrent carpal tunnel syndrome. Hand Clin 12:389–395
63. Rose EH, Norris MS, Kowalsky TA et al. (1991) Palmaris brevis turnover flap as an adjunct to internal neurolysis of the chronically scarred median nerve in recurrent carpal tunnel syndrome. J Hand Surg 16A:191–201
64. Rydevik B, Lundborg G, Nordborg C (1976) Interneural tissue reactions induced by internal neurolysis. Scand J Plast Reconstr Surg 10:3–8
65. Soutar DS, Tanner NSB (1984) The radial forearm flap in the management of soft tissue injuries of the hand. Br J Plast Surg 37: 18
66. Spokevicius S, Kleinert HE (1996) The abductor digiti minimi flap. Its use in revision carpal tunnel surgery. Hand Clin 12:351–355
67. Steichen JB, Goitz RJ (1999) Omental transfer for severe recalcitrant carpal tunnel syndrome: a long term follow-up study. Paper presented at the ASSH Congr, sept 1999, Boston
68. Strickland JW, Idler RS, Lourie GM et al. (1996) The hypothenar fat pad flap for management of recalcitrant carpal tunnel syndrome. J Hand Surg 21A:840–848
69. Sunderland S (1973) Nerve and nerve injuries. Churchill Livingstone, 2nd edn, Edimburgh-London-New York
70. Sunderland S (1976) The nerve lesion in the carpal tunnel syndrome. J Neurol Neurosurg Psychiatry 39:615–26
71. Taleisnik J (1973) The palmar cutaneous branch of the median nerve and the approach to the carpal tunnel. J Bone Joint Surg 55A: 1212–1217
72. Tham SKY, Ireland DCR, Riccio M et al. (1996) Reverse radial artery fascial flap: a treatment for the chronically scarred median nerve in recurrent carpal tunnel syndrome. J Hand Surg 21A: 849–54
73. Timmons MJ (1986) The vascular basis of the radial forearm flap. Plast Reconstr Surg 77:80–92
74. Urbaniak JR (1991) Complications of treatment of carpal tunnel syndrome. In: Gelberman RH (ed) Operative nerve repair and reconstruction. JB Lippincott, Philadelphia, pp 967–979
75. Van Beek A, Kleinert HE (1977) Practical microneurorrhaphy. Orthop Clin North Am 8:357
76. Wadstroem J, Nigst H (1976) Reoperation for carpal tunnel syndrome: a retrospective analysis of 40 cases. Ann Chir Main 5:54–8
77. Weinzweig N, Chen L, Chen ZW (1994) The distally based radial forearm fasciocutaneous flap with preservation of the radial artery: an anatomic and clinical approach. Plast Reconstr Surg 94:675–83
78. Wilgis EFS (1984) Local muscle flaps in the hand. Anatomy as related to reconstructive surgery. Bull Hosp Jt Dis 44:552–557
79. Wintsch K (1983) The gliding tissue flap. Paper presented at the 7th Symposium of the International Society of Reconstructive Microsurgery, New York
80. Wintsch K, Helaly P (1986) Free flap of gliding tissue. J Reconstr Microsurg 2:143–150
81. Wulle C (1996) The synovial flap as treatment of the recurrent carpal tunnel syndrome. Hand Clin 12:379
82. Yang G, Chen B, Gao Y et al. (1981) Forearm free skin flap transplantation. Natl Med J China 61:139
83. Zancolli EA, Angrigiani C (1986) Colgajo dorsal de antebrazo ("on isola") (Pediculo de vases interoseos posteriores). Rev Assoc Arg Orthop Traumatol 51: 161–8
84. Zancolli EA, Angrigiani C (1988) Posterior interosseous island forearm flap. J Hand Surg 13B:130–5

The Ulnar Fascial-Fat Flap for the Treatment of Scarred Median Nerve in Recalcitrant Carpal Tunnel Syndrome

A. Vigasio, I. Marcoccio

Introduction

Carpal tunnel syndrome remains the most frequently recognized peripheral nerve entrapment syndrome and, even if the majority of patients are relieved from their symptoms by the surgical carpal tunnel release, the incidence of failure in open carpal tunnel decompression varies in large clinical series from 7% to 25% [2, 10, 11, 15, 17, 18] despite Phalen's famous statement according to which "there are few operations that are as successful and rewarding as the operation for carpal tunnel syndrome" [14].

The most commonly cited causes of failure include incomplete release of the transverse carpal ligament, postoperative nerve adhesions, intraneural fascicular scar [6, 10, 16], devascularization of the nerve [6], tenosynovitis [10, 16], Sudeck's reflex sympathetic dystrophy, infections, painful scars, hand stiffness, nerve lesions (partial or total section of the median nerve or one of its branches) [10].

Langloh and Lindscheid stated that the most common pathological finding at re-exploration of the median nerve was incomplete release of the transverse carpal ligament [9]: conventional treatment in these cases is re-exploration of the nerve with external neurolysis followed by immediate motion, which provides relief of symptoms for most patients (Fig. 47.1).

However, in a small groups of patients, above all those that undergo a prolonged period of nonsurgical treatment with persistent symptoms such as dysesthetic wrist pain, grasp weakness, sensory disturbances, and the focal irritability of the median nerve [15], at the re-exploration the most common pathological findings are fibrous proliferation within the carpal tunnel, various adherences of the median nerve to the adjacent structures [17], and/or intraneural fibrosis of the nerve (Fig. 47.2).

In these cases, the use of conventional microsurgical techniques, such as extensive internal neurolysis, which theoretically improves neurological function, may fail to relieve the symptoms of most patients. The failure is due to the inability to reverse the adhesive scar phenomena, resulting in a farther fixation of the nerve to either the overlying transverse carpal ligament and the skin, or to the underlying flexor tendons, causing the progression of its interfascicular scar and segmental devascularization [6].

This scar process is termed neurodesis [16], or traction neuritis [6], or adhesive median neuritis [20], or epineural fibrous fixation [5] and its symptoms are generally debilitating with dysesthetic pain, exacerbated by direct pressure over the surgical incision or by flexion and extension of the adjacent joints [6] and may be associated to the recurrence of the carpal tunnel syndrome disturbances.

Etiology of the adherence between the nerve and the surrounding tissues is multifactorial, but the most important factor may be identified in the concurrence of the ligamentous scar formation over the median nerve course and the concomitant formation of hematoma, or the prolonged postoperative splinting, or the delayed or inadequate mobilization of the adjacent joints in the immediate postoperative period [10].

A multicentric study realized by the Switzerland Hand Surgery Society shows that in case of failure of carpal tunnel release, decompression and external neurolysis improves the symptoms in the 94% of patients affected by epineural fibrosis, but if internal fibrosis is found and internal neurolysis is then performed, the improvement of neurological function decreases to the 67% [3, 10].

Internal neurolysis, indeed, enhances axonal regeneration of the chronically compressed nerve with only transient relief of symptoms. This is the reason why it may farther induce an increase of the fascicular scar with segmental devascularization [6] and recurrence of neurodesis with disappointing results.

Coverage of the median nerve with soft tissue flap following internal neurolysis improves the positive results from 67% up to 81% [3, 10].

A soft tissue flap has the following advantages [1, 5, 6, 13, 15–17]:

- It acts as a barrier between the nerve and the surrounding structures, protecting the nerve from external pressure, traction forces, and the adjacent sliding tendons.
- It covers the nerve with a soft unscarred and well-

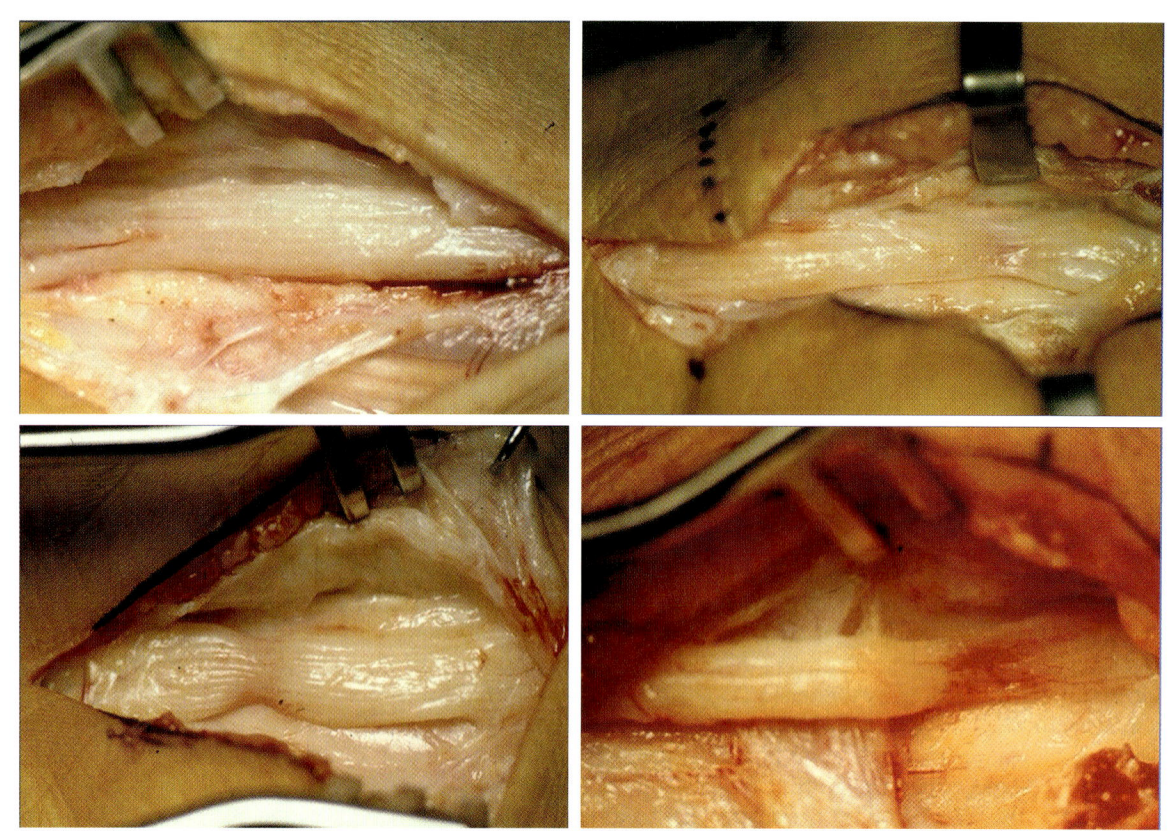

Fig. 47.1. Four different clinical cases of re-exploration of failed median nerve decompression. The lesion is represented by an incomplete release of the transverse carpal ligament with various degrees of median nerve impressions. A simple decompression of the nerve improves the symptoms

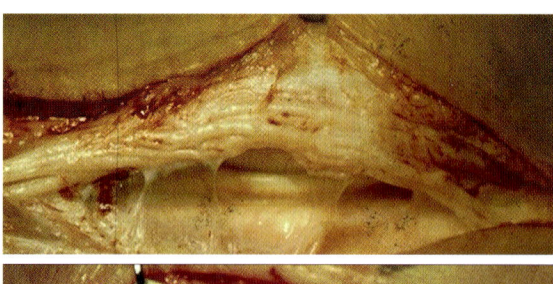

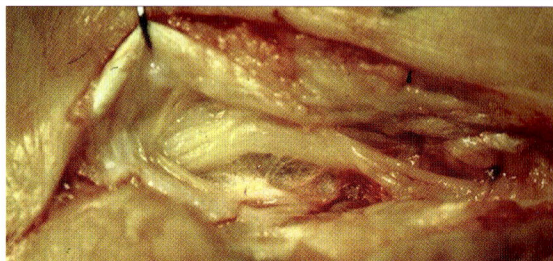

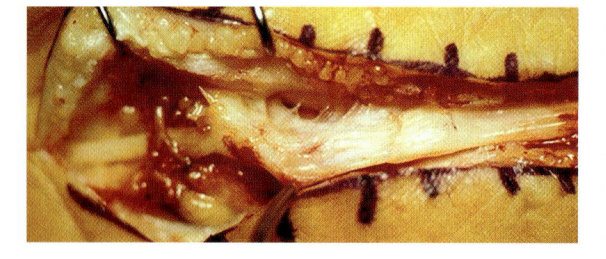

vascularized tissue, improving blood supply into a region of chronic ischemia.
- It prevents readherences and it restores the longitudinal gliding bed of the median nerve.

Several surgical procedures have been described to cover the median nerve within the carpal tunnel with soft and healthy vascularized tissue flap. They include palmaris brevis muscle flap [15], pronator quadratus muscle flap [16], ulnarly based pedicle synovial flap [22], abductor digiti minimi muscle flap [13], lumbrical flap [19], radial forearm flap [17], hypothenar fat pad flap [16], and various free flaps including thoracodorsal and omental transfers [12, 21].

We present our experience with a subcutaneous flap based on a dorsal branch of the ulnar artery.

This flap was first described in 1988 by Becker and Gilbert [1]: it is vascularized by the median branch of the cubital-dorsal artery, which arises constantly (99% of cases) at the forearm from the ulnar artery between 2 and 5 cm proximally to the pisiform bone, then

◁
Fig. 47.2. Three different clinical examples of adherences of the median nerve after failed surgical carpal tunnel release. The nerves are extensively scarred and fixed to the overlying transverse carpal ligament and/or to the surrounding tendons

reaches the deep face of the flexor carpi ulnaris tendon, where it divides into two subcutaneous branches defined descending and ascending branches.

The flap is vascularized by the ascending branch that, lying under the antebrachial fascia, goes towards the medial epicondyle and vascularizes the ulnar side of the antebrachial fascia and the corresponding skin for a maximum extension of 20 cm in length and 9 cm in width, allowing easy and safe dissection of a subcutaneous retrograde fascial-fat flap 13–14 cm long and 3 cm wide. The distal point of rotation, between 2 and 5 cm proximally to the pisiform, permits the flap to reach the distal side of the carpal tunnel covering completely the median nerve with a soft fat tissue. The arc of rotation of this reverse pedicle flap is complete.

Surgical Technique

Dissection begins under loupes magnification exploring widely the median nerve along its tunnel, then working through the reconstituted carpal ligament which must be largely opened ensuring adequate decompression (Fig. 47.3). Then follows the identification of the median nerve from the surrounding scar tissues, particularly the inferior surface of the radial half of the transverse carpal ligament (Fig. 47.4).

Under the operating microscope an external neurolysis, associated if necessary with epineurectomy, is performed with particular care with the respect to the median nerve motor branch, identifying associated lesions of the cutaneous branches which are frequent in multi-operated patients (Fig. 47.5).

In those patients presenting clinical hypersensitivity of the median nerve at the wrist, with intraoperative findings of neurodesis and significant interfascicular scar (Fig. 47.6), requiring internal neurolysis, a fascioadipose pedicle flap is performed.

The incision is outlined longitudinally on the skin overlying ulnar artery extending proximally up to the medial third of the forearm. The pisiform bone is marked as the pivot point and starting from there, the length of the incision is about 15 cm. A sharp dissection is done just under to the subdermal plexus between the skin and the underlying adipose surface, exposing an adipose plane 13–14 cm long and 4–5 cm wide (Fig. 47.7). Care must be taken to avoid too thin a cutaneous flap, in order to not to devascularize the skin.

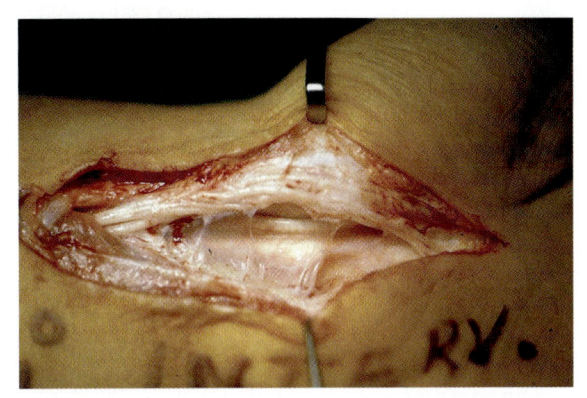

Fig. 47.4. Same clinical case: the extensive adhesions between the nerve and the overlying transverse carpal ligament. The lesion is increased by an evident intraneural scar

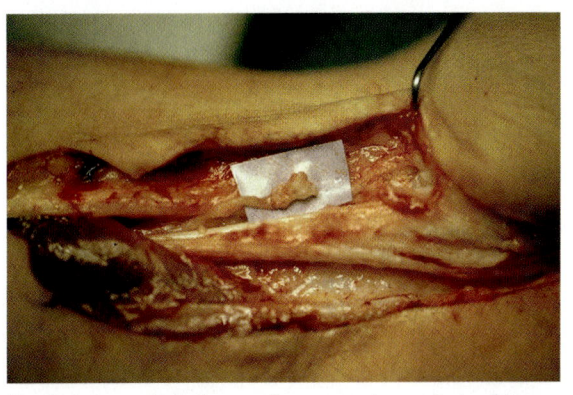

Fig. 47.5. Same clinical case: after external neurolysis a big amputation neuroma of the cutaneous median nerve branch is found

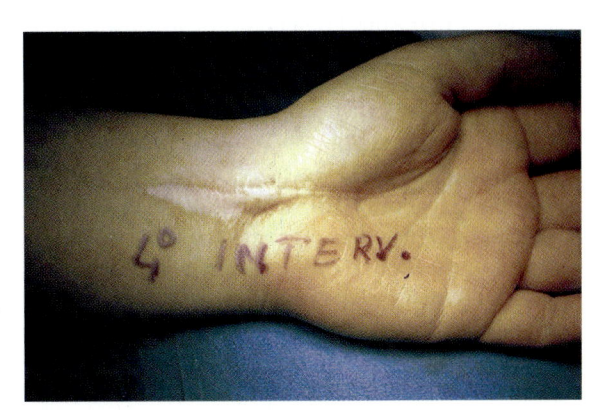

Fig. 47.3. Clinical case: keloid skin scar in patient that underwent three median nerve decompressions

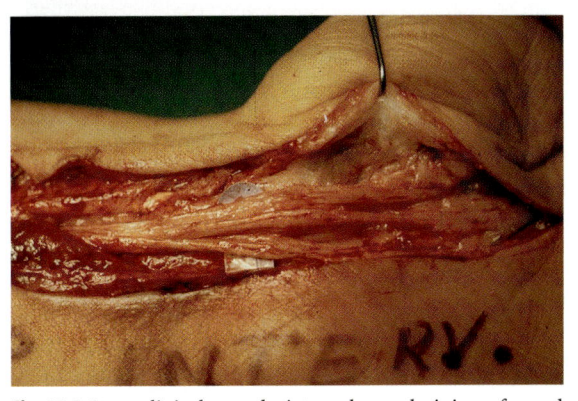

Fig. 47.6. Same clinical case: the internal neurolysis is performed and the nerve may be covered with the ulnar fascial-fat flap

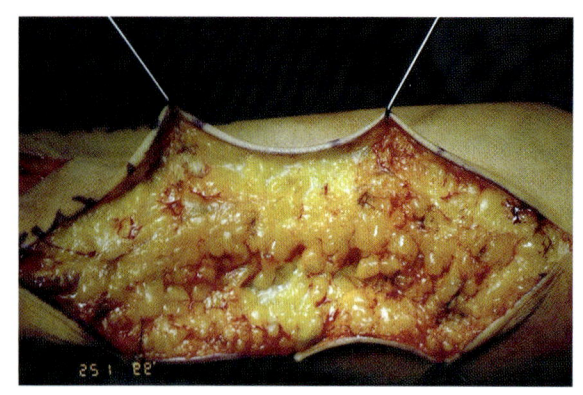

Fig. 47.7. A sharp dissection is done just deep to the subdermal plexus between the skin and the underlying adipose surface, exposing an adipose plane 13–14 cm long and 4–5 cm wide. Care must be taken to not make the cutaneous flap too thin, so as to not devascularize the skin

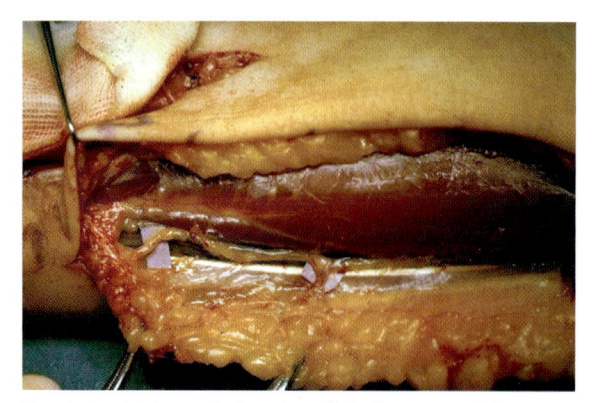

Fig. 47.8. Division and elevation of the flap is carefully prosecuted in a distal direction and easily identifies in the deep plane the ulnar neurovascular bundle and numerous small vascular branches moving from the ulnar vessels to the fascio-adipose flap which are cauterized

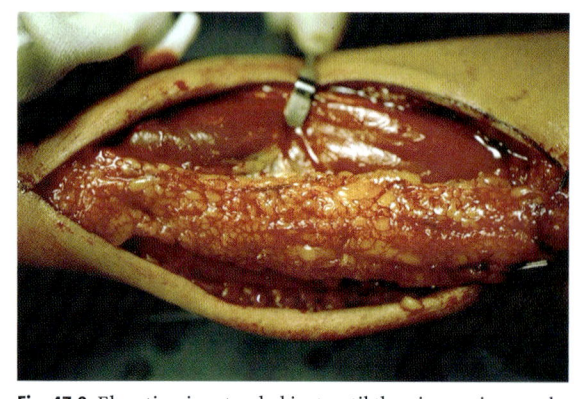

Fig. 47.9. Elevation is extended just until the pivot point, so obtaining a flap 3 cm wide and 13–14 cm long

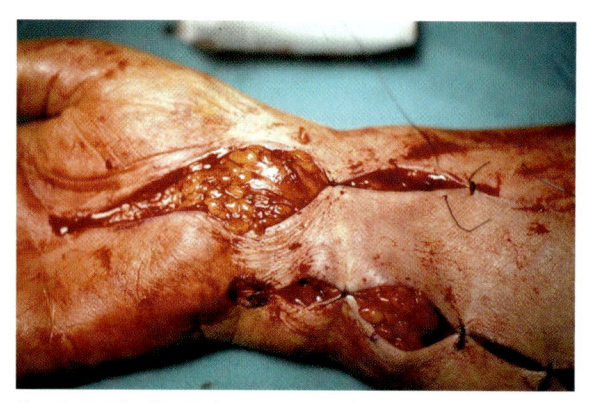

Fig. 47.10. The flap is then overturned in a distal direction and passed subcutaneously under a small skin bridge that separates the ulnar from the carpal incisions, covering the median nerve for the entire carpal tunnel length

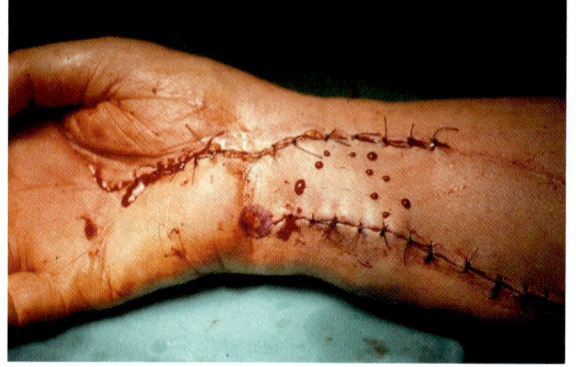

Fig. 47.11. Primary skin closure is possible, in spite of a mild bulk of the flap

Dissection of the flap is started proximally in the forearm at its distal edge: the adipose tissue and the underlying antebrachial fascia are incised transversally in a plane just above the epimysium of the forearm muscles, following both radial and ulnar distal direction, elevating a flap 3 cm wide.

The distal dissection of the flap easily identifies in the deep plane the ulnar neurovascular bundle and numerous small vascular branches moving from the ulnar vessels to the fascio-adipose flap which are cauterized (Fig. 47.8).

Division and elevation of the flap is carefully prosecuted just until the pivot point 2–5 cm proximally from the pisiform bone where the vascular pedicle can be identified. The fascial-fat flap obtained measures 3 cm wide and 13–14 cm long (Fig. 47.9). 2.5 cm proximally from the rotational point, the flap may be turned in a distal direction over the median nerve up to the distal part of the carpal tunnel, passed subcutaneously under a small skin bridge that separates the ulnar from the carpal incision, so to cover the median nerve for the entire carpal tunnel length (Fig. 47.10).

Mattress sutures are placed through the radial and ulnar walls of the tunnel and through the flap distal edge, thereby fixing it over the nerve.

Skin over the donor flap is closed primarily (Fig. 47.11). Despite a mild bulk of the flap, primary skin closure in the carpal region is possible (Fig. 47.10), just applying gentle transverse compression over the flap.

The wrist is splinted in slight extension with the fingers free for immediate postoperative motion. The splint is removed after 7 days to start the active mobilization of the wrist, scar gentle massage, and desensitization.

Results

Between January1993 and November 2001, 26 hands in 24 patients affected by persistent or recurrent carpal tunnel symptoms after previous open surgical decompression were operated on by the senior author (A. Vigasio). There were 22 women and 4 men, aged 24–74 years.

All 26 patients suffered from referred pain proximal to the wrist (Table 47.1).

Twenty-four patients out of 26 presented hypersensitivity at the wrist.

Nocturnal symptoms along the median nerve distribution was present in 20 patients.

Tinel's and Phalen's signs were both equivocal in 1 patient, elicited in 22.

All patients suffered from a decreased grip strength.

Four hands had severe decrease at two-points static discrimination test in the median innervated digits. Twenty hands had mild decrease at two-points static discrimination test (greater than 6 mm), while 2 were normals.

Thenar atrophy was present in 3 hands, while 4 hands presented evidence of damage at the palmar cutaneous branch of the median nerve.

Electrodiagnostic studies showed persistent median nerve compression in 20 hands.

The average time between last failed open carpal tunnel decompression and the re-exploration was 10 months (from 3 to 24 months). The average number of previous open carpal tunnel release was 2.2 (maximum 4 decompressions).

At re-exploration in all cases the median nerve was found entrapped in severe restrictive scar tissue and often adherent to the radial leaf of the divided transverse carpal ligament or to the adjacent flexor tendons. In all cases the nerve was thickened by diffuse epineural fibrosis and in most cases interstitial scarring was severe.

Inadequate release of the carpal ligament was found in 3 cases (1 case at the distal level and 2 cases at the proximal one).

Neuroma of the palmar cutaneous branch of the median nerve was present in 4 cases.

The median nerve motor branch was found avulsed from the thenar muscles in 1 case.

In all cases external neurolysis and fascio-adipose pedicle flap were performed.

Twenty-two nerves underwent internal neurolysis.

Results are presented in Table 47.2. The follow-up varied from 20 to 71 months (average follow-up 42 months):

- Hypersensitivity of the median nerve at the wrist present in 24 patients before surgery, was absent in 16 cases and decreased in 6. Symptoms worsened in 2 subjects.
- Proximal pain from the wrist, found in all patients before surgery, was absent in 23 and decreased in 1. In 2 patients the pain worsened.
- Nocturnal symptoms, present in 20 patients before surgery, were absent in 17, decreased in 1, unmodified in 1 and worsened in another one.
- Phalen's sign present before surgery in 22 patients, was absent in 19, decreased in 1 and worsened in 2.
- Tinel's sign present before surgery in 22 patients, was absent in 20, unmodified in 1 and worsened in another one.
- Grip strength decreased in all patients before surgery, increased in 24 patients and worsened in 2.
- Twenty-two out of 24 patients with abnormal two-points static discrimination test in the median nerve digits showed improvement of their sensibility parameters. Only 2 patients of 4 with severe diminution at two-points static discrimination test showed persistent sensory deficit.
- Thenar atrophy grossly improved in 2 hands, unmodified in 1.

Table 47.1. Preoperative clinical findings

	Hands
Proximal wrist pain	26/26
Wrist hypersensitivity	24/26
Nocturnal symptoms	20/26
Phalen's sign	22/26
Tinel's sign	22/26
<2pDS	24/26
Grip strength decrease	26/26
Thenar atrophy	3/26

Table 47.2. Results

	Absent	Improved	Unmodified	Worsened
Proximal wrist pain	23/26	1/26	–	2/26
Wrist hypersensitivity	16/24	6/24	–	2/24
Nocturnal symptoms	17/20	1/20	1/20	1/20
Phalen's. sign	19/22	1/22	–	2/22
Tinel's sign	20/22	–	1/22	1/22
2pDS	–	22/24	–	2/24
Grip strength	–	24/26	–	2/26
Thenar atrophy	–	2/3	1/3	–

366   V Complications

- Twenty-one patients were satisfied at the final follow-up, 3 were fairly satisfied, and 2 were unsatisfied.
- Of 10 patients in the worker compensation group, 8 went back to work, 6 returning to their original job and 2 retraining to less strenuous occupations.
- The average disability time was 3.2 months (from 62 days to 14.3 months).
- No complications were encountered in this study. Please see Figs. 47.12 – 47.16 for an overview of a selection of other clinical situations in which different presentations of the pathology are shown.

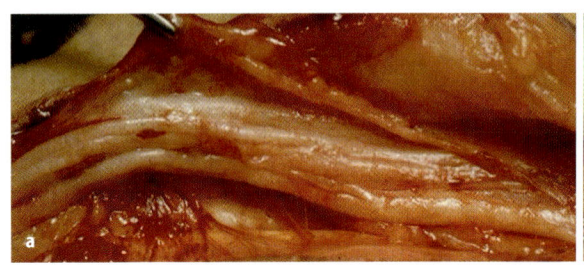

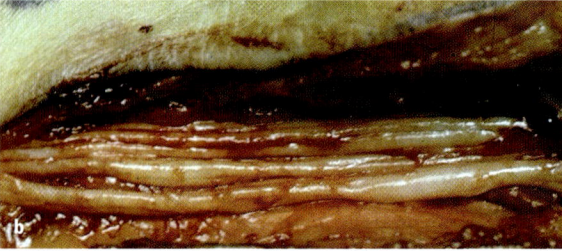

Fig. 47.12. a, b Clinical case: **a** extensive epineural and intraneural fibrosis. **b** the nerve after internal neurolysis and before coverage with the flap

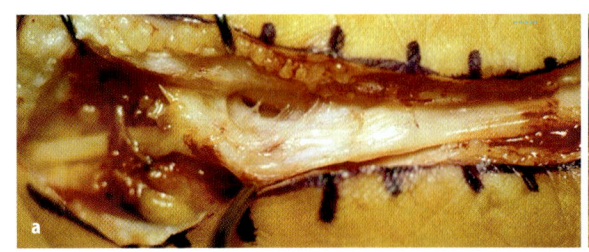

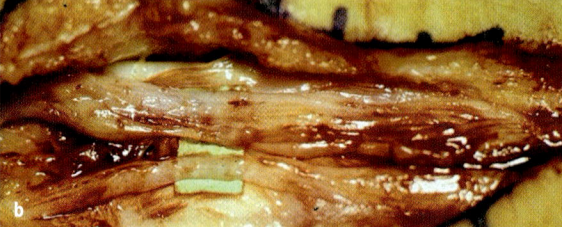

Fig. 47.13. a, b Clinical case: **a** another example of severe scar **b** treated by internal neurolysis and pedicle flap

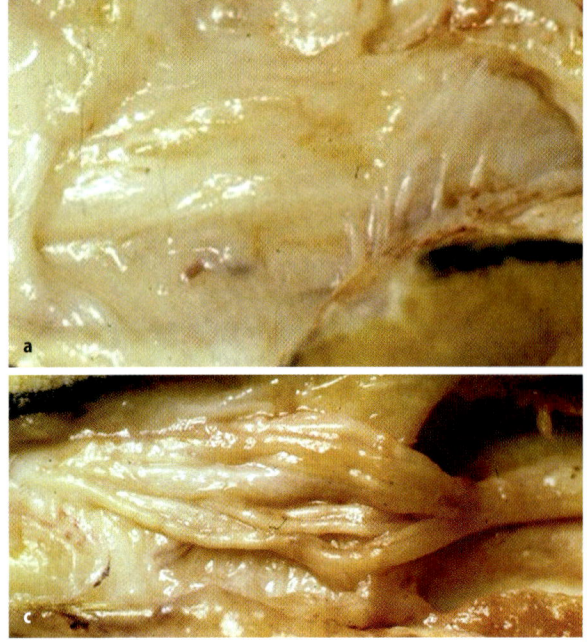

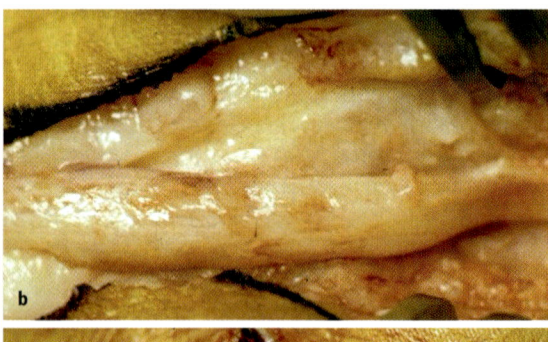

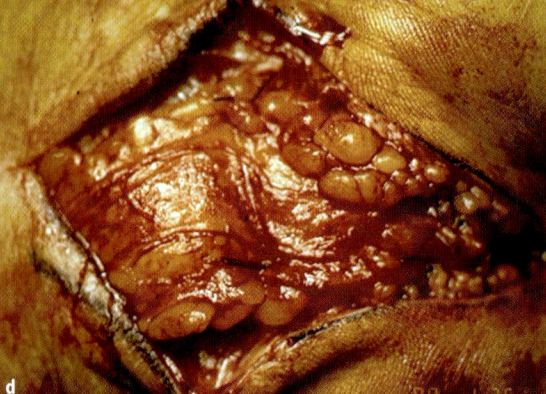

Fig. 47.14. a–d Clinical case: **a** the nerve is largely scarred with the surrounding tissues, **b** after external neurolysis, the nerve presents intraneural scar, **c** internal neurolysis is performed, **d** the flap is placed over the median nerve

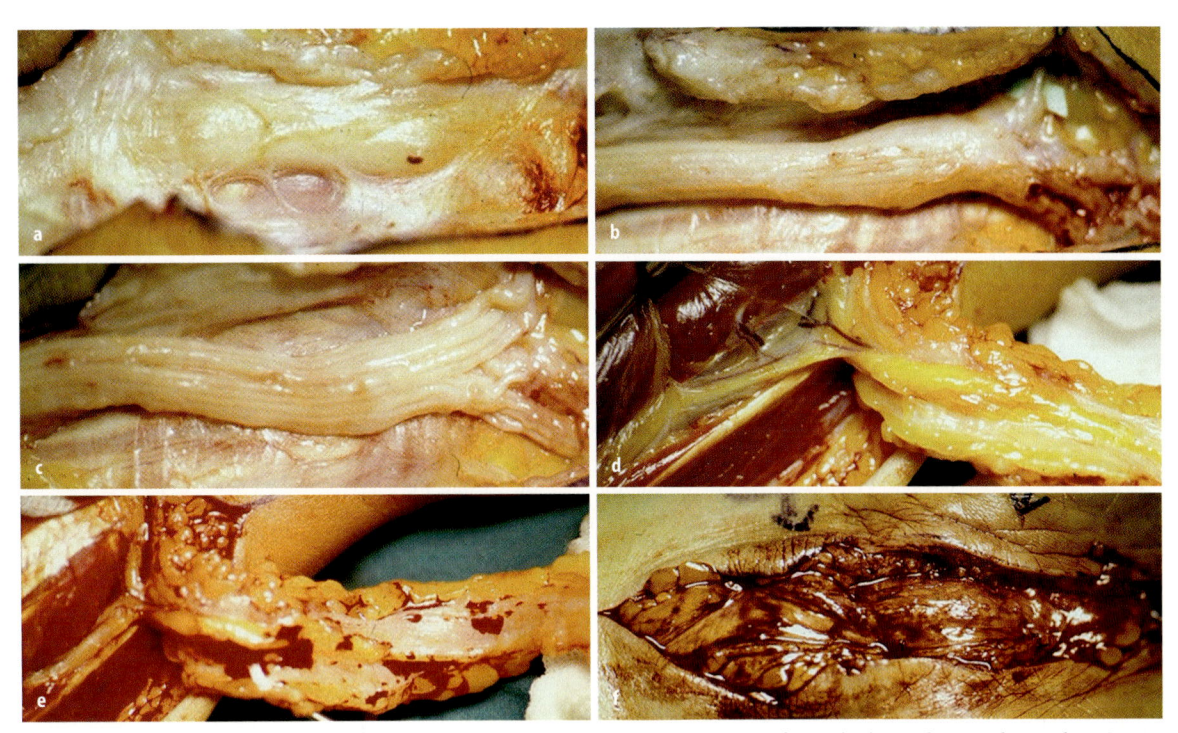

Fig. 47.15. a–f Clinical case: **a** the extensive epineural scar, **b** external neurolysis is performed, **c** limited internal neurolysis is executed, **d** the flap is dissected and the vascular pedicle is visible, **e** good vascularization of the flap after the removal of the tourniquet, **f** final result

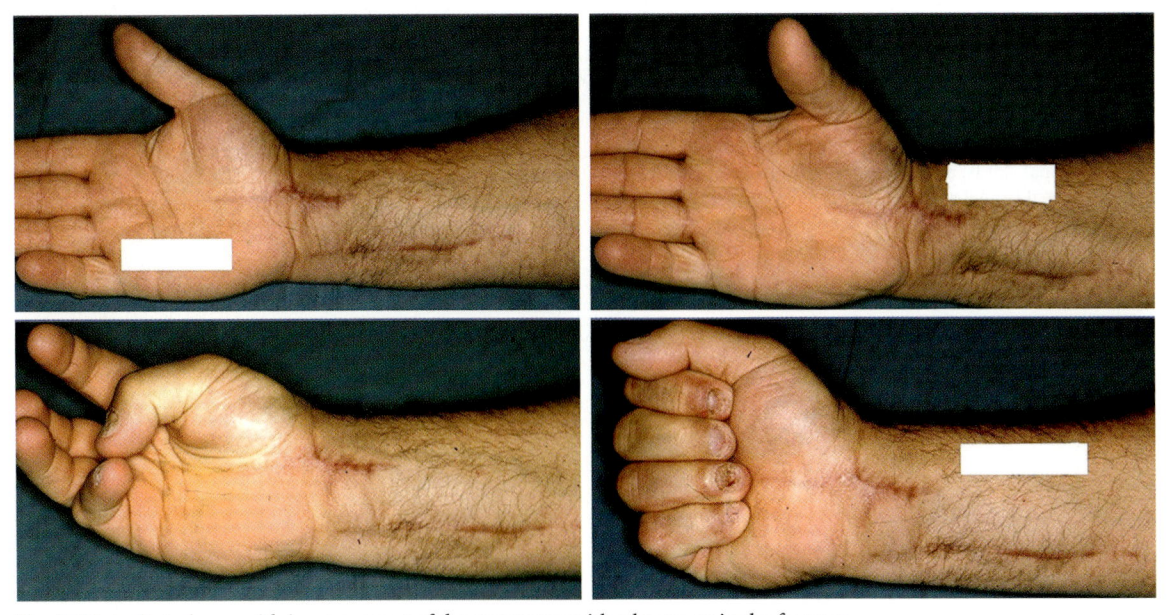

Fig. 47.16. A clinical case with improvement of the symptoms with a long scar in the forearm

Conclusions

In conclusion, only 2 out of 26 patients, operated for nerve decompression, 4 and 3 times respectively, complained of deterioration of their signs and symptoms requiring continuous analgesics drugs treatment with no improvement of their status.

The results of the treatment in patients with chronic pain due to an end-stage neurodesis of the median nerve, treated by neurolysis and subsequent coverage with the Gilbert-Becker's pedicle fascial-fat flap demonstrate that this is a good procedure in the management of recurrent carpal tunnel syndrome.

The major advantages are:

- This pedicle flap is a local flap.
- It can be performed in locoregional anesthesia.
- Its size and arc of rotation is significant, allowing adequate coverage of the median nerve in the carpal tunnel.
- It doesn't sacrifice major vessels of the hand.
- It can be easily performed.

The major disadvantage is the residual long scar in the forearm.

References

1. Becker C, Gilbert A (1988) The ulnar flap. In: Tubiana R. The hand Vol 3. Saunders, Philadelphia pp 149–151
2. Bonnard C, Papaloizos M (1990) Annual Congress of the Swiss Society for Surgery of the Hand (Lausanne, 23–24 March 1990), Proceedings. Ann Hand and Upper Limb Surg 9:388–391
3. Chang B, Dellon L (1993) Surgical management of recurrent carpal tunnel syndrome. J Hand Surg 18B:467–470
4. Dellon AL, Mackinnon SE (1984) The pronator quadratus muscle flap. J Hand Surg 9A:423–427
5. Hunter JM (1991) Recurrent carpal tunnel syndrome, epineural fibrous fixation and traction neuropathy. Hand Clin 7:491
6. Jones NF, Shaw WW, Katz RG (1997) Circumferential wrapping of a flap around a scarred peripheral nerve for salvage of end-stage traction neuritis. J Hand Surg 22A: 527–535
7. Jones SM, Stuart PR, Stothard J (1997) Open carpal tunnel release: does a vascularized hypotenar fat pad reduce wound tenderness? J Hand Surg 22B:758–760
8. Katz JN, Fossel KK, Simmons BP, et al. (1995) Symptoms, functional status, and neuromuscular impairment following carpal tunnel release. J Hand Surg 20A:549–555
9. Langloh ND, Linscheid RL (1972) Recurrent and unrelieved carpal tunnel syndrome. Clin Orthop 83:41–47
10. Luchetti R. (1993) Trattamento delle complicanze della sindrome del tunnel carpale. Riv Chir Riab Mano Arto Sup 30(2):155–161
11. Mackinnon SE, Murray JF, Kin BK, et al. (1991) Internal neurolysis fails to improve the results of primary carpal tunnel decompression. J Hand Surg 16A:211–218
12. Millesi H, Rath T, Reishner R, et al. (1993) Microsurgical neurolysis: its anatomical and physiological basis and its classification. Microsurgery 14:430–439
13. Milward TM, Stott WG, Kleinert HE (1977) The abductor digiti minimi muscle flap. Hand 9:82–85
14. Phalen GS (1986) The carpal tunnel syndrome: seventeen years experience in diagnosis and treatment of six hundred fifty-four hands. J Bone J Surg 48A:211–228
15. Rose EH, Norris MS, Kowalsky TA, et al. (1991) Palmaris brevis turnover flap as an adjunct to internal neurolysis of the chronically scarred median nerve in recurrent carpal tunnel syndrome. J Hand Surg l 6A:l91–201
16. Strikland JW, Idler RS, Lourie GM, et al. (1996) The hypotenar fat pad flap for management of recalcitrant carpal tunnel syndrome. J Hand Surg 21A:840–848
17. Tham SKY, Ireland DCR, Riccio M, et al. (1996) Reverse radial artery fascial flap: a treatment for the chronically scarred median nerve in recurrent carpal tunnel syndrome. J Hand Surg 21A:849–854
18. Wadstroem J, Nigst H (1986) Reoperation for carpal tunnel syndrome. Ann Chir Main 5(1):54–58
19. Wilgis EFS (1984) Local muscle flaps in the hand anatomy related to reconstructive surgery. Bull Hosp Joint Dis 44:552–557
20. Wilgis EFS, Murphy R (1986) The significance of longitudinal excursion in peripheral nerves. Hand Clin 2:761
21. Wintsch K, Helalay P (1986) Free flap gliding tissue. J Reconstr Microsurg 2:143–151
22. Wulle C (1987) Traitement des récidives du syndrome du canal carpien, Ann Chir Main 6(3):203–209

Protective Covering of the Nerve by the "Vela Quadra" Flap

A. Pagliei, F. Catalano, F. Fanfani

Introduction

The "vela quadra" (square sail) flap was initially used for the management of posttraumatic neuromas of the median nerve of the wrist: it is a vascularized fascio-adipose flap aimed at covering the median nerve in the particularly critical area of the wrist which is anatomically more exposed to traumatic and iatrogenic lesions. We subsequently extended this technique to the management of recalcitrant neuropathies following surgical neurolysis of the median nerve.

Anatomy

A study of the vascular anatomy of the upper limb was performed in order to show the arrangement of minor branches of the anterior interosseous artery and anastomotic branches between the vascular interosseous system and the major vascular axes of the forearm at wrist level [5, 6]. The study also pointed out the constant presence of a vascular axis supplying the pronator quadratus fat pad.

The study was performed on thirty upper limbs of fresh cadavers at the Laboratoire d'Anatomie of the René Descartes University of Paris. In 28 upper limbs, an injection of the humeral artery was performed with colored latex, followed by an anatomical dissection. The two remaining upper limbs were subject to an anatomical and radiological study before and after dissection following an arterial injection with latex-lead.

Anatomical data showed that it is possible to harvest the fat pad lying ventrally on the pronator quadratus muscle (Fig. 48.1) and having its own autonomous vascularization (Fig. 48.2). The latter consists of a constant vascular axis of reduced caliber (the mean value of the external diameter of the vessel at its origin is 0.5 mm) originating from the transversal anastomotic confluence between the terminal palmar branch of the anterior interosseous artery and the palmar branches of the ulnar and radial arteries. From this transversal vascular axis, situated just distally to the distal edge of the pronator quadratus muscle, originates the above-mentioned small artery which goes up proximally within the fat pad. The latter consists of an areolar tissue with a weak texture occupying the most distal portion of the Parona space. Despite of its constant presence, this pad may show individual variations which depend neither on the particular habitus of each person nor on sex. The fat pad may be easily harvested, even when it is scarce, by anchoring its more proximal edges to the pronator quadratus fascia on which it lies and which can be used as a supporting structure.

It is thus possible to sculpt a fascio-adipose vascularized flap with an antegrade flow (Fig. 48.2b). By lifting it as a "vela quadra" (square sail) [13] with a hinge point on the distal edge of the pronator quadratus muscle, it can be folded over distally on 2.5–3 cm of the median nerve in the very critical portion where the nerve is more exposed to microtraumas. These can stimulate neuromatous formations which bring about causalgic and pain syndromes. The flap usually provides an adequate covering of the nerve just proximally to its entry in the carpal tunnel and in the initial portion of its intracanalar course. Practically, the length of the flap is the same as that of the pronator quadratus muscle (the fat pad being anchored to the muscle fascia): its mean value according to our observations and to the literature [3, 12] is about 48 mm and the pivot point cannot go beyond the radio-carpal level.

Surgical Technique

When treating recurrent carpal tunnel syndromes following surgical neurolysis, the surgical technique consists of the proximal widening of the surgical scar allowing an adequate neurolysis and a correct evaluation of anatomo-pathological local conditions (Fig. 48.3). The neurolysis is performed after incising the skin and the forearm fascia; the flexor carpi radialis tendon and the median nerve are then divaricated radially, thus giving access to the deep levels by careful dissection of the superficialis and profundus flexor tendons. One must be careful not to damage the intertendinous ramifications of the fat pad situated between the muscle belly and the myotendinous junction of the above-mentioned muscles. By so doing, a good exposition of the

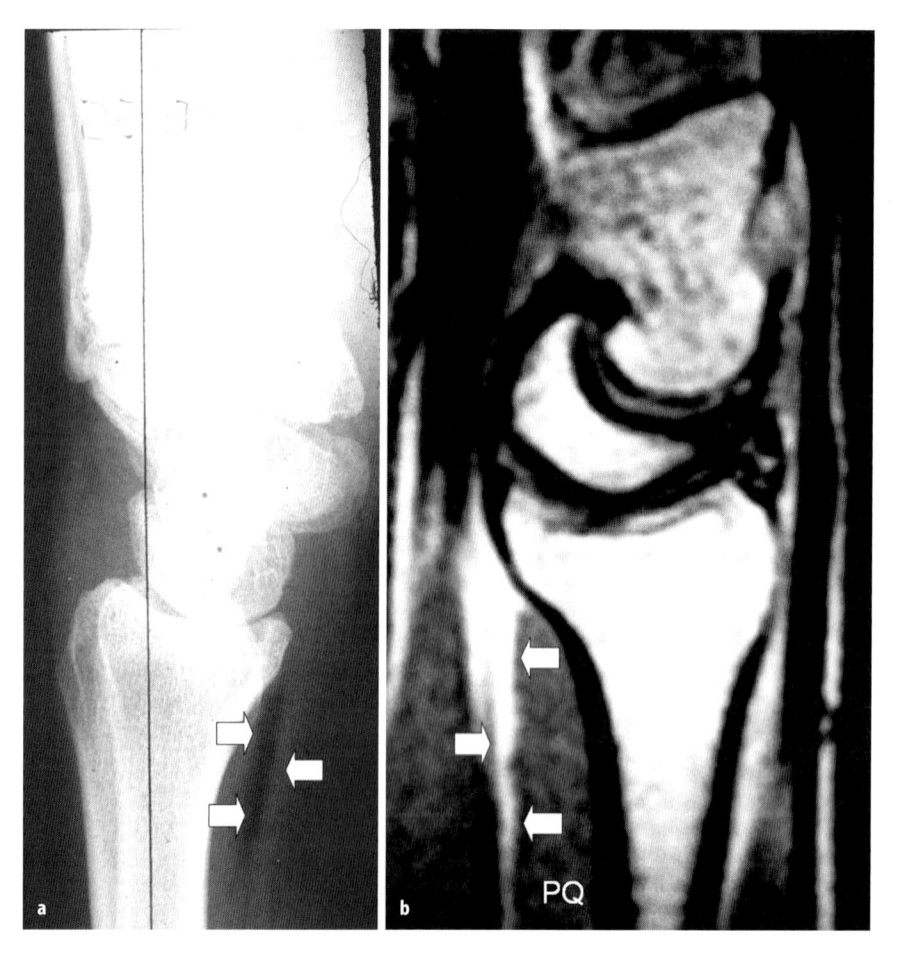

Fig. 48.1. a The pronator quadratus fat pad is partly accountable for the sickle-shaped x-ray image usually observed in lateral projections of the wrist (*arrows*). **b** The MR mirror image clearly shows the position of the fat pad (*arrows*) lying on the pronator quadratus muscle (*PQ*) on a deeper level than the flexor tendons and median nerve (from [9], with publisher's permission)

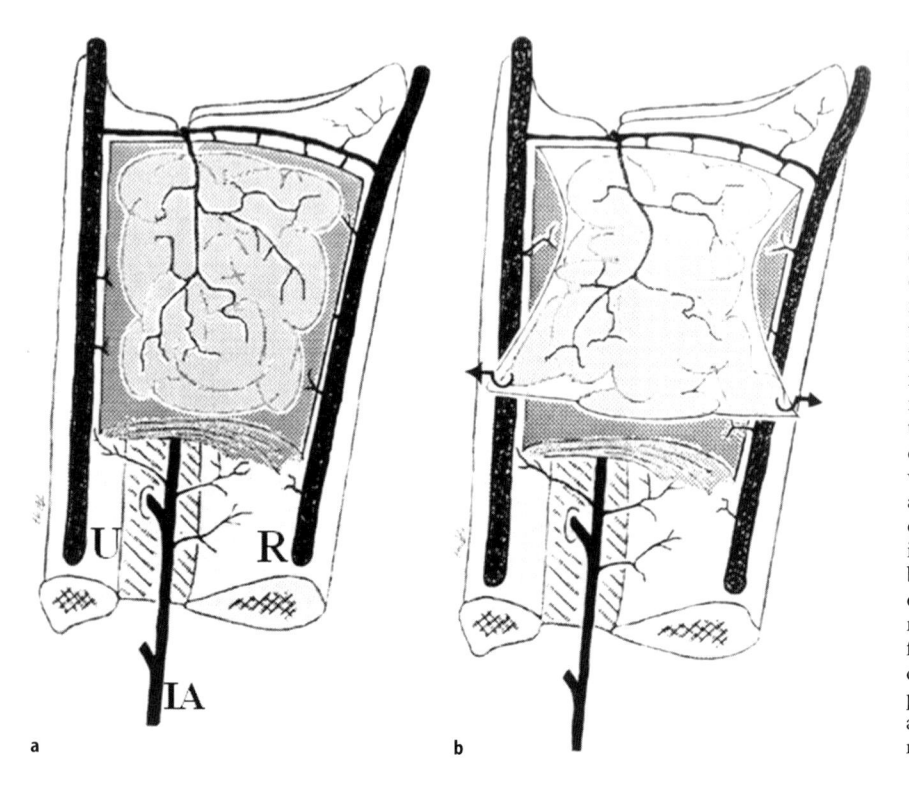

Fig. 48.2. a The vascular anatomy of the distal forearm. We can see the ulnar (*U*), radial (*R*), and interosseous anterior (*IA*) arteries. The latter runs first on the interosseous membrane and then under the pronator quadratus muscle, after originating its dorsal terminal branch which perforates the interosseous membrane in order to reach the posterior compartment. On the radio-carpal level, we see the anastomotic vascular crossing between the main vascular axes of the forearm and the interosseous anterior artery. From this crossing originates the recurrent branch of the fat pad lying on the pronator quadratus muscle. **b** By anchoring the fat pad to the pronator quadratus fascia, the adipose tissue is provided with an adequate support for its mobilization

Fig. 48.2. c The flap is lifted like a square sail after cutting the fascia on the ulnar and radial sides of the pronator quadratus muscle. Being folded distally over the nerve, the flap provides a protecting vault and a septum ensuring the reciprocal gliding between the nerve and the surrounding tendons. The flap also provides a vascularized bed for the damaged segment of the nerve, with positive effects on trophic local conditions. **d** A further dissection shows, after detaching the radial insertion of the pronator quadratus, the terminal course of the anterior interosseous artery under the muscle (from [9], with publisher's permission)

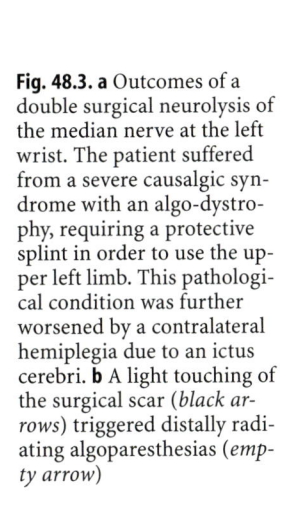

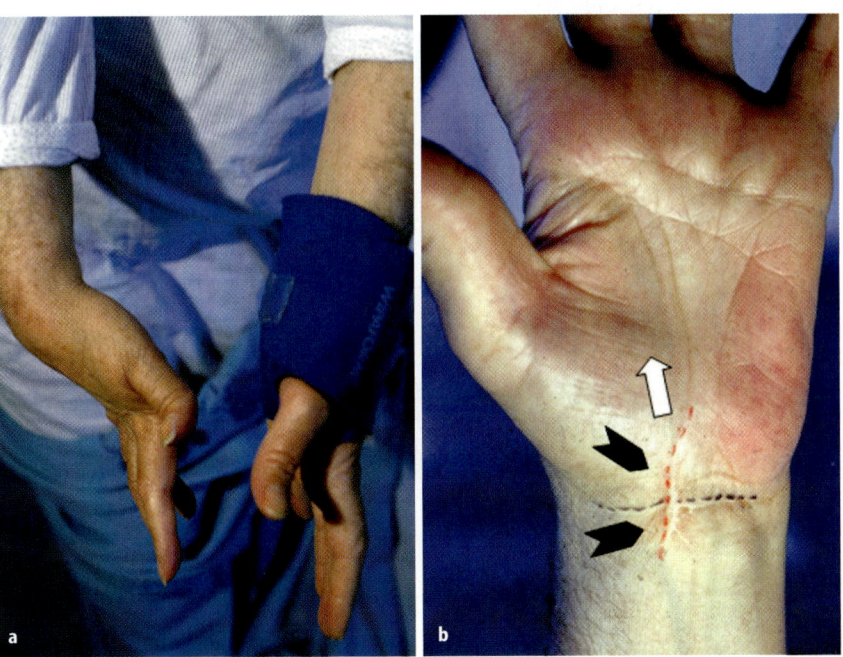

Fig. 48.3. a Outcomes of a double surgical neurolysis of the median nerve at the left wrist. The patient suffered from a severe causalgic syndrome with an algo-dystrophy, requiring a protective splint in order to use the upper left limb. This pathological condition was further worsened by a contralateral hemiplegia due to an ictus cerebri. **b** A light touching of the surgical scar (*black arrows*) triggered distally radiating algoparesthesias (*empty arrow*)

fat pad is possible: the flexor pollicis longus on the radial side and the flexor digitorum profundus on the ulnar side are kept divaricated and the proximal edges of the pad are anchored to the pronator quadratus fascia. The muscle fascia must then be cut on the radial and the ulnar sides, thus providing the fat pad with an adequate support for its mobilization.

The sculpted flap may then be detached, lifted as a square sail and folded over distally on the median nerve which maintains its radial position to the pad,

372 V Complications

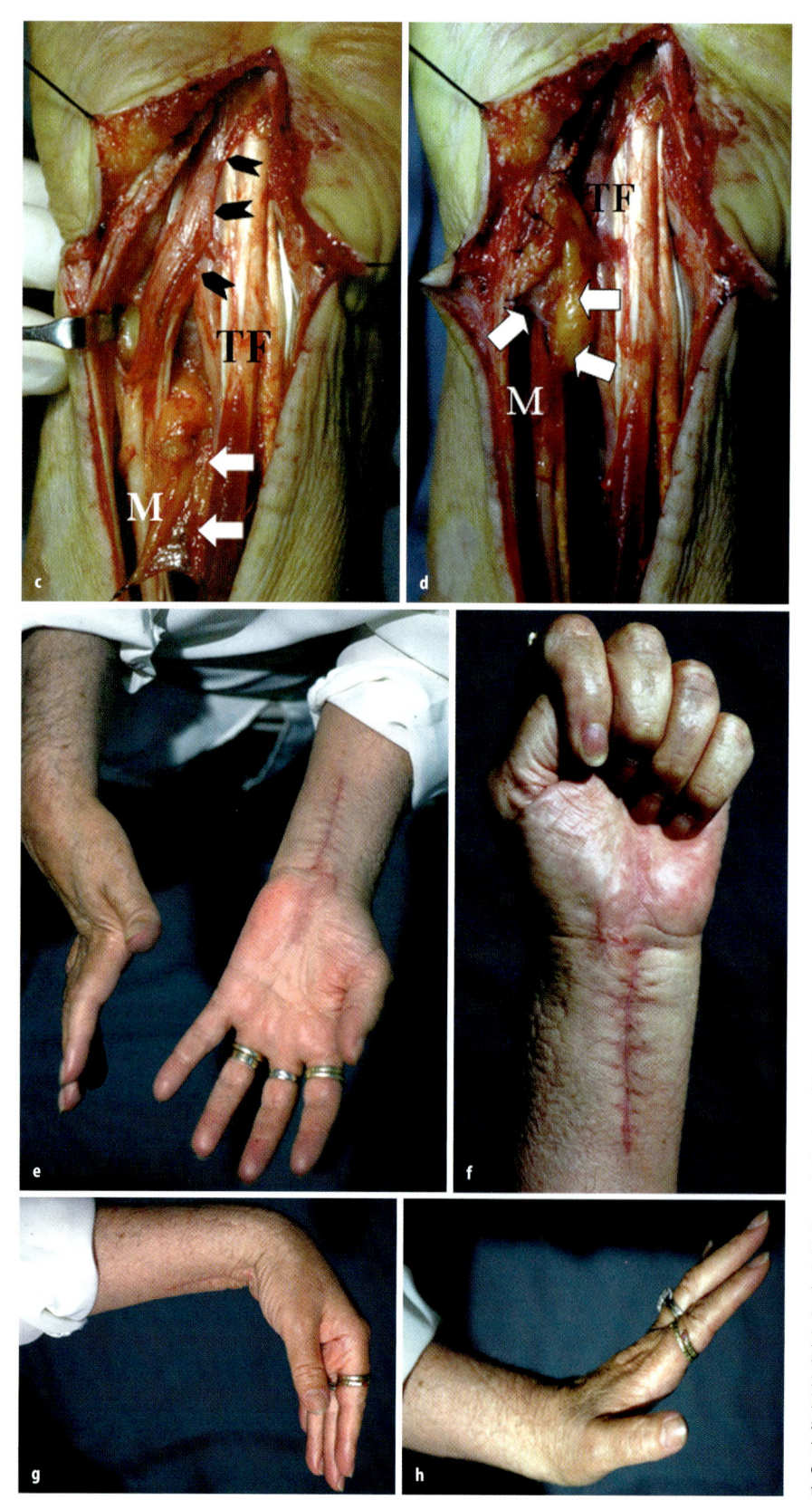

Fig. 48.3. c Surgical view of the lesion showing, at the level of the "trigger" segment of the nerve, local adhesions of the nerve (*M*) to the flexor tendons (*TF*) and to the radial portion of the transverse carpal ligament (*black arrows*), outcomes of epineurotomy with a perineural fibrosis and a persistent compression neuropathy. *White arrows* indicate the square sail flap emerging from below between the median nerve (*M*) and the flexor pollicis longus on the radial side, and the remaining flexor tendons of fingers (*TF*) on the ulnar side. **d** The square sail flap (*white arrows*) is folded over the median nerve (*M*). **e–h** Clinical result 3 months postoperatively showing a clear improvement of the algodystrophic syndrome (the patient was able to wear her rings again), with a good functional recovery of the range of motion of the fingers and the wrist (Fig. 42.3 a–h from [9], with publisher's permission). **i** (see p. 373) Six months postoperatively control: the MR image of the wrist shows the new position of the pronator quadratus fat pad surrounding the damaged segment of the median nerve (*white arrow*, see Fig. 42.1). The MR also shows the good vascularization of this "protective covering nerve flap." *PQ*, pronator quadratus muscle

ciate by see-through observation the vascular axis supplying it and at the same time, by gentle dissection of the more distal fibers of the pronator quadratus muscle from the free edge of the distal radial epiphysis, one can also appreciate the anastomotic crossing from which the vascular pedicle of the flap originates. The direct vision of this pedicle is necessary in order to perform a partial incision of the distal edge of the pronator fascia at the hinge point for a further mobilization of the flap.

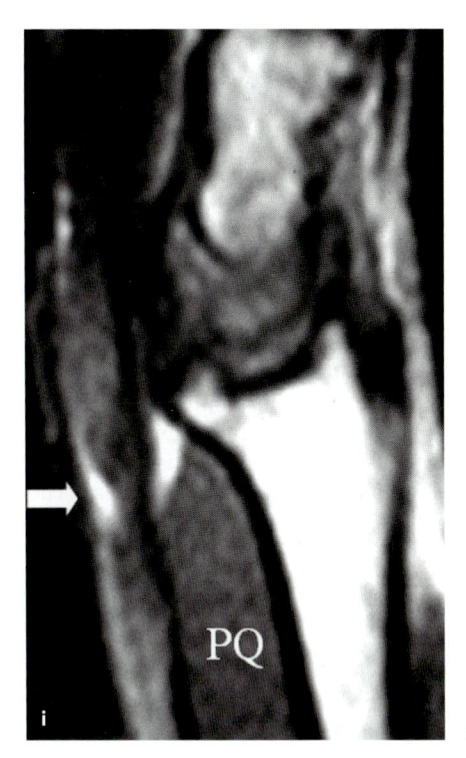

Clinical Applications

Twenty patients suffering from the outcomes of a median nerve lesion at the wrist were treated, of which 11 were subsequent to traumatic lesions and 9 following iatrogenic pathologic conditions [9, 10]. In 8 of the latter patients, the painful causalgic syndrome appeared after surgical neurolysis of a carpal tunnel syndrome.

In all these cases, the mainly causalgic and algo-dystrophic neuralgic syndrome was characterized by intense local pain due to an underlying neuroma and a consequent "non-use" syndrome. This neuralgic syndrome prevailed on the neurological residual deficit.

In posttraumatic cases, we performed a simple neurolysis with covering of the nerve by a "square sail" flap. In one case, the neurological damage was due to an incontinuity neuroma not requiring nervous grafting; in the other cases, the damage was due to an intraneural fibrosis following complex cut lesions of the wrist,

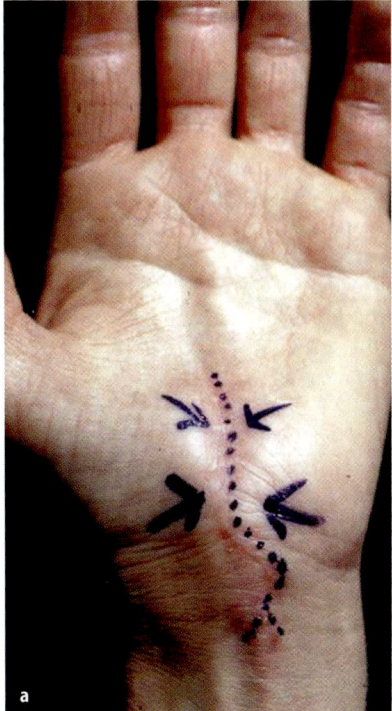

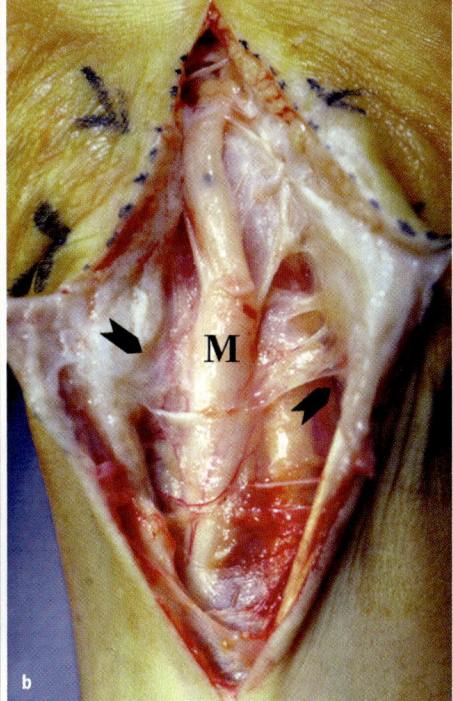

thus avoiding its contact with the flexor tendons. By anchoring the flap by means of two points on the radial edge of the previously cut transverse carpal ligament, the flap can be kept in this position and continue to protect the nerve. While lifting the flap, one can appre-

Fig. 48.4. a Postneurolysis causalgic syndrome of the median nerve at the wrist, with a marked hyperesthesia along the surgical scar. **b** Surgical view of the lesion at the beginning of the neurolysis: we can see strong adhesions of the nerve (*M*) to the surrounding structures and to the skin (*black arrows*)

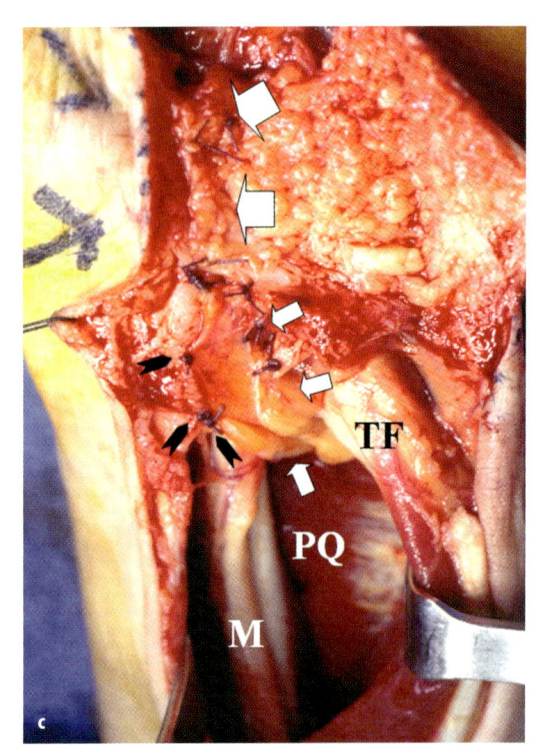

Fig. 48.4. c In order to provide a more extensive covering of the median nerve (*M*) in its pre- and intracanalar course, it was necessary to associate the square sail flap (*small white arrows*) with an hypothenar flap (*big white arrows*). The *black arrows* show the anchoring of the square sail flap to the radial portion of the cut transverse ligament. The flexor tendons (*TF*) were divaricated on the ulnar side in order to see the pronator quadratus muscle (*PQ*). (from [9], with publisher's permission)

with unsuccessful neurorrhaphies, in a fibro-sclerotic perineural environment with scar adhesions of the surrounding tissue which did not allow successful nervous grafting.

Painful syndromes following a neurolysis of entrapment neuropathies of the median nerve were due, in most cases, to a local fibrosis with scar adhesions of the nerve on the surrounding tissue. Only in two cases following an endoscopic neurolysis, we furthermore identified major iatrogenic lesions of the nerve on a great portion of its intracanalar course; because of these lesions and the age of the patient (over 70 years), a nerve reconstruction was not advisable.

In all postneurolysis cases, we simply performed a neurolysis together with a square sail flap. Most of the time, an early and clear improvement of local pain and algo-dystrophic syndrome was obtained, with a progressive sensible reduction of the already existing neurological deficit, conditioned by anatomo-pathological findings of the nerve lesion.

In posttraumatic cases, patients were all satisfied with the results. Two patients suffering from outcomes of a cut lesion and treated by a simple neurolysis together with a square sail flap, refused reconstruction by nerve grafting as a further treatment which we suggested given the considerable improvement of the causalgic and algo-dystrophic syndrome.

The same did not apply to postneurolysis cases where results were not as constant. Besides the different anatomo-pathological findings characterizing the nerve lesion in posttraumatic and postneurolysis cases, the extent of the damaged nerve segment plays a major role as well as that of the protective covering, which the nerve requires. If the covering needs to be extended to the whole intracanalar course of the nerve, as often occurs in postneurolysis cases, a square sail flap only is not sufficient. In these cases, a so-called spinnaker variation of the technique was applied, associating an "adipose hypothenar" flap [4, 11] to a square sail flap. The results obtained were encouraging (Fig. 48.4).

Conclusions

Experimental studies showed that a vascularized adipose tissue can, more than other vascularized tissues, not only have a protective function, but also act as a supplying and gliding tissue for a damaged segment of a peripheral nerve surrounded by adhesion scars [1, 2].

The square sail flap which we described and used [7, 8, 10] is an easily harvested and well-vascularized pedicled flap, which does not sacrifice important structures and does not imply functional and cosmetic deficits. Given the nature of harvested tissue, which is mainly adipose, this technique adequately satisfies treatment requirements in this particular pathology.

Acknowledgements. The Authors wish to thank Prof. Jean Pierre Lassau, Director of the Laboratoire d'Anatomie of the "René Descartes" University of Paris, who made it possible for us to perform the anatomical study underlying this work.

References

1. Bertelli JA, Tumilasci O, Mira JC et al. (1993) L'excursion longitudinale du nerf sciatique: étude expérimentale chez le rat adulte. Ann Chir Main 12: 73–76
2. Brunelli G, Battiston B, Brunelli F (1988) Free greater omentum transfer in ionizing radiation lesions of the brachial plexus. In: Brunelli G (ed)Textbook of Microsurgery, Masson, Paris, pp 825–31
3. Fontaine C, Millot F, Blancke D, Mestdagh H (1992) Anatomic basis of pronator quadratus flap. Surg Rad Anat 14: 295–99
4. Giunta R, Frank U, Lanz U (1998) The hypotenar fat pad flap for reconstructive repair after scarring of the median nerve at the wrist joint. Ann Chir Main 17(2):107–10
5. Pagliei A, Brunelli F, Gilbert A (1991) Anterior interosseous artery: anatomic bases of pedicled bone grafts. Surg Rad Anat 13:152–54

6. Pagliei A, Brunelli F, Gilbert A (1991) Artère interosseuse antérieure: bases anatomiques de la réalisation des greffons osseux pediculés. Bull Soc Anat Paris 15:3–9.
7. Pagliei A, Taccardo G, Tulli A et al. (1997) "Vela Quadra" flap: a new fascio-adipose flap in hand surgery. J Hand Surg 22-B (Suppl):34
8. Pagliei A, Taccardo G, Tulli A et al. (1997) Wrist median nerve neuromas. A new treatment technique. Gastr Intern / Orth Surg 10(3):651–52
9. Pagliei A, Catalano F, Fanfani F (2002) Copertura-protezione del nervo con "lembo a vela quadra." In: Luchetti R (ed) Sindrome del tunnel carpale. Verduci, Roma, pp 290–96
10. Pagliei A, Tulli A, Rocchi R (2003) square sail flap in median nerve injuries at the wrist. Anatomy and review of twenty cases. Chir Main 22: 125–30
11. Strickland JW, Idler RS, Lourie GM et al. (1996) The hypotenar fat pad flap for management of recalcitrant carpal tunnel syndrome. J Hand Surg 21-A:840–46
12. Stuart PR (1966) Pronator quadratus revisited. J Hand Surg 21-B 6:71
13. Ucelli G (1983) Le navi di Nemi. Istituto Poligrafico e Zecca dello Stato, Roma

49 Free Vascularized Omental Transfer for the Treatment of Recalcitrant Carpal Tunnel Syndrome

R. J. Goitz, J.B. Steichen

Introduction

Patients with recurrent or persistent carpal tunnel syndrome (CTS) despite a properly performed carpal tunnel release (CTR) can be quite difficult to manage and classically have poor outcomes [1–3]. Multiple etiologies may be responsible for their persistent symptoms including excessive scar formation around the median nerve resulting in limited nerve mobility otherwise known as adhesive median neuritis or neurodesis (Fig. 49.1) [4–7]. In addition, patients with persistent symptoms may have irreversible nerve injury from internal fibrosis secondary to chronic compression or even iatrogenic causes resulting in a neuroma. These patients may also have a limited incentive for improvement or issues of secondary gain such as workman's compensation or ongoing litigation.

Many surgical procedures have been described to treat patients with persistent symptoms of CTS including the use of local tissue for transposition including the hypothenar fat pad, [4] pronator quadratus, lumbricals, [8] abductor digiti minimi [9], and palmaris brevis [10]. Each of these tissues are limited in their extent of coverage. For instance, the hypothenar fat pad flap has been reported to provide reasonable long-term results but is limited to providing coverage to the median nerve over a 1.5 to 2-in length and only on the volar surface of the nerve. It is not able to be circumferentially wrapped around the nerve to prevent recurrent scar adherence and cannot be used for coverage proximal to the wrist crease. Vein wrapping as been advocated to provide more extensive coverage and uses readily expendable tissue [11]. However, it does not provide padding to the nerve or any known trophic factors for nerve recovery.

Omentum has been shown to be an ideal tissue to treat scarred or injured nerves. The endothelium of omentum produces fibroblast growth factor which has been shown to enhance nerve regeneration through the stimulation of axon and neurite growth [12]. Adipose tissue has long been used to prevent perineural fibrosis especially around the spinal cord [13] and has been shown to be beneficial for the treatment of actinic brachial plexitis [14]. In addition, omentum has significant angiogenic potential and has been used clinically to revascularize the brain [15], myocardium [16], bone [17], and extremities [18]. The additive effects of omentum to potentiate neurotrophism and angiogenesis, but limit perineural fibrosis makes its use optimal for recalcitrant median neuritis especially associated with significant cicatrix. In addition, omentum is readily available, expendable, and able to be harvested laparoscopically with minimal potential donor site morbidity. In addition, it may provide extensive coverage and be wrapped circumferentially around the entire median nerve (Fig. 49.2).

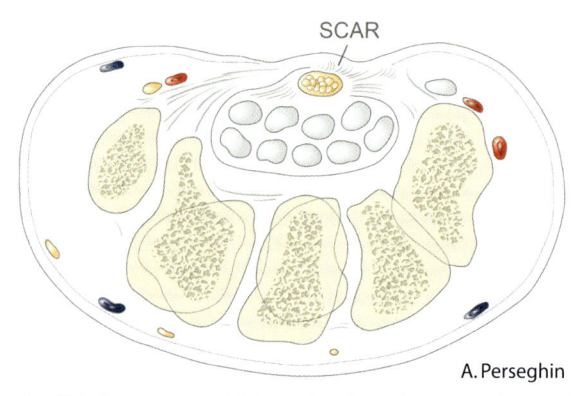

Fig. 49.1. Cross-sectional illustration through the carpal tunnel depicting scar tissue surrounding the median nerve

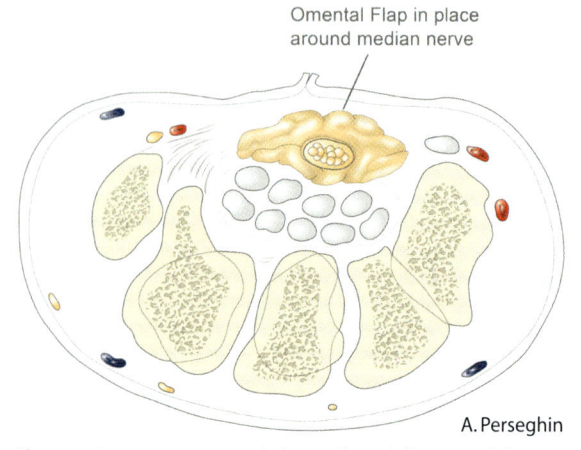

Fig. 49.2. Omentum wrapped circumferentially around the median nerve

However, it does require microvascular technique and a proficient laparoscopist.

Technique

An extended carpal tunnel approach is first performed from at least 7 cm proximal to the wrist crease to the superficial arch to assess the extent of perineural fibrosis. An external neurolysis is performed of the median nerve and its palmar cutaneous branch. An internal neurolysis is initiated if there is any evidence for a neuroma or internal nerve derangement. A flexor tenosynovectomy is performed to reduce the bulk of tissue in the carpal tunnel and facilitate primary closure. The radial artery and cephalic vein are exposed in the proximal part of the wound (Fig. 49.3).

Since 1997, all omentum has been harvested laparoscopically even in patients with previous abdominal surgery. The omentum is harvested on the gastroepiploic artery and vein for microvascular anastomosis. The amount of omentum is determined based on the extent of perineural fibrosis but generally includes at least a 10-cm length. The gastroepiploic vessels are prepared and the omentum is thinned without disrupting its vascularity.

The omentum is then inset and placed circumferentially around the median nerve. The gastroepiploic vein is directly anastomosed in an end-to-end fashion to the cephalic vein and the gastroepiploic artery is anastomosed in an end-to-side fashion to the radial artery (Fig. 49.4). The wound is primarily closed if possible but if excessive tension exists, the closure is supplemented with a split thickness skin graft. A wrist splint is placed with a window available for direct monitoring of the flap both clinically and with a Doppler.

Postoperative management includes low-molecular weight dextran for 5 days, aspirin for 4 weeks, immediate digital motion and wrist motion commencing at 3 weeks postoperatively.

Results

We reported on the first 10 vascularized omental flaps performed in 7 patients between 1989 and 1993 at an average follow-up of 6.6 years (range, 4.5–8.75 years) [19]. All patients had a minimum of 2 previous CTRs and after the 5th patient, all had a hypothenar flap pad flap (HTFPF) preoperatively. All patients exhibited

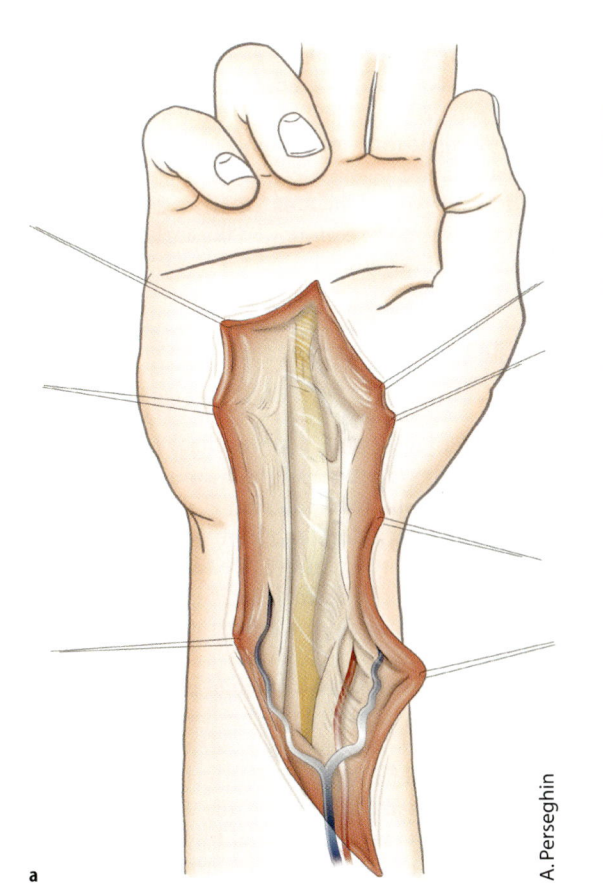

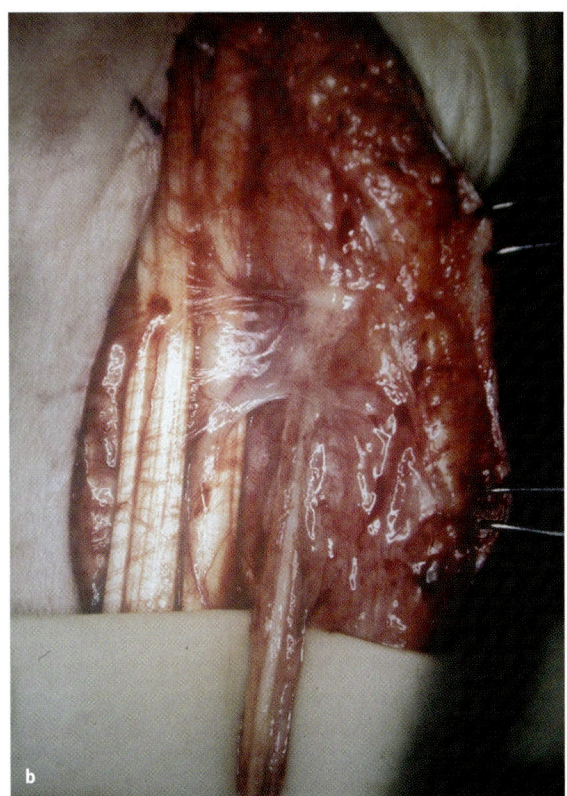

Fig. 49.3. a Median nerve in a scarred bed. **b** Clinical photograph of a extensive scar around the median nerve proximal to the wrist crease

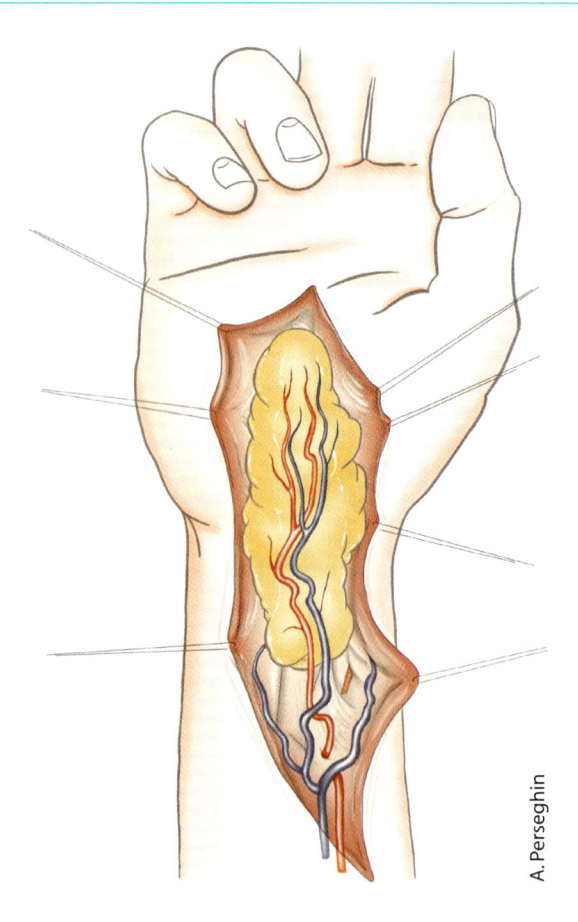

Fig. 49.4. Median nerve wrapped with omentum with proximal anastomosis

similar findings at surgery. The transverse carpal ligament was reformed. Thick scar tissue often encased the median nerve and extended proximal to the wrist crease and distal to the proximal palmar flexion crease. The median nerve was often found in a more superficial position than expected, scarred to the undersurface of the radial leaf of the transverse carpal ligament. If the patient had a HTFPF, the median nerve was often scarred to the reformed ulnar leaf of the transverse carpal ligament and deep to the fat pad flap. There were seven neural abnormalities in six extremities including four neuromas-in-continuity involving the common digital nerves, two involving the main median nerve, and one neuroma of the palmar cutaneous branch of the median nerve. There were two patent median arteries and one aberrant palmaris longus muscle belly which traveled obliquely across the median nerve.

Most patients reported improvement in symptoms except one who had complete relief of symptoms for 5 years following omental transfer but reported recurrence at 5 years following surgery. Despite the improvement in symptoms, patients' overall Symptom Severity Index and Functional Status Index were only slightly better than previous author's reports of patients with primary CTS prior to CTR but not as good as their postoperative results [20–22]. Five of six patients were satisfied with their results and felt the surgery improved their quality of life. Four of six patients reported that they would have the surgery again. Most physical findings had improved at final evaluation, including two-point discrimination which normalized in seven of nine extremities compared to three of nine preoperatively. Grip strength increased 73% in seven of nine extremities and key pinch increased 101% in four of nine extremities. Electrophysiologic results did not correlate with clinical outcome and all motor and sensory latencies increased at final follow-up possibly due to the nature of the test and the increased thickness of tissue between the skin and nerve.

To date, the senior author has performed 19 free vascularized omental transfers for recalcitrant carpal tunnel syndrome in 15 patients. There have been 17 women and 2 men with 4 bilateral omental transfers. Their average age was 41 years (range, 20–52). Since 1997, all omentum have been harvested laparoscopically. There was one ventral wall hernia in the initial 10 that were harvested via a laparotomy. There have been no complications in the laparoscopic group despite multiple patients having had previous abdominal surgery. Patients reported improvement in 15 of 19 extremities over their preoperative symptoms although only one patient reported complete relief. Only three patients were working at final follow-up. There has been only one failed flap. The most common complication has been delayed wound healing in five extremities although this was more common in the early series prior to primary wound closure.

Discussion

The results following revision CTR have been historically poor with up to 40% poor results [3] and 95% residual symptoms [2]. As was found in our patient population, there are multiple potential reasons for continued symptoms including excessive scar surrounding the nerve limiting its mobility as well as previous nerve injury as evidenced by a high incidence of neuroma. Patients with nerve injury would not be expected to have normalization of symptoms and may be akin to patients treated with actinic brachial plexitis [14].

Multiple tissue transfers have been proposed to minimize the scar tissue to improve median nerve glide [4, 9–11]. Omentum has both angiogenic and neurogenic properties that make it ideal for this purpose and has been shown to prevent perineural fibrosis [13, 18]. In addition, omentum is expendable and unlimited in its ability to provide extensive circumferential coverage to the median nerve. With limited goals of symptom improvement in this patient population, there was a high rate of patient satisfaction despite reports of continued median nerve irritability and dysfunction.

The ideal candidate for a vascularized free omental transfer would be the patient who has been recalcitrant to multiple previous carpal tunnel releases including the use of a hypothenar fat pad flap who has evidence of excessive scar formation surrounding the median nerve. The omentum can be used to circumferentially wrap the median nerve to prevent scar adherence. It can be used in any length necessary to cover the median nerve from the midforearm out to the digits. In addition, the omentum provides some additional padding to the nerve which is often lacking in the palm of patients with previous multiple incisions to minimize scar sensitivity. Although patients can expect improvement in symptoms with the omental transfer, complete relief is often not possible. With reasonable expectations by the patient through a thorough preoperative discussion, a high rate of patient satisfaction can be expected.

References

1. Mackinnon SE (1991) Secondary carpal tunnel surgery. Neurosurg Clin North Am 2: 75–91
2. Strasberg SR, Novak CB, Mackinnon SE, Murray JF (1994) Subjective and employment outcome following secondary carpal tunnel surgery. Ann Plast Surg 32: 485–489
3. O'Malley MJ, Evanoff M, Terrono AL, Millender LG (1992) Factors that determine reexploration treatment of carpal tunnel syndrome. J. Hand Surg 17A; 638–641
4. Strickland JW, Idler RS, Lourie GM, Plancher KD (1996) The hypothenar fat pad flap for management of recalcitrant carpal tunnel syndrome. J Hand Surgery 21A: 840–848
5. Szabo RM (1996) Carpal tunnel syndrome. In Szabo RM (ed): Nerve compression syndromes: Diagnosis and treatment. Thorofare, NJ, Slack Inc pp 101–120
6. Wilgis EFS, Murphy JR (1986) The significance of longitudinal excursion in peripheral nerves. Hand Clin North Am 2: 761–766
7. Hunter JM (1991) Recurrent carpal tunnel syndrome, epineural fibrous fixation, and traction neuropathy. Hand Clin 7: 491–504
8. Urbaniak JR (1991) Complications of treatment of carpal tunnel syndrome. In Gelberman RH (ed): Operative Nerve Repair and Reconstruction. Philadelphia, JB Lippincott, pp 967–979
9. Spokevicius S, Kleinert H (1996) The abductor digiti minimi: Flap. Hand Clinics 12: 351–355
10. Rose EH (1996) The use of the palmaris brevis flap in recurrent carpal tunnel syndrome. Hand Clinics 12: 389–395
11. Varitimidis SE, Vardakas DG, Goebel F, Sotereanos DG (2001) Treatment of Recurrent compressive neuropathy of peripheral nerves in the upper extremity with an autologous vein insulator. J. Hand Surgery 26A: 296–302
12. Bikfalvi A, Alteiro J, Inyang AL et al. (1980) Basic fibroblast growth factor expression in human omental microvascular endothelial cells and the effect of phorbol ester. J Cell Physiol 144: 151–8
13. MacMillan M, Stouffer ES (1991) The effect of omental pedicle graft transfer on spinal microcirculation and laminectomy membrane formations. Spine 16 (2): 176–180
14. Brunelli G (1980) Neurolysis and free microvascular omentum transfer in the treatment of post actinic palsies of the bracheal plexus. International Surgery 65 (6): 515–519
15. Goldsmith HS, Chen WF, Duckett SW (1973) Brain vascularization by intact omentum. Arch Surg 106: 695–8
16. O'Shaughnessy I (1936) An experimental method of providing a collateral circulation to the heart. Br J Surg 23: 665–70
17. Azuma H, Kondo T, Mikami M (1976) Treatment of chronic osteomyelitis by transplantation of autogenous omentum with microvascular anastomosis. Acta Orthop Scand 47: 271–5
18. Brunelli GA, Brunelli F, DiRosa F (1988) Neurolized nerve padding in actinic lesions: Omentum versus muscle use. An experimental study. Microsurgery 9: 177–180
19. Goitz RJ, Steichen JB (2005) Microvascular Omental Transfer for the Treatment of Severe Recurrent Median Neuritis of the Wrist: A Long-Term Follow-Up Study. Plastic and Reconst Surg 115(1):163-171
20. Levine DW, Simmons BP, Koris MJ et al. (1973) A Self-administered questionnaire for the assessment of severity of symptoms and functional status in carpal tunnel syndrome. J Bone and Joint Surgery 75A: 1585–92
21. Amadio PC, Silverstein MD, Ilstrup DM et al. (1996) Outcome assessment for carpal tunnel surgery: The Relative Responsiveness of Generic, Arthritis-Specific, Disease-Specific, and Physical Examination Measures. J Hand Surgery 21A: 338–346
22. Cobb TK, Amadio PC, Leatherwood DF et al. (1996) Outcome of re-operation for carpal tunnel syndrome. J Hand Surgery 21A 347–356

Part VI

Evaluation of Results

VI

Outcomes Assessment Protocols

R. Padua, E. Romanini, R. Bondì

Introduction

A critical reconsideration of outcome research in the orthopedic scientific community has been in progress for a few years. With the development of the concepts of quality of life and patient satisfaction, the traditional model of health, considered before to be a lack of disease, has now changed to the more representative "complete physical and psychic well-being condition," formulated by The World Health Organization in 1948.

With this new approach and this new attention to the patient as the center of the treatment, there arose the need for tools able to assess the final outcome of a medical or surgical treatment, based on patient's perspective, which had previously been ignored.

Many tools of analysis were introduced: they make it possible to incorporate the patient's perspective through valid statistical analysis and to compare the physician's perspective with the patient's perspective in outcome measurement, and to evaluate the different role between objective and subjective factors [2, 12].

Moreover, these tools can measure the outcome efficacy correlated to cost (cost-efficacy analysis); diffusion of clinic epidemiology together with analysis of centralized archives underlined marked differences in clinical practice.

The lack of uniformity in the utilization of diagnostic and therapeutic procedures (*practice variation*), gave rise to many questions. Actually, the conception of health is going through a so-called third revolution, based on cost control [14]: efficiency cannot allow contradictory behavior, as has been shown in the literature, where a high practice variation in the field of orthopedics has been reported.

The concept of *Evidence-Based Medicine* (EBM) was was created in an attempt to address research and clinical practice on the following principles: it was born on the fundamental idea of clinical practice based on procedures documented with rigor, controlled and continuously checked [15]. The direct consequence of this revised approach include the greater attention paid to study design and the more and more frequent diffusion of randomized controlled trials (RCTs), the development of new quantitative analysis techniques of the outcomes (meta-analysis), and the increasing dissemination of the idea of systematic revision and guidelines. These principles, albeit belatedly, are disseminating in orthopedics as well [12, 21]. With a higher quantity and quality of data, and a more rigorous outcome analysis procedure, an evolution in orthopedic surgery will be possible.

Outcome Analysis

The issues regarding study design, clinical epidemiology evolution, and quantitative outcome analysis techniques are outside the scope of this paper. Nevertheless, it's undeniable that an outcome assessment that is methodologically correct and universally recognized is necessary. As a result, modern research will concentrate, on one hand, more on outcomes analysis [16, 17] to reveal common features of overall methods about benefits, and on the other hand, on complications and on the differences between single centers and institutions [6].

As a consequence, multicentric studies, even international ones, and national register organizations [10] are increasing, even if they entail many difficulties. To achieve such studies, valid assessment tools are necessary: an outcome analysis method (instrumental and clinical exam or a questionnaire) is valid if it's able to satisfy necessary parameters such as reliability, reproducibility, sensitivity, and responsivity [13].

It is known that the last decade was characterized by outcome analysis techniques based on patient perspective [12]. Such systems answer the need for measuring patients' Health-Related Quality of Life (HRQoL), a concept which expands on the old one of "state of health" and the influence from a specific pathologic condition. In recent years, with the development of clinimetry and psychometry, many point systems, able to quantify a concept surely as abstract and subjective as HRQoL, were developed: autofilled *patient-oriented* questionnaires, in agreement with English language literature, which can measure function and pain, rather than employing the traditional clinical and radiographic scores. The attention moved from the assessment through clinical and radiographic scores to the patient's own perception of his state of health, in relationship with the pathology he is affected by and in which way it can change after a treatment, whether conservative or surgical [1]. Such attitude is not only based on the unexceptionable principle to obtain some data from the patient which only he himself can furnish, but it can provide a valid measure, as reported in many studies, more reliable than the traditional scores; these, usually collected by the surgeon, who effected the treatment, are potentially vitiated by personal factors correlated to the physician-patient relationship and demonstrated to be less "objective" than commonly believed [8]. Similar analyses performed in different places (USA, France) showed, for example, how a widespread outcome index measure such as the *Harris Hip Score*, before considered an unquestionable standard, provides only a partial assessment of patient perspective on his pathology and on the surgical procedure: the questionnaire examines only some of the patient's major disabilities and passes over others (night pain, sexual activity, etc.) which play an important subjective role.

In light of these considerations briefly reported above, the *patient-oriented* questionnaires have to be considered, at the moment, the most valid instrument for outcomes measure for surgical or conservative orthopedic treatment and represent many advantages whether correlated to the practicality in employment (an interview can be conducted via mail or telephone) or to the large diffusion (it guarantees the reference data availability) or to the high collaboration you can obtain from the patient.

Subjective Assessment Questionnaires (Patient-Oriented)

General State of Health can be analyzed in a quantitative way through "generic" questionnaires: the *Short Form 36* (SF-36, see appendix) [20] belongs to this group and represents a standard. This questionnaire, in its actual form, results from a study (MOS, Medical Outcomes Study) began in the 1980s and finished with the publication of SF-36 in 1992 [20]. Later, an international project (IQOLA, *International Quality of Life Assessment*) led to the validation of equivalent versions of questionnaires in 10 different languages: these versions have made it possible to collect data related to health and suffering of patients with various pathologies from all over the world [19]. It's important to emphasize that the use of different language questionnaires requires a complex and rigorous transcultural adaptation to assure uniformity, thereby enabling outcome comparison [5]. As to the SF-36 questionnaire, an Italian validated version, healthy population data regarding different ages and pathologies, and many studies that provide different data for comparative analysis are available. Generic questionnaires can be used to evaluate any morbid condition, but they have some limitations, in particular the potential confusion due to associated pathologies (comorbidity). Then, the use of "specific pathology" questionnaires and "specific-procedure" questionnaires spread: the first is different from the others in that it offers more sensitivity in revealing typical details of the individual pathologic picture; the second is different in that it collects data on patients undergoing a specific treatment, based on more precise questions. Usually they are shorter questionnaires that focus the different questions on two principal domains, pain and function; nevertheless, they are limited in that they do not allow a comparison to be made between different pathologies, interest, or opportunity to make economic/health analyses. Another kind of questionnaire, typical of orthopedic pathology, is the "sectorial" or "regional" questionnaire. An ideal compromise between the two types described above, it was created to surpass the limits of a too generic or too specific measurement; assuming that different pathologies cause similar dysfunction in the same anatomical district, specific regions questionnaires were elaborated upon, reducing the number of systems and favoring the standardization of outcome measurement. In this way, the American Academy of Orthopedic Surgeons changed its approach, with a booklet of questionnaires recently subjected by GLOBE to a transcultural process in Italian [11].

Assessment Protocol in Carpal Tunnel Syndrome

After these preliminary remarks, it's clear there is a problem with more appropriate tools selection to measure a pathology symptomatology such as carpal tunnel syndrome (CTS),which may seem easy to diagnose and treat.

We have many different options, each with advantages and disadvantages: we should carefully evaluate the context and our objectives to select the tool best able to provide the greatest amount of data with the least amount of time and effort. We can differentiate two different situations, defined by English-speaking authors: *Outcomes Assessment* and *Outcomes Research*. These two English terms are not easily translated. In *Outcomes Assessment*, the aim is to control clinical practice to collect one's outcomes with a specific procedure. These kinds of projects require a short system. *Outcomes Research* is characterized by its more scientific approach to solve a clinical problem which is aimed at a precise *end-point*incorporated in the design and driving force of the study. Sometimes, such types of research could be used to employ many different measurements to obtain relevant data. Obviously it limits the study to a restricted group of patients for a circumscribed period; it's clear this second hypothesis permits a greater involvement of the single patient.

Given the continuing development of this area of research as outlined above, it is not very easy to select an assessment protocol.

In recent years, the scientific community has recognized the *carpal tunnel syndrome questionnaire* (or *Boston Carpal Tunnel Questionnaire* – BCTQ, from the city of the authors). Proposed by Levine and the Harvard Medical School Group of Boston in 1993 [7], its the measurement standard for patients affected by CTS. Many papers on the features and capabilities of this tool and many clinical trials based on its use exist. They compared the different questionnaires on their capacity to study the subjective symptoms. All papers analyzing BCTQ concluded it presents the best features as a measurement tool. The comparison with generic questionnaires, reported in the literature, showed a capacity for measurement, in terms of both sensitivity and specificity, better than any other instrument considered. In particular, Bessette showed how, using the BCTQ, it is possible to confirm statistically a phenomenon with a smaller population than is requested by SF-36, with a ratio of 1:4 [3]. The literature provides extensive justifications on the use of this questionnaire in all the studies of the Carpal Tunnel Syndrome Study Italian Group (Gruppo Italiano di Studio per la Sindrome del Tunnel Carpale) [9, 10]. Therefore, the choice of the BCTQ is almost obligatory according to many authors, including those in our group who worked in the field of CTS.

The BCTQ analyzes sensitive symptoms (pain, numbness, etc.) and hand function (capability to perform an action) in patients affected by CTS, providing two different types of data: "symptoms" and "function." The questionnaire consists of multiple choices questions. This system represents the gold standard in modern questionnaires formulation; in fact, even if the filling in phase and data extracting phase are more difficult, it's able to provide data capable of reflecting the natural phenomenon variability and to satisfy in the best way the features asked of a measuring tool like this [1, 7].

A possible alternative to the BCTQ is the DASH questionnaire (Disability Arm, Shoulder and Hand questionnaire; see appendix), classified as a "district questionnaire" because it studies a bodily district (in this specific case the upper limbs). This kind of tool represents a sort of compromise between specific-pathologies questionnaires and generic ones, with the aim of obviating the defects described above. The DASH belongs to the sectorial booklet of questionnaires put out by the American Academy of Orthopedic Surgeons. The system, elaborated upon by the AAOS Outcome Studies Committee, presided over by Peter Amadio, together with specialist orthopedic societies provides a booklet which includes the SF-36, the Charlson Comorbidity index [4], and a district questionnaire. These tools utilize a specific software for filing and elaborating on the final score. The only actual limit of the AAOS system is the poor availability of reference data, in fact, the data relative to a large multicentric study in the USA have not yet been published (P.C. Amadio, personal presentation). We would like to discuss the use of the SF-36 in CTS. In the beginning, the literature paid a lot of attention to the analysis of the general health measuring tools used most frequently in orthopedics as applied to CTS; however, after some studies described its limits in such applications, now it's clear that the SF-36 has a secondary role. In particular, in a recent paper, Vaile et al. established its poor efficacy in CTS [18].

For the most part, the relevant literature doesn't reduce "objective" assessment to a secondary role; despite much criticism regarding its poor reliability, it continues to play a fundamental role in pathology assessment.

Data collection, if carried out rigorously and methodically, always results in useful data, if those data play a fundamental role in the pathology itself.

Conclusion

Data collection on our patients should be fundamental to our professional approach. Unfortunately, reality sometimes precludes us from carrying out this important phase. Data analysis and consequent outcome assessment, obtained with the various treatment procedures, could enable us to check the quality of our work and eventually to modify our practice.

Quality control has been used in industry for many years; it's not clear why this model has not yet been applied to medicine. The evidence-based medicine movement promotes medicine based on facts and efficacy testing through a continuous outcome check, both individual and universal. It's clear that each patient would be treated with the quicker treatment, through the best procedure. Nevertheless, this is not always possible; instead it's possible to check that a treatment results in the hoped-for outcome. Our fundamental concern is the patient's health and quality of life; that's why we cannot ignore scientifically obtained, subjective data collection. The formulation of a serious outcome analysis protocol is the starting point of this quality control program and, believing in a precise and methodical approach to medicine, it should be fundamental to every physician's approach to treating a patient affected by any pathology.

Appendix: The SF-36 Questionnaire

In general, would you say your health is:
1 Excellent / 2 Very Good / 3 Good / 4 Fair / 5 Poor

Compared to **one year ago,** how would you rate your health in general now?

1. Much better now than one year ago
2. Somewhat better now than one year ago
3. About the same as one year ago
4. Somewhat worse now than one year ago
5. Much worse now than one year ago

Current Health Assessment
The following items are about activities you might do during a typical day.
Does your health now limit you in these activities? If so, how much? (Circle one response on each line.)
1 Yes, limited a lot / 2 Yes, limited a little / 3 No, not limited at all

a. Vigorous activities, such as running, lifting heavy objects, or participating in strenuous sports   1 2 3
b. Moderate activities, such as moving a table, pushing a vacuum cleaner, bowling or playing golf   1 2 3
c. Lifting or carrying groceries   1 2 3
d. Climbing several flights of stairs   1 2 3
e. Climbing one flight of stairs   1 2 3
f. Bending, kneeling or stooping   1 2 3
g. Walking more than one mile   1 2 3
h. Walking several blocks   1 2 3
i. Walking one block   1 2 3
j. Bathing or dressing yourself   1 2 3

During the **past four weeks,** have you had any of the following problems with your work or other regular daily activities as a result of your physical health? (Circle one response on each line.): 1 Yes / 2 No

a. Cut down the amount of time you spent on work or other activities   1 2
b. Accomplished less than you would like   1 2
c. Were limited in the kind of work or other activities   1 2
d. Had difficulty performing the work or other activities (for example, it took extra effort)   1 2

During the **past four weeks,** have you had any of the following problems with your work or other regular daily activities as a result of any emotional problems (such as feeling depressed or anxious)? (Circle one response on each line.): 1 Yes / 2 No

a. Cut down the amount of time you spent on work or other activities   1 2
b. Accomplished less than you would like   1 2
c. Did not do work or other activities as carefully as usual   1 2

Current Health Assessment
These questions are about how you feel and how things have been with you during the **past four weeks**.
For each question, please give the one answer that comes closest to the way you have been feeling.
How much of the time during the **past four weeks**... (Circle one response on each line.)
1 All of the time / 2 Most of the time / 3 A good bit of the time / 4 Some of the time / 5 A little of the time / 6 None of the time

a. Did you feel full of pep?   1 2 3 4 5 6
b. Have you been a very nervous person?   1 2 3 4 5 6
c. Have you felt so down in the dumps nothing could cheer you up?   1 2 3 4 5 6
d. Have you felt calm and peaceful?   1 2 3 4 5 6
e. Did you have a lot of energy?   1 2 3 4 5 6
f. Have you felt downhearted and blue?   1 2 3 4 5 6
g. Did you feel worn out?   1 2 3 4 5 6
h. Have you been a happy person?   1 2 3 4 5 6
i. Did you feel tired?   1 2 3 4 5 6

During the **past four weeks,** to what extent has your physical health or emotional problems interfered with your normal social activities with family, friends, neighbors or groups? (Circle one response.)
1 Not at all / 2 Slightly / 3 Moderately / 4 Quite a bit / 5 Extremely

During the **past four weeks,** how much did pain interfere with your normal work (including both work outside the home and housework)? (Circle one response.)
1 Not at all / 2 A little bit / 3 Moderately / 4 Quite a bit / 5 Extremely

How much bodily pain have you had during the **past four weeks**? (Circle one response.)

1 None / 2 Very mild / 3 Mild / 4 Moderate / 5 Severe / 6 Very severe

During the **past four weeks,** how much of the time has your physical health or emotional problems interfered with your social activities (like visiting with friends, relatives, etc)? (Circle one response.)
1 All of the time / 2 Most of the time / 3 Some of the time / 4 A little of the time / 5 None of the time

Current Health Assessment
During the past week, how often have you taken pain medication, including narcotics or over-the-counter medications? (Circle one response.)
1 Three or more times a day / 2 Once or twice a day / 3 Once every couple of days / 4 Once a week / 5 Not at all

If you had to spend the rest of your life with the symptoms you have right now, how would you feel about it? (Circle one response.)
1 Very dissatisfied / 2 Somewhat dissatisfied / 3 Neutral / 4 Somewhat satisfied / 5 Very satisfied

THE DASH

INSTRUCTIONS

This questionnaire asks about your symptoms as well as your ability to perform certain activities.

Please answer *every question*, based on your condition in the last week, by circling the appropriate number.

If you did not have the opportunity to perform an activity in the past week, please make your *best estimate* on which response would be the most accurate.

It doesn't matter which hand or arm you use to perform the activity; please answer based on your ability regardless of how you perform the task.

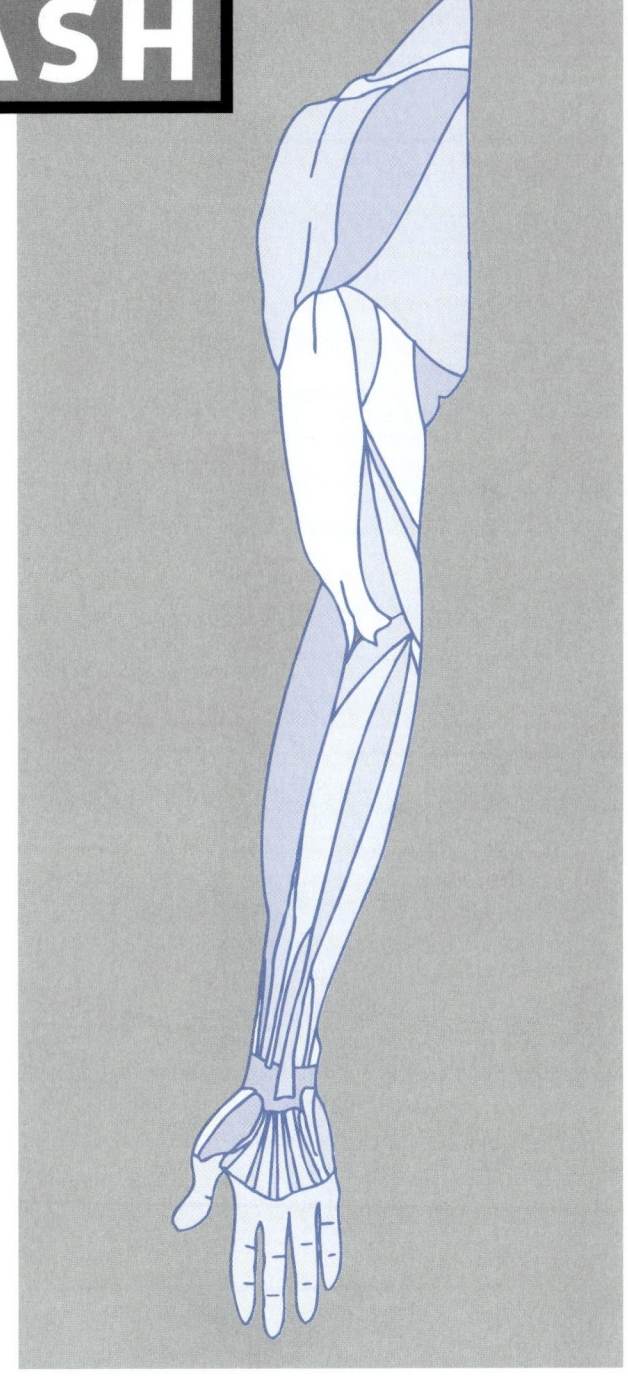

Disabilities of the Arm, Shoulder and Hand

Please rate your ability to do the following activities in the last week by circling the number below the appropriate response.

	NO DIFFICULTY	MILD DIFFICULTY	MODERATE DIFFICULTY	SEVERE DIFFICULTY	UNABLE
1. Open a tight or new jar.	1	2	3	4	5
2. Write.	1	2	3	4	5
3. Turn a key.	1	2	3	4	5
4. Prepare a meal.	1	2	3	4	5
5. Push open a heavy door.	1	2	3	4	5
6. Place an object on a shelf above your head.	1	2	3	4	5
7. Do heavy household chores (e.g., wash walls, wash floors).	1	2	3	4	5
8. Garden or do yard work.	1	2	3	4	5
9. Make a bed.	1	2	3	4	5
10. Carry a shopping bag or briefcase.	1	2	3	4	5
11. Carry a heavy object (over 10 lbs).	1	2	3	4	5
12. Change a lightbulb overhead.	1	2	3	4	5
13. Wash or blow dry your hair.	1	2	3	4	5
14. Wash your back.	1	2	3	4	5
15. Put on a pullover sweater.	1	2	3	4	5
16. Use a knife to cut food.	1	2	3	4	5
17. Recreational activities which require little effort (e.g., cardplaying, knitting, etc.).	1	2	3	4	5
18. Recreational activities in which you take some force or impact through your arm, shoulder or hand (e.g., golf, hammering, tennis, etc.).	1	2	3	4	5
19. Recreational activities in which you move your arm freely (e.g., playing frisbee, badminton, etc.).	1	2	3	4	5
20. Manage transportation needs (getting from one place to another).	1	2	3	4	5
21. Sexual activities.	1	2	3	4	5

DISABILITIES OF THE ARM, SHOULDER AND HAND

	NOT AT ALL	SLIGHTLY	MODERATELY	QUITE A BIT	EXTREMELY
22. During the past week, *to what extent* has your arm, shoulder or hand problem interfered with your normal social activities with family, friends, neighbours or groups? *(circle number)*	1	2	3	4	5

	NOT LIMITED AT ALL	SLIGHTLY LIMITED	MODERATELY LIMITED	VERY LIMITED	UNABLE
23. During the past week, were you limited in your work or other regular daily activities as a result of your arm, shoulder or hand problem? *(circle number)*	1	2	3	4	5

Please rate the severity of the following symptoms in the last week. *(circle number)*

	NONE	MILD	MODERATE	SEVERE	EXTREME
24. Arm, shoulder or hand pain.	1	2	3	4	5
25. Arm, shoulder or hand pain when you performed any specific activity.	1	2	3	4	5
26. Tingling (pins and needles) in your arm, shoulder or hand.	1	2	3	4	5
27. Weakness in your arm, shoulder or hand.	1	2	3	4	5
28. Stiffness in your arm, shoulder or hand.	1	2	3	4	5

	NO DIFFICULTY	MILD DIFFICULTY	MODERATE DIFFICULTY	SEVERE DIFFICULTY	SO MUCH DIFFICULTY THAT I CAN'T SLEEP
29. During the past week, how much difficulty have you had sleeping because of the pain in your arm, shoulder or hand? *(circle number)*	1	2	3	4	5

	STRONGLY DISAGREE	DISAGREE	NEITHER AGREE NOR DISAGREE	AGREE	STRONGLY AGREE
30. I feel less capable, less confident or less useful because of my arm, shoulder or hand problem. *(circle number)*	1	2	3	4	5

DASH DISABILITY/SYMPTOM SCORE = $\left[\dfrac{(\text{sum of n responses})}{n} - 1\right] \times 25$, where n is equal to the number of completed responses.

A DASH score may <u>not</u> be calculated if there are greater than 3 missing items.

Disabilities of the Arm, Shoulder and Hand

WORK MODULE (OPTIONAL)

The following questions ask about the impact of your arm, shoulder or hand problem on your ability to work (including homemaking if that is your main work role).

Please indicate what your job/work is:_____

❏ I do not work. (You may skip this section.)

Please circle the number that best describes your physical ability in the past week. Did you have any difficulty:

	NO DIFFICULTY	MILD DIFFICULTY	MODERATE DIFFICULTY	SEVERE DIFFICULTY	UNABLE
1. using your usual technique for your work?	1	2	3	4	5
2. doing your usual work because of arm, shoulder or hand pain?	1	2	3	4	5
3. doing your work as well as you would like?	1	2	3	4	5
4. spending your usual amount of time doing your work?	1	2	3	4	5

SPORTS/PERFORMING ARTS MODULE (OPTIONAL)

The following questions relate to the impact of your arm, shoulder or hand problem on playing *your musical instrument or sport or both*.
If you play more than one sport or instrument (or play both), please answer with respect to that activity which is most important to you.

Please indicate the sport or instrument which is most important to you:_____

❏ I do not play a sport or an instrument. (You may skip this section.)

Please circle the number that best describes your physical ability in the past week. Did you have any difficulty:

	NO DIFFICULTY	MILD DIFFICULTY	MODERATE DIFFICULTY	SEVERE DIFFICULTY	UNABLE
1. using your usual technique for playing your instrument or sport?	1	2	3	4	5
2. playing your musical instrument or sport because of arm, shoulder or hand pain?	1	2	3	4	5
3. playing your musical instrument or sport as well as you would like?	1	2	3	4	5
4. spending your usual amount of time practising or playing your instrument or sport?	1	2	3	4	5

SCORING THE OPTIONAL MODULES: Add up assigned values for each response; divide by 4 (number of items); subtract 1; multiply by 25.
An optional module score may **not** be calculated if there are any missing items.

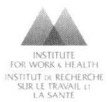

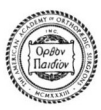

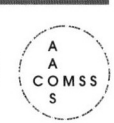

©IWH & AAOS & COMSS 1997

References

1. Amadio PC, Silverstein MD, Ilstrup DM et al. (1996) Outcome assessment for carpal tunnel surgery: the relative responsiveness of generic, arthritis-specific, disease-specific, and physical examination measures. J Hand Surg [Am] 21: 338–46
2. Amadio PC (1993) Outcomes measurements. J Bone Joint Surg Am 75: 1583–1584
3. Bessette L, Sangha O, Kuntz KM et al. (1998) Comparative responsiveness of generic versus disease-specific and weighted versus unweighted health status measures in carpal tunnel syndrome. Med Care 36: 491–502
4. Charlson ME, Pompei P, Ales KL, McKenzie CR (1987) A new method of classifying prognostic comorbidity in longitudinal studies: development and validation. J Chron Dis 40(5):373–383
5. Guillemin F, Bombardier C, Beaton D (1993) Cross-cultural adaptation of health-related quality of life measures: literature review and proposed guidelines. J Clin Epidemiol 46(12):1417–32
6. Keller RB, Soule DN, Wennberg JE, Hanley DF (1990) Dealing with geographic variations in the use of hospitals. The experience of the Maine Medical Assessment Foundation Orthopedic Study Group. J Bone Joint Surg Am 72(9): 1286–93
7. Levine DW, Simmons BP, Koris MJ et al. (1993) A self-administered questionnaire for the assessment of severity of symptoms and functional status in carpal tunnel syndrome. J Bone Joint Surg Am 75:1585–92
8. Lieberman JR, Dorey F, Shekelle P et al. (1996) Differences between patient's and physician's evaluations of outcome after total hip arthroplasty. J Bone Joint Surg 78A: 835–838
9. Padua L, Padua R, Lo Monaco M et al. (1999) Multiperspective assessment of carpal tunnel syndrome: A multicenter study. Neurology 53:1654–9
10. Padua L, Padua R, Lo Monaco M et al. (1998) for the "Italian CTS Study Group." Italian Multicentric study of carpal tunnel syndrome: study design. It J Neurol Scien 19:285–289
11. Padua R, Padua L, Romanini E et al. (1998) Versione italiana del questionario Boston Carpal Tunnel: valutazione preliminare. Giornale Italiano di Ortopedia e Traumatologia 24:123–129
12. Padua R, Romanini E, Zanoli G (1998) L'analisi dei risultati nella patologia dell'apparato locomotore. Guerini e Associati, Milano
13. Pynsent PB, Fairbank JCT, Carr A (1993) Outcome measures in Orthopedics. Butterworth-Heinemann, Oxford
14. Relman A (1988) Assessment and Accountability. The third revolution in medical care. N Engl J Med 319: 1220–1222
15. Sackett DL, Richardson WS, Rosenberg W, Haynes RB (1998) Evidence-based Medicine. Churchill Livingstone
16. Simmons BP, Swiontkowski MF, Evans RW et al. (1999) Outcomes assessment in the information age: available instruments, data collection, and utilization of data. Instr Course Lect 48:667–85
17. Swiontkowski MF, Buckwalter JA, Keller RB, Haralson R (1999) The outcomes movement in orthopedic surgery: where we are and where we should go. J Bone Joint Surg Am 81(5):732–40
18. Vaile JH, Mathers DM, Ramos-Remus C, Russell AS (1999) Generic health instruments do not comprehensively capture patient perceived improvement in patients with carpal tunnel syndrome. J Rheumatol 26:1163–6
19. Ware JE Jr, Gandek B (1998) Overview of the SF-36 Health Survey and the International Quality of Life Assessment (IQOLA) Project. J Clin Epidemiol 51(11):903–12
20. Ware JE, Sherbourne CD (1992) The MOS 36-items Short-Form health survey (SF-36) Med Care 30: 473–483
21. Wright JG, Swiontkowski MF (2000) Introducing a New Journal Section: Evidence-Based Orthopedics. J Bone Joint Surg 82 (6): 759

51 Carpal Tunnel Syndrome: Multicenter Studies with Multiperspective Assessment – Results of the Italian CTS Study Group

L. Padua

Introduction

Although CTS is frequent (there is a 10% risk of developing this pathology during one's lifetime according to the American Academy of Neurology) [4, 30] few clinical/neurophysiological studies are available on wide populations [22, 28, 35, 58, 61].

Clinical diagnosis of CTS is usually easy and sensitive, so it is therefore considered the "gold standard" evaluation. CTS assessment and management involve many different aspects which is why CTS is well defined as a complex challenge, even though it is such a simple condition [30, 54].

Multiperspective and multicenter studies may sometimes be appropriate tools for the CTS challenge. Multicenter studies are commonly accepted as providing a more representative population. Multiperspective studies provide a more comprehensive assessment of disease because they are assessed from different points of view and through different tools. In September 1996, the Italian CTS Study Group was founded. This group designed strict clinical and neurophysiological protocol for performing a wide multicenter study on idiopathic CTS hands. In addition to the traditional clinical and neurophysiologic evaluations, the group also adopted a validated patient-oriented measurement to obtain more comprehensive and consistent data for the clinical picture [63]. Patient-oriented evaluation has recently gained more importance as a scientific approach and is now considered very important in assessing the clinical picture of disease.

The choice to adopt a patient-oriented evaluation makes it possible to obtain a standardized clinical picture which is one of the most important advantages of this kind of measurement. In turn, this standardized clinical picture facilitates wide and multicentric studies and helps to compare clinical-instrumental objective findings with those of the "voice of the patient."

Study Design

A careful review of clinical and neurophysiological studies allowed the Italian CTS group to develop a unique methodology. An extensive and complete description of the study's design has been reported previously [48]. All centers adhere strictly to this protocol. The collaboration is performed according to the recently proposed guidelines for multicenter collaboration and clinical research in neurology [7, 24]. The study of CTS is achieved following the Literature Classification Criteria proposed by the American Association of Electrodiagnostic Medicine (AAEM) and the American Academy of Neurology (AAN) [1, 4].

Definition of Cases and Data Collection

Diagnosis of CTS is based on previously reported [35] and diagnostic criteria proposed by the AAN [4]. The criteria are: paresthesia, pain, swelling, weakness or clumsiness of the hand provoked or worsened by sleep, sustained hand or arm position, repetitive action of the hand or wrist that is mitigated by changing posture or by shaking of the hand, sensory deficits in the median innervated region of the hand, and motor deficit or hypotrophy of the median innervated thenar muscles. The minimum duration of symptoms is 2 months.

A detailed clinical history and a careful clinical examination and extended neurophysiological evaluation (described later) must always be performed to exclude the presence of other diseases that could be related to CTS (e.g., diabetes, polyneuropathy, endocrine diseases, etc.).

Patient-Oriented Data – Boston Carpal Tunnel Questionnaire

A patient-oriented validated measurement is used which is the Italian version of the Boston Carpal Tunnel Questionnaire (BCTQ) [23, 40, 41]. The BCTQ evaluates two domains of CTS, namely "symptoms" (SYMPT, patient-oriented symptom) assessed with an 11-item scale, and "functional status" (FUNCT, patient-oriented function) assessed with an 8-item scale (each item has 5 possible responses). Each score (SYMPT and FUNCT) is calculated as the mean of the responses of the individual item.

Personal Data and Clinical Examination

Before the examination, the physician acquires personal data by asking each patient to complete a case form. Some questions concern specific activities of the patient to evaluate whether hand stress is present (hobby or work with repetitive hand/wrist action, hard manual labor, etc.). An extended clinical neurologic examination must be performed for all patients (tendon reflexes of the four limbs, cutaneous sensitivity, muscle strength, etc.). Examination of the hand includes the Phalen test, performed by a prolonged (1-min) passive forced flexion of the wrist; trophism of the thenar eminence; motor function of the median innervated muscles; and sensory function (cotton wool is used as a standard material for skin stimulation). For clinical examination, a historic and objective scale (Hi-Ob) of CTS is used. This scale is a modified version of a previously reported scale [13] and it includes two measures. The first measure is a score (Hi-Ob) determined by clinical history and objective findings: (1) nocturnal paraesthesia only; (2) nocturnal and diurnal paraesthesia; (3) sensory deficit; (4) hypotrophy or motor deficit of the median innervated thenar muscles; and (5) plegia of median thenar eminence muscles. The second measure of the scale evaluates, by patient-oriented measurement, the presence or absence of pain as a dichotomous categorical score obtained from the patient with a forced-choice answer (yes or no). Therefore, the Hi-Ob score is composed of a number (Hi-Ob) with or without the pain variable (PAIN; e.g., a patient with nocturnal and diurnal paraesthesia also complaining of pain is scored as 2P).

The BCTQ and Hi-Ob scales have different ways of quantifying the clinical picture, but some common features may be found: both SYMPT and PAIN assess symptoms. Moreover, Hi-Ob is in some ways analogous to FUNCT. In fact, although Hi-Ob is a historic and objective measurement, in the more severe scores (scores 3 through 5) it indirectly regards hand function as FUNCT.

Electrodiagnostic Evaluation

Electrodiagnostic (EDX) studies are performed according to a protocol [34, 48] inspired by the AAN and AAEM recommendations [1, 2]. The following median nerve studies, considered standard, are always performed: (1) median sensory nerve conduction velocity in two digit/wrist segments (e.g., the first and the third); and (2) median distal motor latency from wrist to thenar eminence. Moreover, when the standard tests yielded normal results, segmental (over a short distance of 7–8 cm) or comparative studies (e.g., median/ulnar comparison or disto-proximal ratio) are always performed [31]. Sensory conduction studies of the radial or ulnar and sural nerves and motor conduction studies of the peroneal nerve are performed to exclude concomitant polyneuropathy. The patients with abnormal findings in nerves other than the median nerve are excluded from the study.

The severity of neurophysiologic CTS impairment is assessed by a previously reported neurophysiologic classification [32, 35]. CTS hands are divided into six groups on the basis of the neurophysiologic findings (see Table 51.1).

The adopted neurophysiological protocol and classification may easily be used in any needle electromyography (EMG) laboratory because every laboratory can use its own normal neurophysiological ranges. During electrophysiological examination, skin temperature must be greater than 31 °C. Through this protocol, the Italian CTS Study Group performed several studies focused on different aspects of CTS. Further items are assessed in each study as well.

Table 51.1. Neurophysiological classification – median nerve findings

	Sensory conduction study	Motor conduction study
Negative (NEG)	Normal	Normal
Minimal (MIN)	Abnormal segm.-comp test only	Normal distal motor latency
Mild (MILD)	Abnormal digit-wrist	Normal distal motor latency
Moderate (MOD)	Abnormal digit-wrist	Abnormal distal motor latency
Severe (SEV)	Absence of response	Abnormal distal motor latency
Extreme (EXT)	Absence of response	Absence of response

segm.-comp; segmental and/or comparative test

Dissociation Between Clinical-Neurophysiological Findings and Patient Symptoms

Background

The symptoms reported by the patient are important to the diagnosis, but the patient's subjective picture is not always in agreement with the objective findings of the physician [48].

Clinical-neurophysiologic studies were suggested by the AAN and the AAEM [5]. To assess the clinical and neurophysiologic dissociation that is often observed in clinical practice, 1,123 idiopathic CTS hands were studied consecutively in 20 centers distributed equally throughout Italy during 1997. In this study [47], a wide and well-represented population of idiopathic CTS hands were assessed by a large, multi-perspective and multi-measurement evaluation of nerve impairment to compare clinical and neurophysiological objective findings to the "voice of the patient."

Consideration of Results Provided by the Study

Because of the frequent occurrence of dissociation between patient symptoms and clinical-neurophysiological findings, CTS was one of the first pathologies to have a validated patient-oriented measurement: the BCTQ [23]. Data [47] has shown that the clinical-neurophysiological relationships are strong when one evaluates the clinical picture by the functional scores (FUNCT and Hi-Ob, Fig. 51.1) with an exponential increase in functional impairment as the classification of neurophysiological severity progresses. Conversely, the clinical-neurophysiological relationship is not so clear and simple when one evaluates the symptoms. In fact, after observation, symptoms (SYMPT) and pain (PAIN) have similar behavior and do not increase significantly as the classification of neurophysiological severity progresses. Interestingly, all findings related to the sensory function (Phalen sign, SYMPT, and PAIN) decrease in the extreme group (neurophysiologically assessed by the absence of detectable motor and sensory responses). In the more severe patients (assessed by clinical objective findings and neurophysiological evaluation), the function and symptoms have different behavior (worsening of functions and improvement of symptoms, Figs. 51.2–51.5) according to an intuitive effect of the reduction in nerve fiber function. Conversely, a large part of the CTS population complains of severe symptoms, although minimal functional impairment and minimal or no electrophysiological abnormality are observed. This finding was previously observed [39] and could be explained by a low pain and discomfort threshold in the first phase of nerve entrapment, which later becomes higher.

In previous studies, the severity of CTS was age related [28, 35]. In the same way, in this author's population, age is positively related to the severity of hand-function impairment (both referred-FUNCT and ob-

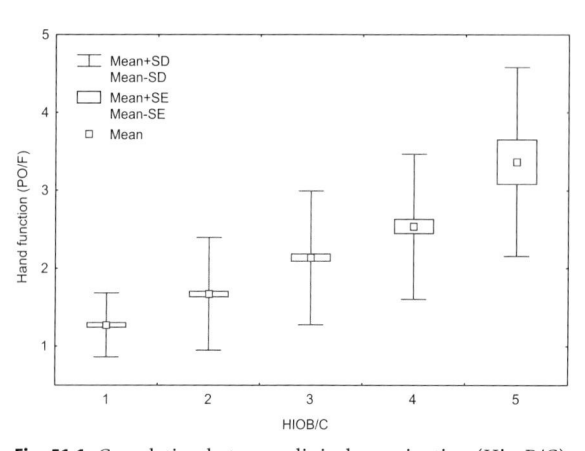

Fig. 51.1. Correlation between clinical examination (Hi-oB/C) and hand function (PO/F)

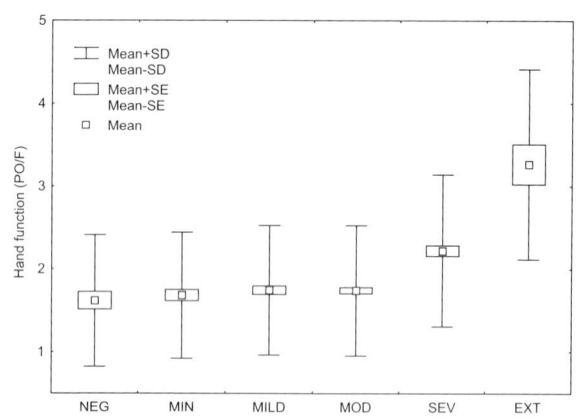

Fig. 51.2. Correlation between hand function (PO/F) and neurophysiological severity

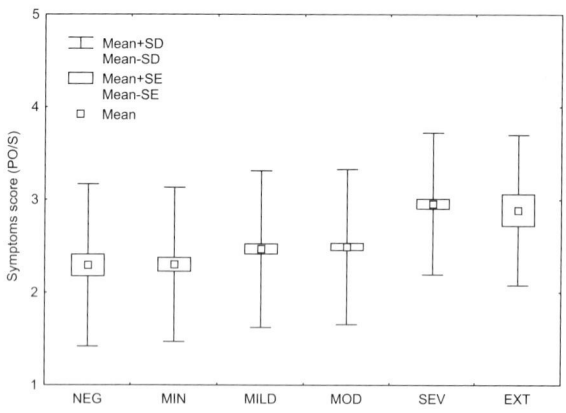

Fig. 51.3. Correlation between symptoms (PO/S) and neurophysiological severity

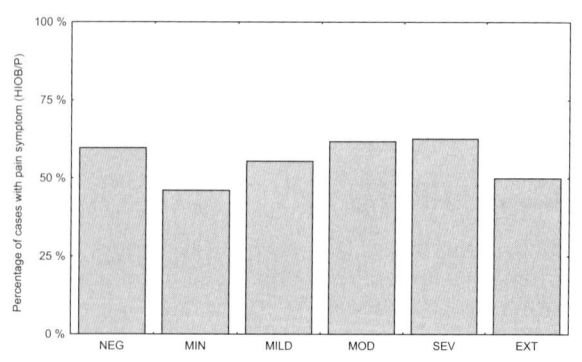

Fig. 51.4. Correlation between presence of pain (Hi-oB/P) and neurophysiological severity

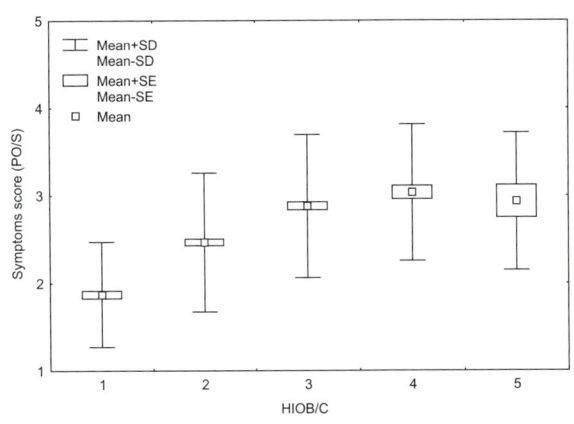

Fig. 51.5. Correlation between clinical examination (Hi-oB/C) and symptoms (PO/S)

jective-Hi-Ob); age is not related to the severity of the symptoms (SYMPT and PAIN).

This explains the frequent observation of young patients with striking symptoms, but without sensory and motor function impairment, as well as elderly patients with mild discomfort and severe sensory and motor function impairment.

Evolution of Untreated Carpal Tunnel Syndrome

Background

Steroid treatment and noninvasive physical therapy may provide temporary benefit for CTS, but surgical decompression is considered the only definitive cure [1, 2, 4, 5, 39, 58]. Many studies focus on the evolution of treated CTS and there is little data on the course of untreated CTS [8, 27, 29, 45, 46]. During 1997, the Italian CTS Study Group studied idiopathic CTS hands enrolled in 20 Italian centers [47]. Of the 20 centers that participated in the first study, 8 adhered to the follow-up study of the same sample [36]. The aim of the study was to evaluate the natural history of CTS and to look at the predictive value of EDX assessment, and the clinical picture at the time of the first diagnosis.

During the initial evaluation, each patient was exhaustively informed about of the knowledge of the management of CTS: surgical decompression provides a definitive cure in the majority of cases, but the real evolution of untreated CTS is not well known [30]. The Italian CTS Study Group showed that in cases where the clinical picture does not indicate immediate surgical decompression and where the hand surgeon does not consider that surgery should be performed immediately, a re-evaluation could be useful. The initial and follow-up evaluations were based on the protocol, which was reported in the study design paragraph (see Sect. "Study Design"). In addition, the following data was acquired.

Follow-up. Each center had to re-evaluate at least 75% of the initially enrolled CTS hands, with a latency between 10 and 15 months from the first evaluation. The evaluation of the evolution was based on the following CTS severity measurements: SYMPT, FUNCT, PAIN, Hi-Ob, and neurophysiological class. In other words, the evolution was assessed by the perspective of the patient (FUNCT, SYMPT, and pain), and the physician/neurophysiology assessment (Hi-Ob and neurophysiological class). When the patient was not able to come to the neurophysiological laboratory, the patient was given a telephone interview in which historical follow-up data, and SYMPT and FUNCT scores (by BCTQ patient-oriented evaluation performed on the phone) were acquired. For multiple regression statistical analysis, SYMPT, FUNCT, PAIN, Hi-Ob, and neurophysiological class were considered as dependent variables.

Statistical Analysis. In this case, a complex statistical analysis was performed and has been extensively reported [36].

Consideration on Results Provided by the Study

Therapeutic recommendations on CTS are not available, especially because of the absence of data on the natural history. In fact, to evaluate and standardize the therapeutic approach of any disease, the course of untreated cases must be known. Many authors are now emphasizing the importance of gaining information on the untreated course of CTS [30, 47, 54]. In other words, from CTS literature, one knows well what can be expected after therapy (especially after surgical decompression) [1, 2, 4, 5, 15, 58], but not when the patient is not treated.

In this study, a varied and well-represented untreated sample of idiopathic CTS hands were assessed using a large, multi-perspective and multi-measurement evaluation of nerve impairment to determine the natural history of CTS. None of the few previous studies on the evolution of untreated CTS [27, 29, 46] is comparable with the current follow-up: none is prospective, and none evaluates a patient-oriented picture using validated measurements.

The limitation of studies on untreated pathologies, especially when the diseases are curable (so randomized controlled trials are not conceivable), is that there is usually a high risk of sampling bias. In the current study, the risk of bias is low. The only problem is that a minority of the sample underwent surgery (the operated sample was demographically similar to the untreated sample, although more impaired). Unexpectedly, the data indicate that some CTS hands improve spontaneously in the absence of therapy. When the evolution was analyzed according to the initial picture, it was observed that CTS hands with initial low severity tend to get worse while CTS hands with initial high severe impairment tend to improve (this is observed in all CTS measurements – either patient-oriented or neurophysiologic).

In the author's study, multiple regression analysis showed a strong dependence of each severity measurement at T1 with its T0 value. Severe baseline pictures were associated with a higher odds of improvement at follow-up (one additional point on neurophysiological class increase by 1.7 the odds to neurophysiologically improve; similarly, the "risk" of improving in CTS symptoms for a patient with a SYMPT score of 3 is 2.8 greater than for a patient with SYMPT score of 2). Moreover, the factor that is most predictive of untreated CTS evolution is the duration of symptoms. In particular, a long duration of symptoms is a negative prognostic factor according to all patient-oriented measurements (FUNCT, SYMPT, and PAIN). For example, for each additional year of duration of symptom the odds of FUNCT improvement is reduced of 23%. Conversely, a long duration of symptoms is not significantly associated with a bad neurophysiological or clinical examination outcome. With regard to the positive prognostic value of hand stress at the baseline evaluation, note that this value is probably due to the interruption of the stress. This could be an interesting topic and a more focused study might provide important information for deciding on a therapeutic approach. As expected, the clinical examination had a lower sensitivity in measuring the outcome of CTS. This is not surprising, as findings from clinical examination have a low sensitivity in CTS diagnosis (clinical examination is normal in many CTS patients even if they complain of severe symptoms) [54].

Symptoms and Neurophysiological Picture of Carpal Tunnel Syndrome in Pregnancy
Background

Usually CTS is idiopathic. Nevertheless, sometimes CTS is considered related to certain physiological [62] (menopause, pregnancy) and pathological (polyneuropathies, Colles fracture, disease of thyroid, etc.) conditions [59]. One of the most frequent physiological conditions associated with CTS is pregnancy. Some papers focus on the incidence of CTS in pregnancy. Nevertheless, the data reported are discordant [12, 17, 26, 60, 66]. Note that in these studies the neurophysiological evaluation was performed using techniques with low sensitivity. At that time the neurophysiological evaluation had a low sensitivity for CTS; recently, the sensitivity of EDX tests increased [1, 2].

During 2000, the Italian CTS Study Group studied the occurrence of CTS in women enrolled in seven Italian centers during the last trimester of their pregnancy [49]. The aim was to evaluate the occurrence of CTS during pregnancy and the predictive value of the clinical picture and lifestyle before and during pregnancy. In addition to the usual protocol adopted by the Italian CTS Study Group, data on pregnancy and concomitant conditions was acquired.

Consideration of Results Provided by the Study

In the author's study 59% of CTS cases complained of paraesthesia in at least one hand (85% of these had positive EDX findings for CTS in at least in one hand). Clinical CTS was diagnosed in more than half of women (62%). Neurophysiological evaluation provided diagnosis of CTS in approximately half of women (43% were positive in at least one hand). Some authors previously reported the correlation between edema in pregnancy and CTS symptoms [12, 66, 67]. This author's study confirms this association and provides evidence, never before reported, of the correlation between edema and neurophysiological picture. Similarly, this study provides a correlation between validated patient-oriented measurement and edema. In conclusion, these observations confirm that the edema of the tissues in the carpal tunnel, as a result of the tendency for fluid retention, could induce a mechanical compression of the nerve and could be an important factor of CTS in pregnancy.

Evolution of Carpal Tunnel Syndrome in Pregnancy
Background

All seven of the centers that participated in the first study adhered to the follow-up study of the same sample [53]. The goal of the follow-up study was to evaluate the evolution of CTS after delivery and lactation and to evaluate the predictive value of EDX assessment and clinical picture at the time of the first diagnosis. Along with the usual protocol, the following additional data was acquired.

Consideration of Results Provided by the Study

As expected, the data showed that in the sample with CTS at initial evaluation, clinical (Hi-Ob) and patient-oriented (PAIN, SYMTP, and FUNCT) measurements significantly improved 1 year after delivery. Conversely, the neurophysiologic picture did not improve, but most patients who improved refused the neurophysiologic evaluation at follow-up; therefore neurophysiologic evaluation at follow-up was performed in a smaller sample and usually in women with CTS symptoms [36]. Although the CTS severity measurements improved at follow-up, more than half of the women who had CTS symptoms during pregnancy complained of CTS symptoms 1 year after delivery [3].

In the author's study, multiple regression analysis showed a strong dependence on each severity measurement at T1 with its T0 value. Severe baseline pictures were associated with a higher probability of improvement at follow-up. Moreover, the factor that was most predictive of untreated CTS evolution was the onset of CTS symptoms during pregnancy. An earlier onset of symptoms was a negative prognostic factor according to all patient-oriented and clinical measurements. According to the neurophysiologic evolution, weight gain appeared predictive – a higher gain implies a lower probability of improvement at follow-up.

Diagnostic Pathway and Differences Between the Populations Enrolled in the Northern, Central, and Southern Regions of Italy

Background

The economic trend in Italy, as in other countries, now requires physicians to pay more attention to the social and economic aspects of health; therefore, it is important to evaluate the diagnostic pathway and the socioeconomical aspect of the pathologies. The Italian CTS Study Group performed a wide multicenter and multidimensional study to assess the clinical-neurophysiological picture and the diagnostic pathway on a large idiopathic CTS population, and to evaluate the differences between the populations enrolled in the neurophysiological centers of the northern, central, and southern regions of Italy [51]. Recently, many studies focused on evaluating differences in the approach of the pathologies between small areas of the country [21].

Consideration of Results

The diagnostic pathway appeared inversely related to the patient's education. In the less-educated group, the time from the onset of symptoms and the first medical visit was longer, while the second part of diagnostic pathway of CTS (the period from the visit to the first EDX evaluation) was not related to education. The less-educated groups were affected by more severe nerve impairment at their clinical and neurophysiological examinations. This was due mainly to their manual jobs (higher percentage of stressed hands). Despite the more severe clinical and neurophysiological impairment, the less educated groups did not complain of major involvement of the hands (SYMPT and FUNCT scores are not related to education). This could be due to a greater tolerance of discomfort in these groups. This greater tolerance would explain the delay in going to the physician for CTS symptoms. Nevertheless, other factors must be considered. In regard to the symptoms, they are not clearly related to the neurophysiological nerve impairment. (Often, cases affected by more severe neurophysiological CTS complain of lower symptoms than cases with mild neurophysiological impairment). In regard to hand function, the hand might not be excessively impaired in less-educated groups because of the strength of the hand due to manual jobs.

In regard to the cost of the pathology, the data showed that nonsuitable and unnecessary investigations (often invasive and costly) were sometimes performed. The analysis of the differences between the populations enrolled in Italy showed that the northern and central regions have a similar clinical-neurophysiological picture, while the southern region's population appears significantly different. In fact, the southern region's CTS population is characterized by a higher frequency of hard manual laborers and less education. This is most likely the cause of the more severe nerve impairment observed in this population.

The diagnostic pathway in the northern, central, and southern regions appears similar in its first phase, while in the southern region, the latency from first medical visit to electrodiagnosis is shorter than in the northern region. In conclusion, analysis of clinical-neurophysiological impairment related to the educational data provided new and interesting information that may have important clinical and social relevance.

Occurrence of Carpal Tunnel Syndrome in Males and Females

It is well known that women are more frequently affected by CTS than men. Nevertheless, results from certain studies [6, 25], including this author's [52, 47, 38], provide data against this accepted opinion.

The Italian CTS Study Group studied 740 patients (a total of 1,123 hands with CTS, 383 affected bilaterally) [50] in 20 centers distributed throughout Italy. Comparing clinical and neurophysiological results and patient responses, it was found that men complained less of discomfort and had better hand function than women, although by neurophysiologic assessment showed that men had more severe nerve impairment [52]. Thus, as had been previously hypothesized by Nathan and colleagues [28], this data indicates that men have a greater tolerance for CTS symptoms than women.

At the time the author's paper was published, Atroshi and colleagues [6] reported findings from a registry-based population study of CTS in southern Sweden. These investigators observed that "the prevalence of CTS recorded in men (male-female ratio, 1:1.4) was higher than previously reported." They did not have a definite explanation for the observation.

Gorsche and colleagues [16] observed similar CTS prevalence rates among men and women working in a meat packing plant, but different incidence rates (for men and women it was 9.7 and 18.4 cases/100 person-years, respectively). From a study of workers in the USA, McDiarmid and colleagues [25] found that men had lower CTS prevalence rates than women in most occupations, except for those who worked in a data entry position. In contrast with other occupational groups, data entry workers perform one single physical task regardless of gender [25].

The author's findings [52], together with those of other investigators [6, 16, 25], indicate that fewer men than women are diagnosed with CTS in population-based surveys, while prevalence rates among men and women who perform the same tasks are similar. Men may seek medical attention only when CTS symptoms become severe, thus, less severe cases remain undiagnosed and recorded prevalence rates remain lower, or physicians may interpret symptoms related to CTS differently in men and women. Hence, this author postulates that the occurrence of CTS in the male population is underestimated.

The Usefulness of Segmental and Comparative Tests

Background

Neurophysiological evaluation is now considered fundamental to confirm the clinical diagnosis of CTS and to assess the severity of the nerve entrapment [1, 2, 5]. Nevertheless, it must be noted that the sensitivity of neurophysiological evaluation strictly depends on the techniques used. Standard EDX tests (median digit-wrist sensory conduction velocity and wrist-thenar distal motor latency) usually have good sensitivity, but in some cases (approximately 20%) they do not show abnormal findings despite the presence of typical CTS symptoms. This may be explained because the median nerve conduction abnormalities in CTS are focal and, at least in the initial phases, restricted to the proximal segment that lies within the carpal tunnel. For this reason, more rapid conduction in the distal segment may mask mild proximal slowing. Hence, segmental studies (which evaluate the involved segment of the median nerve) are more sensitive for detecting mild abnormalities. Another approach involves comparison of median conduction with that of other nerves in the same hand. Because the patient serves as his own control, comparative studies reduce the problem of inter-subject variability in conduction velocity. In 1993, the AAN and the AAEM carried out an extensive study and provided the recommendation for EDX evaluation suggesting segmental or comparative studies to be performed when standard tests yield normal results [1, 44, 55]. In 2002, they roughly confirmed the previous observation [1].

Consideration of the Results Provided by the Study

The author's data [44] demonstrated that digit-wrist sensory nerve conduction studies play a leading role in CTS diagnosis. In spite of the good sensitivity showed by standard tests, the author was unable to neurophysiologically diagnose CTS using these techniques in patients with typical, often severe, CTS symptoms. The use of "more sensitive" tests (comparative and/or segmental) allowed for the disclosure of abnormal findings in an additional 11.4% of cases. The sensitivity of segmental or comparative tests appeared similar, providing CTS electrodiagnosis in approximately 7 out of 10 "standard negative" cases. Note that more sensitive tests allow diagnosis mostly in younger patients. The minimal group, which was neurophysiologically diagnosed by more sensitive tests, had a clinical picture characterized by a high percentage of pain, severe discomfort, but no limitation in functional daily activity. Conversely, severe functional impairment was observed when neurophysiological evaluation showed loss of sensory and motor responses. This data confirmed the usefulness of a complete neurophysiological assessment by using segmental or comparative tests when standard tests yield normal results [9, 10, 14, 31, 33, 42, 43, 54, 56–58, 64, 65].

Electrodiagnosis is a sensitive tool if AAN-AAEM recommendations are followed. It must be noted that recently an increased awareness of CTS by physicians has lead to early clinical and neurophysiological diagnosis [37], confirming that a complete EDX assessment has important clinical and economical implications [2, 8]. In cases where neurophysiological diagnosis is not carried out because nonsensitive EDX protocols are used, the diagnostic path is usually diverted and the patient undergoes other investigations which are unnecessary as well as invasive and costly.

Italian CTS Study Group – Participating Members

Investigators, centers: *Bertin L*, Padova; *Carboni T*, Neurologia, Ospedale Civile S.Benedetto del Tronto (AP); *Di Pasqua*, PG Neurologia, Ospedale pediatrico "Bambin Gesù" Palidoro (RM); *Eleopra R*, Divisione Neurologia, Arcispedale S. Anna Ferrara; *Giannini F*, Istituto Clinica delle Malattie Nervose e Mentali Università di Siena; *Ghirlanda P*, Clinica Neurologica – Univ. Messina; Giunchedi M, Laboratorio Neurofisiologia, Ospedale di Lavagna (Ge); *Grippo A*, Neurofisiopatologia Ospedale Civile Viareggio (Lu); *Insola A*, Neurofisiopatologia Centro traumatologico Ortopedico Roma; *Liguori R*, Neurologia Università Bologna; *Lori S*, Neurofisiopatologia ASL 10 Firenze; *Luchetti R*, Chirurgia della mano Ospedale di stato S. Marino; *Mariani E*,

Neurofisiopatologia Istituti Clinici di perfezionamento Milano, Massi S, Institute Valdarno, San Giovanni Valdarno-Arezzo: Mondelli M, EMG service, ASL 7 – Siena. Morini A, Operative Unit of Neurology Ospedale Santa Chiara-Trento; *Murasecco D*, Neurologia Univ. Perugia; *Padua L*, Neurologia Università Cattolica Roma; *Giuseppe Picciolo*, Clinica Neurologica 2 – Univ. Messina; *Pisano F*, Neurofisopatologia Fondazione S. Maugeri IRCCS Veruno (NO); *Romano M*, Neurofisopatologia Villa Sofia CTO Palermo; *Speranzini C*, Neurologia Ospedale A. Murri Fermo (AP); *Tironi F*, Neurofisopatologia Ospedali Riuniti Bergamo; *Uncini A*, Centro regionale malattie neuromuscolari Ospedale SS Annunziata Chieti

Acknowledgements. Thanks to Pietro Caliandro and Alessandro Calistri for technical support.

References

1. American Academy of Neurology, American Association of Electrodiagnostic Medicine, American Academy of Physical Medicine and Rehabilitation (1993) Practice parameter for carpal tunnel syndrome (summary statement). Neurology 43:2406–2409
2. American Academy of Neurology, American Association of Electrodiagnostic Medicine, American Academy of Physical Medicine and Rehabilitation (1993) Practice parameter for electrodiagnostic studies in carpal tunnel syndrome (summary statement). Neurology 43:2404–2405
3. American Association of Electrodiagnostic Medicine Quality Assurance Committee (1993) Literature review of the usefulness of nerve conduction studies and electromyography for the evaluation of patients with carpal tunnel syndrome. Muscle Nerve 16:1392–1414
4. American Association of Electrodiagnostic Medicine, American Academy of Neurology, American Academy of Physical Medicine and Rehabilitation (2002) Practice parameter: electrodiagnostic studies in carpal tunnel syndrome. Neurology 58:1589–1592
5. Al Qattan mm, Manktelow RT, Bowen CV (1994) Pregnancy-induced carpal tunnel syndrome requiring surgical release longer than 2 years after delivery. Obstet Gynecol 84:249–251
6. Atroshi I, Gummesson C, Johnsson R et al. (1999) Prevalence of carpal tunnel syndrome in general population. JAMA 282:153–158
7. Barker A, Powell R (1997) Guidelines exist on ownership of data and authorship in multicentre collaboration. BMJ 314:1046
8. Boniface SJ, Morris I, MacLeod A (1994) How does neurophysiological assessment influence the management and outcome of patients with carpal tunnel syndrome? Br J Rheumatol 33:1169–1170
9. Buchthal F, Rosenfalck A (1971) Sensory conduction from digit to palm and from palm to wrist in the carpal tunnel syndrome. J Neurol Neurosurg Psychiatr 34:243–252
10. Carroll GJ (1987) Comparison of median and radial nerve sensory latencies in the electrophysiological diagnosis of carpal tunnel syndrome. Electroencephalogr Clin Neurophysiol 68:101–106
11. Devinsky O (1995) Outcome research in neurology: incorporating health-related quality of life. Ann Neurol 37:141–142
12. Ekman-Ordeberg G, Salgeback S, Ordeberg G (1987) Carpal tunnel syndrome in pregnancy. A prospective study. Acta Obstet Gynecol Scand 66:233–235
13. Gorsche RG, Wiley JP, Renger RF et al. (1999) Prevalence and incidence of carpal tunnel syndrome in a meat packing plant. Occup Environ Med 56:417–422
14. Giannini F, Passero S, Cioni R et al. (1991) Electrophysiologic evaluation of local steroid injection in carpal tunnel syndrome. Arch Phys Med Rehabil 72:738–742
15. Giannini F, Cioni R, Mondelli M et al. (2002) A new clinical scale of carpal tunnel syndrome: validation of the measurement and clinical-neurophysiological assessment. Clin Neurophysiol 113:71–77
16. Girlanda P, Quartarone A, Sinicropi S et al. (1998) Electrophysiological studies in mild carpal tunnel syndrome. Electroencephalogr Clin Neurophysiol 109:44–49
17. Gould JS, Wissinger HA (1978) Carpal tunnel syndrome in pregnancy. South Med J 71:144–154
18. Guyatt GH, Feeny DH, Patrick DL (1993) Measuring health-related quality of life. Ann Intern Med 118:622–629
19. Hobart JC, Freeman JA, Lamping DL (1996) Physicians and patient-oriented outcomes in progressive neurological disease: which to measure? Curr Opin Neurol 9:441–444
20. Keller RB, Rudicel SA, Liang MH (1993) Outcome Research in orthopaedics. J Bone Joint Surg 75-A:1562–1574
21. Keller RB, Soule DN, Wennberg JE, Hanley DF (1990) Dealing with geographic variations in the use of hospitals: the experience of the Maine Medical Assessment Foundation Orthopaedic Study Group. J Bone Joint Surg Am 72:1286–1293
22. Kimura I, Ayyar DR (1985) The carpal tunnel syndrome: electrophysiological aspects of 639 symptomatic extremities. Electromyogr Clin Neurophysiol 25:151–164
23. Levine DW, Simmons BP, Koris MJ et al. (1993) A self-administered questionnaire for the assessment of severity of symptoms and functional status in carpal tunnel syndrome. J Bone Joint Surg Am 75:1585–1592
24. Marshall FJ, Kieburtz K, McDermott M et al. (1996) Clinical research in neurology. From observation to experimentation. Neurol Clin 14:451–466
25. McDiarmid M, Oliver M, Ruser J, Gucer P (2000) Male and female rate differences in carpal tunnel syndrome injuries attributes or job tasks? Environ Res 83:23–31
26. Melvin JL, Burnett CN, Johnson EW (1969) Median nerve conduction in pregnancy. Arch Phys Med Rehabil 50:75–80
27. Mühlau G, Both R, Kunath H (1984) Carpal tunnel syndrome – course and prognosis. J Neurol 231:83–86
28. Nathan PA, Meadows KD, Doyle LS (1988) Relationship of age and sex to sensory conduction of the median nerve at the carpal tunnel and association of slowed conduction with symptoms. Muscle Nerve 11:1149–1153
29. Nathan PA, Keniston RC, Myers LD et al. (1998) Natural history of median nerve sensory conduction in industry: relationship to symptoms and carpal tunnel syndrome in 558 hands over 11 years. Muscle Nerve 21:711–721
30. Olney RK (2001) Carpal tunnel syndrome. Complex issues with a "simple" condition. Neurology 56:1431–1432
31. Padua L, Lo Monaco M, Valente EM, Tonali PA (1996) A useful electrophysiologic parameter for diagnosis of carpal tunnel syndrome. Muscle Nerve 19:48–53
32. Padua L, Lo Monaco M, Gregori B et al. (1996) Double-peaked potential in the neurophysiological evaluation of carpal tunnel syndrome. Muscle Nerve 19:679–680
33. Padua L, Lo Monaco, Aulisa L et al. (1996) Surgical prognosis in carpal tunnel syndrome: usefulness of a preopera-

tive neurophysiological assessment. Acta Neurol Scand 94:343–346
34. Padua L, Lo Monaco M, Gregori B et al. (1997) Neurophysiological classification and sensitivity in 500 carpal tunnel syndrome hands. Acta Neurol Scand 96:211–217
35. Padua L, Lo Monaco M, Padua R et al. (1997) Neurophysiological classification of carpal tunnel syndrome assessment of 600 symptomatic hands. Ital J Neurol Sci 18:145–150
36. Padua L, Lo Monaco M, Moretti C, Tonali P (1997) Increase of early clinical diagnosis of carpal tunnel syndrome over the last years. Muscle Nerve 20:1045–1046
37. Padua L, Lo Monaco M, Gregori B et al. (1998) Bilateral clinical-neurophysiological assessment of median nerve in carpal tunnel syndrome patients. Muscle Nerve 21: 264–265
38. Padua L, Padua R, Lo Monaco M et al. (1998) Natural history of carpal tunnel syndrome according to the neurophysiological classification. Ital J Neurol Sci 19:357–361
39. Padua L, Padua R, Lo Monaco et al. (1998) Italian multicentre study of carpal tunnel syndrome: study design. Ital J Neurol Sci 19:285–289
40. Padua L, Padua R, Nazzaro M, Tonali P (1998) Incidence of bilateral symptoms in carpal tunnel syndrome. J Hand Surg 23:603–606
41. Padua L, Padua R, Lo Monaco M, Tonali P (1998) Postoperative outcome related to preoperative symptomatology. Clin Orthop 346:284–285
42. Padua R, Padua L, Romanini E et al. (1998) Versione italiana del questionario Boston Carpal Tunnel: valutazione preliminare. Giornale Italiano di Ortopedia e Traumatologia 24:123–129
43. Padua R, Romanini E, Zanoli G (1998) Analisi dei risultati nell'apparato locomotore. Guerini editore, Milano
44. Padua L, Aprile I, Lo Monaco M et al. (1999) Italian multicentre study of carpal tunnel syndrome: clinical-neurophysiological picture and diagnostic pathway in 461 patients and differences between the populations enrolled in the northern, central and southern centres. Italian CTS Study Group. Ital J Neurol Sci 20:309–313
45. Padua L, Giannini F, Girlanda P et al. (1999) Usefulness of segmental and comparative tests in the electrodiagnosis of carpal tunnel syndrome: the Italian multicenter study. Italian CTS Study Group. Ital J Neurol Sci 20:315–320
46. Padua L, Padua R, Aprile I, Tonali P (1999) Italian multicentre study of carpal tunnel syndrome: differences in the clinical and neurophysiological features between male and female patients. J Hand Surg Br 24:579–582
47. Padua L, Padua R, Lo Monaco M et al. (1999) Multiperspective assessment of carpal tunnel syndrome: a multicenter study. Italian CTS Study Group. Neurology 53: 1654–1659
48. Padua L, Padua R, Lo Monaco M et al. (1999) Multiperspective assessment of carpal tunnel syndrome: a multicenter study: Italian CTS Study Group. Neurology 53: 1654–1659
49. Padua L, Aprile I, Caliandro P et al. The Italian Carpal Tunnel Syndrome Study Group (2001) Symptoms and neurophysiological picture of carpal tunnel syndrome in pregnancy. Clin Neurophysiol 112:1946–1951
50. Padua L, Aprile I, Caliandro P et al. Gruppo Italiano Studio Sindrome Tunnel Carpale (2001) Is the occurrence of carpal tunnel syndrome in men underestimated? Epidemiology 12:369
51. Padua L, Padua R, Aprile I et al. Italian CTS Study Group (2001) Multiperspective follow-up of untreated carpal tunnel syndrome. A multicenter study. Neurology 56:1459–66
52. Padua L, Padua R, Aprile I et al. The Italian CTS Study Group. Carpal tunnel syndrome (2001) Multiperspective follow-up of untreated carpal tunnel syndrome: a multicenter study. Neurology 56:1459–1466
53. Padua L, Aprile I, Caliandro P et al. Italian Carpal Tunnel Syndrome Study Group (2002) Carpal tunnel syndrome in pregnancy: multiperspective follow-up of untreated cases. Neurology 59:1643–1646
54. Pease WS, Cannell CD, Johnson EW (1989) Median to radial latency difference test in mild carpal tunnel syndrome. Muscle Nerve 12:905–909
55. Preston DC, Logigian E (1992) Lumbrical and interossei recording in carpal tunnel syndrome. Muscle Nerve 15: 1253–1257
56. Rosenbaum R (1999) Carpal tunnel syndrome and the myth of El Dorado. Muscle Nerve 22:1165–1167
57. Rossi S, Giannini F, Passero S et al. (1994) Sensory neural conduction of median nerve from digits and palm stimulation in carpal tunnel syndrome. Electroencephalogr Clin Neurophysiol 93:330–334
58. Seror P (1998) Pregnancy-related carpal tunnel syndrome. J Hand Surg Br 23:98–101
59. Sheean GL, Houser MK, Murray NM (1995) Lumbrical-interosseus latency comparison in the diagnosis of carpal tunnel syndrome. Electroencephalogr Clin Neurophysiol 97:285–289
60. Stevens JC (1987) AAEE Minimonograph #26: The electrodiagnosis of carpal tunnel syndrome. Muscle Nerve 10: 99–113
61. Stevens JC, Beard CM, O'Fallon WM, Kurland LT (1992) Conditions associated with carpal tunnel syndrome. Mayo Clin Proc 67:541–548
62. Stolp-Smith KA, Pascoe MK, Ogburn PL (1998) Carpal tunnel syndrome in pregnancy: frequency, severity, and prognosis. Arch Phys Med Rehabil 79:1285–1287
63. Thomas JE, Lambert EH, Cseuz KA (1967) Electrodiagnostic aspects of the carpal tunnel syndrome. Arch Neurol 16:635–641
64. Tobin SM (1967) Carpal tunnel syndrome in pregnancy. Am J Obstet Gynecol 15:493–498
65. Tonali P, Padua L, Sanguinetti C et al. (1999) Outcome research and patient-oriented measures in the multiperspective assessment of neurological and musculoskeletal disorders. Consensus Conference: Third Roman Neurophysiology day, Outcome Research in Neurology and in Musculoskeletal Disorders – 24 October 1998. Ital J Neurol Sci 20:139–140
66. Tonali P, Padua L, Sanguinetti C et al. (1999) Outcome research and patient-oriented measures in the multiperspective assessment of neurological and musculoskeletal disorders. Consensus Conference: Third Roman Neurophysiology day, Outcome Research in Neurology and in Musculoskeletal Disorders – 24 October 1998. Ital J Neurol Sci 20:139–140
67. Uncini A, Lange DJ, Solomon M et al. (1989) Ring finger testing in carpal tunnel syndrome: a comparative study of diagnostic utility. Muscle Nerve 12:735–741
68. Uncini A, Di Muzio A, Awad J et al. (1993) Sensitivity of three median-to-ulnar comparative tests in diagnosis of mild carpal tunnel syndrome. Muscle Nerve 16:1366–1373
69. Voitk AJ, Mueller JC, Farlinger DE, Johnston RU (1983) Carpal tunnel syndrome in pregnancy. Can Med Assoc J 128:277–281
70. Wand JS. Carpal tunnel syndrome in pregnancy and lactation (1990) J Hand Surg Br 15:93–95
71. Ware JE Jr, Kosinski M, Keller SD (1994) SF-36 physical and mental health summary scales: a user's manual. New England Medical Center, Boston

Subject Index

abductor digiti minimi muscle flap 316, 324
abductor pollicis brevis muscle 11, 67, 71, 313
Achilles' tendon 315
acromegaly 21, 23, 98
acroparesthesia 3, 4, 6
– nocturnal 63
actinic brachial plexitis 376, 378
adductor pollicis muscle 15
adipofascial
– flap 350
– vessel 350
adipose
– hypothenar flap 374
– tissue 123
adrenalin 149
Adson forceps 131
Agee technique 241, 291
algodystrophy 284, 286, 295, 371, 373
algoparesthesia 371
Allen test 96, 214, 346, 351, 355
amyloidosis 23, 98, 116
amyotrophy 168, 241
anastomosis 31, 126, 353
anatomic anomaly 95
anesthesia nerve block 317
anesthetic liquid 50
angiogenesis 45, 376
angioma 77
annular
– anterior carpal ligament 166
– ligament 169
– release 126
antebrachial fascia 121, 131, 172, 221, 339, 346, 351
– incomplete sectioning 272
– transverse incision 222
anticoagulant 99
aponeurosis 10
apophysis of the hamatus 180
arachidonic acid 44
arteriole 31
arterio-venous fistula 23
arthritis 22
arthroscope 181
aspecific tenovaginitis 21, 22
atrophy 67
– of the thenar muscle 149
axial X-ray 177
axillary block anesthesia 119
axon 28, 29
– growth 39

– loss 70
axonal
– degeneration 37
– transport 29, 33
axonotmesis 39, 316
axoplasm 33

bands of Fontana 314
B-cell lymphoma 99
Bedeschi sign 272
Bier block 186
Blix curve 227
blood-nerve barrier 31
blunt dissection 137, 187
body diagram 358
bone callus fracture entrapment 38
bone marrow edema 77
Borrelia 23
Boston Carpal Tunnel Questionnaire (BCTQ) 84, 385, 392
bowstringing 280, 310
brachial plexus 5
– anesthesia 115, 128
brachydactyly 97
bupivacaine 141

Camino catheter 56
Camitz transfer 242
carbocaine 214
carpal annular ligament 290
– incomplete section 291
carpal bone 10
– mobilization 107
carpal canal
– deformity 24
– infection 23
– pressure 51, 52
– – segmental study 57
– stenosis 24
carpal fracture 92
carpal ligament, cutting technique 160
carpal transverse ligament, abnormalities 79
carpal tunnel
– anatomy 10
– decompression 127, 204
– endoscopic release 130
– median nerve 13
– open release (OCTR) 130, 214, 244
– persistence 338
– release 111
– – endoscopic 171

– – neurologic complications 310
– syndrome (CTS)
– – diagnosis 63
– – differential diagnosis 90
– – during breastfeeding 23
– – during pregnancy 23
– – history 3
– – idiopathic forms 21
– – in children 25
– – in pregnancy 396
– – pathogenesis 6
– – postoperative symptoms 269
– – questionnaire 385
– – rare causes 95
– – surgical complications 269
CAT scan 226, 274, 280
catheter fiber optic 58
causalgia 276, 285, 286, 295, 374
cellular
– flap 331
– ischemia 44
centimetric pressure measurement 52
central nervous system (CNS) 31
cervical
– disc disease 309
– radiculopathy 90
– syringomyelia 90
cervico-brachialgia 39
Charcot-Marie-Tooth disease 90
Charlson Comorbidity Index 385
Chiena technique 220
Chinese flap 350
chondromalacia 277
Chow's technique 226
chromatolysis 29, 34
chronic nerve compression 37
Churg-Strauss syndrome 91
clepsydra 201
closed compartment syndrome 34
closed field technique 269
collagen disease 21
Colles fracture 3, 4, 24, 49, 51, 96, 145, 247, 248, 396
compartment syndrome 171
complex regional pain syndrome 247, 250
compound motor action potential (CMAP) 71
compression test 65
compressive trauma 32
constrictive stenosis 127
corticosteroid injection 108

Subject Index

cost control 383
cost-efficacy analysis 383
Cotton-Loder position 3, 24, 49, 51, 247, 248
cubital-dorsal artery 362
cumulative trauma disorder 46
cutaneous
- nerve branch 275
- scar pathology 174, 282
cyst 79
cystic ganglia 77
cytokine 44

DASH
- questionnaire 84, 385
- score 341, 387
data
- analysis 385
- collection 385
De Quervain syndrome 21, 23
deep flexor tendon 75
Dejerine-Sottas syndrome 22, 97
Dellon test 356
demyelination 70
dentrites 28, 29
dexamethason 108
diabetes mellitus 21–23, 91, 99, 116, 164, 392
diastase 167
direct flap vascularization 349
disease of thyroid 396
distal
- motor latency (DML) 71
- radial epiphysis 373
- radius fracture 247
- wrist crease 53, 54
dorsal splint 256
double crush syndrome 37, 40, 164, 206
Dupuytren's
- contracture 229
- palmar fasciotomy 24
dysesthesia 292, 319, 322

eburnation osteosis 96
edema 23, 42, 148, 257, 260, 284, 292
- control 255
electrodiagnosis 89, 299, 365, 393, 397, 398
electromyography 63, 69, 89, 105, 177, 341, 393
endocrine disease 392
endoneural
- edema 35
- hypoxia phenomenon 36
- vessel 32
endoneurium 30, 39
endorphin 261
endoscopic
- carpal tunnel release 171
- release 156, 244
- technique (ET) 135, 147
endothelial anoxia 38
endothelium 32
entrapment
- neuropathy 310, 333
- syndrome 96
eosin staining 45

epicondylitis 21
epimysium 364
epinephrine 122
epineural fibrosis 361
- fixation 361
epineurectomy 363
epineurium 30, 39, 122, 316
epineurotomy 127, 128, 132, 339, 346, 258
ergonomic keyboard 105
ETCR technique 218
evicence-based medicine 383
extensor pollicis longus muscle 71, 353
extensor proprius indicis 353
external neurolysis 138, 366
extraligamentous thenar branch 17
extrinsic tumor 99

familiar hypertrophic neuropathy 22
Farabeuf retractor 196, 197
fascia axial vessel 346
fascial flap 351
fat-pad flap 321, 326
ferritin 29
fiber receptor 82
fiber-optic catheter 55
fibroplasia 42
fibrosis 45, 235, 316, 324, 339
fist test 106
flexor
- carpi radialis
- – muscle 11, 213, 236, 249
- – tendon 14
- digitorum profundus
- – muscle 12
- – tendon 227
- digitorum superficialis 313
- – tendon 227
- – muscle 10, 12, 16
- neo-retinaculum 184
- pollicis brevis muscle 11, 12, 15, 151
- pollicis longus
- – muscle 12
- – tendon 75, 285
- retinaculum 6, 7, 10, 13, 16, 49, 151, 152, 189, 201, 308, 333, 338
- – abnormalities 79
- – reconstruction 226
- – tendon
- – hypertrophic tenosynovectomy 273, 274, 291
- – hypertrophic tenosynovitis 272, 273
- – subcutaneous anterior subluxation 280
- – tenosynovectomy 200, 377
- – tenosynovitis 177, 207
fluidotherapy 163
focal dystonia 235
Foley catheter 49
forearm radial artery flap 345
Freer elevator 142, 143, 214
Fröhse arch 28
FUNCT score 86, 393–395
Functional Status Index 378

geyser effect 148
giant cell tumor 23
Gilbert technique 166
Gilbert-Becker's pedicle fascial fat flap 367
Gilliatt and Wilson test 272
gliding surface wrap 347
glycosaminoglycan 43, 97, 98
gonococcal tenovaginitis 25
gout 23
- tenosynovitis 205
granulomatous tenosynovitis 98
greater omentum flap 345
grip strength 190, 239, 245, 280, 365, 378
- evolution 243
- loss 228
- recovery 282
- testing 235
groin flap 333
guide positioning 215, 216
guided release system (GRS) 211
Guillain Barré 22
Guyon's
- canal 112, 152, 167, 202, 203, 213, 279, 294, 319, 329
- – decompression 127
- compartment 232–234

hamartoma 97
hamulus 172
hand
- diagram 84, 133
- edema 24
- pain 93
- prehension strength 295
- strength recovery program 262
- table 187, 188
hand/arm vibration syndrome 92
Hansen's disease 98
Harris Hip Score 384
Health-Related Quality of Life (HRQoL) 383
hematoma 171, 206, 273, 279, 285
hematoxylin 45
hemophilia 99
hemostasis 123, 285, 347
Henry approach 249
heparin 99
histoplasmosis 98
Historical-Objective (Hi-Ob) score 85–87, 393, 395
Hoffmann-Tinel sign 321
homeostasis 220
hook of the hamate 151, 152, 157, 172, 203, 226
hyaluronan 42
hydrocodone 192
4-hydroxy-2,3-alkenal (HAK) 43
4-hydroxy-2,3-nonenal (HNE) 43
hyperalgesia 315, 327
hyperechogenicity 78
hyperemia 119
hyperesthesia 119
hyperexcitability 85
hyperostosis 96
hyperreflexia 90
hypertension 37

Subject Index

hyperthyroidism 23
hypertrophic scar 292
hypertrophy of synovial tissue 132
hypoanesthesia 66, 293
hypoesthesia 90, 357
hypoparesthesia 199
hyposthenia 67
hypothenar
– fat pad flap 316, 321, 334, 341, 376, 377
– hammer syndrome 91
– muscle 76
– pain 276, 277, 282, 292
hypothyroidism 21, 23, 164
hypotrophy 76
– of the thenar muscle 83

iatrogenic
– lesion 206
– nerve injury 317
– – during CTS surgery 289
idiopathic brachial plexitis 90
inching technique 55
Indiana tome 140, 142, 144
indication mistake 290
infection 282, 295
innervation density test 65
intenal neurolysis 127
interdigital nerve apraxia 183
interfascicular neurolysis 349, 358
interleukin (IL)
– IL-1 45
– IL-6 44, 45
internal neurolysis 115, 135, 314, 315, 366
International Quality of Life Assessment (IQOLA) 384
interobserver reproducibility 87
interthenar
– depression 313
– fascia 189, 191, 192, 200, 201, 291
– – integrity 191
intracranial neoplasm 90
intrafascicular fibrosis 39
intraneural edema 35
intrinsic tumor 99
inverted double crush syndrome 40
iontophoresis 260
ischemia 34, 36, 37, 194, 338, 362
ischemic monomelic neuropathy 91

Jakab's ligamentoplasty 239
Jamar
– dynamometer 186, 207, 228, 242, 322
– hydraulic pinch gauge 186

Kaplan's line 145, 147, 178, 213
keloid skin scar 274, 363
Kimura technique 131
knife assembly 188
Kuhlmann-Tubiana-Lisfranc incision 194

laparotomy 378
lateral
– arm flap 333
– neuroma 127

Leri's disease 25
lidocaine 122, 141, 202, 260
ligament injury 92
ligamentoplasty 239
– reconstruction 244
lignocaine 108
limb movement 28
Linburg's syndrome 92
lipofibroma 119
lipofibromatous hamartoma 77, 90
lipoma 77, 79, 118
local anesthesia 156
locking device 188
Loge de Guyon 14
L-shaped incision 198
lunate
– dislocation 4
– excision 4
lupus 164
lymph drainage massage 258
lymphedema 24

macrodactyly 97
Madelung's disease 24, 97
magnetic resonance images 75
malondialdehyde (MDA) 43
manometer 49
marcaine 214
margin effect 35
Martin-Gruber anastomosis 72
mastectomy 24
Mayo Wrist score 341
median artery 18
– thrombosis 22, 25
median nerve 13, 15, 46, 112, 171, 198, 310
– anterior dislocation 310
– compression 21, 314
– – incomplete/complete lack 269
– – test 64
– conduction velocity 72
– decompression 69, 127, 255
– entrapment 231
– fork anomaly 118
– hypersensitivity 365
– iatrogenic injury 278, 313
– incomplete decompression 291
– innervation 275
– muscle branch 278
– palmar cutaneous branch 111
– sensory latency 71
– subluxation 276
– terminal branch 17
– trauma 58, 91
– ultrasound 78
median neurolysis 200
median neuropathy 3, 6, 7
Medical Outcome Survey Short Form-36 (see also SF-36 questionnaire) 84
medication 107
melorheostosis 96
Menon's technique 177
mepivacaine 195
– hydrochloride 149
meta-analysis 383
metabolic conduction block 38
metacarpophalangeal joint 106, 257, 353

metacarpophalanx pulley system 281
methylprednisolone 108
microcurrent stimulation 260, 261
microsurgery 135
midazolam hydrochloride 156
midpalm tenderness 245
miniature compartment syndrome 51, 357
mini-invasive technique 136
minineuroma 274, 282, 286
Moberg pick-up test 263
motor branch anomaly 118
motor function testing 83
motor nerve fiber compression 73
Motta disease 21
mucolipidosis 97, 98
mucopolysaccharidosis 22, 25, 97, 98
multiple neurofibromatosis 116
muscle
– flap 326
– recruitment 264
muscular atrophy 334
myelin damage 37

needle electromyography 72
neoangiogenesis 357
nerve
– conduction study 89, 105
– entrapment 28, 309, 361, 398
– fiber 30, 32
– grafting 315
– injury 32, 199
– of Henle 112
– protector 142
– scar entrapment 357
– trunk 29
– – compression 34
– tumor 205
nerve-gliding
– exercise 107
– mechanism 343
neuralgia 343
neuralgic amyotrophy 90
neurapraxia 192
neurectomy 339
neurinoma 77
neuritis 248, 376
neuroapraxia 38, 39
neurodesis 361, 363, 376
neurofibroma 119
neurofibromatosis 97
neurolysis 128, 241, 319, 320, 369
neuroma 127, 229, 274, 293, 315, 333, 339, 376
neuron 28
neurophysiology 70
neuropraxia 140
neurosensory testing 299
neurotmesis 39
neurotrophism 376
Nissl substance 34
non-reflux phenomenon 34, 35
nonsteroidal anti-inflammatories (NSAIDs) 107, 186
non-use syndrome 373
Nottingham Health Profile (NHF) 84
numbness 89, 91

Subject Index

obesity 24
omentum 376, 377
opponens pollicis muscle 11, 66
oral steroid 108
orthodromic stimulation 71
osteoarthritis 92
osteopetrosis 24, 96
outcome analysis technique 383
Outcomes Assessment 384
Outcomes Research 384
oxidative stress 46

Padua EMG evaluating system 341
pain 84, 89, 292, 315, 322
– questionnaire 358
PAIN score 85, 86, 394, 395
Paine technique 202, 205
– safety 206
palindromia 168
palmar
– aponeurosis 14, 115, 141, 145, 215, 329
– carpal ligament 13, 202
– cutaneous anatomy 113
– cutaneous branch 311, 339
– – injury 275
– – sectioning 275
– cutaneous nerve 128
– fasciectomy 229
– incision 121
– longus muscle 96
– perithenar incision 269
– scar pain 228
– skin incision 235
– soreness 244
– thermoplastic band 256
palmaris brevis
– muscle 132, 162, 327
– – flap 329
– – turnover flap 324
palmaris longus
– muscle 13
– tendon 172, 195, 213
palpatory test 213, 216
pancoast tumor 90
paraproteinemia 23
paresthesia 5, 6, 36, 38, 63, 73, 84, 85, 89, 183, 199, 214, 241, 313, 357
Parona space 369
Parsonage-Turner syndrome 90
partial nerve injury 285
patient
– education 397
– selection 87
patient-oriented questionnaire 384
peak sensory latency 70
pedicled hypothenar fat flap 324
perinervous fibrosis 272
– scar proliferation 273
perineural fibrosis 377
perineuritum stratum 34
perineurium 29, 343
peripheral nerve 29
– function 306
– injury 22
peroneal compression 38
Phalen
– sign 84, 274, 355, 356, 365, 394

– test 49, 64, 66, 107, 272, 322, 393
– – reverse 83
pharmaco-resistent pain syndrome 357
phlebotomy 335
physical therapy 258
pillar
– pain 111, 168, 174, 181, 226, 229, 235, 244, 276, 277, 292, 294, 312
– syndrome 207
– tenderness 191
pinch strength 190, 191, 245
piso-triquetral pain syndrome 226, 229, 277, 293, 312
plethysmography 91
plexopathy 5, 72
plexus anesthesia 338
polyneuropathy 21, 22, 72, 392, 393, 396
posterior interosseous flap 333, 353, 356
postmyocardial infarction syndrome 99
postneurolysis 374
– causalgic syndrome 373
postoperative
– infection 282
– rehabilitation 133
prednisolone 108
prednisone 108
pregnancy 396
pressotherapy 292
pressure
– monofilament 314
– provocation test 83, 313
pressure-specified sensory device (PSSD) 299, 306
probe knife 160, 161
pronator quadratus 321
– fascia 371
– fat pad 370
– muscle flap 327
pronator syndrome 91, 299, 306, 309
prono-supination 55, 58
proper digital nerve 11
prostaglandin (PGE) 44
provocation test 63, 83, 84
proximal uniportal incision technique 186
pseudoarthritis 96
pseudomonas aeruginosa 283
pseudoneuroma 5, 76, 78
psoriatic arthritis 97
Purdue pegboard test 263
pus 171
pyogenic synovitis 168
pyridoxine 23

Quick-DASH questionnaire 356

radial neuropathy 91
radical tenosynovectomy 273
radius fracture 309
Ragnell retractor 131, 132
Rainer node 34, 38
randomized controlled trial (RCT) 383
range of motion (ROM) 211

– exercises 260
Raynaud syndrome 21, 91
reactive oxygen intermediates (ROI) 43
reconstruction ladder 324
rectangular adipofascial flap 350
recurrent focal neuropathy 97
reflex sympathetic dystrophy (RSD) 192, 242, 284, 312, 333, 344, 357
rehabilitation 264, 325
retinaculotome 200, 201, 204, 207
– modified 207
– spatula 200
retinaculum release 126
retrograde
– knife 161
– massage 257
– radial forearm flap 349
revascularization 344
reverse
– blade technique 131, 132
– pedicle flap 363
rheumatic polymyalgia 22
rheumatoid arthritis 21, 22, 116, 121, 127, 130, 141, 164, 168, 205, 274, 291, 338
ring finger axis 112

Salter-Harris II fracture 248, 249
salvage procedure 325
saphenous vein 335, 344
scaphoid
– pseudoarthrosis 22
– tubercle 275
scaphotrapezial arthritis 92
scar
– hypersensibility 259, 260
– keloid formation 259
– pain 276
– sensitivity 111
– tenderness 356
– tissue 309
Schwann cells 32, 40
– necrosis 34
sciatic function index (SFI) 333
sciatic nerve 333
scleroderma 97
Semmes-Weinstein monofilament 65, 299
– test 83, 263
sensibility 322
– testing 82
sensory
– action potential (SAP) 70
– nerve fiber compression 73
sepsis 206
SF-36 questionnaire 384–386
short palmar incision 133, 138
shoulder exercise 258
silicone barrier 344
single distal incision technique 186
single-port technique 291
skin incisions 115
sleeve assembly 188
sliding flap technique 230
slit catheter 52
Smith fracture 248
soft tissue edema 277

spin-echo T1/T2-weighted sequence 75
spinnaker variation 374
splint 132
sporotrichosis 92
sprouting nerve fiber 319
square sail flap 369, 372, 374
staphylococcus aureus 283
steroid injection 8
streptozotocin 33
stress test 52
Struther's ligament 72
superficial flexor tendon 75
superficial palmar
– aponeurosis 245
– arch injury 280
sympathetic maintained pain syndrome (SMPS) 344
SYMPT score 86, 394–396
Symptom Severity Index 378
synovectomy 127, 132, 135, 194, 338
synovial flap 324, 339
– technique 338
synovitis 147, 167, 274
syringomyelia 72
systemic
– lupus erythematosus 97
– sclerosis 97

tadpole lesion 37
tarsal tunnel syndrome 334
T-cell lymphoma 99
tendon adhesion 255
tenosynovectomy 115, 116, 141, 279
tenosynovitis 77, 79, 149, 193
tenosynovium 42, 44, 46
– edema 42
tenotomy scissors 159
thalidomide 98
thenar
– atrophy 365
– crease 122, 192, 338
– hypotrophy 177
– muscle
– – atrophy 67, 85, 149
– – hypotrophy 67, 83
– neuritis 3, 5, 6
– pain 276, 277, 282, 292

– plica 178
Thera-Putty 262
thoracic outlet syndrome 90, 164
threshold test 65
thrombosis 345
Tinel
– sign 63, 64, 84, 272, 313, 355, 356, 365
– test 63, 83, 107, 291
tissue
– fluid pressure 35
– gliding 345
– interpolation flap 315
tourniquet test 65
traction
– neuritis 361
– neuropathy 333
transcutaneous electric stimulation (TENS) 260, 231
transillumination 167
transport velocity 29
transverse carpal arch 227
transverse carpal ligament (TCL) 10, 54, 121, 124, 135, 140, 187, 203, 211, 239, 269, 291, 307, 357
– incomplete distal sectioning 272
– pulley system 282
trauma 50
traumatic lesion 96
triamcinolone 108
trigger
– finger 21, 92, 281, 294, 313
– thumbs 92
t-test 191
tuberculous tenosynovitis 205
two-point discrimination test 263

ulnar
– artery 198, 233, 362
– – flap 350, 351, 356
– – thrombosis 91
– fracture 309
– nerve 14, 66, 112, 233
– – iatrogenic injury 278
– – innervation 275
– – muscle branch 278
– – palmar cutaneous branch 111
– neuropathy 91

– sensory latency 71
ultrasound 78
– axial scan 79
– longitudinal scan 78, 79
– therapy 107

Van Frey's pressure test 65, 66
VAS test 356
vascular injury 79, 198, 312
vascularization 331
vein
– autograft 334
– grafting 333–335
– stripper 335
– wrapping 376
vela quadra flap 369
Velcro closure 105
Venn diagram 358
venous
– drainage 346
– thrombosis 99
venule 31
vibrometry testing 82
video equipment 140
video-assisted instrument 218
vitamin B6 108
volar plating 250

warfarin 99
Weber's test 65, 66, 356
Weil-Marchesani syndrome 25, 97, 198
Weitlaner retractor 131
wick catheter 36, 49, 50, 55
Will-Leri pleonosteosis 97
word hardening program 263, 264
wrist
– crease 121, 130, 164
– extension pressure 49
– fracture 3, 24, 49
– pain 92, 312
– rest position 56
– splint 55, 58, 105, 256, 377

xylocaine 131, 156, 159

Yellowstone sign 218
yoga 107